Anterior Hip Replacement

Joel M. Matta • Alexander P. Sah
Editors

Anterior Hip Replacement

From Origin to Current Advanced Techniques

Springer

Editors
Joel M. Matta
Steadman Clinic
Vail, CO, USA

Alexander P. Sah
Sah Orthopaedic Associates
Institute for Joint Restoration
Fremont, CA, USA

ISBN 978-3-030-91895-8 ISBN 978-3-030-91896-5 (eBook)
https://doi.org/10.1007/978-3-030-91896-5

This Springer imprint is published by the registered company Springer Nature Switzerland AG
The registered company address is: Gewerbestrasse 11, 6330 Cham, Switzerland

Preface

The growth of anterior approach total hip arthroplasty (AATHA) has been an evolutionary phenomenon. Undoubtedly, no one saw it coming. It has been facilitated by innovative and influential surgeons, but it probably does not owe its growth entirely to any individual(s). And yet, the growth may have been an inevitability.

Like many innovations, however, AATHA was not immediately recognized as an advantageous approach, but in fact was "sleeping" and used by only a few surgeons for over 50 years before its dramatic growth began.

What is the background that set these events in motion? The initial efforts related to prosthetic hip arthroplasty were logically directed toward developing a workable prosthesis that met several criteria. It needed to be biologically inert, represent longevity in relation to material fatigue and wear, maintain a stable bond to the host bone, and allow physiologic motion without dislocation. Sir John Charnley is credited with the first design that could meet the above criteria for a very high percentage of diseased hips. After a big leap by Charnley, there followed incremental improvements over the following years. The majority of new prostheses following Charnley's, however, were probably worse than Charnley's original design. The US FDA has over 1000 approved designs for hip prostheses on file, but only a minority have met or exceeded the results of Charnley. There were also steps to improve the surgical procedure. The original Charnley technique of greater trochanter osteotomy led to problems which necessitated the adoption of the posterior approach as well as the lateral trans-gluteal approach. Overall, for the majority of surgeons, the functional results improved with posterior and lateral approaches. There was always the argument, however, between surgeons that "I don't use posterior approach because patients dislocate" or "I don't use lateral approach because patients limp."

I believe that as the results of prosthetic improvements started to plateau, the attention of hip surgeons turned more toward improving the result by improving the surgical procedure. In 1996, I was 16 years into my hip practice and abandoned posterior approach in favor of anterior in order to prevent hip dislocation. By the early 2000s, there was widely prevalent advocacy of "minimally invasive" hip replacement as a means to improve clinical results. At this point, the discussion around technique became more passionate. Technologies such as computer guidance also started to emerge to address the recognized problems with prosthesis accuracy.

When I conducted my first course on AATHA in 2003, there was a wide array of technical courses available: minimally invasive two-incision technique, mini-posterior, mini-lateral, and others. Over the past 17 years, however, AATHA has been the technique that has garnered the largest growth and is emerging as the dominant technique.

Several years ago, I concluded that "anterior approach has won." The initial efforts that have been spent demonstrating that it is safe and efficacious, as well as showing benefits over other techniques, have been fruitful. Not to say that the majority of hip experts would agree with the above statement. I would say they do not! But I felt that further efforts to convince long-established hip experts was a questionable use of time. Time could be better allocated to developing the best AATHA methodologies and technologies as well as surgeon education. Max Planck said, "A new scientific truth does not triumph by convincing its opponents and making them see the light, but rather because its opponents eventually die, and a new generation grows up that is familiar with it." Certainly, we do not wish for an early death of AA opponents, but the new generation's influence is evident with the wide adoption of AA by young orthopedic surgeons completing residency and fellowship.

With this background, the emphasis of this book will not be on convincing surgeons that anterior approach is better. The benefits are addressed in the results section, but rather the emphasis is on how to do anterior approach in the best way.

Though AATHA refers only to implanting the hip prosthesis through AA, there is significant variation in the methodologies. To simplify, one group of anterior approach surgeons advocates continuing with intuitive and experience-based techniques that have been used for years with posterior and lateral approaches, while changing the incision to anterior. Another group advocates changing the incision to anterior and additionally abandoning many previous methods for exposure and confirming accuracy as well as integrating new technologies. My sentiments lie with the latter group.

Historically there have been significant differences in THA results based on surgeon skill and experience. The emphasis has therefore been to improve surgeon skill. I am completely in favor of maximizing surgeon skill, but surgeon skill will always vary and there is a limit. I think the ideal is to seek to limit the variability of results between the "virtuoso" surgeon and "average" or "normal" surgeon. The variability of results among hips done by a single surgeon should also be limited. The results of hips operated by high-volume vs low-volume surgeons should also have limited variability. In order to achieve the above consistent results, education is important, but, additionally, the technique that is taught must be consistent, proven by many surgeons and repeatable. The final factor is that we need technologies to support and validate our surgical skills. I like to say, "don't do AA like you did posterior or lateral approach. You can, but you won't achieve the best results possible."

I think of four basic surgical approaches to the hip as: anterior = Hueter or Smith-Petersen, antero-lateral = Watson-Jones, lateral = Harding, and posterior = Kocher-Langenbeck. Though some surgeons have referred to Watson-Jones and even Harding as "anterior" approaches, I believe that doing so confuses understanding and definitions. I also do not advocate the term "direct anterior approach" or "DAA." Using the term "DAA" implies that there are other types of anterior approach which again confuses terminology. Also, historically, Judet in France and Keggi in the USA referred to the anterior approach; therefore, modifying the name to "DAA" gives a false impression that "DAA" may be a new approach, which it is not.

The initial section of this book details an established methodology that has evolved and been taught at surgeon courses for over 15 years and is supported by innovative technology that has developed to facilitate the repeatability of this technique.

Following will be descriptions of other variations of AATHA and direct point and counterpoint discussions that highlight differences and invite the reader to draw their own conclusions.

The dynamic field of treating unusual hip problems and revision surgery is presented in its current state of the art.

Finally, as a hip surgeon, I think it is best that, in addition to thoroughly knowing hip, pelvis, and femur anatomy, one should also be facile with all surgical approaches to the hip and be able to apply them when indicated.

I was asked at the conclusion of a lecture on AATHA if I thought what I just presented was the final best way to perform THA. Thankfully, I had the presence of mind to reply, "I certainly hope not."

Vail, CO, USA — Joel M. Matta
Fremont, CA, USA — Alexander P. Sah

Contents

Contributors

Kris Alden Hinsdale Orthopedics Associates/Illinois Bone and Joint Institute, Hinsdale, IL, USA

Kenoma Anighoro Arthroplasty & Value-Based Health Care Delivery, University of Texas at Austin—Dell Medical School, Austin, TX, USA

Steven L. Barnett Hoag Orthopedic Institute, Irvine, CA, USA

William P. Barrett Proliance Orthopedic Associates, Renton, WA, USA

Paul E. Beaulé Division of Orthopaedic Surgery, The Ottawa Hospital, University of Ottawa, Ottawa, ON, Canada

Michael J. Bellino Department of Orthopaedic Surgery, Stanford University Medical Center, Stanford, CA, USA

Friedrich Boettner Hospital for Special Surgery, New York, NY, USA

Samuel W. Carlson Mayo Clinic, Rochester, MN, USA

Anthony T. Carter Hampton Roads Orthopaedics & Sports Medicine, Newport News, VA, USA

Michael J. Chen Department of Orthopaedic Surgery, Stanford University Medical Center, Stanford, CA, USA

Andrew J. Cooper Orthopaedic Associates of West Florida, Clearwater, FL, USA

Jonathan R. Dattilo Anderson Orthopaedic Research Institute, Alexandria, VA, USA

Charles A. DeCook Northside Hospital, Arthritis and Total Joint Specialists, Cumming, GA, USA

Dimitri E. Delagrammaticas Central Coast Orthopedic Group, San Luis Obispo, CA, USA

Tania A. Ferguson Nashville Hip and Pelvis, Nashville, TN, USA

William G. Hamilton Anderson Orthopaedic Research Institute, Alexandria, VA, USA

Matthieu Hanauer Department of Orthopaedic Surgery and Traumatology, University of Fribourg, HFR Cantonal Hospital, Fribourg, Switzerland

Thierry Judet Professor Honoris Causa Paris 5 University, Paris, France

Anna Jungwirth-Weinberger Hospital for Special Surgery, New York, NY, USA

Kantonsspital Baden AG, Baden, Switzerland

Atul F. Kamath CCLCM, CWRU SOM, Hip & Knee Reconstruction, Department of Orthopaedic Surgery, Cleveland Clinic Foundation, Cleveland, OH, USA

Center for Hip Preservation, Orthopaedic and Rheumatologic Institute, Cleveland Clinic, Cleveland, OH, USA

Raymond H. Kim Department of Orthopaedic Surgery, The Steadman Clinic, Vail, CO, USA

Philip James Kregor The Hughston Clinic, HCA TriStar Skyline Medical Center, Nashville, TN, USA

Stefan W. Kreuzer INOV8 Orthopedics, Houston, TX, USA

Frédéric Laude Clinique du sport, Paris, France

Jonathan Laurençon Department of Orthopaedic Surgery and Traumatology, University of Fribourg, HFR Cantonal Hospital, Fribourg, Switzerland

Michael Leunig Hip Surgery - Schulthess Clinic, Zürich, Switzerland

Timothy P. Lovell Providence Orthopedics & Sports Medicine, Spokane, WA, USA

Daniel March Norton Orthopedic Institute, Louisville, KY, USA

John L. Masonis OrthoCarolina Hip & Knee Center, Atrium Musculoskeletal Institute, Charlotte, NC, USA

Nicholas H. Mast The Hip and Pelvis Institute, San Francisco, CA, USA

Joel M. Matta Steadman Clinic, Vail, CO, USA

Niall P. McGoldrick Division of Orthopaedic Surgery, The Ottawa Hospital, University of Ottawa, Ottawa, ON, Canada

Brandon H. Naylor Northside Hospital, Arthritis and Total Joint Specialists, Cumming, GA, USA

Michael Nogler Department of Orthopaedic Surgery, Medical University of Innsbruck, Innsbruck, Austria

John Jay Perry Perry Orthopedics, Melbourne, FL, USA

Amir Pourmoghaddam Memorial Bone & Joint Research Foundation Orthopaedic Research Houston Texas, Houston, TX, USA

Saul Hernandez Rodriguez Miami Orthopedics and Sports Medicine Institute, Baptist Health South Florida, Miami, FL, USA

Joshua C. Rozell Department of Orthopaedic Surgery, NYU Langone Health, New York, NY, USA

Hannes A. Rüdiger Hip Surgery - Schulthess Clinic, Zürich, Switzerland

Robert P. Runner Department of Orthopedic Surgery, Rancho Los Amigos National Rehabilitation Center, Downey, CA, USA

Alexander P. Sah Sah Orthopaedic Associates, Institute for Joint Restoration, Fremont, CA, USA

Linsen T. Samuel Department of Orthopaedic Surgery, Cleveland Clinic Foundation, Cleveland, OH, USA

Joseph M. Schwab Department of Orthopaedic Surgery, Medical College of Wisconsin, Milwaukee, WI, USA

Jeremy Statton Northside Hospital, Arthritis and Total Joint Specialists, Cumming, GA, USA

Vera M. Stetzelberger Department of Orthopaedic Surgery and Traumatology, University of Fribourg, HFR Cantonal Hospital, Fribourg, Switzerland

Juan C. Suarez Miami Orthopedics and Sports Medicine Institute, Baptist Health South Florida, Miami, FL, USA

Moritz Tannast Department of Orthopaedic Surgery and Traumatology, University of Fribourg, HFR Cantonal Hospital, Fribourg, Switzerland

Jakub Tatka White Plains Hospital, White Plains, NY, USA

Michael J. Taunton Hip & Knee Reconstructive Surgery, Mayo Clinic, Rochester, MN, USA

Martin Thaler Helios Klinikum München West, Arthroplasty Center, München, Germany

Maria-Roxana Viamont-Guerra Hip Surgery Unit, Hospital Israelita Albert Einstein, São Paulo, SP, Brazil

Jonathan Yerasimides Norton Orthopedic Institute, Louisville, KY, USA

Corinne A. Zurmühle Department of Orthopaedic Surgery and Traumatology, University of Fribourg, HFR Cantonal Hospital, Fribourg, Switzerland

Part I

The Origins of the Anterior Hip Surgical Approach

The French Beginning and Judet School of the Anterior Approach

1

Thierry Judet

Introduction

Hip replacement is undoubtedly the leading procedure of today's orthopedic surgery.

It provides a solution to the frequent situations of disabling hip pathology, degenerative, post-traumatic, or of any cause. It is caricaturally a winning-winning procedure, highly standardized, and reproducible, with a low impact on patient general condition, which allows indication in extreme situations of age or associated pathology. The result is predictable, close to a 100% functional recovery in most of the cases, the recovery period is easy and short, and the actual design of the implant provides a long-term stability of these results. This allows considering hip prosthetic replacement even for young and active patients.

These amazing qualities of hip prostheses are the result of more than 70 years of evolution since the first attempt of articular replacement and improvements went step by step thanks to the contribution of orthopedic surgeons and manufacturers, mainly in Europe and North America.

Among the multitude of contributors, a special place must be given to the Judet, world initiators of hip replacement with the acryl Judet prosthesis, involved in most of the evolutions of implant, and moreover users and defenders since the first day of the anterior approach.

It is worthwhile to remember Judet and Judet School contribution to hip prosthetic surgery and, simultaneously, the evolution of the anterior approach as the gold standard.

We shall successively give a short review of hip surgery in the last century, point the contribution of Judet school in that evolution, and point out the place and evolution of the anterior approach when it was a "confidential" procedure as well as when it became a widely used world practice.

The Long Road of Hip Surgery

Like most of the bone and joint surgeries, hip surgery began with the advent of anesthesiology and asepsis and was initially devoted to trauma and some septic situations.

Planned surgery appeared in the first half of the last century, mainly for correction of hip dysplasia in children and progressively to improve the function of adult patients with degenerative changes.

Many types of surgery have been tried, such as soft tissue release, head and neck resection of Girdlestone, femoral osteotomies, shelf procedure, or acetabular remodeling without or with interposition as described by Smith Petersen.

T. Judet (✉)
Professor Honoris Causa Paris 5 University, Paris, France
e-mail: thierry@judet.com

J. M. Matta, A. P. Sah (eds.), *Anterior Hip Replacement*,
https://doi.org/10.1007/978-3-030-91896-5_1

All these procedures variously indicated regarding the local anatomical status, the degree of degenerative changes, age of the patient, and importance of functional impacts. Their results were obviously moderate and, moreover, widely unpredictable.

A new era began in 1947 when Robert and Jean Judet imagined, finalized, and applied a completely new concept based on a femoral head resection and replacement by a mechanical device [1]. The initial design was a kind of acrylic mushroom stabilized by a short stem axially implanted in the femoral neck (Fig. 1.1). This opened the door to hip arthroplastic surgery and had a tremendous impact on the international orthopedic community immediately after the presentation of the initial series.

The first design was imperfect, with weaknesses of the material being wear of the acrylic and stem fracture, failure of bone fixation and implant migration, and unpredictable tolerance of the acetabulum.

So appeared from everywhere a lot of new options, such as the use of metallic implants, initially stainless steel or chrome-cobalt alloy, and long stem design for a better stability in femoral diaphysis.

Bone fixation was a concern, which found an initial answer in the systematic use of acrylic cement.

The acetabular wear and suffering found a solution in the early sixties with the concept of total hip replacement with initially two options, metal on metal, following Mac Kee or metal on polyethylene as promoted by John Charnley.

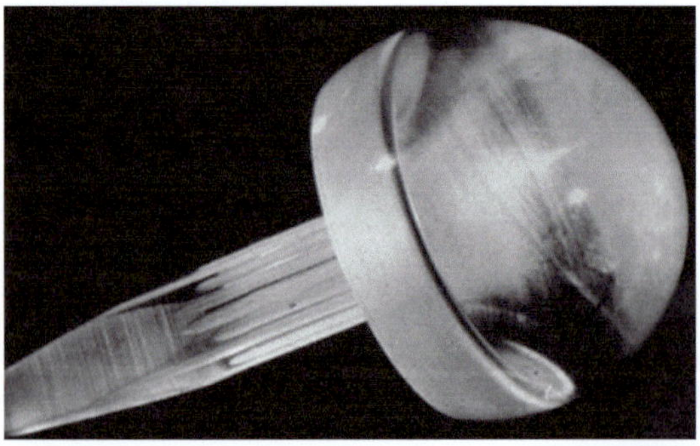

Fig. 1.1 Judet acryl prosthesis 147

The seventies also gave place to completely new concepts, among which remain the dual mobility acetabular component of Gilles Bousquet (St Etienne France), the use of ceramics proposed by Pierre Boutin (Pau France), and an alternative way to obtain a long-lasting implant fixation to the host bone: it was the concept of direct fixation by active bone ingrowth in the intentionally porous surface of the metal. This idea of cementless prosthesis was initiated by Robert Judet and applied in 1970 in the so-called Judet Poro-metal Prosthesis [2]. The prerequisites for bone ingrowth were described, irregular surface, strong impaction of a double tapered square section stem to provide a perfect initial stability, mandatory to obtain long-term stability due to bone ingrowth. This prosthesis also introduced the modularity concept by a Morse taper, the world's first application in prosthetic surgery, which is now a standard of modern prostheses (Fig. 1.2).

During this decade, following Robert Judet implant, many authors worked on this concept of cementless implantation, initially mainly in France and Europe. Some of them relied only on mechanical stability; as an acetabular screwed ring, this concept has been abandoned.

Most of them tried to obtain active bone ingrowth in a devoted surface, surface treatment, and adjunction of plasma to obtain macro- or microscopic porosity.

In the following years, while cementless implantations began in the USA, new options were studied; Use of different materials such as titanium or new polyethylene, discussion of the ingrowth zones, full stem or only proximal in the metaphyseal area, to prevent the possible effect of stress shielding, new hemispheric press-fit acetabular component.

Hydroxyapatite coating was developed in Europe and is now widely used to enhance ingrowth phenomena in a metallic surface adapted, irregular, or covered by a titanium plasma.

In those decades of intense evolutions, some options have been tried, and partially or totally abandoned, such as screwed acetabular components or, more recently, double cup metal on metal arthroplasties. The same is for a partial femoral head replacement for AVN in young patients [3].

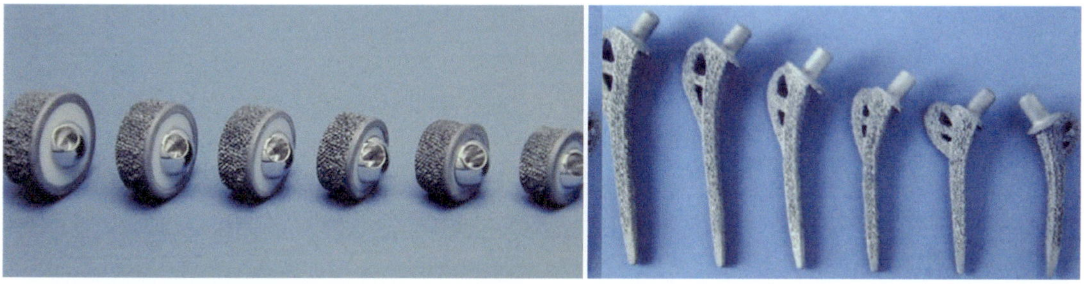

Fig. 1.2 Robert Judet Poro-Metal cementless prosthesis

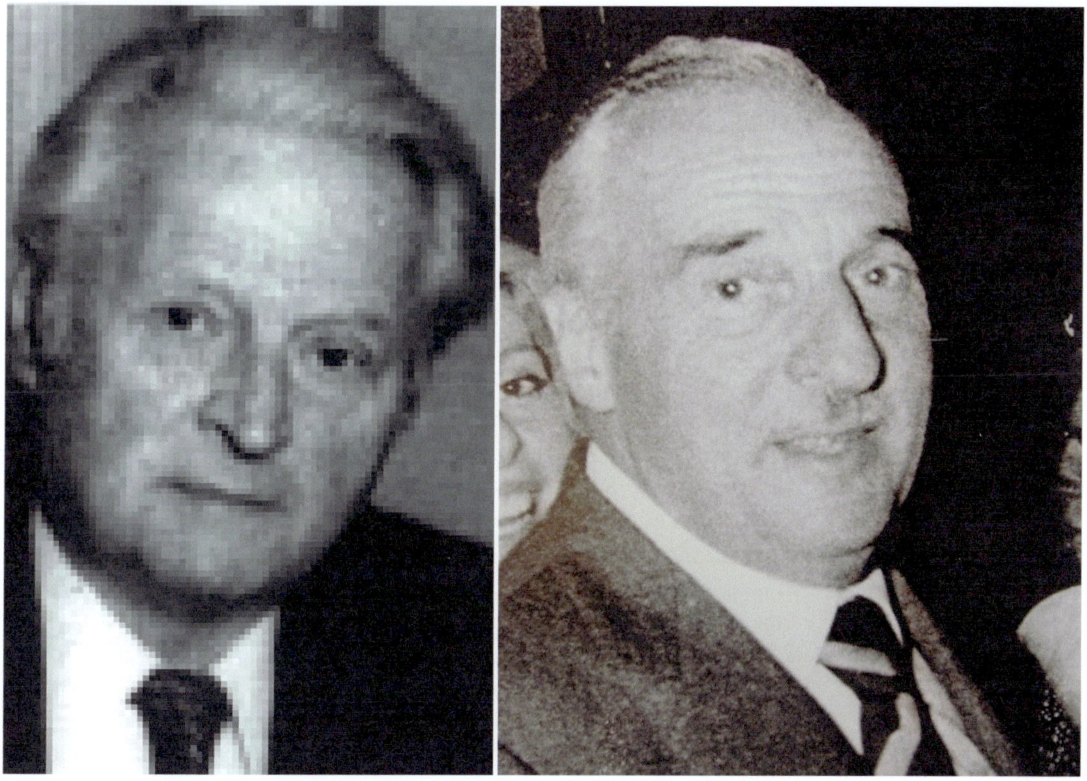

Fig. 1.3 The Judet Brothers, Jean and Robert

The advantages of the recent option of short stem prostheses have to be evaluated.

Judet School in the Hip Arthroplasty Surgery

It is hardly possible to make a border between Judet Family and Judet School so close and similar were the relations between the members of the family and all the surgeons who cooperated within the framework of the university's orthopedic and traumatology department led by some members of the family. In the family, the first surgeon was Henri (1880–1942), son of a peasant, doctor in medicine and in sciences; among the first surgeons specialized in bone and joint, he published in his thirties a reference book on traumatology. His two sons Jean (1905–1989) and Robert (1909–1980), known as the Judet Brothers (Fig. 1.3), have been major actors of the world's great development of the orthopedic and trauma surgery of the second half of the last century. Besides hip surgery, they have been at the origin of many new concepts and techniques, simultaneously in their private clinic and in their public hospital activity. Jean had his public activity in an orthopedic pediatric department and Robert, as head of a big orthopedic and trauma department in Garches university hospital, involved a lot of his assistants in the national and international recognition of Judet's school.

There innovative technics concerned all fields of trauma surgery, polytraumatized patients, all articular and acetabular fractures with Letournel, spine surgery with Roy-Camille, trauma sequelae such as osteo-muscular decortication for long bone malunion and nonunion, quadriceps release for knee stiffness, biological arthroplasties by bone remodeling, and external distraction to treat articular fusions and major stiffness.

Among this school and this surgical team, both Jean and Robert had successors in their families, Henri (1939–), Jean's son, had a private practice, Robert's son-in-law, Marc Siguier (1939–), took a great place in cementless hip prosthesis development and, with his son Thierry, in the promotion and evolution of the hip anterior approach. Myself, Thierry (1948–), Robert Judet's son, has been his assistant and has had a public career as head of a university's orthopedic and trauma department, with a wide range of activities concerning hip, knee, ankle, and elbow.

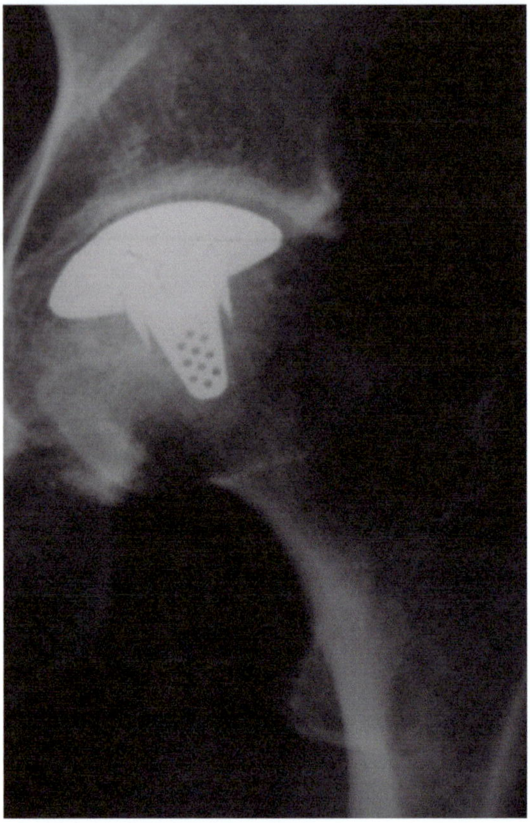

Fig. 1.4 Partial head replacement for AVN

Judet School's Place in the Hip Replacement History

We have seen the major place in two founding periods: the first attempt of mechanical replacement of the femoral head in 1946 with the acryl prosthesis and the first attempt of direct bone implant fixation by microscopic living bone ingrowth in the prosthetic surface with the poro-metal Robert Judet prosthesis in 1970. Both were widely imperfect, but both opened the way for a new era of hip surgery and were totally innovative: moreover, the poro-metal brought the concept of modularity with the Morse taper.

Between and after those two dates, a lot of attempts, modifications, or adoptions have been made. Some have been abandoned, such as the original technique partial head replacement for avascular head necrosis (Fig. 1.4) and metal-on-metal double cup arthroplasties. On the other hand, techniques of reconstruction for massive acetabular bone defects have been experimented and evaluated.

Everything has changed in 70 years except a double common thread: the anterior approach and the use of an orthopedic table.

The anterior approach has been adopted till the first hip replacement because of the comfort it could provide. For the record, the anterior approach has been described a long time before by Carl Hueter from Leipzig in 1878 [4]. Smith-Petersen used this approach with a proximal extension by release of the anterior part of the iliac crest and external fossa [5]. The same extension was used for shelf procedure. Anatomical considerations led the Judet brothers to adopt this anterior approach: anterior position of the hip, anteversion of both femoral neck and acetabulum, preservation of anatomical structures, no proximity of the vulnerable structure, and vascular or nervous.

They were regular users of the orthopedic table for trauma or planned surgery because of the stability and comfort it gave. They had already developed with their father Henri Judet a fracture table, which gave a wide range of possibilities, and they did not consider operating without this help.

This orthopedic table is still in use for all the surgeon members or successors of Judet School, with minor or no modification. It is considered as the carpenter's bench, which helps all maneuvers, stabilizes bone pieces when preparing, and, for most of the surgeons, allows a sufficient positional control to get rid of X-ray control during the procedure.

The approach itself was a standard Hueter with a proximal debridement of the anterior part of the iliac wing. The anterior approach in hip prosthetic surgery was a specificity of Judet School with a diffusion limited to the surgeons trained in it. For years and years, there has been no or only minor evolution of this approach. In the 1970s, the incision line was shifted laterally, from the anatomic interval between Sartorius and facia iliaca tensor, to facia iliaca belly itself to minimize the risk of superficial femoral nerve involvement: this new incision line was called Hueter-sheet incision.

One must say that in the first period of hip replacement, there were so many questions and problems to solve that the approach was not really considered as a key point. Surgeons, as well as companies, had to make decisions about design, material, friction couple, and type of bone-implant fixation, cemented or cementless. None or little interest was given to surgical procedure, except for John Charnley, who was a strong advocate of the trans-trochanteric approach.

Implant designs and concepts reached some maturity in the last eighties and early nineties, with a few options for cemented or cementless bone fixation, the material of friction couple, and there were more and more similarities between the companies' products.

That is probably one of the reasons for which a growing interest began to be given to the approach, with, at the beginning, excesses. For exemple a double approach has been described and made the buzz as the most minimal invasive procedure: beyond the poor prosthetic design it imposed, this double approach quickly demonstrated to be dangerously aggressive [6].

The same period was marked by an evolution of the anterior approach, led by Marc Siguier [7]. Schematically he limited the approach to the original Hueter, in the interval between gluteal and femoral nerves, without any debridement of the tendon. Previously the proximal debridement of the anterior part of the iliac wing was part of the technic, as well as the trans section of the reflected tendon of the rectus femoris and a frequent section of piriformis and external obturator tendons to facilitate femoral exposure. Siguier showed that all those tendons could be preserved with the help of a good muscular relaxation by general or spinal anesthesia and allowed minimal cutaneous incision. The results in terms of recovery and stability, despite the use of a 22.2-mm prosthetic head, gave a worldwide interest to the anterior approach. Moreover, the ectopic bone formation, frequently observed in the iliac debridement of the traditional Smith-Petersen approach, did not occur anymore.

From this period, all companies found a commercial interest to this approach, which became a promotional support to sell prostheses. They provided orthopedic tables, more or less efficient, dedicated ancillary tools, presented as being essential, and planned training sessions for new customers.

This sudden enthusiasm for a new approach happened to have adverse consequences due to insufficient training and practice. This very precisely anatomic technique, with new anatomic landmarks and a totally different spatial evaluation of the hip joint, requires a real training, particularly for new customers, previously users of posterior or lateral approaches. Noncompliance with a sufficient learning curve led some surgeons to become very reluctant toward the anterior approach. There has been a trend to highlight the cutaneous incision length as a criterion of mini-invasiveness: anyone must keep in mind that the anterior approach is anatomically noninvasive and can be performed through a relatively short cutaneous incision, 6–10 cm, but under that, excessive skin traction often leads to unsightly hypertrophic healing.

Under these reserves, with the advent of short hospital stage and ambulatory surgery, the anterior approach proved to be the more efficient and secure technique.

In the case of revision surgery, the anterior approach is the royal road for acetabular reconstruction [8, 9] at the price of a limited or large proximal extension on the iliac wing. Distal access on the femoral shaft is less comfortable but possible by the extension described by Zarad-Nicek. The concept is to contour the distal extremity of the facia-lata tensor and reach the femoral shaft by a classical postero-lateral approach. This procedure allows a full preservation of neurologic territories, femoral medially and gluteal laterally.

Conclusion

In modern orthopedic surgery, quite a few techniques have a prolonged lifetime. The anterior approach was at the origins of hip replacement more than 70 years ago. For decades, it has had unconditional supporters, but they were only a happy few, all coming from the Judet School. With the extension of a more and more performing hip prosthetic surgery, appeared a demand for a more secure and less invasive surgery, with a quicker recovery. The old anterior approach proved to be the most efficient for that purpose, especially after minor adaptations, most of them proposed by Judet School surgeons. It became in the last years the most trendy and widely used procedure in hip replacement, but anyone must keep in mind that before being a sales pitch for companies and surgeons, it is a highly precise and anatomic technique that requires real training.

References

1. Judet J, Judet R. The use of an artificial femoral head for arthroplasty of the hip joint. JBJS. 1950;32 B.
2. Judet R, Siguier M, Brumpt B, Judet T. A noncemented total hip prosthesis. Clin Orthop Relat Res. 1978;137:76–84.
3. Siguier T, Siguier M, Judet T, Charnley G, Brumpt B. Partial resurfacing arthroplasty of the femoral head in avascular necrosis. Methods, indications, and results. Clin Orthop Relat Res. 2001;386:85–92.
4. Grundiss der Chirurgie Vogel ECN 1883.Hueter Carl.
5. Smith-Petersen MN. Arthroplasty of the hip: a new method. J Bone Joint Surg Am. 1939;21:269–88.
6. Bal BS, et al. Early complications of primary total hip replacement performed with a two-incision minimally invasive technique. J Bone Joint Surg Am. 2005;87(11):2432–8.
7. Siguier T, Siguier M, Brumpt B. Mini-incision anterior approach does not increase dislocation rate: a study of 1037 total hip replacements. Clin Orthop Relat Res. 2004;426:164–73.
8. Piriou P, Norton M, Marmorat JL, Judet T. Acetabular reconstruction in revision hip surgery using femoral head block allograft. Orthopedics. 2005;28(12):1437–44.
9. Piriou P, Sagnet F, Norton MR, de Loubresse CG, Judet T. Acetabular component revision with frozen massive structural pelvic allograft: average 5-year follow-up. J Arthroplast. 2003;18(5):562–9.

My French and American Beginning and Evolution of the Anterior Approach

2

Joel M. Matta

My first exposure to Anterior Approach primary hip was in 1981 with Professor Emile Letournel, a former resident of Robert Judet, at his hospital in Paris at Port de Choisy. At the time, Letournel had international notoriety for his pioneering work with surgical treatment of acetabular and pelvic fractures. I was a junior faculty member, beginning in 1980, Assistant Professor in the Department of Orthopedic Surgery at the University of Southern California. My Chairman/Chief was Augusto Sarmiento, MD, another internationally recognized orthopedist and hip surgeon.

My main interest and clinical focus at the time was fractures of the pelvis and acetabulum. I had met Prof Letournel in Los Angeles in Dec 1980, when he was a visiting lecturer to our department. I was awestruck by Letournel who was the recognized leading world expert on the subject that I was focused on, and he granted my request to visit him at Port de Choisy in May 1981. My visit was limited to a few weeks; however, it was informative and inspirational. Emile gave freely of his time, allowed me to observe him in the operating room, and reviewed x-rays of my cases, and some of his that were particularly instructive. He also took the opportunity to show me an anterior hip replacement as he performed it on the Judet orthopedic table.

Letournel was among the most impressive surgeons I had observed. His command of pelvic and acetabular fracture surgery was unmatched. He also performed anterior THA with the patient supine on the Judet orthopedic table, efficiently and with minimal tissue trauma through a small incision. On this first visit with Letournel, however, my focus was acetabular fracture surgery, and I did not seek to adopt the Judet-Letournel anterior THA. Furthermore, my Chief at USC, Sarmiento was the surgeon who did most to lead the world to use of posterior as the most common approach for THA [1]. So, at the time, I was following my two mentors, Letournel for acetabular fractures and Sarmiento for THA. Sarmiento had been a Charnley fellow and learned the trans-trochanteric approach for the Charnley prosthesis. Prior to this, however, he had been Austin Moore's resident and learned to implant the Austin Moore femoral prosthesis through a posterior approach. Probably, it was difficulties with Charnley's trochanteric osteotomy that was a major factor in the worldwide trend to the posterior approach.

The posterior approach was an improvement with less soft tissue trauma and respect of the greater trochanter; however, it was not without problems. The approach disrupted the hip's external rotators. Also, the patient was now necessarily placed lateral, which made the pelvis and

J. M. Matta (✉)
Steadman Clinic, Vail, CO, USA

J. M. Matta, A. P. Sah (eds.), *Anterior Hip Replacement*,
https://doi.org/10.1007/978-3-030-91896-5_2

acetabular component position harder to judge. The combination of these issues made the possibility of post-operative dislocation higher.

Though I did not initially see the advantages and adopt anterior THA, my focus on acetabular fractures laid the basis. For the operation of acetabular fractures, there were many surgeons who attempted to stay with the posterior approach and lateral position and make extensions of this approach to increase access to the innominate bone (proximal extension, trochanteric osteotomy, triradiate extension). My initial acetabular fracture surgeries followed this posterior approach extension method, which included operating the patient in a "floppy lateral" position, which allowed the surgeon to roll the pelvis during surgery to hopefully increase access. Following Letournel's protocol, however, the surgeon operated acetabular fractures with the patient either supine, lateral, or prone through the ilioinguinal, iliofemoral, or posterior approaches, respectively. I found this protocol to be clearly superior [2].

An important part of Letournel's protocol was also operating the patient on the Judet orthopedic table. As I moved toward Letournel's protocol, I initially did not appreciate how valuable the Judet Table was for maximizing the capability of each surgical approach. Further experience, however, showed the advantages of the orthopedic table: enhancing exposure, control of the femur and pelvis, limiting soft tissue trauma, and access to a wider skin area. The standard flat top table technique was possible for the operation of acetabular fractures but more likely to lead to the necessity for second incisions and difficulties with fracture reduction.

This Letournel acetabular fracture background taught me hip and pelvis anatomy and radiology. It also made the concept and practice of considering the relative advantages of different surgical approaches natural and logical. The advantages and ease of use of the orthopedic table also became evident and as a natural facilitator for anterior THA (Fig. 2.1).

In 1996, I was 16 years into my orthopedic practice and focused on hip and pelvis fractures, hip preservation, and primary plus revision THA. I had left the full-time faculty at USC in 1990 and was granted a semi-academic position as the John C Wilson, Jr Chair of Orthopedics at Good Samaritan Hospital, Los Angeles. Charles Munger, Chairman of the Board at good Samaritan Hospital, had the vision to encourage academics and innovation at a private hospital without the politics, bureaucracy, and loss of intellectual property ownership that typically was present in a University setting. I was contacted by a patient from Washington State who wished to have a THA. The unusual part about his request is that he wanted his THA done through the anterior approach. He told me that he had had his right hip replaced while he was living in Paris and was extremely happy with the result. He had been searching the United States for someone who had trained with Letournel and who could replace his left hip through AA and he had found me. I explained that despite my past contact and instruction from Letournel, I had continued with Sarmiento's posterior method. I was however very familiar with the anterior approach and performed it frequently for peri-acetabular osteotomy, and I did use the Judet orthopedic table at my hospital for acetabular fracture surgery. I told the patient that if he wished, I would perform his THA through AA on the Judet table though he would be my first anterior THA. The anterior THA was performed, and the patient and I were very pleased with the outcome.

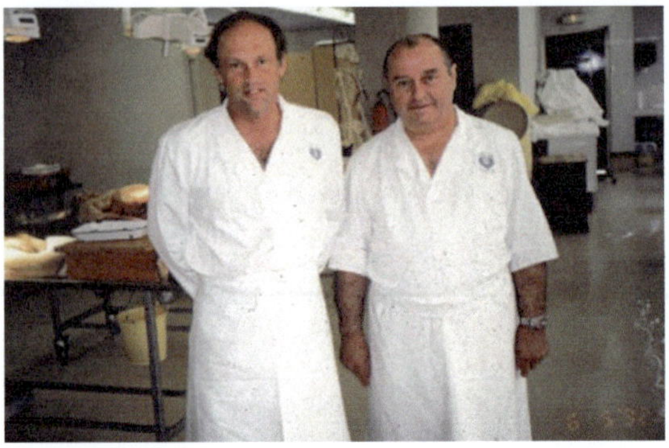

Fig. 2.1 The author with Prof. Emile Letournel and the Fer a' Moulin Paris anatomy institute in 1992

Paradoxically, beginning at least 10 years earlier, I had used AA for selected cases of revision THA. In some instances requiring extensive reconstruction for acetabular bone loss, I chose AA over PA for revision because of the proximal extensile capabilities of AA. The posterior approach is extensile distally for the femur; however, it is not extensile for the innominate bone because proximal extension is limited by the inferior and superior gluteal nerves. An extensile approach to an extremity is classically and correctly described by Arnold Henry as following the inter-nervous plane, which makes AA the extensile approach to the hip [3] (Fig. 2.2).

At this point I thought that maybe I had missed something by following Letournel's guidance regarding acetabular and pelvic fracture surgery and not adopting AA for primary THA. Using PA I was also not able to prevent the problem of hip dislocation in a small but significant percentage of my patients. I thereby began my series of primary anterior THAs that have been a consecutive and unselected series of ATHAs from 1996 to the present. I operated with the patient supine on the Judet table. I used a cemented stem and uncemented cup, which was a common construct in 1996. To my dismay, I struggled with the operation. A procedure (posterior THA) that I knew well from Sarmiento's tutelage and easily performed in one hour had been replaced with a 2- to 3-hour struggle, and because of Letournel's passing in 1993, I could not go to him for instruction.

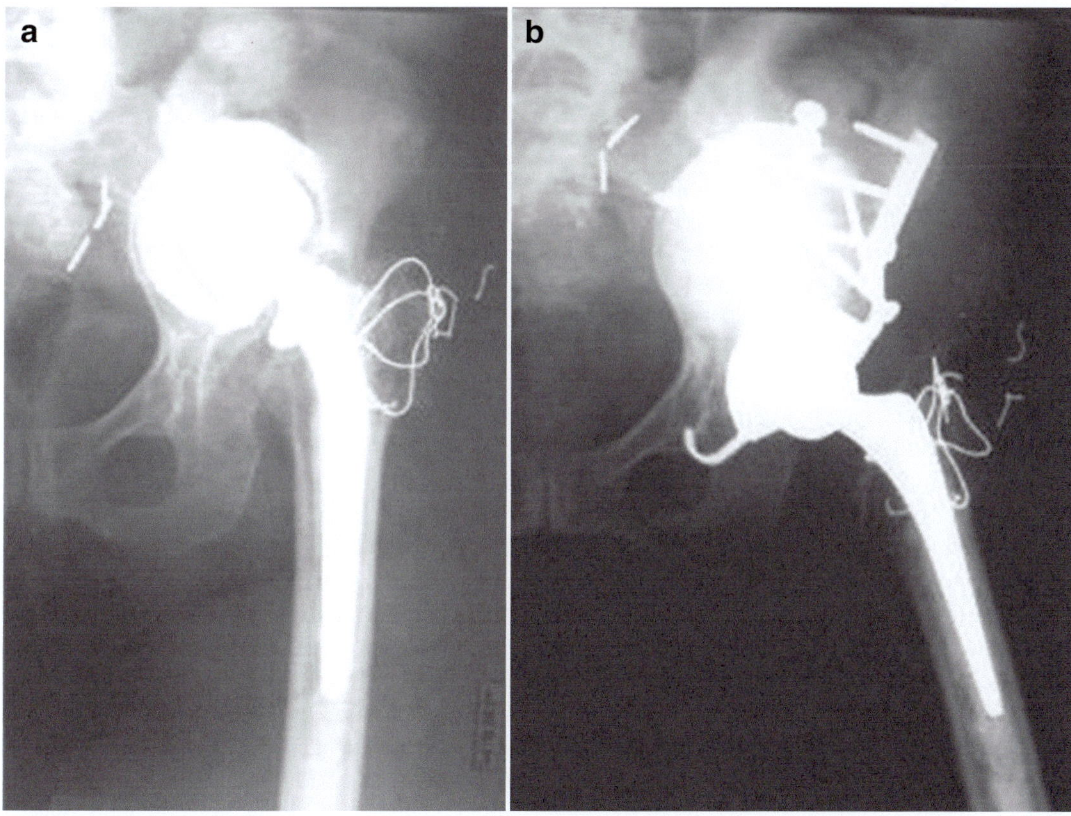

Fig. 2.2 (**a**) Painful left THA. Acetabular component has migrated medial and anterior with large anterior column defect. (**b**) Revision surgery performed in 1986 utilizing an anterior approach with access to internal iliac fossa and then the lateral aspect of innominate bone and acetabulum. The cup and associated fractured cement were surrounded by a thin bony shell in the internal iliac fossa and along the pelvic brim. A window was made in this shell and the cup was removed from inside the pelvis. The window was replaced and plated. The cavity was filled with impacted morselized allograft bone, and a custom cup-cage device with an obturator foramen hook and iliac plate was used to bridge the defect and load the allograft

During this initially difficult surgery, I would vow to abandon AA; however, following surgery, I was consistently impressed by the patient satisfaction and rapid recovery. I did remember, however, the ease and efficiency I saw when Letournel performed AA and I thought "there must be a way!" My spatial perception of factors such as neck cut, cup position, leg length, and offset was impaired at the beginning, so I utilized the C-arm for confirmation, which was easy with the patient supine and radiolucent orthopedic table. Later, it became evident that the use of the C-arm greatly enhanced the accuracy of cup position, leg length, and offset. My command of AA improved, surgical times dropped, and my confidence improved. My surgical exposure was also improved by observing Kristaps Keggi in Waterbury, CT, and especially Thierry Judet, in Paris, France.

An interesting technical development for AA as I performed it came about when I was presented with a very challenging hip/patient, "Coach." Coach had been a professional heavyweight boxer and was now a boxing instructor. The problem he presented was a bad hip requiring THA and the obstacle of massive gluteal and thigh musculature. The Judet table had a feature of a variable height transverse perineal post for the operation of the patient in the lateral position. This height could be varied during surgery by a crank rotated by the anesthesiologist that drove a vertical "jackscrew." My thought was to solve the problem of femoral access, and I would design a hook that would lift the femur through connection to the upper end of the jackscrew. The jack-hook device would thereby lift the femur anterior to a position where I could access it for broaching, cementing, and stem insertion. To fabricate the necessary steel parts for the job, I would need to utilize Larry at the "race car shop." Larry and son Rick owned and operated a SoCal hot rod and race car shop with extensive metal working capabilities, and I used them for work on my 1963 Lotus 23B vintage race car. Larry made the custom parts according to my design, and I attached them to the Judet table to facilitate Coach's surgery, and his THA was successfully performed.

Following the Coach THA, the custom parts went into a back room in the OR. Some months later however, I thought "if the hook-lift device made a very difficult ATHA possible would it not facilitate more standard surgeries." I began using the femoral hook-lift for all ATHA and saw the benefits. Later, when new tables were designed with OSI, the hook-lift became an integral part of the design.

As the initial months and years went on, I became convinced that ATHA was a superior method. I was, however, consciously not in a rush to start advocating the technique. One reason was that I already enjoyed an international positive reputation for expertise regarding acetabular and pelvic fractures. Looking back, I realized that my career had included me advocating both good and bad ideas, and I wanted to make sure that ATHA was among the good ideas before I risked denigrating my reputation. The other reason was that I felt the orthopedic table was an important part of the procedure and the best table; the Judet table was no longer produced. I had observed the Keggi ATHA technique on a standard table; however, this further convinced me of the importance of the orthopedic table.

On one of my visits to Letournel in Paris, I was introduced to the president of the Tasserit Company, Mr. Axelrod, that produced the most recent Judet type orthopedic table. After beginning ATHA, I spoke with Mr. Axelrod by telephone and encouraged him to restart the production of the table. He told me that the table had been a commercial failure because he only sold a few, primarily at selected locations in France and that he was not interested in further production. I then began a discussion with OSI in Union City, CA, regarding the design and production of a new orthopedic table. The design and manufacture of a special table for a procedure, ATHA, that had hardly any surgeons in the United States performing the procedure was a tough sell. The initial table, the ProFx, was therefore to be a multipurpose table with the application for the operation of pelvic and acetabular fractures, general trauma, and ATHA. ATHA was the "wild card." When the first table was produced, in 2003, I held a course for about 20 surgeons with one table and one cadaver at Good Samaritan Hospital in Los Angeles. Stephan Kreuzer and Anthony Hedley were among the attendees. The ProFx table was also shown at the Letournel course, "Fractures of the Acetabulum and Pelvis."

Following the first courses, however, it became evident that ATHA was driving the sales of the ProFx table. OSI then saw the need for a table designed primarily to facilitate ATHA, and the Hana Table was born, which became a clinical and commercial success.

The journey to the current safe, reliable, and repeatable technique for AA that I currently use and advocate was not entirely smooth! Complications and problems need to be solved, and I will mention a few. As I began the technique, I began the use of a new cemented stem with a new cement. In the initial cases, despite a post-op x-ray showing a very good cement mantle, I saw the early development of radiolucency at the bone–cement interface in a significant percentage of cases, and these cases required revision. This was very disappointing, and the multiple revision surgeries made me consider giving up AA. I finally decided that AA was probably not the cause. I changed to the use of the triple taper polished MS-30 cemented stem, and the radiolucencies and resulting revisions disappeared. The other early discouraging factor was the long OR times and associated increased blood loss compared to my previous posterior approaches though these problems disappeared as I became more technically proficient.

In about 2001, I began using the Zweymuller stem because of its excellent long-term record and the trend toward uncemented stems. Unfortunately, it was not a good fit for the anterior approach with its straight (not offset) insertion tools and proximal lateral flare into the great trochanter. The associated new problems were fractures of the greater trochanter or proximal femur, which I had not seen with the cemented stems. Larry at the race car shop helped mitigate these problems by making me custom broach handles, but a new direction was needed.

After visiting Thierry Judet in 2002, I began dislocating the hip prior to the neck cut. Apparently, I did not dislocate like Thierry recommended, and forceful leg rotation caused three ankle fractures over a 2-month period. After changing the dislocation technique, no more fractures!

Conducting my first course on anterior approach in 2003, we had one ProFx table and one cadaver, and I demonstrated implantation of the Zweymuller. The initial ProFx table was laborious to use, and some participants went away and broke the GT inserting the Zweymuller as I had. Still, the technique went forward!

As I came from the perspective of acetabular and pelvic fracture surgery, complications were expected, reported, and discussed with a focus on solving and limiting them. Possibly as I entered the THA arena, the results were already at a high level and complications low enough that the reporting and discussion of complications created an immediate backlash against the anterior approach. Possibly I was naïve, but I was taken a bit by surprise at the immediate focus of anterior approach critics on complications. Critics seemed to gleefully detail and exaggerate complications, especially the three ankle fractures, even though these complications occurred only during the development phase of the anterior approach. I had made a conscious decision to report all complications from the beginning, including the development phase of the technique [4, 5]. Even though these complications did not continue, I felt it important that others be aware and thereby not go down paths that I tried and abandoned. As far as one's reputation in orthopedics, it is better to be identified as the one who has complications than the one who lies and does not report them. Being identified as a liar is the "kiss of death."

When starting on a new technique, there will be problems and complications; however, these complications and problems are not irrevocably tied to the technique. They are problems to solve. The uncomplicated cases, however, show the results that can be achieved, and if these results are clearly superior, the goal is to solve and eliminate the complications and make the superior results of uncomplicated cases the predicable standard. There are many examples of this as positive change occurred in orthopedics including Charnley's bad results with Teflon bearings and Letournel's initial 30% infection rate with the ilioinguinal approach. Though not true in all cases, having the vision and courage to go forward despite initial complications and problems can lead to an important step forward.

By 2004 I was fully committed to advancing AA as its advantages had become clear. On the other side, the naysayers, mostly the established experts in hip surgery, remained convinced that AA was nonsense if not outright dangerous. In a funny way, I liked all the opposition. I had been through advocating an unpopular point of view before: operative treatment of acetabular fractures, which later became the standard. You can't "win the game" if there is no one to play against!

In 2004, it was also my conclusion that I needed a commercial educational partner to advance AA. After meeting with all of the prominent implant companies, I chose DePuy. DePuy had an uncemented stem, the Corail with a proven long-term record. The Corail was a broach-only stem that was a match for anterior approach as well as a satisfactory broach handle. Also, I thought that among the big implant companies, DePuy was most open to new directions in hip surgery.

In 2004, I began the AA hip educational courses with DePuy that have continued to this day. The courses have provided important education. The courses have also been a catalyst for the evolution and improvement of the technique and its associated technologies. The initial technique that I brought to DePuy (now DePuy Synthes, DPS) has evolved and improved by contributions from faculty members, feedback from course participants, innovative facilitating technologies, and associated clinical research. The current DPS-sponsored courses that I continue to be involved in are conducted in association with the brands: Anterior Advantage® and Matta Method®. The prevalence of AA THA has grown dramatically since my first course in 2003. Probably today, most primary THAs performed in the United States are anterior (Fig. 2.3).

Anterior Approach THA has been criticized by saying that its growth and adoption have been driven primarily by industry marketing. This is

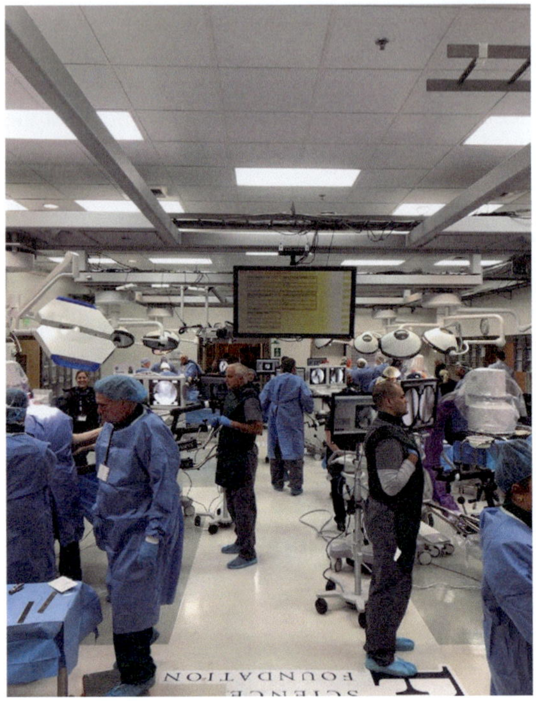

Fig. 2.3 Instructional cadaver lab sponsored by DePuy Synthes associated with contemporary surgeon course on Anterior THA

false. A significant force, however, that has pushed AA forward is "the market," and the market has driven anterior approach marketing (Figs. 2.4 and 2.5).

What is "the market" in relation to the anterior approach? The market is surgeons, and what surgeons want, an improvement they can provide to their patients and thereby satisfy patients and grow their practice. Additionally, the market is the patients in need of hip surgery who want the best possible results. The surgeon and patient-driven market drove the adoption of AA despite often vigorous opposition from known hip surgery authorities.

Marketing of AA by industry followed the market-driven trend. When I started working with DePuy on AA education in 2004, DePuy also conducted courses on mini-posterior and mini-lateral THA. As time went on, however, the surgeon's interest in posterior and lateral education fell while the AA courses were consistently filled. The bottom line for an implant company is

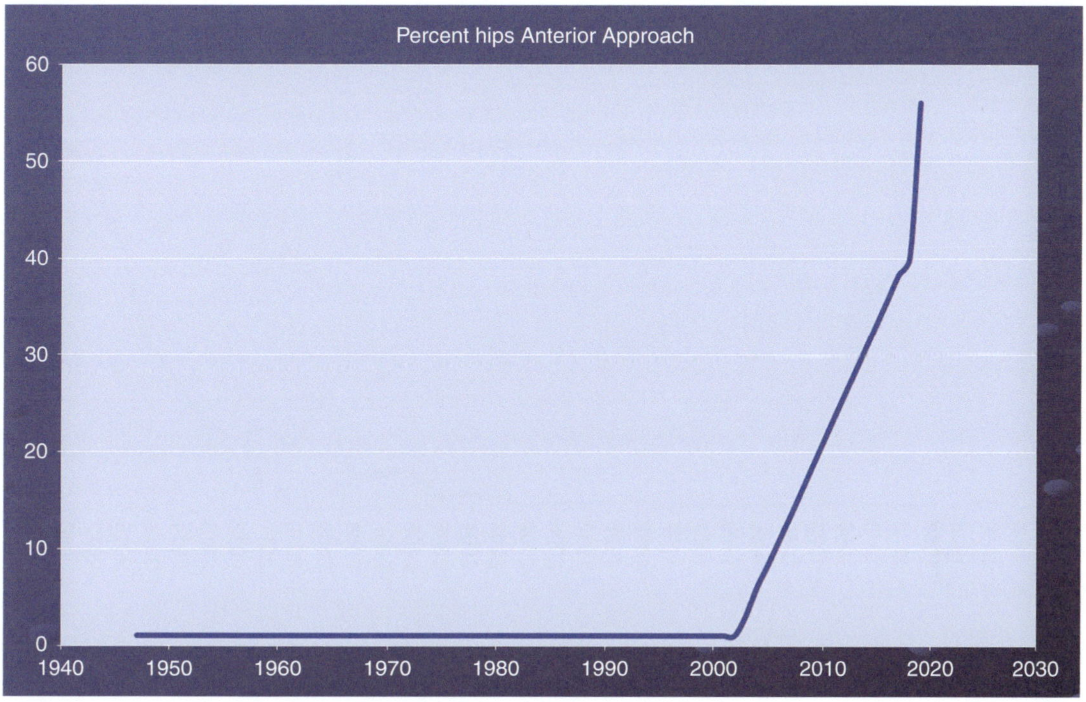

Fig. 2.4 Growth of Anterior THA since the first case by Judet in 1947 to present. (Data based on surveys of surgeon attendees at the Annual Meeting of the American Association of Hip and Knee Surgeons and Ref. [6])

selling implants, and to state the obvious, the company can only effectively show their implants to a surgeon at educational events if the event has consistent surgeon attendance. The market (surgeons and patients) thereby drove the marketing direction of DePuy and other implant companies. Similarly, as surgeons sensed the patient (market) demand for AA hip, those surgeons who had been trained to perform AA adopted marketing. The surgeons through marketing informed patients that they could provide the surgery that the patient wanted.

At this point in time, it is a rare surgeon that does not have a web page that markets himself and his practice regardless of their chosen approach for THA.

During my AA journey, I have learned several general things regarding change and innovation in orthopedics. Authorities in a field are often not open minded and objective. Their impetus is often to look for the best way to advocate and support what they already know and advocate. Scientific journals and publications are influenced by reviewers who can be prejudiced in their judgments. Papers submitted with conclusions that don't meet reviewers' preconceptions are held to a much higher standard than those that do. Finally, the market is a powerful and mostly positive force in influencing directions in orthopedic surgery.

I have heard logical arguments that new techniques and technologies should be tested first in academic settings. If the academics confirm validity through scientific methodology, then these academic authorities can teach them to rank and file orthopedic surgeons who can then provide them to their patients. This all sounds very good, except that it sounds suspiciously like how communism was supposed to work (and didn't): an elite group of experts would decide which products would be provided to the populace in order to bring the populace the greatest benefit. Also, academic institutions are often not where useful orthopedic innovations originate. I am completely in favor of academic institutions, basic and clinical scientific methodology; however, I am a firm believer that

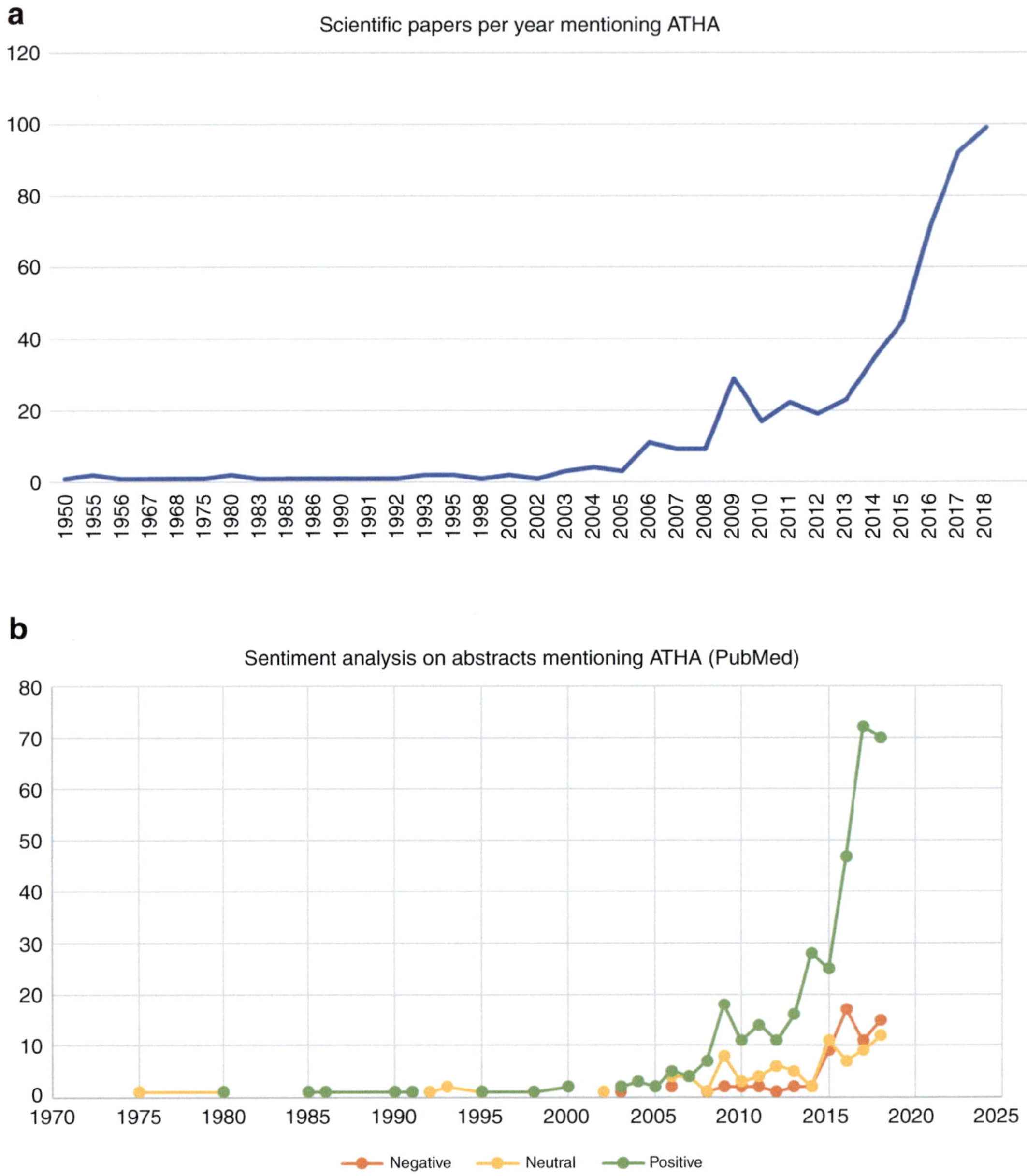

Fig. 2.5 (**a**) Numbers based on the search for keywords "anterior approach hip replacement" in academic papers listed in PubMed. (**b**) Numbers based on subjective analysis of abstracts of papers investigating results of ATHA in PubMed

the mix of many factors that are present in a free information, capitalist society leads to the best products, services, and medical care. This is what has driven AA to its current rightful prominence, the combination of input from medical science and experts, information that is available to professional and laypeople alike, and the positive power of the market.

References

1. Sarmiento A. Hip surgery: an odyssey. 1st ed. New Delhi: Jaypee Brothers Medical Pub; 2011.
2. Letournel E, Judet R. Fractures of the acetabulum. Posterior wall fractures. 2nd ed. New York: Springer-Verlag; 1993.

3. Henry A. Extensile exposure. 2nd ed. Edinburgh: Churchill Livingstone; 1973.
4. Matta JM, Shahrdar C, Ferguson T. Single-incision anterior approach for total hip arthroplasty on an orthopaedic table. Clin Orthop Relat Res. 2005;441:115–24. https://doi.org/10.1097/01.blo.0000194309.70518.cb.
5. Matta JM, Ferguson TA. The anterior approach for hip replacement. Orthopedics. 2005;28(9):927–8.
6. Patel NN, Shah JA, Erens GA. Current trends in clinical practice for the direct anterior approach total hip arthroplasty. J Arthroplast. 2019;34(9):1987–1993.e3. https://doi.org/10.1016/j.arth.2019.04.025.

Part II

Introduction to Part II

How wide are the variations of anterior approach THA? AATHA simply refers to the surgical approach and using it to implant a prosthetic hip. Throughout the world, there is variation in the details of how AATHA is performed. In the USA, since growth began in 2003, the majority of AATHA have been performed with an orthopedic table or table attachment that controls the lower extremity and also with use of the image intensifier (C-arm, fluoroscope) as an aid in confirmation of accuracy. Probably in Europe, operation on a standard OR table with more traditional confirmation of hip biomechanics is more common (hip motion, soft tissue tension, bony landmarks, palpation of extremities to judge leg length).

Within the orthopedic table, C-arm utilizing group of surgeons, I believe that there is enough similarity in methodology to allow this grouping. This section draws on the experience and expertise of this group of surgeons. As such, it is applicable for the reader/learner to combine techniques and technologies from the various chapters in Part II.

I believe that a benefit of the wide US adoption of the orthopedic table and c-arm is a consistent repeatable AA technique that has evolved and improved since 2003.

3 The Anterior Approach Surgical Technique for Total Hip Arthroplasty: The "Matta Method" of 2020

Tania A. Ferguson and Joel M. Matta

The Orthopedic Table

The current technique utilizes the Hana Table (Mizuho OSI, Union City, CA). The table allows unlimited spatial positioning of the lower extremities and unobstructed imaging possibilities with radiolucent leg spars. The extremity may be precisely positioned with extension, abduction, adduction, and internal or external rotation to facilitate various parts of the procedure and enhance surgical access to the acetabulum or femur. Specific increments of traction can be added to facilitate dislocation or reductions and further improve exposure during different steps in the procedure. The Hana Table allows unobstructed fluoroscopic imaging of the hip and pelvis, which allows fluoroscopic guidance during the surgery and navigation of component placement (Fig. 3.1).

The ideal operative experience would be with no operating table at all but with the body suspended and positioned by a yet-to-be-developed body controlling "magnetic field." In this theoretical environment, there would be full access to skin areas with no impediments to sterile draping. Additionally, the impediment that the operating table surface makes to the movement of lower extremities through the plane of its' surface would be gone, allowing extremities to be moved in any direction. The magnetic field would hold the new position or add a traction or rotation active force. The purpose of the Orthopedic Table is to approach the function of the "no table theoretical ideal." The Orthopedic Table contacts and covers only a limited skin area. The Orthopedic Table also positions and holds or applies active force in desired directions and magnitudes. The results are ease of draping and setup, improved sterility, better control of the operated extremity, better exposure, eliminating a human assistant, and consistent and stable positioning for C-arm images.

T. A. Ferguson (✉)
Nashville Hip and Pelvis, Nashville, TN, USA

J. M. Matta
Steadman Clinic, Vail, CO, USA

Room Setup and Draping

The OR is set up such that the instruments are on the operative side of the patient (Fig. 3.2). Generally, the use of two back tables (a), one Mayo stand (b), and one basin stand (c) is sufficient, creating an L-shaped area. The C-arm (d) is positioned on the nonoperative side, perpendicular to the patient. The C-arm monitor (e) and Velys™ Hip Navigation monitor (f) are positioned toward the end of the Hana table on the nonoperative side such that the surgeon can easily see the screens. A typical OR team will consist of the surgeon, assistant, anesthesiologist,

J. M. Matta, A. P. Sah (eds.), *Anterior Hip Replacement*,
https://doi.org/10.1007/978-3-030-91896-5_3

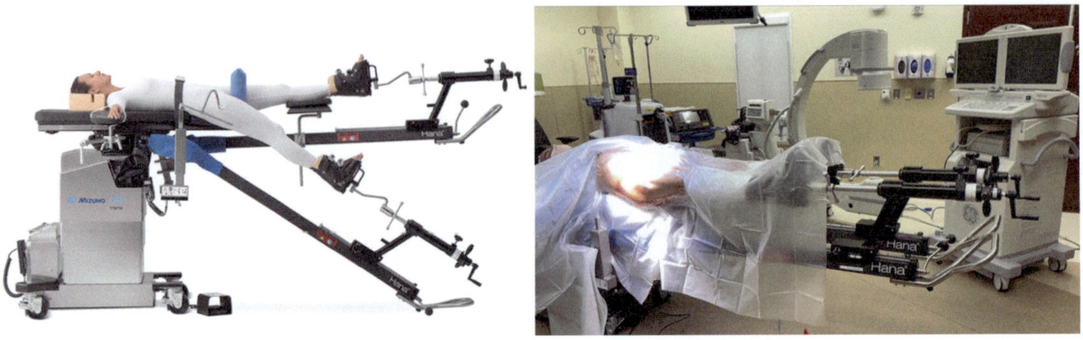

Fig. 3.1 The patient positioned on the Hana Table. The lower body is able to be visualized fluoroscopically without obstruction

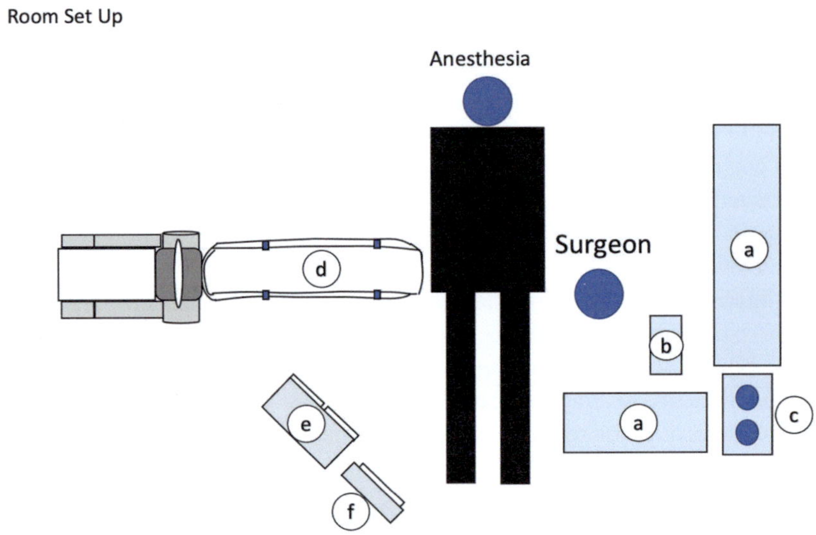

Fig. 3.2 The OR is set up such that the instruments are on the operative side of the patient and the C-arm across from the surgeon. (**a**) Back tables, (**b**) Mayo stand, and (**c**) basin stand create an L-shaped area on the surgeon's side. The C-arm (**d**) is positioned on the nonoperative side, perpendicular to the patient. The C-arm monitor (**e**) and Velys™ Hip Navigation monitor (**f**) are positioned toward the end of the Hana table on the nonoperative side turned to face the surgeon

scrub nurse, circulating nurse/table operator, and X-ray technician.

Instruments and Retractors

The instruments and retractors have been modified over the senior author's experience with the anterior approach total hip replacement. Modifications of angles and vectors have evolved to facilitate the operation and minimize soft tissue injury. Shown in Fig. 3.3 are the current retractors utilized.

Patient Positioning

The patient is prepared for positioning on the hospital bed. Anesthesia is administered, and the Hana boots and sequential compression devices (SCDS) are applied before transferring and remain on during surgery for intraoperative DVT

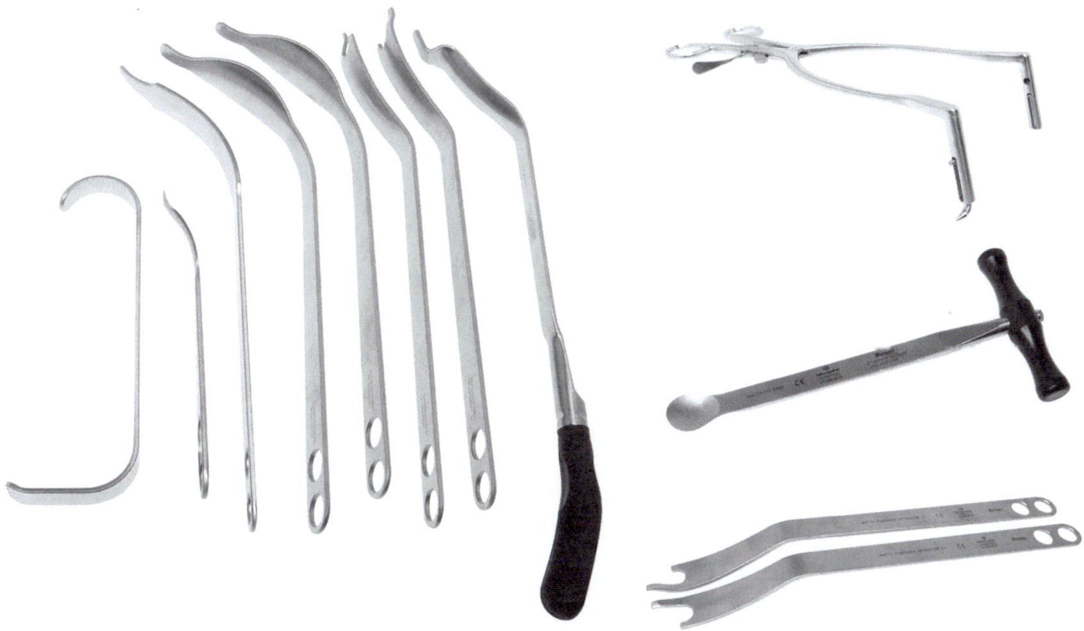

Fig. 3.3 The current anterior approach retractor set includes (**a**) Hibbs, (**b**) Narrow Hohmann, (**c**) Large Hohmann/GT retractor, (**d**) Narrow Cobra retractors, (**e**) Right Posterior Femoral retractor, (**f**) Left Posterior Femoral retractor, (**g**) GT Broaching retractor, (**h**) Capsular retractor, (**i**) Hip Skid, and (**j**) Right and Left Posterior Femoral retractors

prophylaxis. The patient is then positioned on the Hana table with the arms outstretched on the arm boards. The perineal post is placed. The boots are secured into the leg spars. The spars are raised/flexed 3–5 degrees to reduce lumbar lordosis, which eases accurate radiographic interpretation during fluoroscopic navigation. The operative leg is positioned with slight internal rotation to accentuate the landmark of the natural bulge of the tensor fascia lata muscle. The contralateral hip is positioned in slight internal rotation and neutral abduction-adduction to serve as an appropriate radiological control for intra-operative comparison of leg length and offset during the trialing stage of the surgery. A small amount of traction is applied to the contralateral limb to stabilize the pelvis around the perineal post.

Incision and Exposure

The incision landmarks (the anterior superior iliac spine (ASIS) and the profile of the greater trochanter) are marked. The incision is created over the muscle belly of the tensor fascia lata in order to enter the muscular interval between the tensor fascia lata and the rectus femoris. The mistake to be avoided is entering the interval *medial* to the rectus femoris. Thus, the incision begins 0–1 cm distal and 3–4 cm lateral to the tip of the ASIS and avoiding mistakenly proceeding too medially with the exposure. The incision is also initiated laterally to avoid injury to the lateral cutaneous femoral nerve as it exits the pelvis medial to the ASIS and branches out thereafter. The incision extends distally with a trajectory aimed slightly posteriorly (15–25 degrees from the long access of the femur and toward the head of the fibula) for a total of 8 to 10 cm (Fig. 3.4a).

- Some surgeons utilize a "Bikini Line" horizontal incision rather than the traditional vertical limb of the Heuter approach. The muscular intervals and exposure remain the same. This variation will be covered in detail in a later chapter.

Once the skin is incised and subcutaneous fat dissected, the fascia of the tensor will be identi-

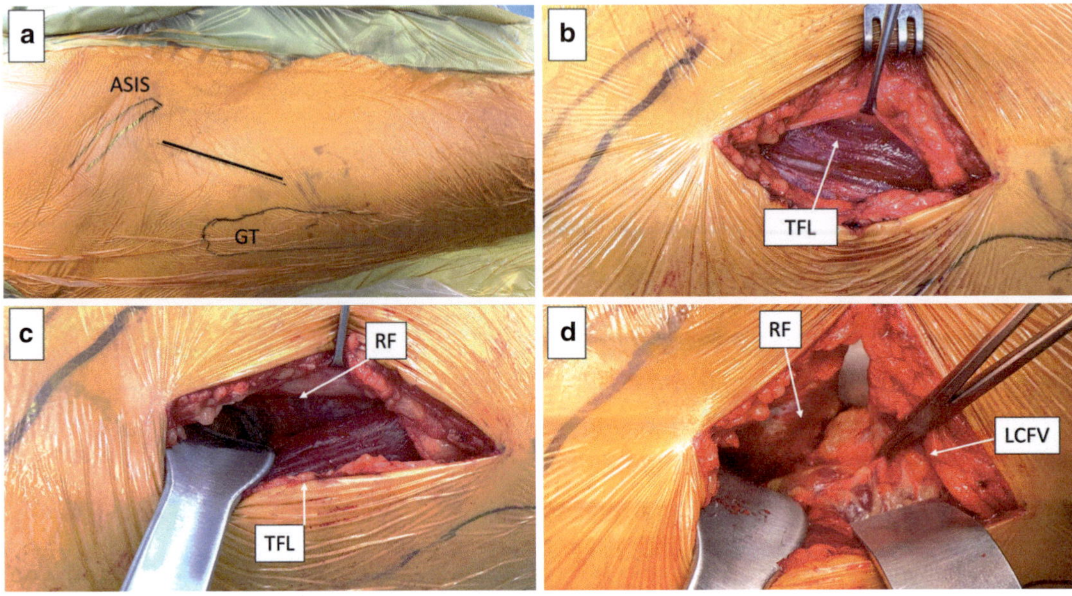

Fig. 3.4 (**a**) The incision starts 0–1 cm distal and 3–4 cm lateral to ASIS, oriented slightly posteriorly. (**b**) The anterior tensor's fascia is grasped with the Allis clamp, and the muscle belly is then mobilized laterally from the sheath. (**c**) A narrow Cobra retractor is placed between the superior/lateral hip capsule and the gluteus minimus. (**d**) The lateral circumflex femoral vessels are seen in the distal wound in the pericapsular fat. ASIS anterior superior iliac spine; TFL tensor fascia lata; RF rectus femoris; LCFV lateral circumflex femoral vessels

fied. The fascia is a translucent, blue appearing layer through which the tensor fibers can be visualized, and commonly has identifiable perforating vessels. The fascia is incised in line with the incision and parallel to the muscle fibers the length of the incision and extended subcutaneously a few centimeters distal and proximal to the skin incision. The lateral location of the fascial incision is between the anterior two-thirds and posterior one-third of the tensor muscle. The iliotibial band lies along the posterior border of the tensor and should not be injured.

The anterior tensors fascia is grasped and elevated with an Allis clamp, and the remaining dissection is performed within the tensor's sheath (Fig. 3.4b). Blunt dissection around the medial aspect of the tensor, pulling it laterally from its medial fascia, develops the interval between the tensor and sartorius superficially and between the tensor and the rectus femoris deeper. Continued blunt dissection around the medial tensor in the proximal region of the wound in the posterior direction will allow palpation of the anterior superolateral hip capsule. For orientation, one can palpate the anterior inferior iliac spine and the interspinous notch. A narrow Cobra retractor is placed in the interval between the superior/lateral capsule and gluteus minimus, retracting the tensor and the gluteus minimus laterally and exposing the hip capsule in the vicinity of the reflected head of the rectus femoris (Fig. 3.4c).

- It is possible to end up anterior and medial to the rectus, inappropriately exposing the interval medial to the rectus femoris.
- The superolateral retractor can perforate the gluteus minimus, which would appear as a muscle interposed between the retractor tip and the hip capsule. This is addressed by moving the tip of the retractor medially onto the capsule and sliding it down such that the muscle is now on the lateral surface of the retractor.

The anterior hip musculature (the sartorius, rectus femoris, and iliocapsularis—or capsular origin of the iliopsoas) needs to be mobilized medially to expose the hip capsule for capsulotomy. The authors' preference is to minimize disturbance of these and to not disrupt their relationship with the anterior hip capsule. A

Hibbs retractor can be used medially to gently retract the rectus and sartorius medially off the hip capsule slightly, and then to insert a narrow Hohmann or short curved Hohmann retractor just under these muscles, exposing the capsule for capsulotomy.

- Alternatively, an elevator may be directed distally and medially to mobilize the musculature from the anterior capsule, making a path for a second narrow cobra to be placed over the inferomedial capsule.

A Hibbs retractor now applied to the distal tensor muscle, retracting it laterally in the distal wound, will expose pericapsular fat and a fascia tethering the tensor to the rectus in the distal wound. The lateral circumflex femoral vessels will be observed as they cross the distal portion of the wound in this pericapsular fat and are cauterized, tied, or clipped (Fig. 3.4d). Care should be taken to ensure that all branches of this leash of vessels, including the ascending branches, be cauterized before cutting. Once the vessels are cut, they will retract.

The innominate fascia between the tensor and the rectus can be released by blunt or sharp dissection from distal to proximal to further retract the rectus and sartorius medically. This fascia/aponeurosis lies just distal to the cauterized vessels. Additional dissection of the aponeurosis that overlies the anterior capsule and at times excision of some of the pericapsular fat will expose the vastus lateralis muscle's origin just distal to the insertion of the hip capsule along the intertrochanteric line. The capsule is now exposed for capsulotomy.

Capsulotomy and Capsular Management

The capsulotomy is performed in an L-shaped fashion (Fig. 3.5). Starting cranially at the proximal capsule just lateral to the AIIS, the capsular incision continues distally parallel to the neck and at the junction of the anterior and lateral/superior capsule. The distal extent of this incision is at the tubercle on the anterior greater trochanter at the most lateral extent of the anterior intertrochanteric line. The second limb detaches the capsule from the intertrochanteric line from lateral to medial, just proximal to the origin of the vastus lateralis. The anterior flap of the capsule is retracted after placing a suture tag into the lateral edge, and a narrow cobra retractor can now be placed inside the capsule around the anteromedial femoral neck. Further mobilization of the anterior capsule can be accomplished aided by external rotation of the femur, and the capsule is elevated further medially off the intertrochanteric line at the base of the femoral neck. Careful vascular control is important as there are commonly several vascular channels along the inferomedial capsule and proximal vastus lateralis at the medial intertrochanteric line.

The lateral/superior capsular limb is also tagged near the greater trochanter and can be elevated off its femoral insertion from the lateral intertrochan-

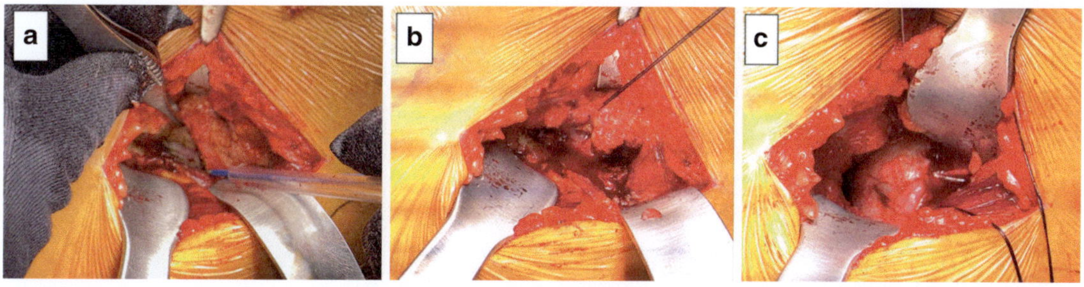

Fig. 3.5 The capsulotomy is performed in an L-shaped fashion. Starting cranially at the proximal capsule just lateral to the AIIS, the capsular incision continues distally parallel to the neck and at the junction of the anterior and lateral/superior capsule (**a**). The distal extent of this incision is at the tubercle on the anterior greater trochanter at the most lateral extent of the anterior intertrochanteric line. The second limb detaches the capsule from the intertrochanteric line from lateral to medial, just proximal to the origin of the vastus lateralis. The anterior flap of the capsule is retracted after placing a suture tag into the lateral edge, and a narrow cobra retractor can now be placed inside the capsule around the anteromedial femoral neck (**b**). Further mobilization of the anterior capsule can be accomplished aided by external rotation of the femur, and the capsule is elevated further medially off the intertrochanteric line at the base of the femoral neck (**c**)

teric line, exposing the base of the lateral neck where it meets the greater trochanter. The narrow cobra retractor previously positioned between the muscles, and the capsule is moved within the capsule over the superolateral head-neck junction of the femur. At this point, the capsular incision/exposure should be sufficient to visualize the acetabular labrum and/or osteophytes as well as the "saddle" of the neck joining the greater trochanter. All further work is done within the capsule, minimizing trauma to the extra-articular musculature.

The articulation now needs to be visualized to prepare for dislocation and removal of the femoral head. The Narrow Hohmann retractor is placed on the anterior acetabular rim and the anterolateral labrum excised to expose the articulation. If part of an osteophyte obscures the articulation, it is removed from this area with an osteotome. Application of traction by applying two to three turns of fine traction through the spar creates a small gap between the femoral head and the roof of the acetabulum. A Hip Skid or 3/4 inch curved osteotome is placed into the gap superiorly to loosen the tissues. It is then directed medially to dissect the ligamentum teres. One to two turns of traction are removed.

Hip Dislocation

We have found that preliminary hip dislocation before the neck osteotomy allows exposure of the posterior and medial neck and improves mobilization of the femur for subsequent preparation. Infrequently, dislocation is made difficult because of protrusio. With only a small amount of traction applied, the Hip Skid is reintroduced to the superomedial joint and the hip externally rotated about 20 degrees. A corkscrew is placed into the femoral head in an anterior to posterior direction, and the T-Handle is applied. The rotation on the leg spar is released, and the rotation wheel is used to guide the limb into external rotation. The force however comes from the surgeon balancing a levering with the Hip Skid and an upwards and lateral pull of the T-Handle. The head is levered laterally with the Hip Skid while an upward and externally rotating force is applied to the T-Handle to dislocate the head anterior and lateral (Fig. 3.6).

After dislocation, the hip is externally rotated as much as possible, and a narrow Hohmann retractor was placed distal to the lesser trochanter and beneath the vastus lateralis origin. The capsule on the medial neck is further reflected medially to expose the medial and posteromedial neck. This also gives the surgeon a nice special understanding of the neck anatomy and location of the lesser trochanter for the femoral neck osteotomy location planning. Once the capsule has been released as medially and posteriorly as desired, the hip is reduced with internal rotation and the cobra retractors are replaced within the capsule at the inferomedial neck and the supero-

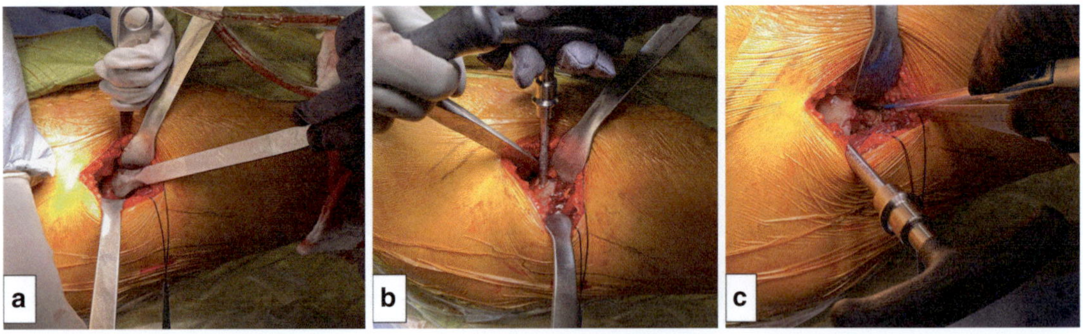

Fig. 3.6 (**a**) The hip dislocation is performed by first inserting the Hip Skid into the superomedial joint after traction has been applied. (**b**) The Cork Screw is placed into the femoral head directly anterior-to-posterior. (**c**) The Hip Skid is used to leaver the head laterally while the surgeon pulls the Cork Screw upward and externally rotates to dislocate the head. The medial and posterior-medial neck proximal to the lesser trochanter is now exposed for further capsular reflection

lateral head–neck junction in preparation for the neck osteotomy.

- The hip dislocation step has been found to gain femoral mobility early in the procedure. With the hip dislocated, the femur has now externally rotated 90 degrees and the femur is also displaced to a lateral position with the head lateral to the superior rim of the acetabulum. The access for release of the capsule from the medial and posteromedial neck is ideal. There is probably another benefit of "stretching" tissues that tether the femur. Following this step, it is observed that both acetabular and femoral exposure later in the procedure is enhanced. The benefits to later femoral exposure are most important.

Femoral Neck Osteotomy and Head Removal

The neck cut is based on the preoperatively templated radiographs. The most identifiable visible landmark in the wound is the anterolateral portion of the base of the neck at its junction with the greater trochanter, often called the saddle of the neck. Fluoroscopy can be used to confirm the location of the neck cut prior to osteotomy. With a Hibbs retractor placed distally to retract the tensor laterally and protect it from the oscillating blade, the osteotomy is performed by first aiming posteromedial to prevent the blade from contacting the posterior greater trochanter. The saw blade cuts the anterior, medial, and posteromedial cortices of the neck while the neck saddle and postero-lateral cortex remain. The neck cut is completed with an osteotome that divides the lateral neck from the medial greater trochanter, directed posterior and slightly medial to avoid injury of the greater trochanter.

Acetabular Exposure

External rotation of the femur of about 45° facilitates acetabular exposure. Light traction also limits femoral interference. Too much traction will tighten the iliopsoas and pull the femur into an anterior obstructing position. If the femoral neck continues to block access to the acetabulum, it is likely to have been cut too high, and a revision osteotomy may be required before proceeding.

A Narrow Hohmann retractor is carefully placed over the distal anterior rim of the acetabulum, taking care to keep the Hohmann tip on the bone to avoid perforation of the capsule or injury to the overlying iliopsoas and extra-articular soft tissues. The tip will lie on the pectineal eminence or just distal to it. A Narrow Cobra retractor is placed posteriorly with the tip on the mid-posterior rim external to the labrum but within the hip capsule (Fig. 3.7a, b). Alternatively, and preferably, the contemporary Capsular retractor can be placed as seen in Fig. 3.7c, d. This retractor has the benefits of being self-retaining, avoiding disruption or trauma to the anterior hip musculature, and providing retraction during the reaming and acetabular component insertion.

The inferomedial capsule is carefully transected to relax this area and ease liner placement medially. This also allows exposure of any osteophytes at the infracotyloid groove and the posteromedial acetabulum. Any remaining native acetabular labral tissue is removed.

Acetabular Reaming

Fluoroscopy Navigation Acetabular reaming proceeds with at least some aid from fluoroscopic navigation to ensure precise positioning of the acetabular component. Some surgeons use fluoroscopy throughout the reaming process, while others use fluoroscopy only for the terminal reaming and component placement. Certainly, when learning the technique, it is useful to check the reamer position with frequent fluoroscopic checks. The ultimate goal is to have the acetabular component placed with its center at the patient's anatomic center of rotation. The fluoroscopic guidance facilitates this goal and also aids in the orientation of the final component.

It is important to standardize your intraoperative fluoroscopy images before relying on

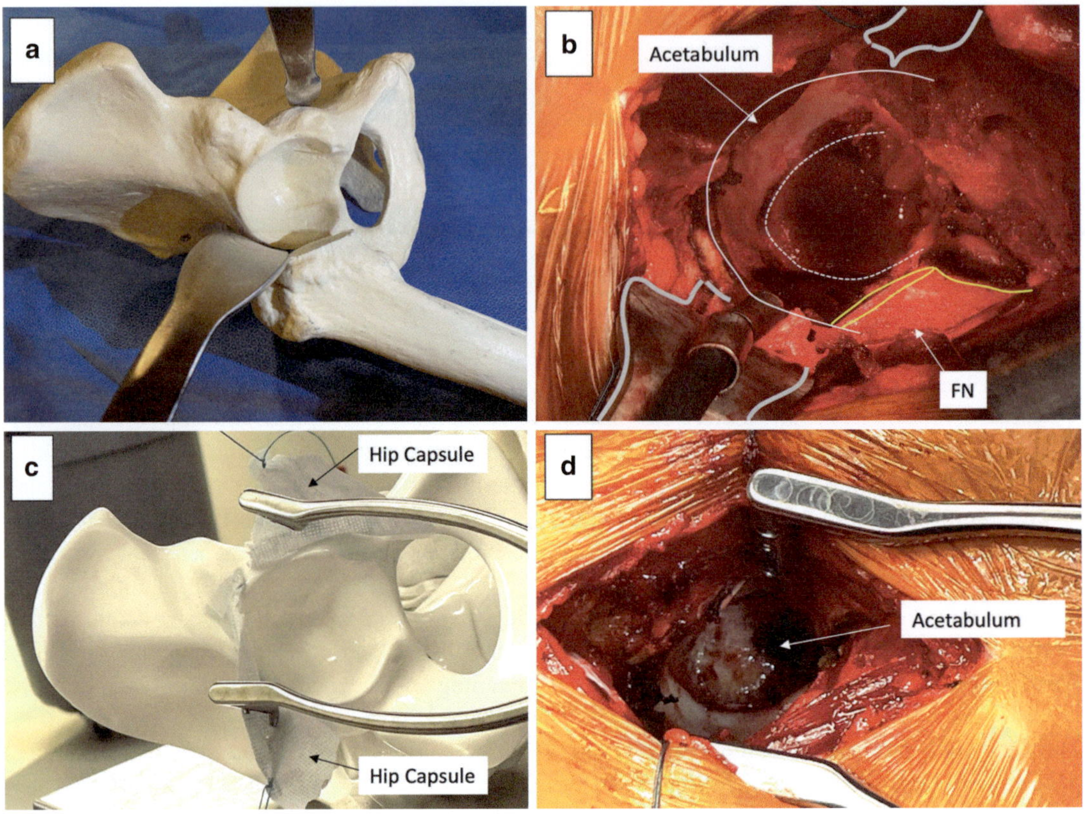

Fig. 3.7 (**a**, **b**) Historically, acetabular exposure includes the Narrow Hohmann retractor placed over the distal anterior rim of the acetabulum, and the Narrow Cobra retractor placed posteriorly with the tip on the mid-posterior rim. (**c**, **d**) The self-retaining Capsular retractor is now preferred in place of the Narrow Hohmann and Narrow Cobra. This retractor is placed between the anterior and posterior capsular flaps, giving excellent exposure of the acetabulum without any violation of the anterior or posterior periacetabular musculature

these images to guide the reaming process and component placement. "Leveling" the pelvis involves ensuring that the pelvis fluoroscopy image is adjusted such that the pelvic orientation and position observed on the C-arm screen is standardized to the preoperative X-ray. We obtain a fluoroscopic view of the pelvis (not hip view) centered at the midline and adjust the following parameters:

- Rotation: Rotate the image on the screen clockwise or counterclockwise until the transverse anatomical line is horizontal and the symphysis perpendicular. If traction has been applied during the procedure, it is not uncommon that the image is rotated toward the operative extremity (Fig. 3.8).
- Tilt: Exceptionally, the lumbar spine may be more lordotic and the pelvic tilt more positive on the orthopedic table than as seen on the pre-op supine AP pelvis. To assess the pelvic tilt, evaluate the height of the obturator foramen compared to the preoperative films as well as the distance from the coccyx to the symphysis. To adjust these parameters, change the "cant" or orientation of the C-arm cranially or caudally (Fig. 3.9).
- Roll: If the patient has rolled on the table (which can occur with traction), one side of the pelvis may appear more as an obturator oblique and the contralateral side more like an iliac oblique (Fig. 3.10). Leveling the table can address this issue, as can repositioning the patient on the table to be more level (if the table has already

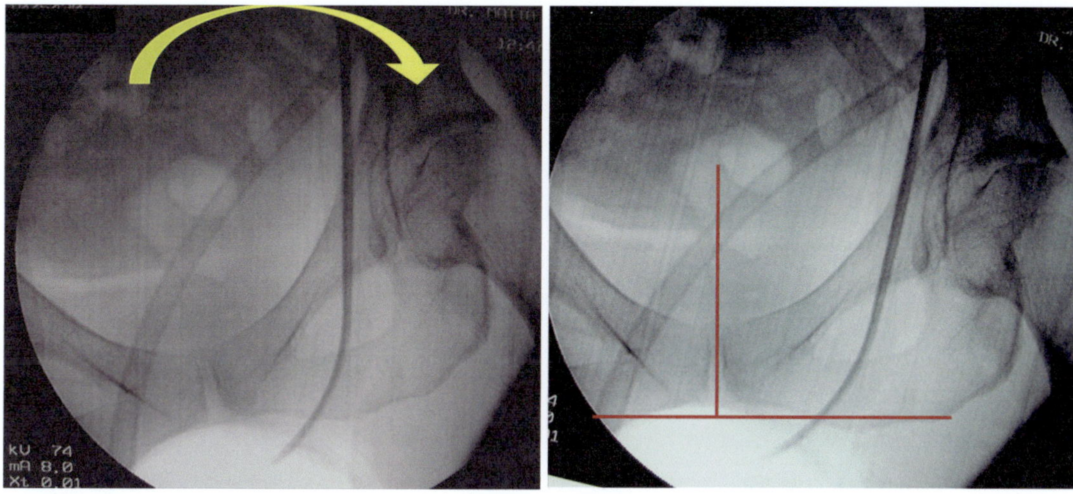

Fig. 3.8 The first step in standardizing the intra-operative C-arm image to the preoperative template is to rotate the image on the screen clockwise or counterclockwise until the transverse anatomical line is horizontal, and the symphysis is perpendicular

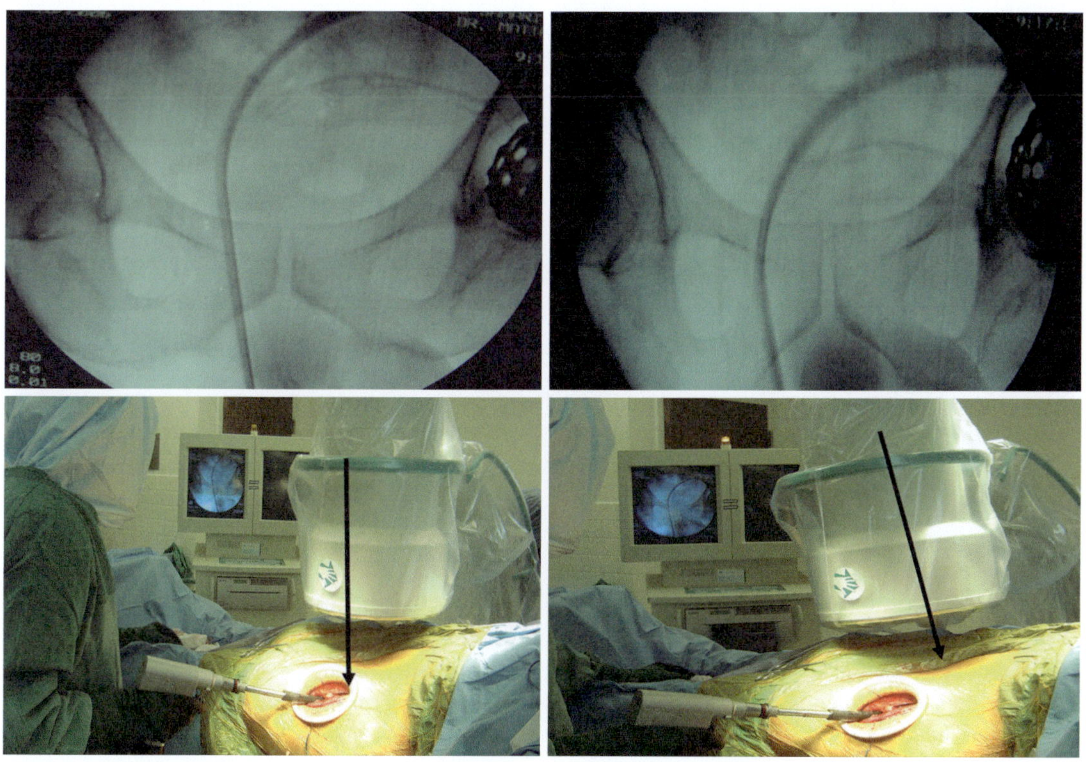

Fig. 3.9 The pelvic tilt, which can change in relationship to the X-ray beam on the Hana table, is then adjusted by changing the C-arm orientation cranially or caudally. We use the height of the obturator foramen as an indicator of the pelvic tilt

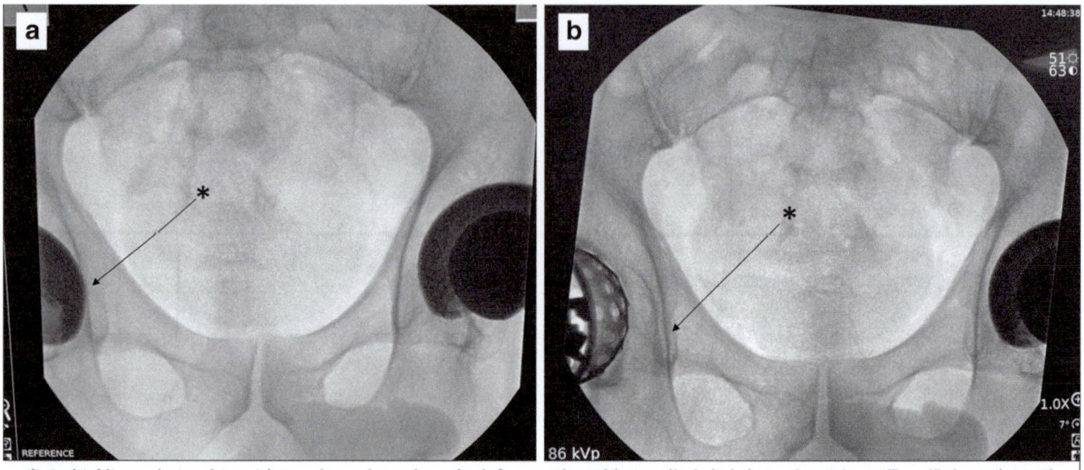

Fig. 3.10 The patient may be rolled slightly with respect to the X-ray beam, as seen with image (**a**) in which the pelvis is rolled to the left. The right hip image is a relative obturator oblique, and the ilioishial line relationship to the tear drop is lateral, compared to the contralateral left hip image that demonstrates a relative iliac oblique image, where the ilioischial line is seen to be medial to the obturator foramen. (**b**) To correct for this, the table is rolled to the left slightly until the ilioischial line is in a similar relationship to the teardrop on both sides

been leveled). If necessary, the c-arm can be "rolled" over or back until the obturator foramen appear equal in the medial-lateral dimension, though this technique will change the magnification of two hips and should not be used as a technique when imaging for the assessment leg length and offset (discussed below).

The pelvis is "level" when the coccyx is pointing at or overlapping the symphysis, the obturator foramen appears symmetrical from side to side, and the relationship of the teardrop and ilioischial line is similar to that of the reference image.

- The authors prefer to reference a pre-op supine AP pelvis, intra-op supine views, and post-op supine check view to maintain a consistent reference. Subsequent chapters on acetabular component insertion position will cover these concepts in detail.

After leveling the image and pelvis, center the image over the center of the operative acetabulum. This minimizes the effect of parallax on the perceived orientation of the acetabular component when positioning.

Reaming the Acetabulum Reaming begins with the reamer aimed about 25 degrees posterior in relation to the horizontal and about 25 degrees proximal. Medialize with the reamer aimed medially and slightly posteriorly and superiorly toward the teardrop (Fig. 3.11). Fluoroscopically, the reamer will appear more vertical and anteverted than desirable for the component positioning. Reaming commences in 1–2 mm increments, and as the reaming proceeds, bring the cup into a more horizontal position.

Progress is checked with fluoroscopic checks, and the reamer's depth and orientation are adjusted appropriately. Digital palpation and/or direct inspection is performed between reamings to ensure that the reamers are successfully removing sclerotic subchondral bone and that the reamers are not too large.

The senior author normally starts with a small reamer, 42–44 mm to penetrate a medial acetabular osteophyte and reach the acetabular fossa. Following this, a reamer 4 mm smaller than the templated size is used, and the depth of reaming is checked with fluoroscopy progressing at 2 mm increments. The final reamer size will match the cup size, and reaming the final size is typically

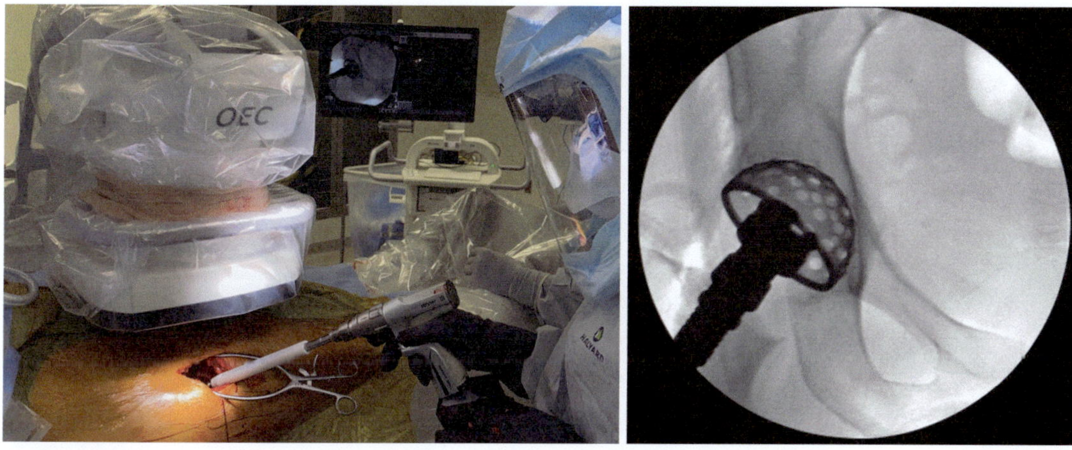

Fig. 3.11 Reaming begins more posteriorly and vertically directed than the desired cup position, and progress is checked with fluoroscopic checks and direct palpation

not with continuous rotation but rather by applying short reamer pulses while applying strong axial pressure to the reamer. There should be a sensation of reamer grip and torque with the final reaming. Continuous rotation of the final reamer as well as changing angles of the final reamer can lead to a reamed cavity that is too big and/or nonspherical and subsequent lack of cup purchase.

Using only the final size reamer for a single reamer technique is also used successfully by some surgeons; however, in this case, a 1-mm under-ream is preferable.

- The authors prefer that the acetabular component not extrude from the acetabular rim, particularly anteriorly, as this can cause irritation of the overlying iliopsoas tendon. At the completion of reaming, there is typically incomplete reaming of the acetabular rim. Reaming of all of the rim cartilage will typically lead to placement of too large an acetabular component. The majority of the subchondral bone of the roof should remain undisturbed at the completion of reaming, and this is seen on fluoroscopy. Reaming away this dense roof bone may impair proximal cup support and typically leads to a too proximal center of rotation.

Acetabular Component Placement

After reaming to the appropriate size, the acetabular component is placed with a goal of placing the cup in the patient's anatomic center of rotation. For surgeons unaccustomed to the supine position, it is common to place the acetabular component too much inclination and with too much anteversion. The correct insertion orientation is typically with the acetabular inserter more parallel to the floor and long axis of the body than expected.

The use of intraoperative fluoroscopic control greatly enhances the accuracy of the acetabular component placement. The authors aim for an orientation of 43 degrees inclination and 23 degrees anteversion for the acetabular component in almost all cases. The angle and proportions of the fluoroscopic image of the ellipse of the rim of the acetabular component indicate inclination and anteversion (Fig. 3.12).

- These angles are the preferred method by the authors. Acetabular component orientation targets vary based on surgeon preference.
- In patients with spinal fusion and no motion at the lumbosacral junction, a target of 45 degrees inclination and 25 degrees of anteversion is chosen to protect against posterior instability during sitting and deep hip flexion.

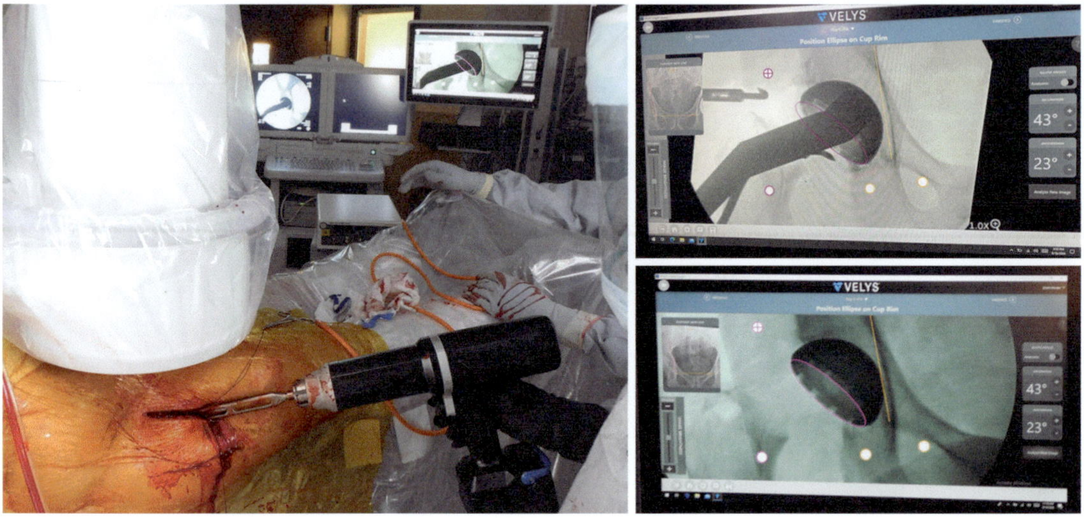

Fig. 3.12 The acetabular component placement facilitated by the Kincise impactor. The VELYS™ Hip Navigation computer navigational software system utilization for assessment of component inclination and anteversion

There are many options to facilitate the surgeon's interpretation of the fluoroscopic image of the acetabular component's orientation and inclination. Historically, a transparency with the desired ellipse drawn on it was placed over the image intensifier's display screen so that one could target the drawn ellipse during implantation. The authors now utilize the VELYS™ Hip Navigation computer navigational software system to more accurately position the acetabular component to their desired orientation (Fig. 3.12).

The acetabular component is impacted into its final position, with fluoroscopic assessment verifying accurate orientation. The authors now utilize the Kincise Automated Impactor, which allows fine adjustments to more precisely achieve the targeted position. It is useful to visualize the acetabular position with fluoroscopy prior to fully seating the cup. The cup position is then "micro adjusted" with small angular forces as the Kincise fully seats the cup. It is the author's preference to not use trial acetabular components. It is also the author's preference to use cups with no screw holes. The stability of the cup will vary from patient to patient, and the cup only needs to be stable enough to resist relatively gentle applications of angular force applied through the inserter. It is the author's experience that if a Pinnacle cup placed without screws is initially stable and remains stable throughout the rest of the procedure, there is a very high probability of osteointegration. If cup stability cannot be obtained, the first response should not be to go to a bigger cup or cup with screws. In this case, if the cup size is 54 mm, ream slightly deeper with a 53-mm reamer (one or a few pulses with pressure) and stability will almost always be obtained.

Once the acetabular component is impacted, the retractors are repositioned to allow placement of the acetabular liner. It is important to visualize the far inferomedial region of the liner-component interface, particularly if hard liners (ceramic or metal) are utilized. The incision in the inferior capsule performed before reaming aids this process by relaxing those far medial tissues. Once the liner is concentric within the acetabular component, it is impacted to lock it into place.

Femoral Exposure

Learning femoral exposure is the key to becoming comfortable with anterior THA. Exposure begins with the initial capsulotomy, is facilitated by the hip dislocation step, and finally is facilitated with the Hana table. The hip capsule release from the proximal femur mobilizes and exposes the femur while the capsule remains attached to the acetabular rim. A minority of femurs may require a tenotomy of the obturator internus tendon and possibly the piriformis tendon if the exposure becomes a problem. The surgeon needs to be patient and systematic during femoral exposure. Effort to force or lever the broach into the proximal femur can lead to proximal femur perforation or fracture.

The Hook Attachment for the Hana Table was designed to facilitate exposure of the femur through the single anterior incision. Once attached to the bracket on the table, the surgeon can use the Hook Attachment to elevate the proximal femur and stabilize the bone for broaching.

The gross traction control on the leg spar is released, and the femur internally rotated to neutral. The femoral hook is placed just distal to vastus tubercle into the interval between the vastus and the tensor, rotating into position around the posterior femur (Fig. 3.13). The rotational control and the gross traction controls on the spar are unlocked, and the surgeon externally rotates the limb by applying a rotational torque to the patient's foot/boot by grasping the foot boot along with the overlying sterile drapes. The surgeon thereby has control over the amount of torque applied to the extremity, and care should be taken, particularly in cases of osteoporosis. We externally rotate only as much as our current soft tissue tensions will allow, and the table operator locks the rotation into place via the spar control. In some cases, initial femoral external rotation is short of 90 degrees, but subsequent soft tissue releases will allow 90 degrees of femoral external rotation. Lifting up on the hook verifies appropriate positioning and starts to loosen the tissues still connected to the proximal femur (the posterior capsule, the piriformis, and obturators). A Mueller, a Hohmann, or a specialized retractor is placed on the posterior calcar region.

The hip is extended as the table operator lowers the spar to the floor. Further external rotation can often be gained by releasing the spar's rotational lock and, again carefully manipulating the foot under the drape, and applying more rotational torque before relocking the rotational control on the spar. Excessive force is never utilized to gain more external rotation of the hip. Force appropriate to the soft tissue tension is applied and locked. Any further rotational goals are accomplished by releasing additional capsules and soft tissues. Ultimately the goal is to have the proximal femur/hip externally rotated about 90 degrees, which commonly appears as 110–120 degrees external rotation at the foot. The leg is then slightly adducted to further enhance the proximal femoral exposure.

The Hook Attachment is placed into the Bracket (which has been attached to the elevator on the Hana Table during draping). Elevation of the jack causes the hook to deliver the proximal femur anteriorly, aiding femoral preparation. The surgeon should monitor the tension on the leg

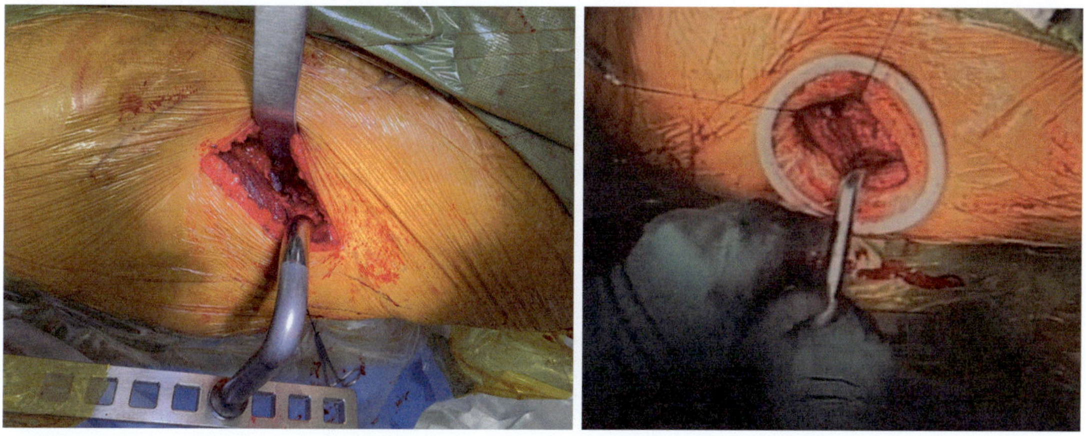

Fig. 3.13 The femoral hook is placed just distal to the vastus tubercle

during the elevation of the hook, as too much tension may cause a fracture of the trochanter.

The large Hohmann/GT retractor or the GT Broaching retractor is applied over the tip of the greater trochanter outside of the hip capsule. The lateral capsule (previously tagged with a suture) is now dissected off of its femoral insertion following the capsule-gluteus minimus interval. This will reflect the capsule off the lateral remnant of the femoral neck and the medial greater trochanter in an anterior to posterior direction, enhancing femoral mobility. Any lateral neck remnant is removed with a Rongeur. It is useful to perform a "prophylactic" cauterization along the areas from where the capsule was mobilized as well as the area of the retinacular vessels along the posterior–superior neck.

If further mobilization of the femur is necessary, it can be accomplished with further release of the posterior capsule and infrequently with sequential releases of the obturator internus and piriformis tendons. The obturator internus tendon inserts on the anteromedial greater trochanter and traverses posterior medial to the greater trochanter. In difficult cases may be released to allow additional mobilization of the femur. Likewise, release of the piriformis (commonly inserting at the anterior superior trochanter) may be done in extreme cases. The release of these rotators is preferred over the release of the obturator externus, which pulls the femur in a medial direction and is considered to exert an important anti-dislocation function and contribute to the hip's stability.

Balancing the releases of the soft tissues and manipulating the extremity ultimately result in adequate exposure of the proximal femur to allow broaching. Some patients require virtually no additional releases while others require more. The ideal visualization of a proximal femur ready for broaching is depicted in Fig. 3.14, with the posterior neck externally rotated 90 degrees and completely visible such that the broach's relationship to the posterior neck is easily appreciated (Fig. 3.14).

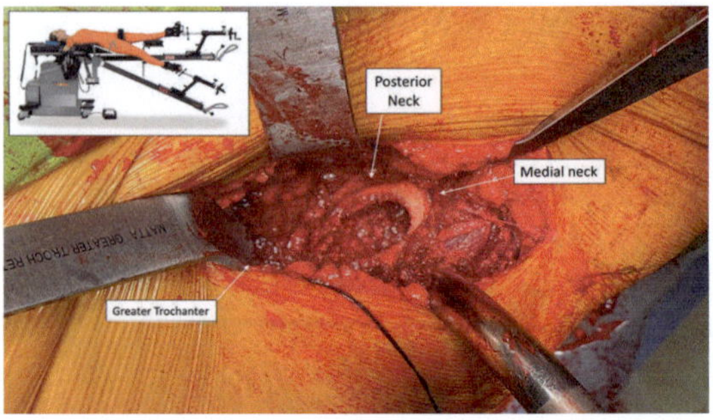

Fig. 3.14 The femur is externally rotated, extended, and slightly adducted. The Posterior Femoral retractor is seen medial at the posterior femoral neck, the GT Broaching retractor is positioned over the greater trochanter and oriented in line with the body cranially, and the Femoral Hook is physically lateral. The posterior femoral neck is seen externally rotated 90 degrees and completely visible, such that one can easily appreciate the relationship of the broach to the posterior neck

Femoral Broaching

Although any stem can be used with this approach, stems requiring straight reamers for canal preparation are more difficult because they require the most anterior mobilization of the femur to allow access down the canal. We prefer systems that utilize a single offset (anterior) broach handle, which facilitates femoral broach insertion while minimizing soft tissue releases.

- Many ATHAs are performed using double offset (anterior plus posterior) broach handles, especially when the orthopedic table is not used as an aid for exposure. It is the author's opinion that the use of the double offset handle poses significant disadvantages over the single offset and indicates a lack of adequate femoral exposure. The double offset handle is associated with an angular broach insertion into the proximal femur that can "hollow out" the proximal femur of its' cancellous bone that should provide a closely fitting envelope for the stem. Also, the nonlinear application of force to the broach leads to unwanted angular and rotational forces, which can further impair the broach/stem envelope.

Before broaching, any remaining lateral neck remnant should be removed. The "Cookie Cutter" osteotome or Ronguer may be used to remove a small area of the metaphyseal region entering near the posterior medial cortex, with the orientation such that the plane of the resection is parallel to the posterior cortex of the neck. The tip of the broach should begin near the calcar and near the posterior cortex, with the plane of the broach parallel to the plane of the posterior cortex. Broaching is then accomplished sequentially, always ensuring that the broach is parallel to this posterior cortex and not excessively anteverted. If this orientation cannot be accomplished, further femoral mobilization is necessary. Broaching continues until complete stability is achieved, with consideration of the size templated preoperatively (Fig. 3.15).

- The authors use the ACTIS stem (DePuy Synthes)—a metaphyseal impaction stem system. Using the Actis broach system, it is preferable to place the initial, smaller than final broaches in varus with regard to obtaining stability. The broach thereby enters the femur next to the calcar, and the broach tip proceeds distal and lateral until its' tip contacts the inner lateral cortex of the proximal femur. A canal finder can be used, but we prefer to begin with the "starter broach." After successfully passing the starter, the surgeon can proceed with a broach 2 sizes smaller than the final, templated size (rather than sequentially broaching in single size increments) and then proceed larger as indicated.
- The fluoroscopic view of the final broach and stem will show the broach/stem to be near the calcar proximal and distally the broach/stem will lie next to the lateral cortex and a radiolucency will be present between the distal broach/stem and the medial cortex.
- Using the Kincise is the preferred method of broaching for the Actis stem. Rotational stability is achieved more reliably, the broach envelope is most consistent, there is less chance of fracture, and the reduced surgeon effort enhances patience and focus. As the final broach size is reached, the broach will progress less than 1 mm with each pulse of the Kincise and will exhibit rotational stability. It is necessary to apply only moderate force during rotational checks for stability.
- The neck cut made earlier during the procedure is an approximation that is typically slightly long and will be adjusted as necessary as trials for leg length and offset are made. The depth of broach insertion is judged by relation of the top of the broach to the tip of the greater trochanter as represented by the

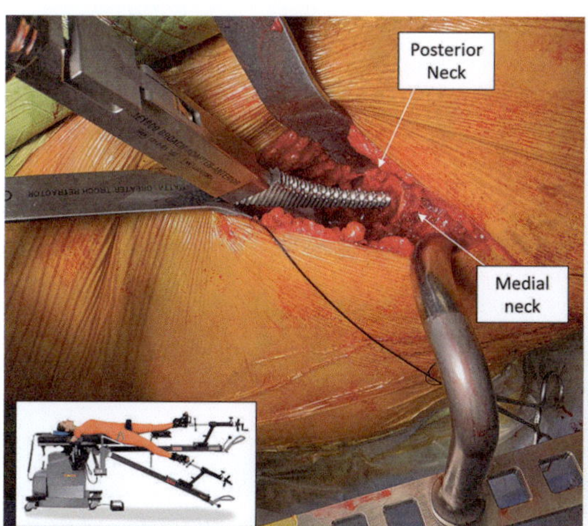

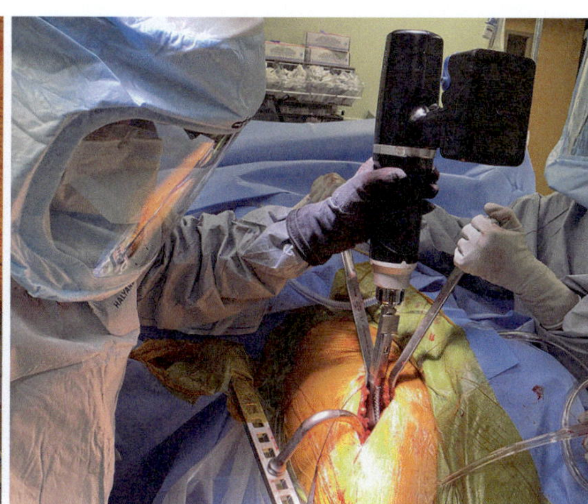

Fig. 3.15 Femoral broaching is performed with the lateral aspect of the broach in close approximation to the GT Broaching retractor. Rotational control is enhanced with the use of the Kincise impactor, and the goal is to position the broach such that the posterior surface is parallel to the posterior neck cortex

pre-op template. Most typically, the top of the broach is distal to the greater trochanteric tip by a few millimeters. However, depending on the femoral anatomy, the broach will be more distal for a short/varus neck and possibly proximal to the greater trochanter in the case of a long valgus neck. In most cases, the top of the broach will not be flush with the neck cut but will be slightly distal to the cut. The neck should not be calcar-planed at this point, but final neck planning should follow the length and offset information from the trial phase.

Once the broach is stable and near or at templated size, we trial the hip and evaluate length and offset.

Trialing and Fluoroscopic Evaluation

A trial reduction is done once broaching is complete. The appropriate neck and head balls are applied per the preoperative templates. To reduce the hip with the trialed components, the hook is lowered with the table jack and then removed. The hip is flexed to neutral, the rotational control is unlocked, and internal rotation is applied to reduce the hip. Hip reduction can be performed either by the surgeon grasping the foot, pushing distally and internally rotating, or by an unscrubbed assistant (operating room nurse) pulling traction and internally rotating. The traction is then released and the hip reduced. Significant traction and force should not be required. If the trial reduction requires excessive traction or force to push the headball into the liner, the construct is likely too long, and the ball head length or depth of broach insertion may need to be adjusted.

- It is typically necessary for the surgeon to push with a finger on the trial ball head during the reduction maneuver to prevent the trial neck and head from disengaging from the broach.

After reduction, the leg length and offset determination is done with the use of an image intensifier. An image of the contralateral hip is obtained (note that traction across the contralateral hip should be released before imaging for comparison). This image is printed and transferred to the right-sided image intensifier screen. A comparable image is then taken of the operated hip, ensuring that the magnification, rotation, abduction, and flexion are all equivalent with the imaged contralateral side. The table is very helpful for making and holding small adjustments of abduction and rotation to maximize the accuracy of comparison X-rays.

Once the position is equal, this image is also printed and the two images were compared by overlying the transparencies on a lightboard. The bony landmarks of the femurs are aligned, and the pelvic landmarks are compared (Fig. 3.16).

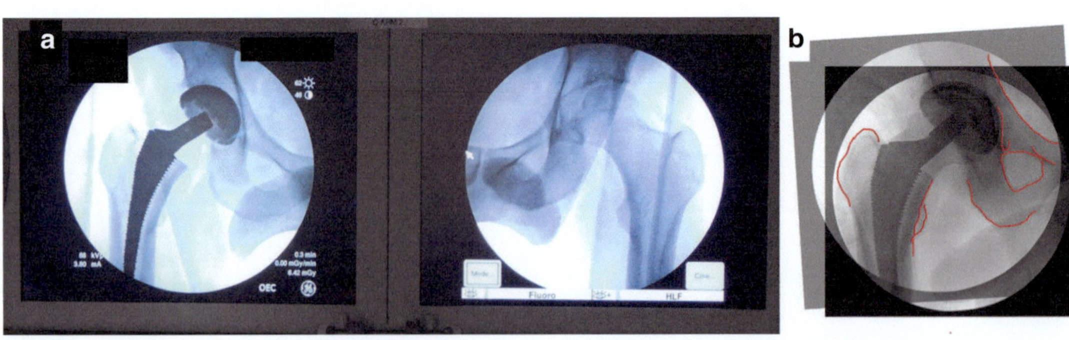

Fig. 3.16 (**a**) The C-arm is utilized to obtain comparable images of the contralateral hip and the reduced operative hip with the trial components. Magnification, rotation, abduction, and flexion must be equivalent in order to line up the landmarks for comparison. (**b**) The images are then both printed on a film (not paper) and transferred to a light board where they are overlapped to assess the length and offset compared to the nonoperative side

- The authors now utilize the Velys Hip Navigation system to evaluate leg length and offset, rather than the overlay technique. With the Velys system, one can compare either the trialed image to the contralateral side or compare the trial to an image of the operative hip taken before the neck cut (Fig. 3.17).
- Additional parameters, including implant size and position, and the varus/valgus position of the stem, depth of the stem seating, and stem sizing are all evaluated and changed if appropriate to allow for precise implant positioning and sizing. Typically, the goal is to match the length and offset to the contralateral side. If the contralateral side is not disease/deformity free, the surgeon can use his or her own "artistic leeway" and precisely alter these parameters to optimize the resultant mechanics of the hip and the prosthesis.

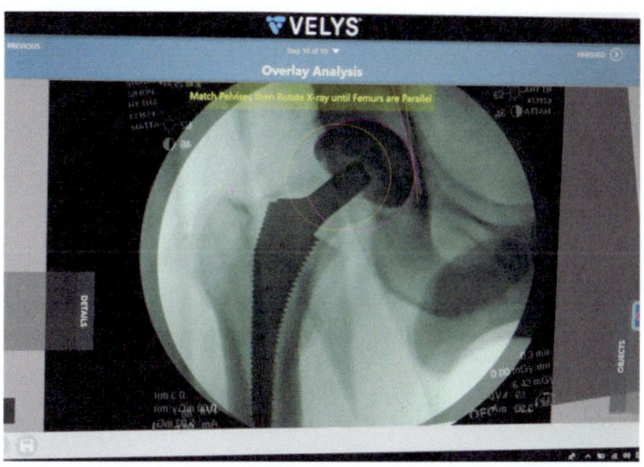

Fig. 3.17 Utilization of the VELYS™ Hip Navigation computer navigational software system for assessment of offset and leg length, in this case compared to the contralateral hip. Alternatively, VELYS™ can utilize an image taken of the ipsilateral/operative hip prior to the neck cut compared to the trialed image

Final Implantation

The femur is then re-exposed. The Hook Attachment is replaced, and the hip is dislocated with traction and external rotation. The traction is released, and the hip is extended and slightly adducted. The femoral exposure is re-established with the retractors and Hook elevation via the bracket and table jack. If the trial reduction was satisfactory, with good broach size and position, and accurate length and offset, then one can plane the calcar and implant the same final components (Fig. 3.18).

- The authors use a collared stem, and thus the stem is impacted until the collar is flush with the neck cut, ensuring the components are at the same height and thus the construct is the same length as the trialed situation.
- If a noncollared stem is to be utilized, measure the height of the trialed neck and impact the collarless stem to the same height to ensure equivalent leg lengths to the trialed situation.

If during trial reduction it was determined that adjustments were needed, make the necessary adjustments to correct broach size, broach inser-

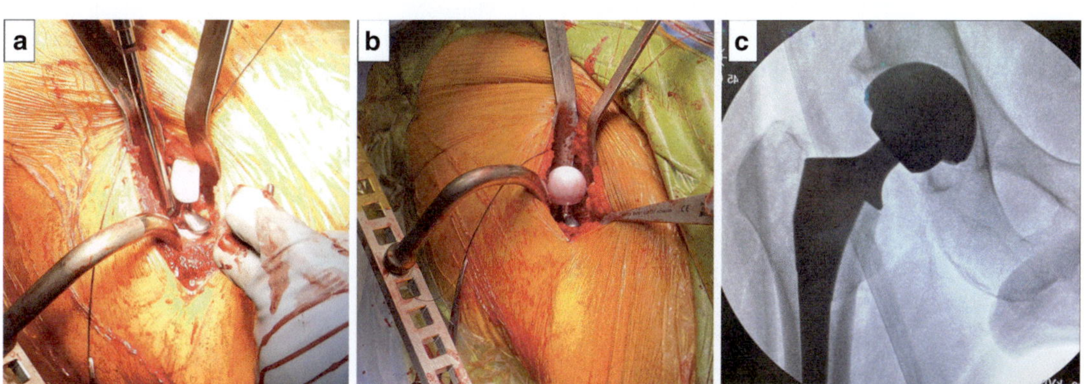

Fig. 3.18 (**a**) The trials are removed and the Actis stem is implanted, (**b**) the head ball is placed and secured, and (**c**) final images are obtained

tion depth, neck length, or offset. In some cases, the necessary correction is easily made and the next step will be stem and ball head insertion. The Velys one trial system is often useful in guiding these corrections. For significant corrections and if there is any doubt, perform another trial and X-ray comparison prior to inserting the final implant. The stem is impacted controlling rotation, and the Kincise Impactor is preferred.

The final headball is impacted onto the stem utilizing Kincise for proper head impaction force. The hip is reduced using the same maneuvers utilized to reduce the trials. Final fluoroscopic checks are made. The authors do not advocate "stability checks", as our practices indicate that accurate component positioning and restoration of the length and offset of the hip leads to stability reproducibly, and that "stability" checks in an anesthetized patient may lead to inappropriate and unnecessary changes. For surgeons who insist on performing a passive hip range of motion with trial or final components in place, the foot boot can be easily disconnected from its table attachment, and the extremity and hip can be moved in any direction.

Wound Closure

There is a lot of diversity as to the use of periarticular blocks, betadine soaking, application of antibiotic powder into the joint, and closure techniques. Certainly, surgeon preference can be applied without restrictions. The authors close the capsule by tying the tag sutures together. The tensor's fascia is closed with great care taken to avoid injury to the lateral cutaneous femoral nerve branches in the cranial medial fascia. Scarpa's fascial layer is closed as is the subcutaneous skin with vicryl sutures. Care is taken to ensure that the knots are deep and don't cause any skin irritation, particularly in the cranial wound. Skin closure is performed with a subdermal monocryl or barbed suture, and skin glue is applied.

Conclusion

While the technique has evolved to involve less tissue dissection and is enhanced by new technologies, the fundamental procedure has not changed significantly since our first publication of the technique in 2005. The tenants of muscular preservation and minimizing muscular trauma ensure dynamic stability of the hip immediately postoperatively and accelerate the patient's functional return. The use of the Hana Table facilitates these goals and allows an atraumatic surgery while assuring unrestricted use of fluoroscopy. Fluoroscopic guidance allows precise acetabular component placement as well as accurate restoration of the leg length and offset, optimizing the hip's mechanical environment further ensuring a stable construct and optimal patient outcomes.

Reference

1. Matta JM, Shahrdar C, Ferguson T. Single-incision anterior approach for total hip arthroplasty on an orthopaedic table. Clin Orthop Relat Res. 2005;441:115–24.

4 Understanding the Modern Surgeon's Transition to Anterior Hip Replacement

Alexander P. Sah

Introduction

The traditional successes of hip arthroplasty are based on a foundation of extensive clinical research and long-term patient outcomes. Conventional teaching and thought processes in arthroplasty are therefore inherently resistant to change and instead are focused more on improving upon these prior successes. This matter of thinking is deeply ingrained in traditional training and education and woven into the mindset of past mentors and trainees. Only in the recent two decades has the arthroplasty community begun to embrace new techniques and thought processes to achieve faster recovery, better pain management, and improved patient outcomes. What was previously thought not possible has recently become nearly universal in modern joint arthroplasty. These changes have not come easily, but the benefits of transitioning to these new procedures will fuel future enthusiasm to challenge prior standards and to adopt novel techniques.

In his 1980s groundbreaking book "Transitions," [1] Bridges maps out the cycle of change into three discrete stages (Fig. 4.1). The main strength of the model is that it focuses on transition, not change. The difference between these is subtle, but important. Change is something that happens to people, even if they don't agree with it. Transition, on the other hand, is internal; it's what happens in people's minds as they go through change. Change can happen very quickly, while transition usually occurs more slowly.

According to Bridges, every transition begins with an ending and ends with a beginning. In between Endings and Beginnings is an unsettling Neutral zone that most people would rather avoid but is essential for personal growth. There will be hurdles and motivators throughout the transition process that may encourage some or overwhelm others. Bridges says that people will go through each stage at their own pace. For example, those who are comfortable with the change will likely move ahead to stage three quickly, while others will linger, or even stall, at stages one or two. In the transition to anterior hip arthroplasty, the surgeon will likewise progress sequentially through these stages. How one navigates through the ensuing obstacles can often determine whether the transition is completed successfully or not. Understanding the expected stages of transition can turn seemingly overwhelming hurdles into opportunities to discover important lessons from each step. Demystifying these stages as it applies to a transition to anterior hip approach surgery can make the journey shorter, safer, more enjoyable, and ultimately successful.

A. P. Sah (✉)
Sah Orthopaedic Associates, Institute for Joint Restoration, Fremont, CA, USA
e-mail: asah@sahortho.com

J. M. Matta, A. P. Sah (eds.), *Anterior Hip Replacement*,
https://doi.org/10.1007/978-3-030-91896-5_4

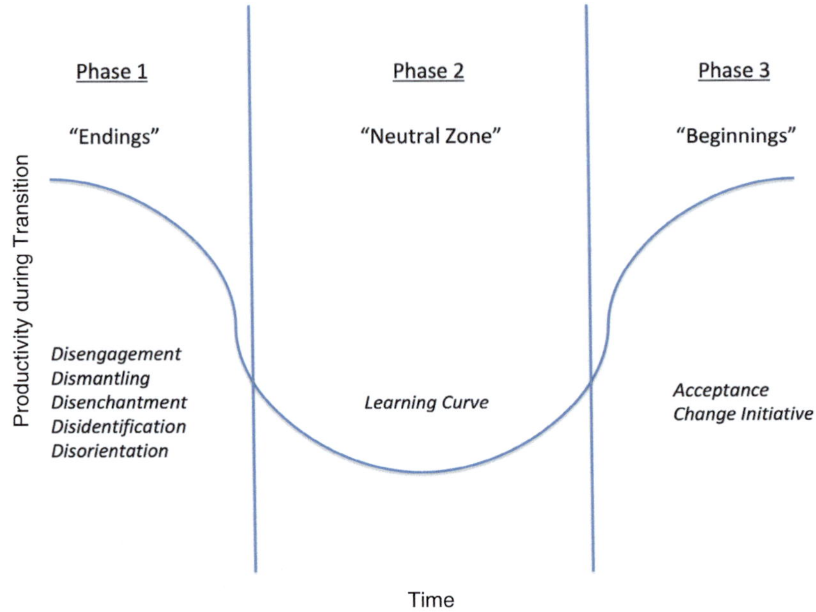

Fig. 4.1 The three stages of Transition, according to Bridges [1]

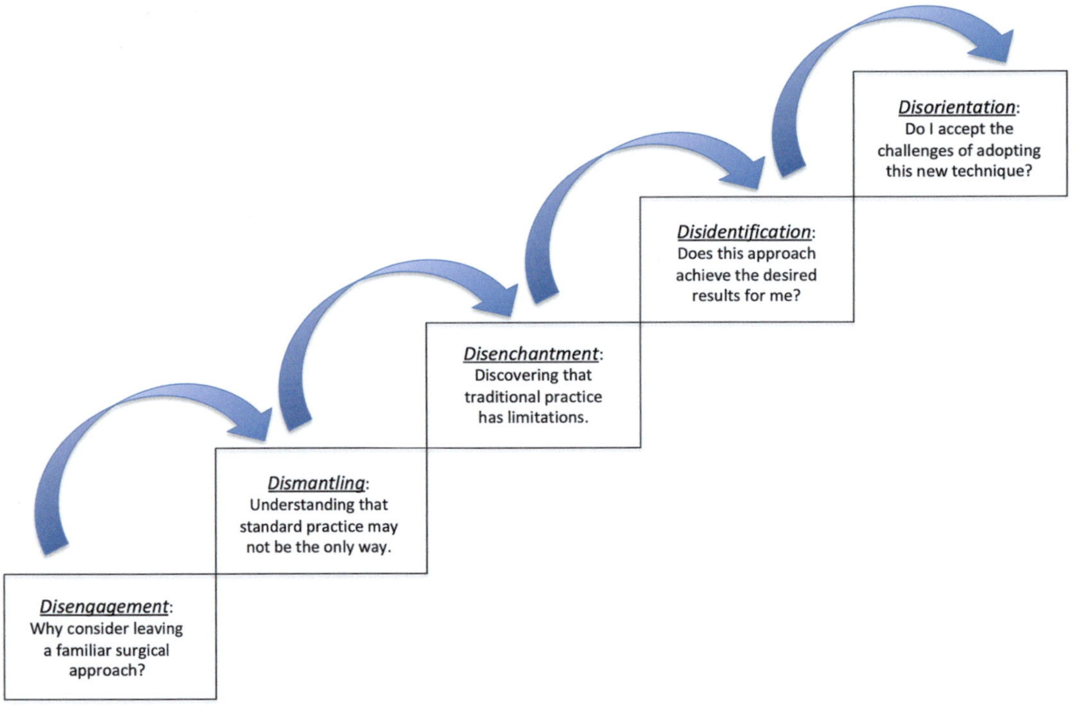

Fig. 4.2 The first stage, Endings, is comprised of five fundamental tasks that must be conquered in succession to move to the next stage

Endings

Within the rubric of Endings, Bridges identifies five fundamental tasks one must master in order to successfully move to the next chapter (Fig. 4.2). They are disengagement (separation from the familiar), dismantling (letting go of what is no longer needed), disenchantment (discovering that certain things no longer make sense), disidentification (reevaluating one's identity), and disorientation (a vague sense of losing touch with one's reality). People enter this initial stage of transition when first presented with the opportunity for change. This stage is often marked with resistance and emotional upheaval because people are being forced to let go of something that they have grown comfortable with. This first, and frequently most challenging, stage of transition often presents the greatest obstacles to a surgeon's adoption of a new technique. In fact, most failures to complete the transition process will occur within this first stage. For this reason, the majority of the focus will be spent on an in-depth exploration of this initial stage of transition to the anterior hip approach.

(i) **Disengagement**—Why consider separating from a familiar surgical approach?

Over the years, there has been long-standing debate over which surgical approach is most effective for total hip arthroplasty. Various techniques have been used, each with their own set of advantages and disadvantages. In prior decades, posterior and lateral approaches have been most commonly used based on national registry reporting, domestic and abroad. The posterior approach has the benefit of not interfering with the abductor mechanism, is familiar to surgeons, is relatively straightforward as a technique, and subsequently it is traditionally the most common approach taught in teaching institutions. In a medical field typically based on convention, this approach has subsequently had the broadest adoption in respect to both time and scope.

However, there is a risk of injury to the sciatic nerve during dissection or retractor placement with the posterior approach. The inferior gluteal artery may be damaged as it leaves the pelvis beneath the piriformis to supply the gluteus maximus muscle. Most significantly, the principal disadvantage of this approach is a dislocation rate of about 3%, as per a meta-analysis of >13,000 THAs [2]. Regardless of capsule repair or external rotator repair or preservation, the modified versions of the posterior approach all remain limited by the persistent risk of early and late hip instability [3].

The direct lateral approach described by Hardinge in 1982 avoids the need for trochanteric osteotomy. This technique asserts better hip stability by avoiding violation of the external rotators and posterior capsules. However, the risks associated with the lateral approaches include injury to the superior gluteal nerve, postoperative limp, and heterotopic ossification. Other variations of less invasive surgical techniques such as minimally invasive posterior, superior posterior approach, modified anterolateral approaches, two-incision, and others have been adopted and popularized by some small groups of users in recent years. However, none of these approaches have gained widespread popularity, nor sustained increased growth, to surpass the usage of the posterior or lateral approaches.

Disengagement, the first step of stage one, is likely the largest hurdle for surgeons attempting to transition from conventional surgical approaches. Because of the tradition and clinical history of standard techniques, it can be a daunting challenge to acknowledge a viable alternative. By nature, and reinforced with traditional training methods, arthroplasty surgeons are typically creatures of habit. From retractors to implants to dressings to medications, surgeons usually imitate what their mentors did, practice how they were trained, replicate what they were exposed to, and emulate the processes they learned. With this history of success, it can be difficult to find the initiative to make a change. In addition, people are often quite uncomfortable with change for many of the reasons outlined in these stages of transition. This apprehension can lead some to have a passionate and instinctive reaction to resist and oppose that change.

Ultimately, there must be a curiosity or motivation to be better than status quo to even entertain the idea of transition. Self-reflection may determine that there is an opportunity for improvement, whether it is faster recovery or minimizing complications and limitations with traditional approaches. Perhaps one realizes that while standard techniques are reliable and predictable, leaving a comfort zone to an alternative approach may be worthwhile to have the opportunity for even greater success. Most frequently, these motivations are internally driven, as the surgeon seeks personal improvement. On some occasions, the change may be driven by external forces such as competitors or patient demand. To successfully pass this first stage, one must at least be open to entertaining the idea of leaving the familiar.

The literature has supported that the anterior approach is associated with a reduced risk of dislocation, faster recovery, less pain, and fewer surgical complications [4]. The perceived shortcoming of the approach has primarily been a steep learning curve, which will be briefly described later in this chapter, and also warrants in-depth examination in dedicated chapters following in this book. Nonetheless, the anterior approach has persevered through initial resistance and opposition to the surgical technique. It has proven to have rapid adoption and continued growth because of its potential advantages over traditional approaches. In the AAHKS annual meeting poll in 2018, the anterior approach was the preferred technique for 40% of attendees, rapidly increasing from 12% in 2009 [5]. In a subsequent survey of nearly 1000 AAHKS members, the anterior approach surpassed other approaches and was performed by the majority of surgeons at 56.2% [6] (Fig. 4.3). Recent history has shown that the early reported clinical benefits and the opportunity to address limitations of traditional approaches by using the anterior approach have provided the motivation for overcoming the largest hurdle to change, disengaging from the familiar.

(ii) **Dismantling**—Understanding that tradition and standard practice may not be the only way to perform hip arthroplasty. Becoming critical of one's own practice and letting go of what's not needed.

Considerable controversy has emerged due to reluctance to abandon standard successful surgical approaches that have shown excellent long-term results and patient satisfaction [7]. While these traditional approaches are indeed clinically successful, they also have consistent, and not insignificant, complications such as dislocation, limp, leg-length discrepancy, muscle injury, or limitations in recovery. Conventional wisdom has accepted that these risks are rare and are acceptable based on the consistency and repro-

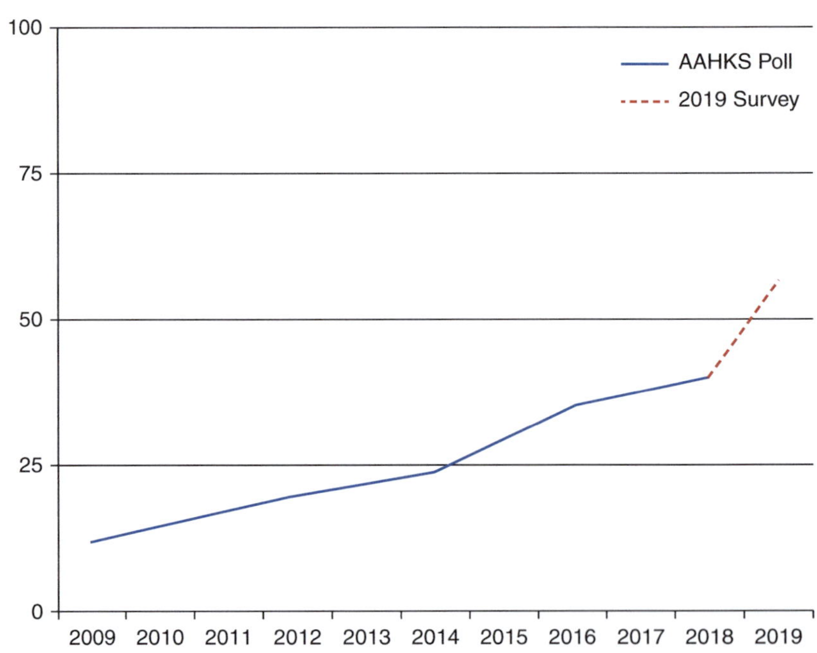

Fig. 4.3 Percentage of AAHKS members surveyed using the anterior hip approach as their primary technique by year. (Adapted from AHHKS Annual meeting symposium and Patel, Current Trend in Clinical Practice for the Direct Anterior Approach [5, 6])

ducibility of positive outcomes in the majority of patients. However, as surgeons become critical of their own results, rather than the reported averages of others, it may become apparent that hip instability, improper component positioning, or unequal leg length restoration is actually occurring more frequently than they would desire in their own practice. This realization can be the seed of dismantling and letting go of the dependence on traditional surgical approaches.

In addition, recent promotion of the two-incision, Watson-Jones, and various alternative surgical paths to the hip joint has created enthusiasm for alternative approaches for hip arthroplasty. In the early 2000s, a two-incision surgical approach gained popularity with reports of earlier functional recovery, faster discharge with a novel muscle-sparing approach [8]. However, this approach was associated with significant complications and difficulty during adoption by other surgeons. Cadaveric studies actually documented substantially more muscle damage to the gluteus medius and minimus through this two-incision approach versus a posterior approach [9]. Similarly, these other approaches may have benefits in the hands of experts, but they also have associated complications or technical challenges that prohibit them from being adopted by the masses.

However, the proposed benefits of these alternative approaches have garnered enough interest to fuel the search for a better technique. Even though most of these surgical approaches have not individually sustained widespread adoption, together they have laid the groundwork for a change of mindset of relying only on traditional approaches to one of enthusiasm to develop and adopt new methods.

(iii) **Disenchantment**—Discovering that traditional thinking no longer makes sense.

While other less invasive surgical approaches have paradoxically shown increased muscle damage compared to traditional approaches, there remains enthusiasm for performing hip arthroplasty with the least invasion possible. Some studies have shown that an alternative approach like the direct anterior technique may have muscle-sparing advantages. A retrospective magnetic resonance imaging study at 1-year postoperatively revealed significantly less frequent detachment of the abductor insertion, partial tears or tendonitis of gluteus medius and minimus, lower presence of peritrochanteric bursal fluid, or fatty atrophy of the gluteus medius and minimus with the anterior approach [10]. Furthermore, inflammation and muscle damage markers were lower in anterior versus posterior approach groups, suggesting significantly less muscle damage with the anterior approach [11]. When comparing trochanteric and groin pain, the anterior approach has a decreased incidence compared to the posterolateral approach [12].

Another deviation from conventional techniques is the movement toward using fluoroscopy or real-time guidance during hip component placement. Unlike spine or orthopedic trauma surgery, hip arthroplasty has traditionally been taught to be performed without the use of image guidance. And yet, it makes sense that using imaging during hip surgery would potentially address improper component positioning, which is a leading cause of hip replacement failure. In fact, studies have shown the benefits of intraoperative fluoroscopy to confirm implant fit and position, leg length, and offset [4]. This higher degree of accuracy of acetabular component position is evident even during the learning curve of the anterior approach compared to the traditional experienced technique [13]. Furthermore, performing hip replacement in a supine position provides the advantage of accurately measuring leg lengths either manually or with fluoroscopy.

Through these first three stages, a surgeon transitioning to the anterior approach has completed the theoretical hurdles to adopting the new technique. At this point, the surgeon is open-minded to entertain an alternative to the traditional, recognizes limitations of the status quo, and realizes that there may be opportunities for improvement. While these initial steps in the first stage of transition are commonly the barriers to change for many, these three steps are generalizations and are conceptual. The last two steps of Endings can prove to be challenging because they involve personal assessments and challenge the individual surgeon's capabilities.

(iv) **Disidentification**—Does this approach achieve the desired results in my hands?

At this stage, the surgeon has entertained that the anterior approach possesses advantages over the traditional approach but now must determine if these benefits can be achieved within their own practice. First, the surgeon must commit to investing the time and the effort to learn the surgical technique. This may involve learning the anatomical approach and the associated pearls and pitfalls. The technique may require a change in implant design used, or retractor and instrument changes. Complicating matters is that it may have been years, if not decades, since the surgeon has learned a new surgical approach.

Next, the surgeon must have the motivation to direct the surgical team in adopting the anterior approach. The surgeon is responsible not only for the surgical procedure itself but also for the coordination of the operating room staff to ensure the procedure is successful. Somewhat unique to this procedure is its dependence on ancillary staff such as a nurse responsible for leg positioning and a radiology technician for fluoroscopy. During this assessment of the team, some surgeons may change staff or modify the surgical steps to accommodate the limitations of their supporting staff. Others may determine that the technique might not be performed efficiently or with enough reproducibility to be worthwhile in their program. Compared to traditional approaches, the anterior approach initially requires more staff and greater coordination directed by the surgeon throughout the procedure.

Leaving a comfort zone can be difficult, and the motivation to try something new must be strong enough to overcome any reservations. However, desire alone will not overcome shortcomings of a team or joint program in anterior hip approach adoption. If the surgeon does deem that the support staff is capable, then the question remains if the surgeon has the individual confidence and ability to perform the procedure with the desired outcomes. Positive results and outcomes of others' experiences do not always translate to the individual. However, the availability of education courses, cadaver training, and virtual reality and multimedia experiences offer abundant opportunities to both improve and assess competency prior to attempting the first case. If the surgeon does pass this self-reflection step, then the last stage of Endings remains.

(v) **Disorientation**—Do I understand, and do I accept, the worst-case scenarios of embarking on this transition?

It is anticipated that there will be challenges and possible complications when adopting a new technique. Understanding and preparing for the worst-case scenarios can make the learning curve shorter and less steep. Therefore, in the final stage of the Endings phase of transition, the surgeon must recognize one's own limitations and understand and accept the possible outcomes to best prepare to avoid them.

Potential complications during the learning curve of anterior approach adoption have been well described in the literature. Complications due to femoral canal broaching are relatively unique to this approach and are of concern [14]. This adverse event is typically a technical error, and the surgeon must acknowledge one's own skills and limitations to avoid this complication. In fact, this unusual complication expectedly tends to lead to slower or failed adoption for those who do not recognize the nuances of the technique. Femoral fracture and nerve injury are the two most recognized risks that differ from the usual instability or component malposition of traditional techniques. Even so, the anterior approach provides significant benefit for patients in the early postoperative period based on pain scores and functional recovery, whether in the first 50 learning curve or in a more established group, compared to posterior approach, and carried through 6 weeks postop [15]. Other hip scores show continued benefit favoring the anterior approach to 3 months [4]. With regard to complications, a recent meta-analysis of only randomized controlled studies comparing direct anterior to posterior approach found no difference in complications [16].

People often fear what they don't understand, so the more education that can be provided about how to successfully navigate the transition, the likelier they are to move on to the next stage. Supporting the rapid growth and adoption of anterior hip replacement has been the development of robust education and training tools available to surgeons. It cannot be emphasized enough that the quality of training courses and availability of mentors to prepare surgeons how to avoid potential pitfalls has supported the rapid expansion of the technique. Educational sessions are available both in person and via multimedia to introduce and to simulate surgery before entering the operating room. Reverse visitation with experienced mentors has been one of the most helpful tools available to surgeons in transition (Fig. 4.4). Cadaveric training, one on one mentoring, and selective implementation minimizes risk in the learning curve [17]. It is suggested that a learning curve in the anterior approach can be accelerated, with proper training and technique, to less than 50 procedures [18]. Once equipped with all of these tools, the surgeon can be confident to be able to apply the skills, experience, and knowledge learned to successfully implement the new technique.

Neutral Zone

Once the Endings stage is complete, people progress to an uncomfortable but growth-filled Neutral zone, which Bridges describes as "an empty in-between time when... everything feels as though it's up for grabs and you don't quite know who you are or how you're supposed to behave." As such, most people would prefer to skip this awkward stage. However, by doing so, one may miss important insights and opportunities, putting them at risk of poor decision-making in the future. Bridges includes suggestions for dealing effectively during this phase, including accepting the need for this time in the Neutral zone, to keep moving forward, and to take the time to discover what one really wants out of this transition.

This stage of transition with anterior hip replacement represents the learning curve of adoption. Think of this phase as the bridge between the old and the new; in some ways, people will still be attached to the old, while they are also trying to adapt to the new. In this stage, people affected by the change are often confused, uncertain, and impatient. It is being in limbo between seeing potential advantages of the anterior approach and possibly being dissuaded by early inefficiencies or less than ideal results. The very advantages the surgeon seeks with a

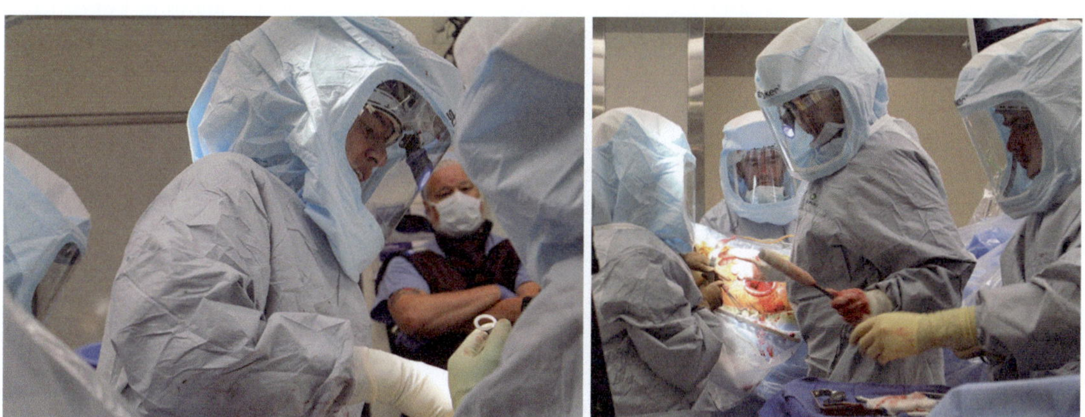

Fig. 4.4 Reverse visitation and supervision by an experienced surgeon can shorten the learning curve of the first cases performed

new surgical approach may not be apparent while beginning to learn the technique. Here, the surgeon or staff might even experience resentment toward the change initiative. But it is important that a true effort is given once transition has started to be able to fully evaluate whether the technique can be successful or not.

The degree of unfamiliarity in the Neutral zone may be overwhelming for some. All surgeons have a learning curve with any new operation, but the more it diverges from established methods, the greater the risk of unanticipated complications [19]. The anterior approach learning curve will be discussed in more detail in later chapters. The anterior approach differs from traditional approaches in patient positioning, the operative table, unfamiliar anatomy, and orientation, among others. Some early studies have subsequently reported a high complication rate and steep learning curve [20]. In contrast, experienced, high-volume surgeons undergoing the learning curve may be as short as only 30 cases, when comparing experienced surgeon's last 30 standard exposure cases to first 30 with the anterior approach [21]. Other high-volume experienced surgeons have reported no significant increase in complications or readmissions from the beginning, when comparing the first 200 anterior hip cases performed to the prior 200 cases performed with the standard approach [22]. Regardless, major complications seem to decrease with increasing experience, with the most dramatic improvements after the first 100 cases [23]. Other studies have suggested a learning curve of only 50 cases. Revision rate can be associated with experience, with 6% and 2% reported for surgeons who performed fewer than 15 or more than 100 procedures, respectively [24]. Australian Registry data also suggests 50 cases for the revision rate to be equal to more experienced surgeons [24]. Learning curves can vary based on surgeon experience and high annual number of surgeries prior to embarking on the learning curve [25].

Depending on how well the team is managing the change, they may experience a higher workload as they get used to new systems and new ways of working. In fact, surgical times are likely to be longer than the prior used approach, as the learning and coordination of the surgery progress. Operating time has been longer in the learning curves, but typically the differences disappear with time [26]. Proficiency improved after only 40 cases, and even more so after 60 cases, with no major complications [21]. Reduced operative and fluoroscopic times occur after the first 100 cases [27]. It was also concluded that the risk of fracture was eliminated with experience. Others report a decrease in operative time and blood loss after the first 37 patients [17]. This can be an uncomfortable time because it can seem unproductive, and it can seem that little progress is being made. Yet gradually the pendulum swings, and the benefits begin to become more apparent and consistent.

Even with a low-volume hip replacement surgeon, muscle-sparing advantages can still be achieved as measured by myoglobin levels postoperatively compared to a lateral approach group and without higher complication rates [28]. Furthermore, when comparing the anterior approach in the learning curve to posterior approach surgeries by high-volume surgeons, the anterior approach still shows a shorter length of stay, shorter procedure time, lower transfusion rate, increased discharge to home, lower minor systemic complication rates, and lower revision rates [29]. Single surgeon studies report no increased complications or revisions associated with the anterior approach compared to the posterior approach during the learning curve [22]. The anterior approach may be associated with a reduced risk of dislocation, faster recovery, reduced pain, and fewer complications. Early meta-analyses showed improved functional scores up to 6 weeks postoperatively [16].

Improvements in instrumentation, surgical tables, and retractor devices have possibly made the approach more accessible to more surgeons [30]. In 2013, it is estimated that the anterior approach accounted for about 10% of all surgical procedures worldwide [31]. Recent surveys have revealed that over 50% of US surgeons are performing the technique. During this learning curve, the surgeon can gradually increase indications, then commonly after the first 100 cases, the overall majority is anterior [23]. With more experience, the surgeon can relate to the growing body of literature reporting advantages of the anterior approach over traditional techniques. Growing mid-term outcomes show that the revision rate is significantly less for anterior versus posterior hip approaches [29]. An analysis of the Norwegian Arthroplasty Register found that the posterior approach was associated with more than twice the risks of revision for dislocation than anterior and other approaches [32].

The most successful teams will navigate through the Neutral zone by building upon new successes and having a solid sense of direction. This phase can cause anxiety for some because they feel uncomfortable in limbo but remind the team of its goals. Providing them encouragement and providing feedback on their performance will keep them motivated during this transition phase. Make sure that the staff see and experience the early benefits of the anterior approach, like faster recovery or earlier ambulation. These samples of early victories will keep the team confident that their efforts to complete the transition are worthwhile and result in positive outcomes. In spite of being a relatively awkward intermediary phase, the Neutral zone can also be one of great creativity, innovation, and renewal. This is an ideal time to encourage and reinforce people's efforts to try new ways of thinking and performing.

Beginnings

In the final stage of transition, it is typically a time of acceptance and energy. The surgeon and staff have begun to embrace the change initiative. They are building the skills they need to work efficiently and successfully with the new technique, and they are starting to see early victories from their efforts. While many may feel invigorated by Beginnings, for others it may take longer to become adjusted to this new identity or situation. Either way, as the Roman poet Horace wrote, "He has half the deed done, who has made a beginning." In other words, moving on to this Beginnings stage is a critically important step in successfully completing the transition process.

Having navigated past the Neutral zone, the surgeon and staff often find a renewed sense of enthusiasm and energy because they are past the prior challenges and hurdles. What was previously difficult and worrisome is now part of standard practice with the new technique. For example, the integration of fluoroscopy or other technology-based guidance is almost second nature at this point and is a routine part of the procedure. The staff has become familiar and comfortable with operating the leg positioner and understanding the leg maneuvers during each step of the procedure. The relief of these prior hesitancies allows energy to be focused on moving forward.

In addition, previous unknowns or apprehensions for safety have been addressed in the early experiences, and now attention can be directed toward an openness to learning how to personalize the approach or improve efficiencies. Skills can be developed and optimized by the surgeon and supporting staff alike. As such, there is a renewed commitment of the group to their respective roles. In this stage, the very advantages of the anterior approach that initiated the surgeon's transition are now starting to be realized. Patients may have faster recovery than prior approaches or have less pain or narcotic requirement. Use of fluoroscopy or technology-based tools may reveal its benefit in optimal component sizing and placement. Contrary to the initial perceived reservations that produced reluctance at the start of this transition, studies have shown shorter length of stay, shorter operating time, and lower revision rates at 1 year compared to the standard posterior approach [33]. In a meta-analysis of anterior versus posterior studies with minimum 1 year follow-up, the anterior approach was associated with a lower risk of reoperation, dislocation, and infection [34]. With a minimum 2-year follow-up, the anterior group achieved superior quality of life outcomes when compared to a matched group of posterior surgeries [35].

Importantly, as people begin to adopt the change, it's essential to help them sustain it. Reminding staff of the challenges they have overcome for the benefit of the team is valuable. Highlighting success stories and realizing the benefits of anterior approach adoption reinforces the importance of making the change. Take time to celebrate the change that the surgeon and entire team have gone through, and reward the staff for all their hard work. However, don't become too complacent—remember that not everyone will reach this stage at the same time, and also remember that people can slip back to previous stages if they think that the change isn't working.

Conclusion

With the continued successful outcomes of the anterior approach, the surgeon can explore applications of the technique to complex primary and revision procedures, as detailed in subsequent chapters of this book. Furthermore, by successfully completing all three stages of transition to adopting the anterior approach, the resulting change in thought processes and the willingness to strive for better outcomes opens the door for new and exciting opportunities. In this case, rather than being an obstacle, the transition process is a springboard to an enriched way of thinking and an enhanced method of performing hip arthroplasty.

References

1. Bridges W. Transitions: making sense of life's changes. Da Capo Press Inc. Massachusetts; 1980.
2. Masonis JL, Bourne RB. Surgical approach, abductor function, and total hip arthroplasty dislocation. CORR. 2002;405:46–53.
3. von Knoch M, Berry DJ, Harmsen WS, Morrey BF. Late dislocation after total hip arthroplasty. J Bone Joint Surg Am. 2002;84-A:1949–53.
4. Barrett WP, Turner SE, Leopold JP. Prospective randomized study of direct anterior versus posterolateral approach for total hip arthroplasty. J Arthroplast. 2013;28:1634–8.
5. Abdel M, Berry DJ. Current practice trends in primary hip and knee arthroplasties among members of the American Association of Hip and Knee Surgeons: a long-term update, 2018 AAHKS Annual Meeting Symposium, Volume 34, Issue 7, Supplement, S24–S27, July 01, 2010.
6. Patel NN, Shah JA, Erens GA. Current trends in clinical practice for the direct anterior approach total hip arthroplasty. J Arthroplast. 2019;34(9):1987–1993.e3.
7. Menghini RM, Pagnano MW, Trousdale RT, Hozack WJ. Muscle damage during MIS total hip arthroplasty- Smith-Petersen versus posterior approach. Clin Orthop Relat Res. 2006;453:293–8.
8. Berger RA, Duwelius PJ. The two0-incision minimally invasive total hip arthroplasty: technique and results. Orthop Clin North Am. 2004;35:163–72.
9. Mardones R, Pagnano MW, Nemanich JP, Trousdale RT. The frank Stinchfield award: muscle damage after total hip arthroplasty done with the two-incision and mini-posterior techniques. CORR. 2005;441:63–7.
10. Bremer AK, Kalberer F, Pfirrmann CW, Dora C. Soft-tissue changes in hip abductor muscles and tendons after total hip replacement: comparison between the direct anterior and the transgluteal approaches. JBJS Br. 2011;93:886–9.
11. Bergin PF, Doppelt JD, Kephart CJ, Benke MT, Graeter JH, Holmes AS, Haleem-Smith H, Tuan RS, Unger AS. Comparison of minimally invasive direct anterior versus posterior total hip arthroplasty based on inflammation and muscle damage markers. JBJS. 2011;93:1392–8.
12. Nam D, Nunley RM, Clohisy JC, Lombardi AV, Berend KR, Barrack RL. Does patient-reported perception of pain differ based on surgical approach in total hip arthroplasty? JBJS Br. 2019;101:31–6.
13. Kobayashi H, Homma Y, Baba T, Ochi H, Matsumuto M, Yuasa T, Kaneko K. Surgeons changing the approach for total hip arthroplasty from posterior to direct anterior with fluoroscopy should consider potential excessive cup anteversion and flexion implantation of the stem in their early experience. Int Orthop. 2016;40:1813–9.
14. Wayne N, Stoewe R. Primary THA: a comparison of the lateral Hardinge approach to an anterior mini-invasive approach. Orthop Rev. 2009;1:27.
15. Zawadsky MW, Paulus MC, Murray PJ, Johansen MA. Early outcome comparison between the direct anterior approach and the mini-incision posterior approach for primary total hip arthroplasty: 150 consecutive cases. J Arthroplast. 2014;29:1256–60.
16. Wang Z, Hou J, Hu C, Zhou Y, Gu X, Wang H, Feng W, Cheng Y, Sheng Z, Bao H. A systematic review and meta-analysis of direct anterior approach versus posterior approach in total hip arthroplasty. J Orthop Surg Res. 2018;13:229–40.
17. Seng BE, Berend KR, Ajluni AF. Anterior-supine minimally invasive total hip arthroplasty: defining the learning curve. Orthop Clin North Am. 2009;40:343–50.
18. Navarro SM, Frey C, Blackwell T, Voges S, Del Schutte H. Clinical results of direct anterior approach with minimal fluoroscopic exposure optimization techniques. Surg Tech Inter. 2018;33:1–4.
19. Goosen JM, Kollen BJ, Castalein RM, Kuipers MB, Verheyen CC. Minimally invasive versus classic procedures in total hip arthroplasty. A double-blind randomized controlled trial. CORR. 2011;469:200–8.

20. Meermans G. The direct anterior approach in total hip arthroplasty- a systematic review of the literature. JBJS Br. 2017;99B:732–40.
21. Goytia RN, Jones LC, Hungerford MW. Learning curve for the anterior approach total hip arthroplasty. J Surg Orthop Adv. 2012;21:78–83.
22. Schwartz BE, Sisko ZW, Mayekar EM, Wang OJ, Godron AC. Transitioning to the direct anterior approach in total hip arthroplasty: is it safe in the current health care climate? J Arthroplast. 2016;31:2819–24.
23. Harford JM, Bellino MJ. The learning curve for the direct anterior approach for total hip arthroplasty: a single surgeon's first 500 cases. Hip Int. 2017;27:483–8.
24. De Steiger R, Lorimer M, Solomon M. What is the learning curve for the anterior approach for total hip arthroplasty? CORR. 2015;473:3860–6.
25. Pogliacomi F, Paraskevopoulos A, Costantino C, Marenghi P, Ceccarelli F. Influence of surgical experience in the learning curve of a new approach in hip replacement: anterior mini-invasive vs standard lateral. Hip Int. 2012;22:555–61.
26. Berend KR, Lombardi AV, Seng BE, Adams JB. Enhanced early outcomes with the anterior supine intermuscular approach in primary total hip arthroplasty. JBJS. 2009;91:107–20.
27. Masonis J, Thompson C, Odum S. Safe and accurate: learning the direct anterior total hip arthroplasty. Orthopedics. 2008;31:128–34.
28. Nistor DV, Caterev S, Bolboaca SD, Cosma D, Lucaciu D, Todor A. Transitioning to the direct anterior approach in total hip arthroplasty. I it a true muscle spearing approach when performed by a low volume hip replacement surgeon? Int Orthop. 2017;41:2245–52.
29. Ponzio DY, Poulsides LA, Salvatore A, Lee Y, Memtsoudis SG, Alexiades MM. In-hospital morbidity and postoperative revisions after direct anterior versus posterior total hip arthroplasty. J Arthroplast. 2018;33:1421–5.
30. Post ZD, Orozco F, Diaz-Ledezma C, Hozack WJ, Ong A. Direct anterior approach for total hip arthroplasty: indications, technique, and results. JAAOS. 2014;22:595–603.
31. Chechik O, Khashan M, Lador R, Salai M, Ama E. Surgical approach and prosthesis fixation in hip arthroplasty worldwide. Arch Orthop Trauma Surg. 2013;133:1595–60.
32. Mjaaland KE, Svenningsen S, Fenstad AM, Havelin LI, Furnes O, Norsletten L. Implant survival after minimally invasive anterior or anterolateral vs conventional posterior or direct lateral approach: an analysis of 21,860 total hip arthroplasties from the Norwegian Arthroplasty Register (2008 to 2013). JBJS. 2017;99:840–7.
33. Balasubramaniam U, Dowsey M, Ma F, Dunin A, Choong P. Functional and clinical outcomes following anterior hip replacement: a 5-year comparative study versus posterior approach. ANZ J Surg. 2016;86:589–93.
34. Miller LE, Gondusky JS, Kamath AF, Boettner F, Wright J, Bhattacharyya S. Influence of surgical approach on complication risk in primary total hip arthroplasty. Acta Orthop. 2018;89:289–94.
35. Maldonado DR, Kyin C, Walker-Santiago R, Rosinsky PJ, Shapira J, Lall AC, Domb BG. Direct anterior approach versus posterior approach in primary total hip replacement: comparison of minimum 2-year outcomes. Hip Intern. 2021;31(2):166–73.

The Learning Curve for the Anterior Approach: Early, Middle, and How It Continues

5

Juan C. Suarez and Saul Hernandez Rodriguez

Introduction

The field of orthopedic surgery has experienced a rapid increase in innovation in an attempt at improving patient care and outcomes. Innovation has been introduced in terms of technology, surgical techniques, implants, and instrumentation. Although hip replacement has been termed the "operation of the century," this has not quenched the thirst for improvement [1]. Although the anterior approach to total hip arthroplasty is not novel, it has recently gained popularity for its superior early functional outcomes, improved component positioning, and lower dislocations rates [2–5]. Nakata et al. published their results comparing the anterior approach to the posterior approach and showed faster recovery, improved gait mechanics, and component positioning with the anterior approach [5]. Matta et al. followed with their consecutive series of patients using a specialized table and fluoroscopy showing accurate component position and low dislocation rates [4]. These early reports, in addition to the growing research, have fueled the enthusiasm for the anterior approach.

The posterior and lateral approaches have been the most popular approaches to hip arthroplasty in the United States and the more commonly taught in residency programs [6]. The adoption of the anterior approach has increased consistently over the last two decades. Sheth et al. reported a 4% anterior approach prevalence on the Kaiser Permanente data from 2001 through 2011 [7]. Subsequently, Maratt et al. showed a 14% on the Blue Cross Blue Shield data in Michigan in 2012 through 2014 [8]. More recently, a survey of the American Association of Hip and Knee Surgeons showed 56.2% usage among the responders [9]. These studies confirm the increased adoption of the approach in the United States.

The recent adoption of the approach along with the educational gaps at teaching institutions has led surgeons to learn the approach outside their formal surgical training. As with any learning process, the introduction of a new surgical technique or approach comes with a learning curve. The same AAHKS survey showed that fear of the learning curve was the main reason for not adopting the technique in 23.6% of the surgeons [9]. The learning curve presents an ethical dilemma where the surgeon must balance the risk of patients with the need to learn innovation aimed at improving patient care.

Surgical Learning Curve

The surgical learning curve is the association between a surgeon's proficiency in a procedure and the times he/she has performed the proce-

J. C. Suarez (✉) · S. H. Rodriguez
Miami Orthopedics and Sports Medicine Institute, Baptist Health South Florida, Miami, FL, USA
e-mail: jcsuarez@me.com

J. M. Matta, A. P. Sah (eds.), *Anterior Hip Replacement*,
https://doi.org/10.1007/978-3-030-91896-5_5

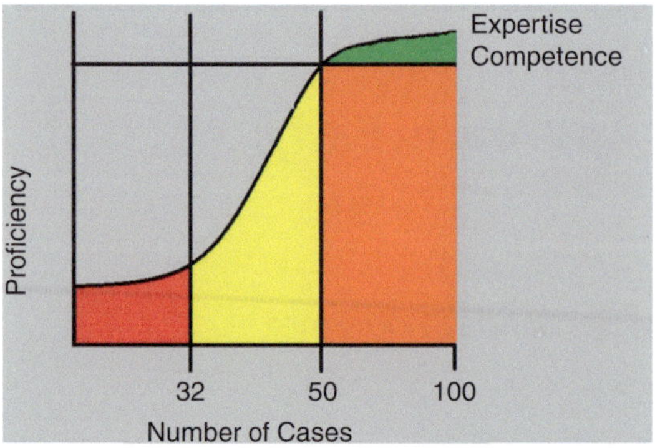

Fig. 5.1 Surgical learning curve example graph. From 0 cases to 32, the area under the curve is the highest risk area for patients and represents the early LC. This flat curve represents a slow gain in proficiency as per case basis and is where initial skills are developed. Bear in mind some skills are already present; that is why the curve inherently starts with some built-in proficiency as a measure of surgeons' training. The steepest part of the curve, between 32 and 50 cases, represents the optimization zone where there is an exponential gain in proficiency per case. There is a rapid progression in the intended measured variables such as blood loss or surgical time. The area under the curve between 50 and 100 cases illustrates the achievement of defined surgical competence and beyond. Once the competence level is achieved, further repetition leads to expertise that is slower to achieve, represented by flattening of the curve

dure. It tries to determine at what point the surgeon has become competent in the procedure. The standard curve has the proficiency outcome on the y axis and the number of cases on the x axis (Fig. 5.1). A steep learning curve has been perceived as negative when its intention is to define the curve by the amount of effort required to overcome it. In fact, a steep learning curve is advantageous since it means that the surgeon reached the proficiency level with a smaller number of cases. As explained in Gofton et al., a steep curve is ideal because only a small number of patients are being exposed to the increased risk of complications that are associated with the early stages of learning (1). The variables used to measure proficiency are numerous and include surgical time, blood loss, complication rate, and patient-reported outcomes. Although incomplete, surgical time has been shown to be an adequate indicator of surgical proficiency within a learning curve [10]. More comprehensive statistics such as a cumulative sum analysis can determine when competency is reached based on specific surgical performances [11]. Inconsistency remains the most effective method of measuring and monitoring an individual surgical learning curve.

The concern of a surgical learning curve was highlighted by the experience of laparoscopic cholecystectomy in which a spike in complications was observed after its early adoption [12]. This experience underlined the importance of proper training and education when implementing a new surgical technique. Other surgical fields such as spine and abdominal robotic surgery have also described this phenomenon. Curiously, 40 cases seem to be a consistent number of procedures required to reach a minimum surgical proficiency in these reports [13].

The literature describing surgical learning curves in the anterior approach is heterogeneous, making interpretation difficult. Study methodology, patient selection, specific technique, implants used, surgeon training, and experience vary significantly. Furthermore, there are single surgeon series, multiple surgeon series, and registry data. Proper interpretation of the data requires understanding of the strengths and weaknesses of each one. Single surgeon series are often the experience of highly skilled surgeons with vast experience and dedicated teams. Furthermore, not infrequently these surgeons are promoting a technique, approach, or implant. These series are often described as "what is accomplishable." Registry data may offer more information that is generalizable to surgeons as long as the data collected is ubiquitous and includes surgical volume and experience so that it can provide comparable benchmarks to individual surgeons.

Let us review the available data looking at various measures of surgical proficiency in the anterior approach to total hip arthroplasty.

Surgical Time

Surgical time is the most common parameter used when reporting learning curves in the literature [14–28]. In general, the surgical time decreases as the number of cases increases along the learning curve, but the number of cases needed to achieve a meaningful reduction varies. Zawadasky et al. reported an initial surgical time of 102.7 min that dropped to 82.4 min after 50 cases [14]. Similar time improvement was reported by Kong et al., where the initial 50 cases took 113.4 min and then dropped to 86.6 min [11]. Masonis and Van den Eeden et al. found that 100 cases were required prior to observing a significant drop in the surgical time [22, 23]. In general, using surgical time as the proxy for surgical proficiency in the anterior approach has shown a wide range of required cases from 20 to 100 [14–24, 26]. Some series have failed to demonstrate decreased surgical time, with a number of cases hinting at the inability to overcome the learning curve with the cases reported. Melman et al. and Woolson et al. reported no significant improvement in time throughout their series [29, 30]. However, when isolating studies that demonstrate robust training prior to the start of the learning curve, we can observe either no significant difference compared to the prior approach or a lower number of cases (32–50 cases) needed to overcome the learning curve in relation to surgical time [17, 21, 25]. Table 5.1 summarizes studies that have used surgical time for measurement of surgical proficiency in the anterior approach.

Table 5.1 Procedure time and number of cases needed to reach steady state

Study	LC surgical time (Min.)	Surgical time past LC (Min.)	No. of cases to reach steady state
Pogliacomi	111	85	30
Berend	99	69	37
Goytia	124	98.1	40
Spaans	84	77	46
Alexandrov	229.5	139	43
Zawadsky	102.7	82.4	50
Kong	113.44	86.66	50
Stone	108.98	88.98	50
Pirrucio	60.45	47.45	100
Masonis	132.8	109.9	100
Van Den Eeden	115	70	100

LC, learning curve

Blood Loss

Various studies have used blood loss as a measurement of surgical proficiency in the learning curve [14–28]. Some studies report it as a per case improvement in surgical blood loss, while others compare the blood loss to their previous approach. In this way, we can evaluate improvement in blood loss either as an absolute decrease or relative to the expected blood loss a particular surgeon has on his traditional approach. Goytia et al. divided his 81-case series into three groups (two groups of 20 and one 21) and showed a decrease in blood loss from 596 ml to 347 ml after the second group [18]. Similarly, but with a smaller number of cases, Alexandrov et al. reported a mean blood loss of 2180 ml (range 600–2600 ml) in the initial 10 cases that decreased to 500 ml (range 250–900 ml) in the following 10 cases [19]. Seng et al. showed an increased blood loss and transfusion requirements in the learning curve of the anterior approach in the initial 37 cases or 6 months since the start of the curve [17]. Other studies have shown a similar trend in blood loss decreasing with progression through the learning curve [17–19, 23]. On the contrary, other authors failed to show an improvement in their blood loss throughout the adoption of the anterior approach. Melman et al. did not find a decrease in blood loss after 120 cases, neither did Spaans et al. after 46 cases [25, 29]. Not surprisingly, studies describing meticulous training prior to the learning showed comparable blood loss to the previous approach even in the learning curve [21, 31]. Other studies have not been consistent in their findings [15, 21, 29].

Complications

The complication rate has also been used as a proxy of surgical proficiency. Reported overall complication rates in the early experience vary from 2% to 44% [11, 32]. Melman et al. reported no change in time or blood loss in their learning curve series but did report a decrease in complications from 11.5% to 2% after the initial 120 cases [29]. Van den Eeden et al. reported 12%

complication rate for the first 100 cases of DA and then 6% for the second 100 cases [23]. Kong et al. reported a 44% complication rate in the initial 50 cases that dropped to 16% in the second 50. Their data was analyzed using CUSUM analysis showing a steady state in complication rate as well as in surgical time after 85 cases [11]. Their study discusses the inconsistency in complication reporting. Their study is more liberal in the definition of complications, and when using the criteria used by Woolson et al. for complications, their overall complication rate was only 6% [30]. Similarly, Seng et al. report an overall complication rate of 5.4%, but only 2.2% clinically relevant complications [17]. The reader is cautioned when interpreting the results of these studies as the inclusion of clinically insignificant complications such as transient lateral thigh numbness, mild heterotopic ossification, or greater trochanteric small avulsion fractures overestimates the true complication rate. Nevertheless, the literature is consistent, demonstrating a higher complication rate in the early learning curve. Table 5.2 summarizes some of these articles reporting on complication rates in the learning curve of the anterior approach.

The majority of intraoperative complications in the anterior hip approach involved proximal femur fractures. Alexandrov et al. reported a 30% complication rate, and more than half were femur fractures [19]. As stated by Horne et al., proximal femur fracture rates using the direct anterior approach are inversely related to experience, and potentially 200 cases are required to decrease the fracture rate [33]. This has been proven in multiple case series like in Yi et al. where they had 8.2% of intraoperative femur fractures that occurred in the first 32 cases and none during the last 29 cases [28]. Masonis et al. reported that femur fractures occurred in the initial 62 cases [22]. Jewett et al. reported that 12/16 proximal femur fractures occurred in the first 200 cases [34]. Others reported a high proximal femur fracture rate that continued throughout their series [25, 30]. In general, there appears to be lessening of the femoral complications with increased experience after 20 to 200 cases [11, 17, 20, 22–24, 25–37, 29–35, 33, 36]. Again, isolating a series of experienced surgeons with healthy volume and rigorous training demonstrates either no increase in early complications or a reduced number of cases to achieve a steady state between 32 and 100 cases [17, 21, 22, 28, 35].

Table 5.2 Complications rates and number of cases needed to reach steady state

Study	LC complication rate	Steady-state complication rate	No. of cases to reach steady state
Muller	10%	2%	20
D'Arrigo	13.30%	6.70%	20
Yi	31.25%	0	32
Alexandrov	40%	30%	43
Kong	44%	16%	50
Van Den Eeden	12%	6%	100
Rathod	6.25%	1.40%	100
Hartford	5%	2%	100
Melman	11.50%	2%	120
Jewett	10%	0.83%	200

LC, learning curve

Revision Rates

The revision rate has also been used as a proxy for the learning curve. Both single surgeon series and registry data provide good insight. De Steiger et al. reported data from the Australian Orthopaedic Association National Joint Replacement Registry. They used a specific implant combination to identify patients undergoing the anterior approach. The cumulative percent revision at 4 years was 6% for surgeons with less than 15 cases and 2% for those with greater than 100 cases. They estimated that at least 50 cases were required in order to achieve the same risk of revision as of those with at least 100 cases [32]. Interestingly, the implant combination analyzed was flagged as a revision outlier in the first 2 years in the registry, most likely due to an anterior approach learning curve. Single surgeon series also corroborates these findings. Müller et al. reported a 5-year survivorship of 78.9% in their initial 20 cases compared to 96.8% for subsequent cases [36]. Hartford et al., with a clinical series of 500 cases, had a mean revision rate of 1.6%. He demonstrated a significant decrease in revision rate from the first 100 cases group to the last 100 cases group from 2% revision risk to 1%. The majority of revisions were due to proximal femoral fractures, 55.5% [37].

Component Positioning Accuracy

Another metric used to describe the learning curve for the anterior approach is the accuracy of component positioning, especially the acetabular component. Hamilton et al. and Rathod et al. demonstrated improved acetabular component positioning with less variance than their previous approach even in the learning curve with greater than 90% mean cup positioning within the safe zone [24, 2]. De Geest et al. and Van den Eeden et al. reported that the majority of their cup outliers occurred within the first 100 cases although their overall accuracy even in the learning curve was above 85% [23, 38]. These studies have shown an initial tendency of increased cup inclination and anteversion during the early experience. Yausa et al. showed a 5.9° increase in anteversion and 2.8° abduction when changing from posterior to anterior approach [35]. These series demonstrate that fluoroscopy helps both with accuracy and consistency in component positioning compared to other approaches even within an early learning curve.

Similarly, restoration of leg length and avoidance of over lengthening have been evaluated. The evaluation of leg length in a specialized table with reliance on fluoroscopic techniques could be more challenging in the early adoption. The utilization of the inferior ischial line has been shown to be inconsistent and affected by distortion and parallax [39]. Measuring leg length on a standard table with contralateral comparison may be less challenging in the early adoption. Van den Eeden reported greater than 1 cm leg length discrepancy in 13% of his initial 100 cases [23]. Hartford reported 7% perceived leg length discrepancy in the initial 100 cases followed by 2% [37]. The use of fluoroscopy appears to mitigate this issue even in the learning curve. Masonis et al. reported 3.5 mm LLD in the initial 100 cases and 1.1 mm after 200 cases [22]. Kong et al. reported greater than 94% within 10 mm with improvement over time, and Goytia et al. reported 87% within 5 mm of the contralateral side even in the learning curve [11, 18]. Newer technologies like standard computer navigation, fluoroscopic navigation, and robotics may improve in our ability to hit our targets.

We can appreciate the influence of fluoroscopy improving the restoration of leg length and reducing cup position outliers. However, proper interpretation of fluoroscopy is required and may present a learning curve of its own. Masonis et al. reported a 32.1 s mean of fluoroscopy time for the initial 100 cases, and then it decreased to a mean of 14.5 s for cases 101–300 [22]. Slotkin et al. evaluated cup positioning for 780 consecutive hips performed by two fellowship-trained surgeons including their learning curve. Primary endpoint was the number of cups that were within the targeted "safe zone" defined by Lewinnek et al. for anteversion and cup inclination [40]. The authors demonstrated high accuracy with a low variance that continued to improve throughout the first 3 years and peaked at 97.4% in the last year [3]. The reader must recognize the challenges of proper imaging interpretation due to the dynamic nature of the pelvic position that affects the appreciated cup anteversion and inclination angles. The authors recommend consistency in the intended pelvic position used to target cup positioning [3, 41–43].

Lessons Learned

Despite the heterogeneity of the literature, consistent findings and learning points can be identified. The literature has been consistent in the fact that early intraoperative complications occur on the femoral side [22, 25, 34, 30]. Intraoperative complications include femoral perforations, calcar fractures, and greater trochanter fractures. Patient-related factors such as bone quality (DORR C), diagnosis (hip dysplasia), gender (female), and BMI contribute to these complications. These findings suggest that the most challenging aspect of learning the anterior approach is adequate femoral exposure. Small incisions, inadequate releases, and compromised femoral exposure can all be contributing factors to these findings. Matta et al. describe their technique that dislocates the hip first, followed by reduction and femoral neck cut. This maneuver is intended at enhancing femoral exposure by traumatically releasing structures that help femoral exposure like the pubofemoral ligament, which is typically under released [4]. After the initial learning curve, the rate of intraoperative femoral fractures appears to be comparable to other approaches [22]. Technical keys for effective releases and femoral exposure should be prioritized in the training of surgeons adopting the anterior approach. Figure 5.2 illustrates the contrast between poor and adequate femoral exposure that would allow for safe and reproducible femoral stem preparation.

Increased blood loss and transfusion requirements can be anticipated in the learning curve as highlighted in the review of the literature [17]. The authors believe that this is a result of the immature understanding of the vascular anatomy through the anterior approach and increased length of surgery. Once the surgeon becomes proficient, blood loss can be equivalent or less than other approaches [17]. Nevertheless, adequate preoperative planning for the learning curve can help mitigate this issue in the beginning. Technology such as bipolar sealers and cell saver should be considered as options along with standard preoperative anemia optimization. The utilization of perioperative tranexamic acid for operative hemostasis, aspirin for VTE prophylaxis, and modification of transfusion thresholds has led to a significant reduction in transfusions across joint arthroplasty including anterior approach THA and should help ease this problem [44, 45].

Patient selection has been shown to influence success in the learning curve. Body habitus as well as radiographic signs can help identify the level of difficulty. Careful evaluation of these features can anticipate the difficulty of femoral exposure that is a critical component in the learning curve. Patients with short varus femoral necks as well as protrusion are more difficult since the periarticular structures such as the capsule and short external rotators are contracted and require more releases to mobilize the femur laterally (Fig. 5.3). A large tensor muscle can also make femoral exposure challenging. On the contrary, long valgus femoral necks with narrow pelvis provide easy mobilization and uninterrupted access to the femur with fewer releases. Typically, females tend to be more lax and easier in the learning curve.

Other factors such as BMI and bone type can influence the difficulty of the learning curve. Lower BMI has been associated with less surgical difficulty and improved component positioning [46]. Bone quality and bone type are also

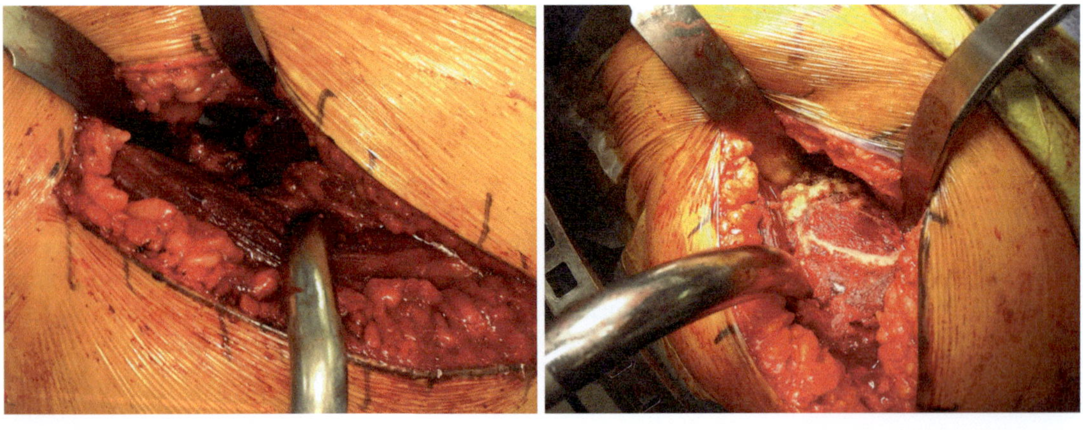

Fig. 5.2 Intraoperative photograph illustrating poor femur exposure (left) compared to generous femoral exposure with easy access to intramedullary canal

important. DORR type B bone provides the ideal balance of bone quality and morphology to prevent femoral complications [18, 27]. Osteoporosis leads to an increased risk of fractures in any

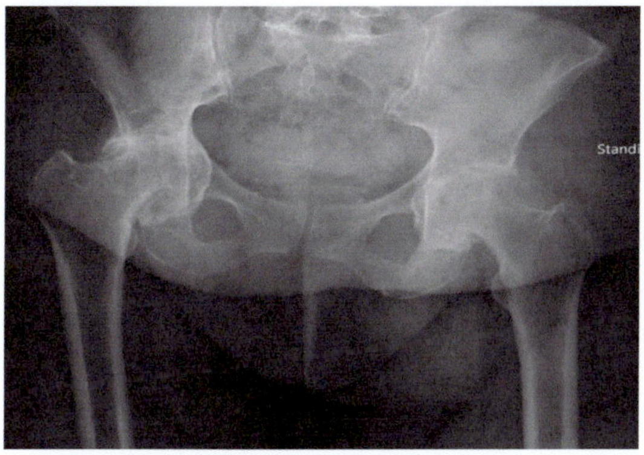

Fig. 5.3 Showing pelvis AP x-ray with right hip protrusio, which makes femoral exposure difficult due to capsule and short external muscle contractures

approach and should be avoided during the learning curve. DORR type C bone presents challenges not only during bone preparation but also in the process of retractor placement and retraction. Cementation of the femoral stem could be more appropriate in these cases. DORR A with its metaphyseal/diaphyseal mismatch presents unique challenges. This type of bone may dictate the type of stems used including straight stems that require reaming and broaching. This would require more generous femoral exposure to enable safe femoral preparation that can be more challenging in the early learning process [15, 29]. Figure 5.4 shows the three types of bone as described by DORR et al. [27].

Although few studies have evaluated the benefits of the anterior approach for arthroplasty treatment of femoral neck fractures, none have analyzed its effect on the learning curve [47]. The

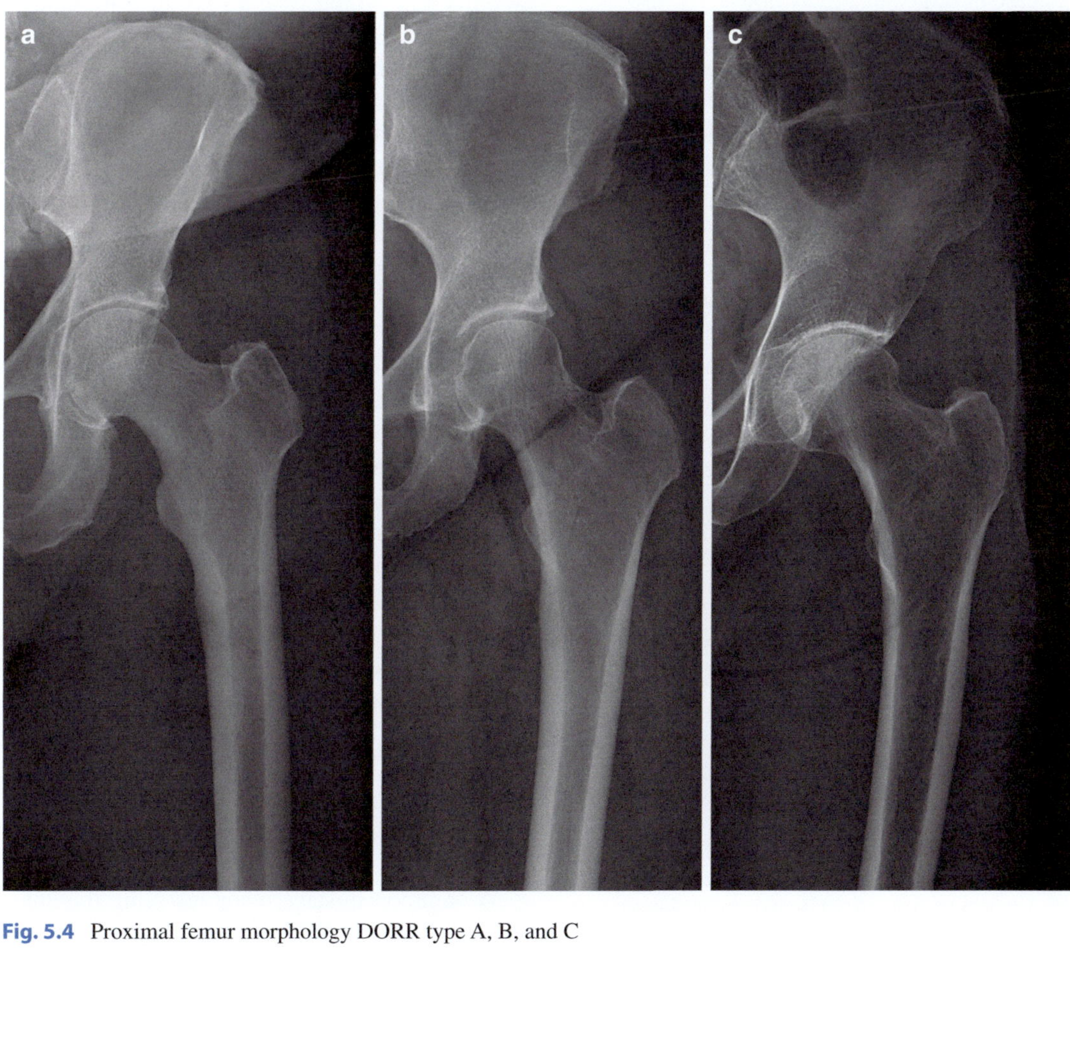

Fig. 5.4 Proximal femur morphology DORR type A, B, and C

authors caution against selecting femoral neck fractures in the learning curve as these patients have demonstrated compromised bone quality and are at high risk of fracture. Clear understanding of generous releases that facilitate femoral exposure is required to avoid femoral complications. Furthermore, the use of the anterior approach for hemiarthroplasty presents unique challenges. Hip reduction with large femoral heads used in hemiarthroplasties can be difficult as the rectus femoris muscle and/or capsule may hinder the ease of the maneuver. Forceful attempts at reduction may lead to femoral fractures. Techniques to mitigate these issues include aggressive femoral releases, anterior capsulectomy, and release of the indirect head of the rectus femoris. Figure 5.5 shows the anatomical location of the indirect head of the rectus femoris; generous release can improve visualization and ease of large head reductions.

There are inherent complications to the anterior approach, which both surgeons and patients need to be aware of. Lateral femoral cutaneous nerve neuropraxia has been commonly reported in the learning curve of the anterior approach [18]. The anatomical location of the LFCN makes it vulnerable to injury as it exits the pelvic region and typically runs over the sartorius muscle. Medialization of the incision or vigorous subcutaneous dissection can place the nerve at risk. Furthermore, the anatomical location of the nerve and the pattern of ramification are variable, making it difficult to avoid consistently [48, 47]. Although true injury to the LFCN with meralgia paresthetica is low, mild peri incisional or lateral thigh numbness is not uncommon and typically resolves over time [18, 48]. Patients should be counseled regarding this possibility of LFCN injury that has been reported with a wide range of incidence from 0.1% to 81% in different clinical case series, but as reported by Goytia et al., the majority of cases resolved in their series where 10 of 12 cases resolved completely [18, 48]. Hartford et al., on their clinical series of 500 cases, reported an overall LFCN deficit of 5.4%, but interestingly the incidence was higher for the first 100 cases with a 7% incidence compared to 2% for the last 100 cases of the clinical series [37].

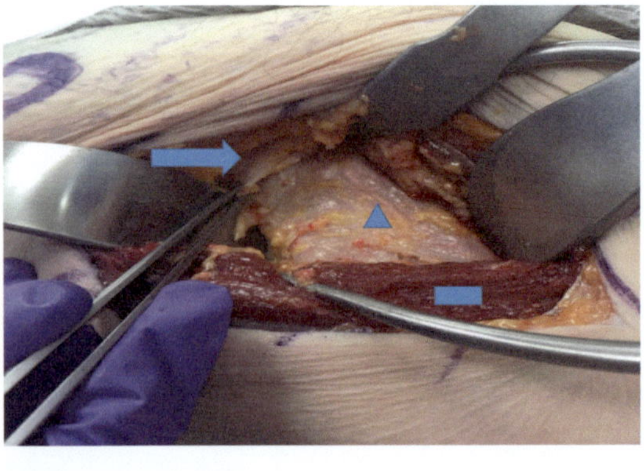

Fig. 5.5 Anterior hip exposure illustrating the hip capsule demarked by a triangle, tensor fasciae latae identified with a rectangle, and indirect head of rectus femoris identified with an arrow

Component positioning is important for the stability and durability of a total hip arthroplasty. Although the anterior approach provides adequate acetabular visualization, there is a tendency of placing cups with high inclination and anteversion angles in the learning curve [23, 24]. The use of intraoperative fluoroscopy helps mitigate component malalignment. In fact, the use of fluoroscopy, even in the learning curve, has shown improved component positioning when compared to other exposures [2]. Proper fluoroscopy interpretation may pose an additional learning curve and should be part of a robust training process [3].

Surgical volume and experience influence the learning curve process as expected. Series from high volume, highly skilled surgeons provide insight of what is accomplishable in the adoption of the anterior approach with a steep learning curve and low complications [21]. In contrast, series from low-volume surgeons show a more challenging route [30]. Registry data is more generalizable and does show a higher early revision rate with lower volume and less experienced surgeons [32]. It is important for surgeons embarking in a surgical learning curve to anticipate the challenges experienced by comparable peers.

A common mistake when adopting the anterior approach is to change more than just the approach to total hip arthroplasty. The anterior approach enthusiasm led to the development of specialized tables, instrumentation, implants, and technology in order to facilitate the procedure. Unfortunately, adoption of other variables may have a learning curve of its own. Broach handle designs highlight this concept. Traditionally, surgeons have been accustomed to using straight broach handles that provide a direct force vector with minimal force dissipation. Offset handles have been designed in order to facilitate femoral preparation with limited exposure through an anterior approach (Fig. 5.6). Single and double offset handles have been popularized [16]. Vertical force transmission decreases as broach handle offset increases, and in double offset handles, there is a 20–60% deflection of the vertical load into the horizontal plane, thus increasing proximal femur stress; even more, if the impaction is inefficient, it can increase up to an 86.9% of deflection [16]. This force transmission can lead to inconsistent femoral bone envelope preparation, potentially resulting in fractures or femoral stem under-sizing, subsidence, and mechanical failures. Fleischman et al. reported a higher incidence of femoral-sided mechanical failures in the anterior approach compared to the posterior or anterolateral approach [42]. Experience with these handles is recommended prior to implementation into a new approach in order to avoid inconsistent femur broaching and compromising the bone envelope. In a similar way, implants and technology such as fluoroscopy may pose an additional learning curve that can lessen with judicious incorporation.

Useful training is paramount when adopting the anterior approach. Proper training may include didactic sessions, cadaveric courses, live surgical demonstrations, and expert surgeon visitations. The industry has taken a leading role in training surgeons and providing valuable cadaveric courses and surgeon visitation opportunities. The effectiveness of limited educational experiences prior to adoption of the anterior approach has shown poor success [30]. However, constant engagement with the educational experience that continues after the commencement of the learning curve is advantageous [21]. The most successful reports describe multiple cadaver sessions, surgeon visitation, and video evaluations prior to starting the learning curve, followed by further cadaver training and surgeon visitations after multiple cases have been performed. The recognition of surgical proficiency gaps and the ability to change behavior accordingly are only possible through repetition and exposure to training opportunities that alert the learner to those gaps. In this manner, the initial part of the curve can be steepened by making the learner aware of the surgical deficiencies in the anterior approach that will effect change and progression through the curve. The senior author did not learn

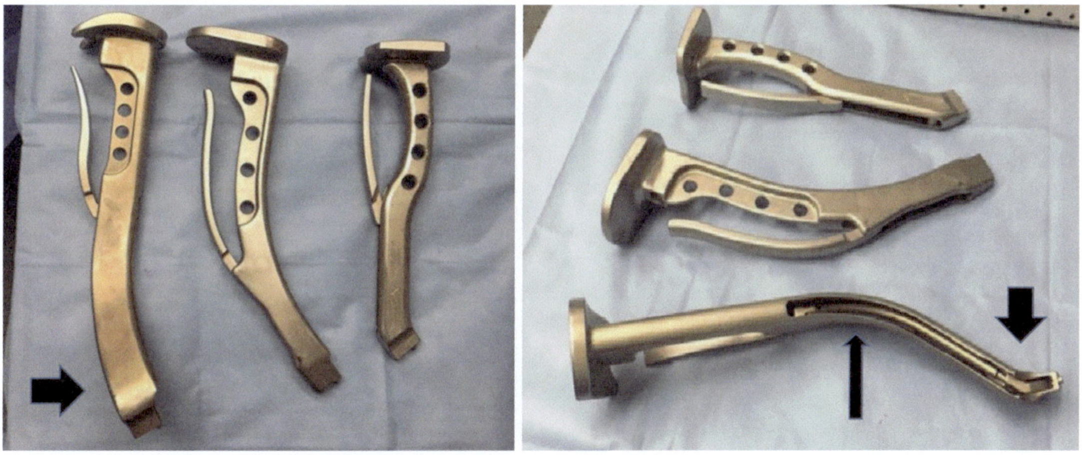

Fig. 5.6 Double offset handles are identified with black arrows. The other two handles are single offset handles

the anterior approach in residency or fellowship. However, he attended multiple cadaver courses, one-on-one cadaver sessions, and expert surgeon visitation prior to starting the anterior approach. The initial 20 cases were done with a peer who was also learning the anterior approach. Further courses and cadaver sessions were attended to work on the gaps and technical challenges identified in the early learning curve. We continue our learning process and challenge ourselves with increased complexity and revision surgery through the anterior approach.

It is our expectation that the anterior approach will continue to grow and infiltrate teaching institutions. Formal training can identify necessary milestones for successful surgical proficiency. This will provide much-needed structured training in the approach to residents and fellows and minimize their learning curve once removed from their training programs. Furthermore, exciting technology such as virtual reality may play a larger role in the future for surgical training. Lastly, the American Joint Replacement Registry will report broad information about the anterior approach, implants utilized, and their survivorships providing useful information to surgeons.

References

1. Learmonth ID, Young C, Rorabeck C. The operation of the century: total hip replacement. Lancet. 2007;370(9597):1508–19.
2. Hamilton WG, Parks NL, Huynh C. Comparison of cup alignment, jump distance, and complications in consecutive series of anterior approach and posterior approach total hip arthroplasty. J Arthroplast. 2015;30(11):1959–62.
3. Slotkin EM, Patel PD, Suarez JC. Accuracy of fluoroscopic guided acetabular component positioning during direct anterior total hip arthroplasty. J Arthroplast. 2015;30(9 Suppl):102–6.
4. Matta JM, Shahrdar C, Ferguson T. Single-incision anterior approach for total hip arthroplasty on an orthopaedic table. Clin Orthop Relat Res. 2005;441:115–24.
5. Nakata K, Nishikawa M, Yamamoto K, Hirota S, Yoshikawa H. A clinical comparative study of the direct anterior with mini-posterior approach: two consecutive series. J Arthroplast. 2009;24(5):698–704.
6. Chechik O, Khashan M, Lador R, Salai M, Amar E. Surgical approach and prosthesis fixation in hip arthroplasty world wide. Arch Orthop Trauma Surg. 2013;133(11):1595–600.
7. Sheth D, Cafri G, Inacio MC, Paxton EW, Namba RS. Anterior and anterolateral approaches for THA are associated with lower dislocation risk without higher revision risk. Clin Orthop Relat Res. 2015;473(11):3401–8.
8. Maratt JD, Gagnier JJ, Butler PD, Hallstrom BR, Urquhart AG, Roberts KC. No difference in dislocation seen in anterior vs posterior approach Total hip arthroplasty. J Arthroplast. 2016;31(9 Suppl):127–30.
9. Patel NN, Shah JA, Erens GA. Current trends in clinical practice for the direct anterior approach total hip arthroplasty. J Arthroplast. 2019;34(9):1987–1993.e3.
10. Sammon J, Perry A, Beaule L, Kinkead T, Clark D, Hansen M. Robot-assisted radical prostatectomy: learning rate analysis as an objective measure of the acquisition of surgical skill. BJU Int. 2010;106(6):855–60.
11. Kong X, Grau L, Ong A, Yang C, Chai W. Adopting the direct anterior approach: experience and learning curve in a Chinese patient population. J Orthop Surg Res. 2019;14(1):218.
12. Shea JA, Healey MJ, Berlin JA, et al. Mortality and complications associated with laparoscopic cholecystectomy. A meta-analysis. Ann Surg. 1996;224(5):609–20.
13. Gofton WT, Solomon M, Gofton T, Page A, Kim P, Netting C, et al. What do reported learning curves mean for orthopedic surgeons? Instr Course Lect. 2016;65:633–43.
14. Zawadasky M, Paulus M, Murray P, Johansen M. Early outcome comparison between the DAA and the mini-incision posterior approach for primary total hip arthroplasty: 150 consecutive cases. J Arthroplast. 2014;29(6):1256–60.
15. D'arrigo C, Speranza A, Monaco E, Carcangiu A, Ferreti A. Learning curve in tissue sparing total hip replacement: comparison between different approaches. J Orthopaed Traumatol. 2009;10(1):47–54.
16. Greenhill DA, Abbasi P, Darvish K, Star AM. Broach handle design changes force distribution in the femur during total hip arthroplasty. J Arthroplast. 2017;32(6):2017–22.
17. Seng BE, Berend KR, Ajluni AF, Lombardi AV. Anterior-supine minimally invasive total hip arthroplasty: defining the learning curve. Orthop Clin North Am. 2009;40(3):343–50.
18. Goytia RN, Jones LC, Hungerford MW. Learning curve for the anterior approach total hip arthroplasty. J Surj Orthop Adv. 2012;21(2):78–83.
19. Alexandrov T, Ahlmann ER, Menendez LR. Early clinical and radiographic results of minimally invasive anterior approach hip arthroplasty. Adv Orthop 2014;2014. Accessed 1 May 2020. Available from: https://www.ncbi.nlm.nih.gov/pmc/articles/PMC3955657/pdf/AORTH2014-954208.pdf; https://doi.org/10.1155/2014/954208.

20. Stone AH, Sibia US, Atkinson R, Turner TR, King PJ. Evaluation of the learning curve when transitioning from Posterolater to direct anterior hip arthroplasty: a consecutive series of 1000 cases. J Arthroplast. 2018;33(8):2530–4.
21. Pirruccio K, Evangelista PJ, Haw J, Goldberg T, Sheth NP. Safely implementing the direct anterior Total hip arthroplasty: a methodological approach to minimizing the learning curve. J Am Acad Orthop Surg. 2020;28:930–6.
22. Masonis J, Thompson C, Odum S. Safe and accurate: learning the direct anterior Total hip arthroplasty. Orthopedics. 2008;31(12 Suppl 2):129–34.
23. Van Den Eeden Y, Van Den Eeden F. Learning curve of direct anterior total hip arthroplasty: a single surgeon experience. Acta Orthop Belg. 2018;84(3):321–30.
24. Rathod PA, Bhalla S, Deshmukh AJ, Rodriguez JA. Does fluoroscopy with anterior hip arthroplasty decrease acetabular cup variability compared with a nonguided posterior approach? Clin Orthop Relat Res. 2014;472(6):1877–85.
25. Spaans AJ, van den Hout JA, Bolder SB. High complication rate in the early experience of minimally invasive total hip arthroplasty by the direct anterior approach. Acta Orthop. 2012;83(4):342–6.
26. Wayne N, Stoewe R. Primary total hip arthroplasty: a comparison of the lateral Hardinge approach to an anterior mini-invasive approach. Orthop Rev (Pavia). 2009;1(2):e27. https://doi.org/10.4081/or.2009.e27.
27. Nash W, Harris A. The Dorr type and cortical thickness index of the proximal femur for predicting perioperative complications during hemiarthroplasty. J Orthop Surg. 2014;22(1):92–5.
28. Yi C, Agudelo JF, Dayton MR, Morgan SJ. Early complications of anterior supine intermuscular total hip arthroplasty. Orthopedics. 2013;36(3):e276–81. https://doi.org/10.3928/01477447-20130222-14.
29. Melman WP, Mollen BP, Kollen BJ, Verheyen CC. First experiences with the direct anterior approach in lateral decubitus position: learning curve and 1 year complication rate. Hip Int. 2015;25(3):251–7.
30. Woolson ST, Pouliot MA, Huddleston JI. Primary total hip arthroplasty using an anterior approach and a fracture table: short-term results from a community hospital. J Arthroplast. 2009;24(7):999–1005.
31. Restrepo C, Parvizi J, Pour AE, Hozack WJ. Prospective randomized study of two surgical approaches for total hip arthroplasty. J Arthroplast. 2010;25(5):671–9.e1. https://doi.org/10.1016/j.arth.2010.02.002.
32. de Steiger RN, Lorimer M, Solomon M. What is the learning curve for the anterior approach for total hip arthroplasty? Clin Orthop Relat Res. 2015;473(12):3860–6.
33. Horne PH, Olson SA. Direct anterior approach for total hip arthroplasty using the fracture table. Curr Rev Musculoskelet Med. 2011;4(3):139–45.
34. Jewett BA, Collis DK. High complication rate with anterior total hip arthroplasties on a fracture table. Clin Orthop Relat Res. 2011;469(2):503–7.
35. Yuasa T, Maezawa K, Sato H, Maruyama Y, Kaneko K. Safely transitioning to the direct anterior from posterior approach for total hip arthroplasty. J Orthop. 2018;15(2):420–3.
36. Müller DA, Zingg PO, Dora C. Anterior minimally invasive approach for total hip replacement: five-year survivorship and learning curve. Hip Int. 2014;24(3):277–83.
37. Hartford JM, Bellino MJ. The learning curve for the direct anterior approach for total hip arthroplasty: a single surgeon's first 500 cases. Hip Int. 2017;27(5):483–8.
38. De Geest T, Vansintjan P, De Loore G. Direct anterior total hip arthroplasty: complications and early outcome in a series of 300 cases. Acta Orthop Belg. 2013;79(2):166–73.
39. Rueckl K, Alcaide DJ, Springer B, Rueckl S, Kasparek MF, Boettner F. Intraoperative measurement of cup inclination using fluoroscopy requires a correction factor. Arch Orthop Trauma Surg. 2019;139(11):1511–7.
40. Lewinnek GE, Lewis JL, Tarr R, et al. Dislocation after total hip arthroplasties. J Bone Joint Surg Am. 1978;60:217.
41. Lembeck B, Mueller O, Reize P, Wuelker N. Pelvic tilt makes acetabular cup navigation inaccurate. Acta Orthop. 2005;76(4):517–23.
42. Fleischman AN, Tarabichi M, Magner Z, Parvizi J, Rothman RH. Mechanical complications following total hip arthroplasty based on surgical approach: a large, single-institution cohort study. J Arthroplast. 2019;34(6):1255–60.
43. DiGioia AM, Jaramaz B, Blackwell M, et al. The Otto Aufranc Award. Image guided navigation system to measure intraoperatively acetabular implant alignment. Clin Orthop Relat Res. 1998;355:8–22.
44. Mitchell MD, Betesh JS, Ahn J, Hume EL, Mehta S, Umscheid CA. Transfusion thresholds for major orthopedic surgery: a systematic review and meta-analysis. J Arthroplast. 2017;32(12):3815–21.
45. Fillingham YA, Ramkumar DB, Jevsevar DS, et al. The efficacy of tranexamic acid in total hip arthroplasty: a network meta-analysis. J Arthroplast. 2018;33(10):3083–3089.e4.
46. Wagner ER, Kamath AF, Fruth KM, Harmsen WS, Berry DJ. Effect of body mass index on complications and reoperations after total hip arthroplasty. J Bone Joint Surg Am. 2016;98(3):169–79.
47. Thürig G, Schmitt JW, Slankamenac K, Werner CM. Safety of total hip arthroplasty for femoral neck fractures using the direct anterior approach: a retrospective observational study in 86 elderly patients. Patient Saf Surg. 2016;10:12. Published 2016 May 6. https://doi.org/10.1186/s13037-016-0100-2.
48. Rudin D, Manestar M, Ullrich O, Erhardt J, Grob K. The anatomical course of the lateral femoral cutaneous nerve with special attention to the anterior approach to the hip joint. J Bone Joint Surg Am. 2016;98(7):561–7.

6 Introducing the Direct Anterior Approach (DAA) at a Swiss University Hospital

Corinne A. Zurmühle, Vera M. Stetzelberger, Joseph M. Schwab, Matthieu Hanauer, Jonathan Laurençon, and Moritz Tannast

Introduction

Introducing the direct anterior approach (DAA) to the hip joint in a university hospital is a multi-level challenge for the whole department, particularly when the previously used technique offered very reliable and reproducible results. The choice of DAA for total hip arthroplasty (THA) should be rooted in superior clinical results such as less muscle damage, improved implant positioning and leg length, and consequently a faster recovery for the patient with improved long-term function [1, 2]. Other, more administrative, advantages of this technique automatically accompany it but should not be the primary motivation for changing a surgical approach. These additional advantages can be reduced costs due to a decreased length of stay in the hospital or the economization of operative assistants.

The introduction of such a technique involves not only the treating orthopedic surgeon but also all responsible hospital stakeholders. This chapter summarizes our experience introducing DAA with the use of an orthopedic table in two orthopedic A1-teaching, university-affiliated hospitals in Switzerland: the Inselspital in Bern and the Cantonal Hospital in Fribourg. The introduction of this new surgical approach is subdivided into three steps: preparation, execution, and evaluation.

Preparation

Surgeon Training

The preparation of the orthopedic surgeon for the introduction of DAA should aim at providing the highest level of care possible while minimizing complications right from the beginning. The reported learning curve for the DAA is approximately 50 cases [3]. We are convinced that with careful preparation by the surgeon and his/her team, the learning curve can be much shorter.

Preparation starts with cadaveric dissections aimed at identifying structures at risk and recognizing topographical relationships to important neurovascular structures (e.g., the femoral neurovascular bundle). Of specific consideration for DAA, the anatomic variations of the lateral femoral cutaneous nerve should be known [4], providing the best basis to protect them intraoperatively (Figs. 6.1 and 6.2). Specific hands-on instructional courses are strongly recommended, whether provided by industry

C. A. Zurmühle (✉) · V. M. Stetzelberger · M. Hanauer
J. Laurençon · M. Tannast
Department of Orthopaedic Surgery and Traumatology, University of Fribourg, HFR Cantonal Hospital, Fribourg, Switzerland
e-mail: corinneandrea.zurmuehle@h-fr.ch; moritz.tannast@h-fr.ch

J. M. Schwab
Department of Orthopaedic Surgery, Medical College of Wisconsin, Milwaukee, WI, USA

J. M. Matta, A. P. Sah (eds.), *Anterior Hip Replacement*,
https://doi.org/10.1007/978-3-030-91896-5_6

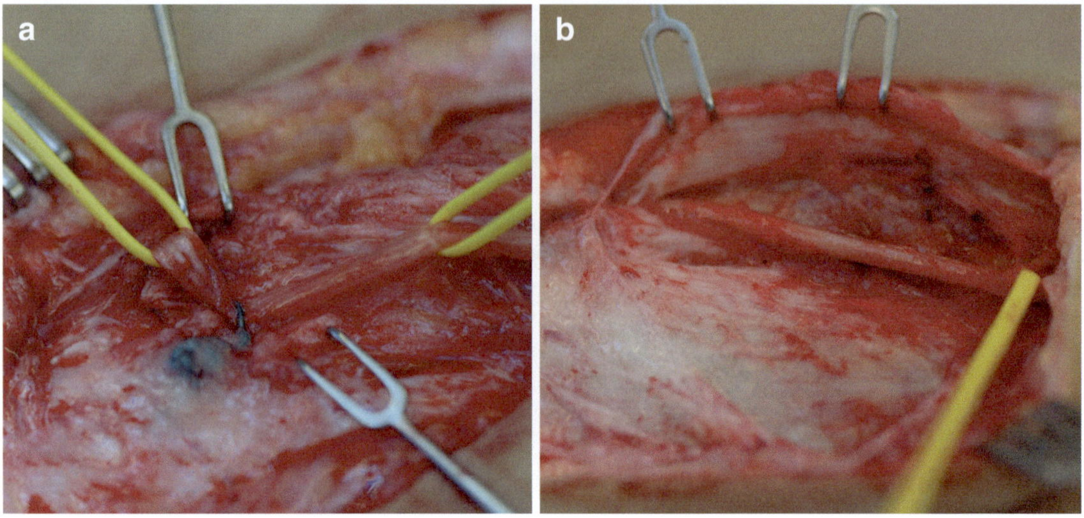

Fig. 6.1 Revision of DAA in a patient with postoperative irritation of the lateral femoral cutaneous nerve. Intraoperatively the nerve was captured by suture during the closure of the tensor fascia (**a**) but fortunately could be released (**b**)

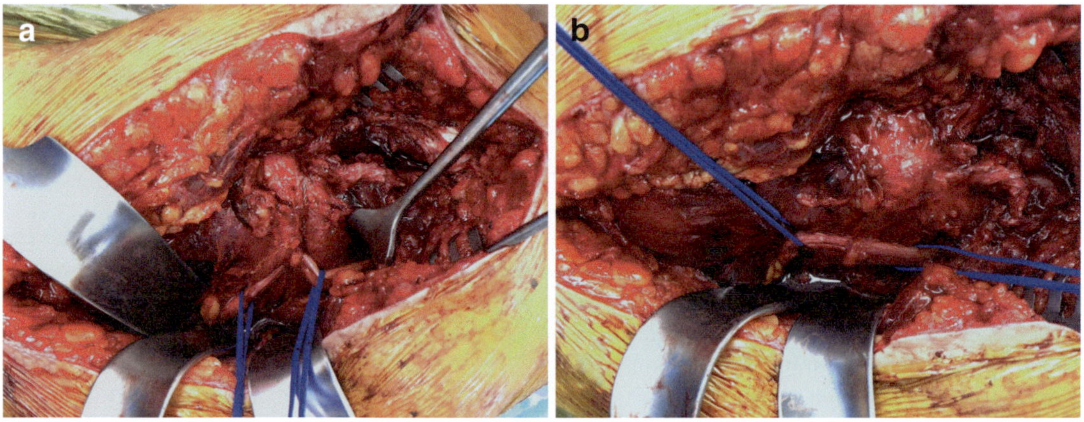

Fig. 6.2 A patient with postoperative sciatic nerve palsy after THA through DAA where an intraoperative periprosthetic fracture was treated with the application of a femoral cerclage cable. The postoperative CT scan was inconclusive. Intraoperative exploration through the posterior approach showed the sciatic nerve entrapped by the cerclage (**a**). An intraoperative complication, which is not visible through DAA. (**b**) The nerve after release was in continuity but showed visible damage

or—as in our case—in combination with self-organized cadaver labs.

When choosing to perform DAA on the orthopedic table, the surgeon should master its use beforehand. In our setup, DAA required a change of patient position on the operating table from the established lateral decubitus position, which was used for the transgluteal approach, to the supine position. Altering patient position may affect surgeon interpretation of, for instance, cup orientation and needs to be approached thoughtfully.

A fellowship at a high-volume DAA center is essential and should be repeated after the first set of cases. Depending on the experience, such a fellowship can last from days, for experienced surgeons, to a year, for beginners. Once a surgeon is familiar with the DAA at their own institution, a coaching system can be set up to disseminate the surgical technique and provide mentorship. In addition, it can be helpful to invite a skilled surgeon for the first set of cases to support the new process.

Operating Room

Transiting to DAA implies multiple changes for the entire operating room staff, which need to be trained specifically before the first implantation.

Placing the patient in the supine position is preferred in many respects to the lateral decubitus position. It is advantageous for anesthesia and reduces prep time. With the use of an orthopedic table, care has to be taken not to overtighten the boots. We did not make any specific changes in the anesthesia protocol. However, pain blocks can easily be applied.

Although DAA can basically be done with standard instruments for THA, we strongly recommend the use of approach-specific instruments for better exposure, particularly of the femur. This involves at least a hook attached to the femoral shaft and a special curved hook behind the greater trochanter (Fig. 6.3). Over time, we have introduced a commercially available self-holding system (Gripper™, MedEnvision, Aarschot, Belgium) and a specific drape (Esysuit™, MedEnvision, Aarschot, Belgium) (Fig. 6.4).

The operating room setup changes substantially with DAA. Fluoroscopy is used as a standard part of the procedure, and the orthopedic

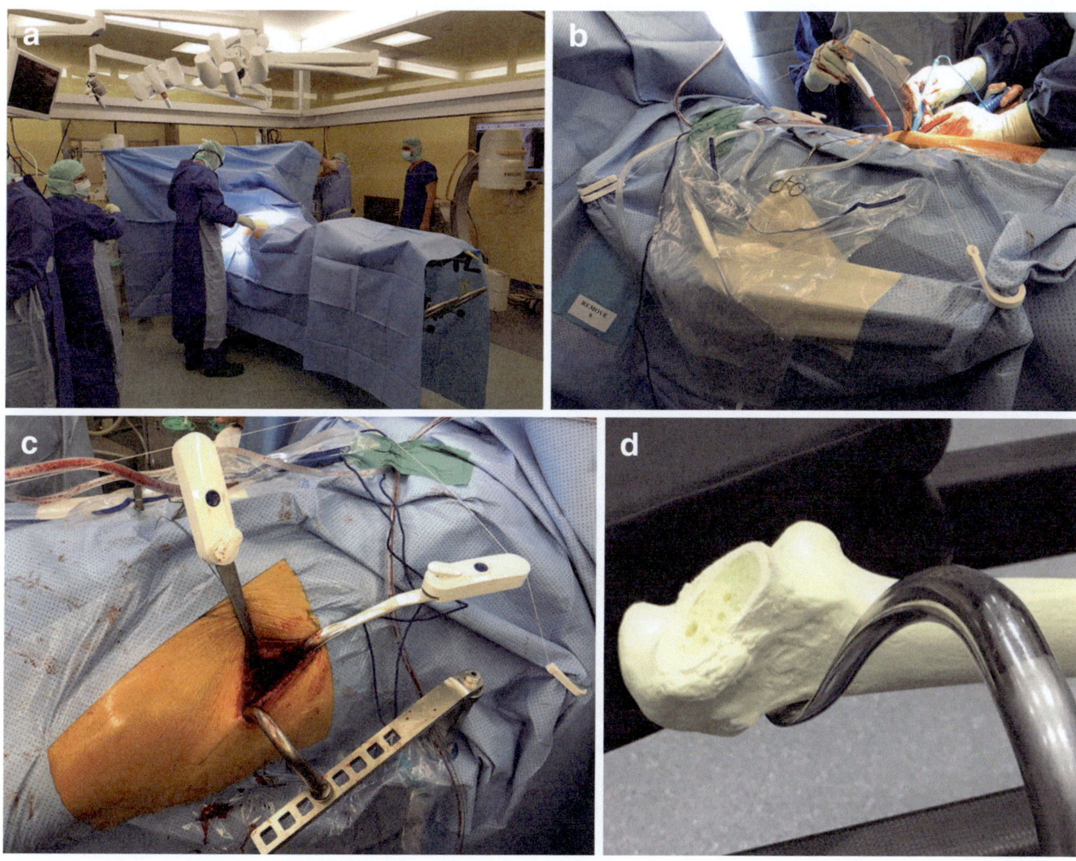

Fig. 6.3 (**a**) Specific drape (Esysuit™, MedEnvision, Aarschot, Belgium). The position of the self-holding system (Gripper™, MedEnvision, Aarschot, Belgium) for the medial and the cranial hook. Laterally, the special curved hook behind the greater trochanter. Surgeon's view (**c**) and opposite view (**b**). Hana Hook position during operation (**c**) and in a femur model slightly inferior to the grand trochanter (**d**)

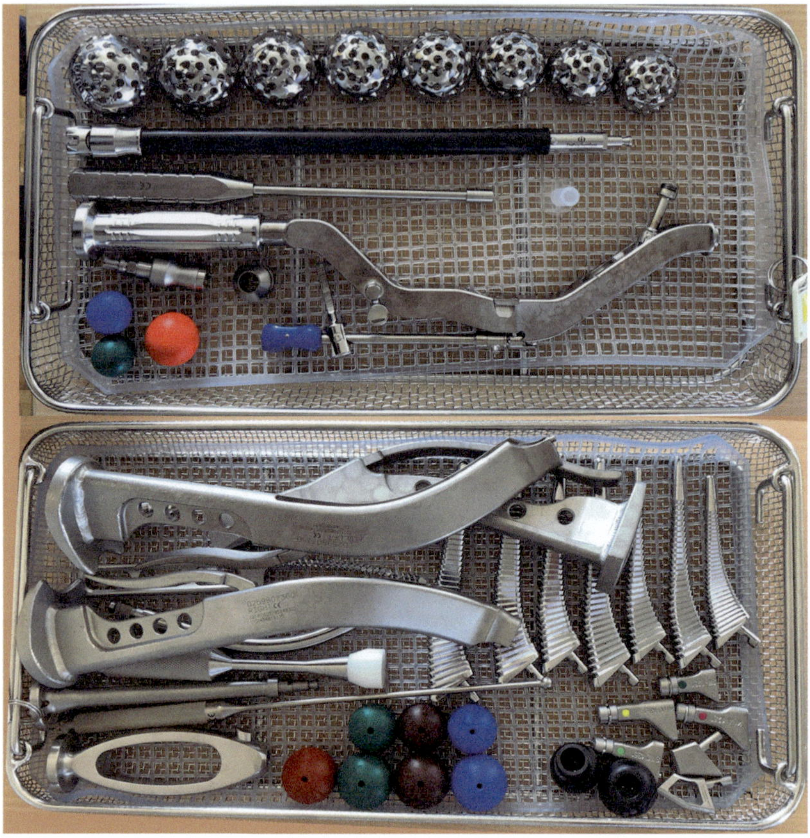

Fig. 6.4 Reduced tray

table requires a trained rotating nurse for manipulation. Pre-training of the individual table-based maneuvers will reportedly decrease the surgical time and radiation exposure [5]. A reduction in the number of opened instrument trays is important (Fig. 6.4). Large-sized, rarely used rasps, and other instruments, can be stowed in a separate tray and opened on demand.

Physical Therapy

The use of this minimally invasive, intermuscular, and internervous procedure facilitates faster rehabilitation with immediate mobilization and weightbearing as tolerated. The introduction of DAA presents a paradigm shift for physical therapists from the restrictive regimen used in the past to a more active protocol with minimal to no restrictions. In our experience, the introduction of DAA will naturally lead to a decreased length of stay and can even be reduced further with a formal "rapid recovery program."

Administration

Case management should be informed that patients are typically able to return home and that expensive rehabilitation and skilled nursing facilities are generally not required.

Patient Information

Patients need to be made aware, ahead of their hospitalization, that DAA leads to a shorter length of stay, immediate mobilization, predictable pain management, and faster rehabilitation. Specific brochures covering preoperative preparation, hospitalization, operative procedure, and rehabilitation prove to be helpful.

Implant Choice

In order to provide a smooth transition to DAA, we recommend not changing the implant at the same time. This minimizes potential sources of error during the transition.

On the femoral side, any femoral implant can be used; however, implants with a low shoulder profile, and short stems, are easier to implant. We used cemented and uncemented stems. Since the exposure of the stem is different from other approaches, offset femoral broaches are recommended. During our initial phase, we used noncollared implants, but subsequently, we switched to a collared stem. Collared stems prevent subsidence, offer better rotational stability, and are associated with improved long-term results [6–8]. On the acetabular side, uncemented press-fit cups were used as a standard, but the approach is extensile, offering the opportunity to use revision implants such as cages or rings.

Execution

Choosing the First Case

For the first DAA cases, patients should be carefully selected. This helps all team members gain familiarity with the new approach and allows indications and levels of difficulty to expand in a controlled manner, minimizing complications. The ideal first patients are nonobese, without previous surgery, and with few morphological changes to the acetabulum and proximal femur apart from the osteoarthritis (Fig. 6.5). Table 6.1

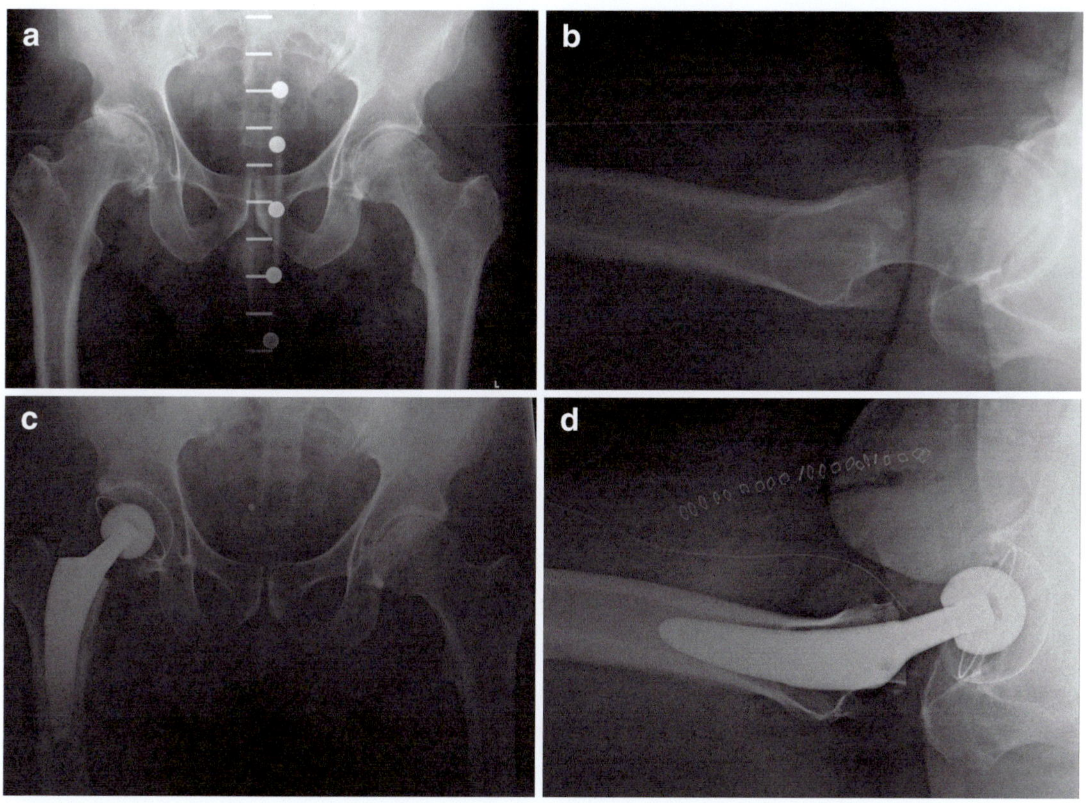

Fig. 6.5 Example of a good starter case. A 71-year old male presented with right-sided, symptomatic hip osteoarthritis. He had no previous hip operations. The radiographs show no relevant varus or valgus deformities or signs of relevant shortening (2C/D). The postoperative radiographs showed a well-inserted stem with anatomically restored leg length and offset. Because of the rather narrow intramedullary space inferior to the lesser trochanter (Dorr Type A morphological femur [9, 10]), a short stem was chosen. The cup orientation is fine according to the target values of Lewinnek [11] (inclination of 30–50°, anteversion 5–25°)

Table 6.1 Lists of challenging conditions, with their problems and potential complications

Figure	Condition	Problem	Potential complications
1	Previous surgery	Difficult identification of anatomic landmarks	Problem with exposure
2	Muscle contractures	Exposure of the femur	Cortical perforation, periprosthetic fracture
3	Severe osteoporosis	Bone quality	Cortical perforation, periprosthetic fracture
4	Short femoral neck	Acetabular and femoral exposure	Malpositioning cup and stem
5	Large acetabulum (>60 mm cup planned)	Acetabular exposure	Cup implantation
6	M. Perthes	High riding greater trochanter, shortening	Femoral exposure, trochanteric fractures, acetabular exposure
7	Hardware in situ	Hardware removal, stress risers	Periprosthetic fractures, osteopenia, greater trochanter, cement leakage
8	Severe joint destruction with joint contractures	Exposure, landmarks	Femoral neck osteotomy with extension into the acetabulum
9	THA for femoral neck fracture	Unexpected extension of the fracture into the greater trochanter Difficult identification of the landmarks	Greater trochanteric fractures
10	Massive varus deformity	Less space to work on the femur	Stem implantation
11	Massive valgus deformity	Less space to work on the acetabulum due to prominent calcar	Cup implantation
12	Severe rotational deformity of the femur	Stem implantation, forced malpositioning through short stems	Dislocations, extraarticular impingement
13	Obesity	Incision in the inguinal fold	Wound/deep infection
14	Severe acetabular dysplasia	Cup positioning, grafting	Cup implantation
15	Severe acetabular retroversion	V-shape pelvis	Femur insertion

lists a number of conditions that can pose a problem for the inexperienced surgeon (Fig. 6.6). Although the way to the hip in DAA may be comparable between obese and nonobese patients, we do not recommend starting in patients with a high body mass index (Fig. 6.7). The incision is exactly in the inguinal fold under the panniculus, which predisposes to wound healing problems and even infection if the wound is not properly protected. Furthermore, exposure of the hip joint in obese individuals is more challenging and often requires more time.

Preoperative Planning

Preoperative routine digital planning is essential. It helps anticipate intraoperative problems with implant sizes and availability, get familiar with the individual patient anatomy, and identify anatomic landmarks for intraoperative referencing.

Helpful landmarks for the acetabulum are the superolateral extent of the acetabulum and the posteroinferior acetabular horn. The obturator externus tendon groove in the area of the greater trochanter serves as a reference for the depth of the stem (Figs. 6.8 and 6.9) [12]. The distance of the broach to the calcar give a hint on varus/valgus malpositioning (Fig. 6.9).

Coaching

It is recommended that an experienced surgeon, familiar with the procedure, acts as a coach for the very first cases.

Intraoperative Fluoroscopy

Although we have never used fluoroscopy for THA prior to starting DAA, it has become a stan-

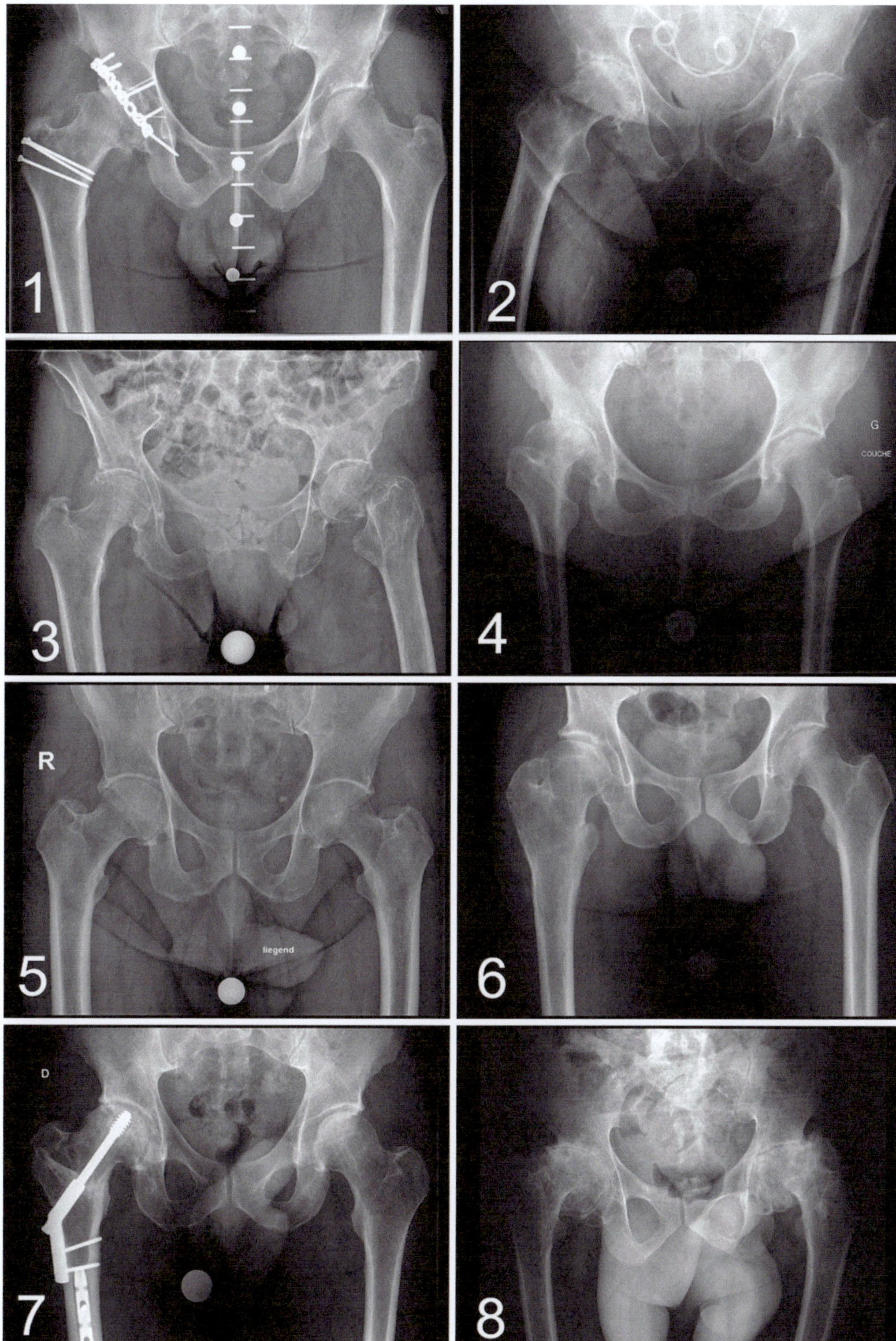

Fig. 6.6 Corresponding examples to the list of conditions (Table 6.1), which pose a problem for the inexperienced surgeon

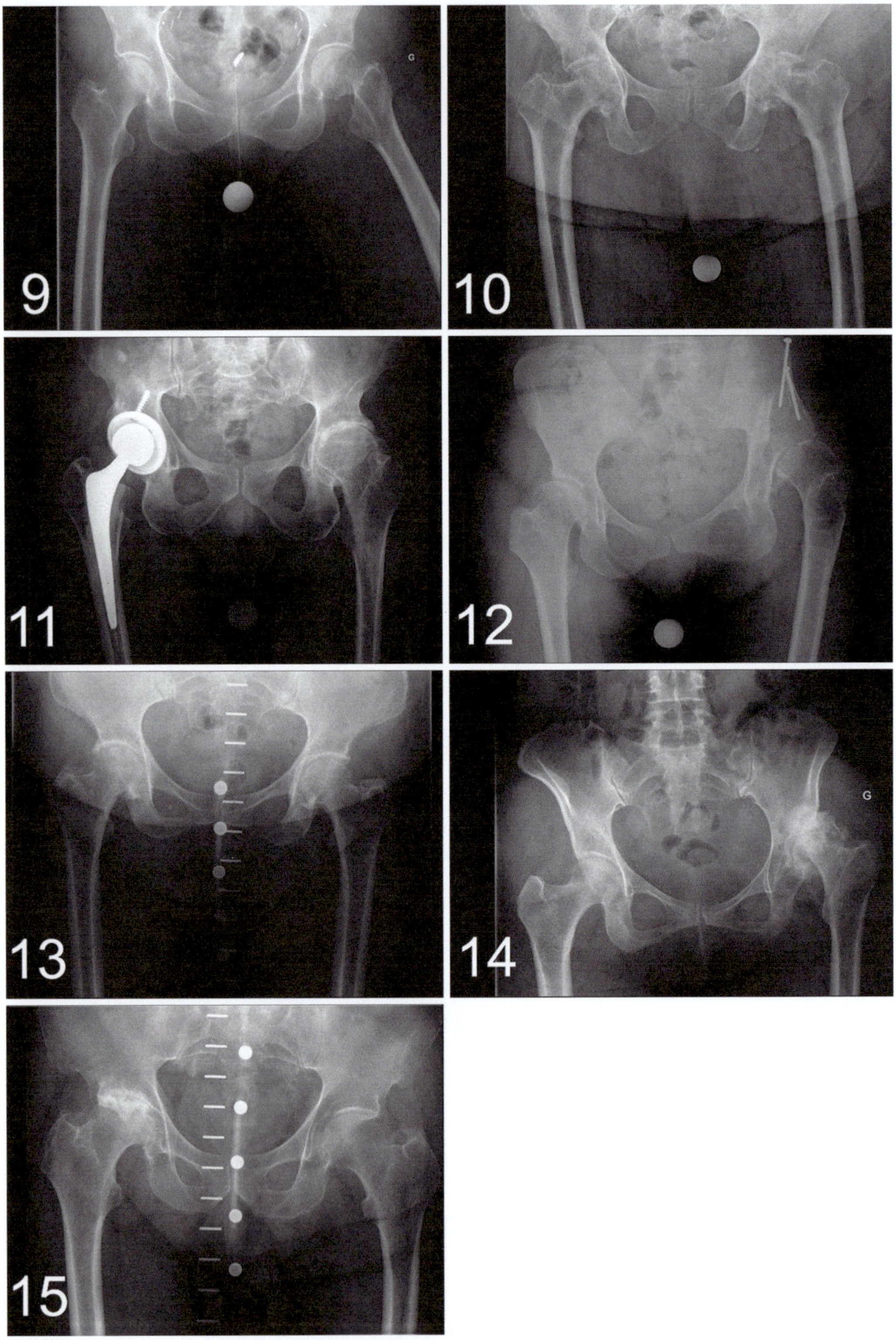

Fig. 6.6 (continued)

dard part of our procedure from the very first case. Acetabular reaming and cup positioning can be performed under direct visualization with immediate radiographic feedback (Fig. 6.10). Use of a fluoroscope enables additional control for femoral leg length and offset. Fluoroscopy also provides immediate visual feedback of the femoral component, including positioning in the femoral shaft (avoiding varus or valgus malposition), appropriate component sizing, and any perforation, fractures, or fissures of the femur. Getting direct feedback during implantation

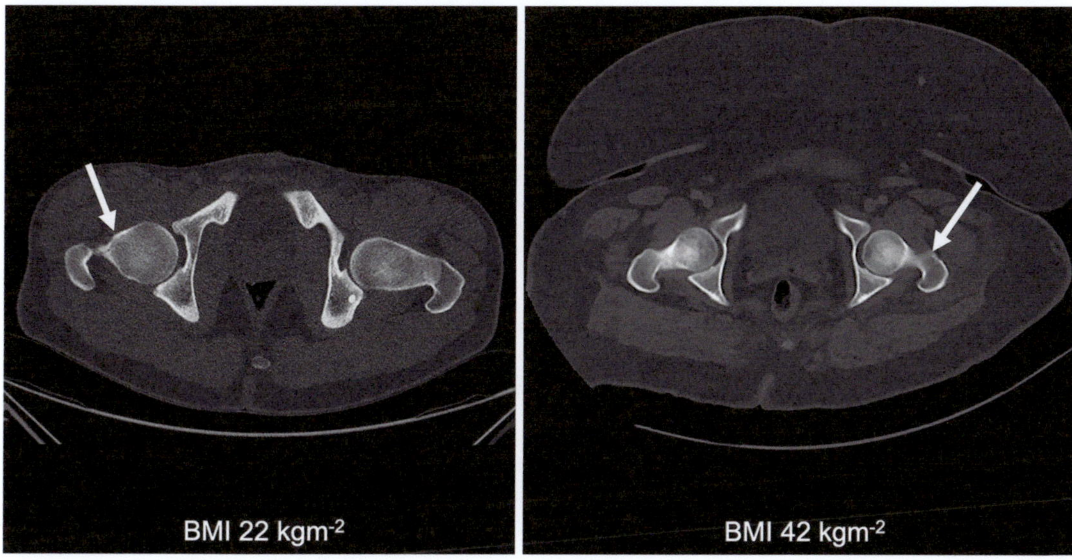

Fig. 6.7 The left patient with a BMI of 22 kg/m^2 is a perfect candidate for a DAA. However, the right patient with a BMI of 42 kg/m^2 shows more or less the same distance to the hip joint, but the abdominal fat will interfere with the surgeon's field of view and potential complications

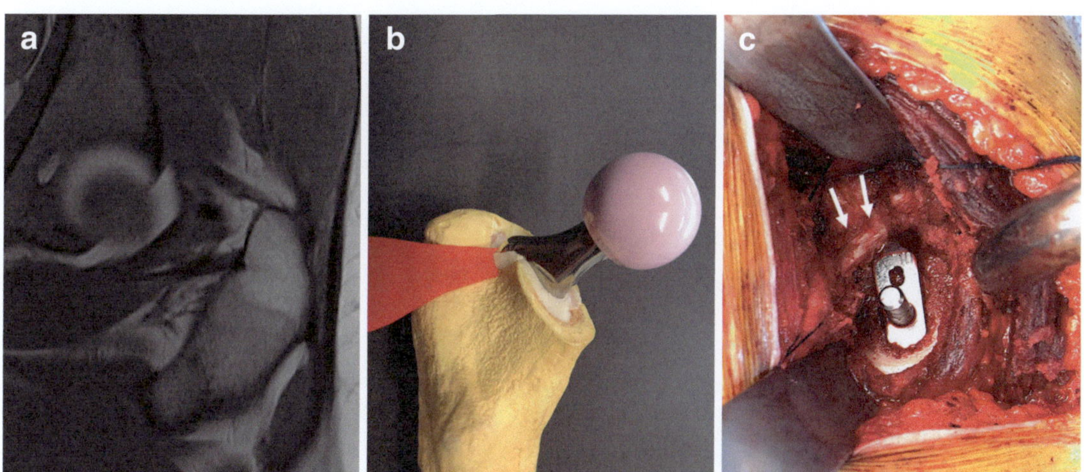

Fig. 6.8 The footprint of the obturator externus muscle functions as a landmark, which is always visible during insertion of the prosthesis. The typical position shown in magnetic resonance imaging (MRI) is located at the base posteromedial border of the greater trochanter (**a**). During stem preparation, the area of the footprint is exposed with maximal external rotation of the hip (**b**/**c**)

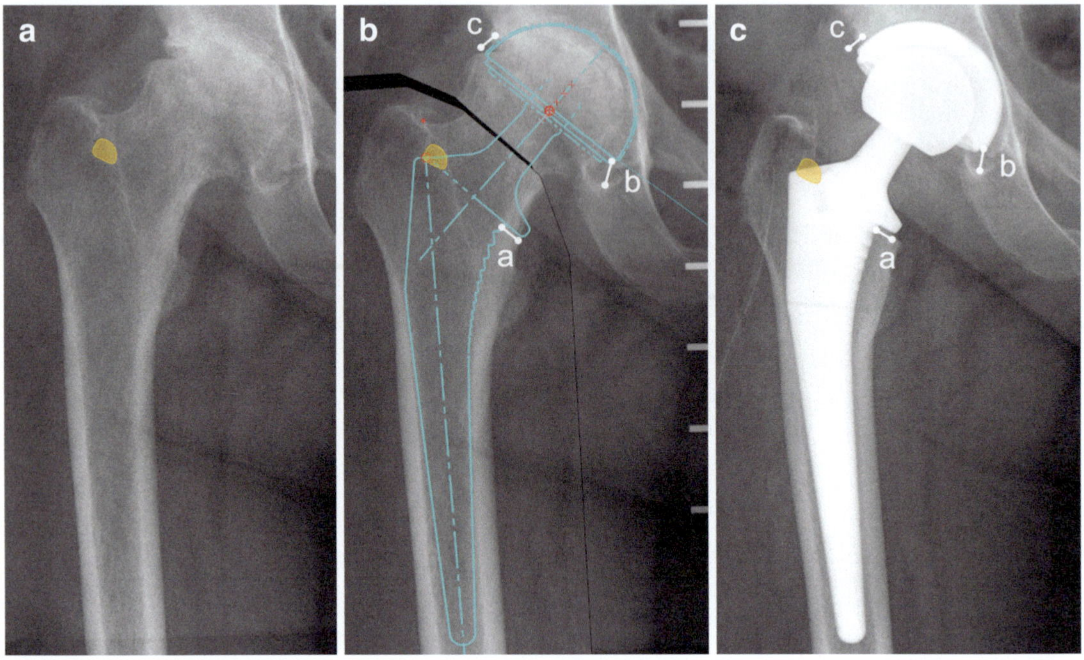

Fig. 6.9 Based on a standard radiograph (**a**), the planning (**b**) was performed. The footprint of the obturator externus muscle is a helpful landmark (yellow). The final postoperative radiograph (**c**) shows the same references with equal distances of the broach to the calcar (a), the cup to the posteroinferior acetabular horn (b), and the superolateral extent of the acetabulum (c)

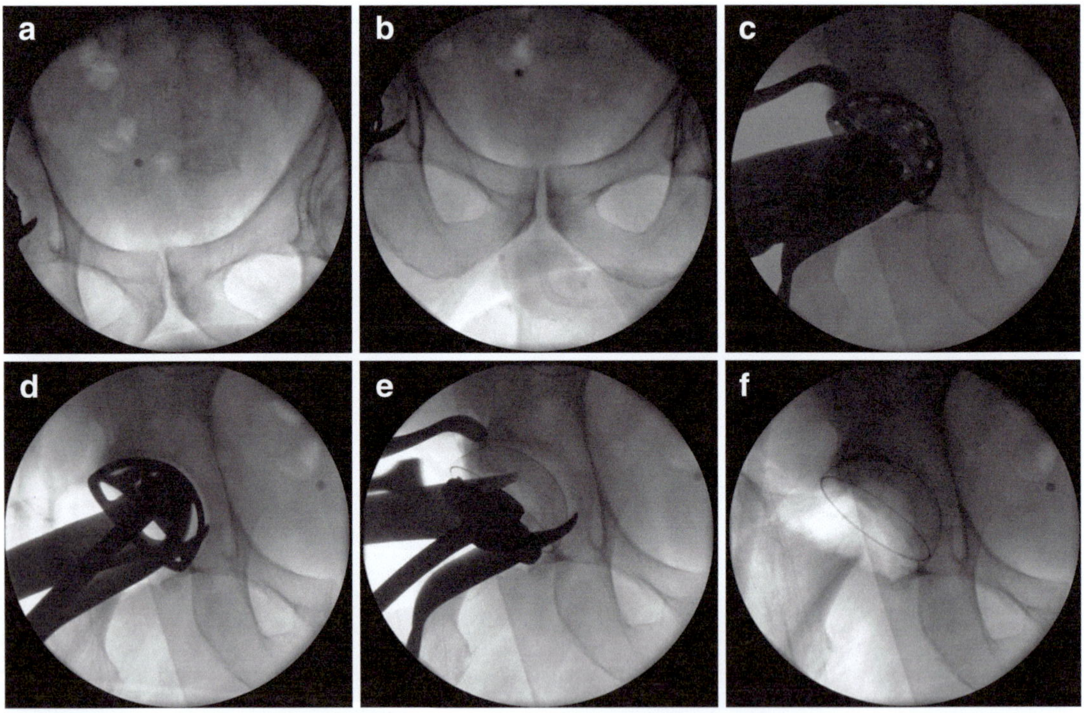

Fig. 6.10 Alignment of the fluoroscopy to the pelvic anatomy (**a**/**b**). Intraoperative reaming with the adaptation of the inclination and anteversion (**c**). Trial component placement (**d**). Insertion of the cup while controlling version, inclination, and depth (**e**/**f**)

helps optimize the learning process of the new technique [13–17], particularly in a training environment.

Capsular Management and Release for Femur Access

In our early experience, we noted that partial capsulectomy of the anterior capsule did not necessarily result in better access to the acetabulum. Instead, an L-shaped capsulotomy with retraction of the capsular flap anteriorly creates a sleeve of soft tissue that facilitates the insertion of reamers and further protects the periarticular musculature.

The capsular release on the inside of the greater trochanter turned out to be the most difficult step of the operation. A straight incision cranially starting from the superior neck osteotomy to the tip of the greater trochanter is usually enough. Levering the femur with the hook lift helps visualize remnants of capsular insertion on the posterior aspects of the greater trochanter. Mobilization of the capsule on the posterior aspect of the proximal femur is rarely necessary but possible (Fig. 6.11).

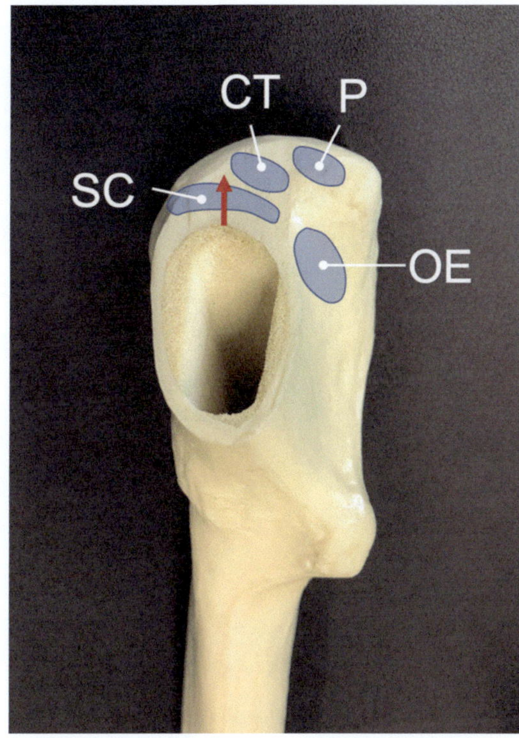

Fig. 6.11 The capsular release starts cranially from the superior part of the femoral neck osteotomy and is performed in the direction of the tip of the greater trochanter. SC, superior capsule; CT, conjoint tendon insertion; P, piriformis tendon insertion; OE, obturator externus tendon insertion. (Adapted according to Chughtai et al. [18])

Evaluation

Patient Selection

In some cases with chronic abductor tears, we observed persistent lateral pain after THA. In those cases, we recommend preoperative magnetic resonance imaging for evaluation of trochanteric bursitis associated with lesions of the M. gluteus minimus and medius (Fig. 6.12). In those cases, we favor the lateral approach, which allows concomitant repair of the abductors.

Complications

Apart from immediate short-term dysfunction of the lateral femoral cutaneous nerve (Fig. 6.1), the most frequent complication in the early phase was avulsion fracture of the posteromedial aspect of the greater trochanter due to insufficient release of the capsule in the trochanteric fossa (Fig. 6.13). This fracture also occurred in osteoporotic cases with a femoral neck fracture where the fracture extended into the greater trochanter. Fissures of the calcar area occurred typically in cases with an abnormal femoral version or previous surgery (Fig. 6.14).

We had three major nerve palsies, two femoral and one sciatic. One femoral nerve palsy occurred in a patient with previous Legg–Calvé–Perthes disease and a lengthening of approximately 2 cm. The only sciatic nerve palsy was caused by a cerclage cable placed for an intraoperative femoral fissure (Figs. 6.2 and 6.15).

A rare and probably underreported complication was the atrophy of the M. vastus lateralis. A patient underwent bilateral staged THA through

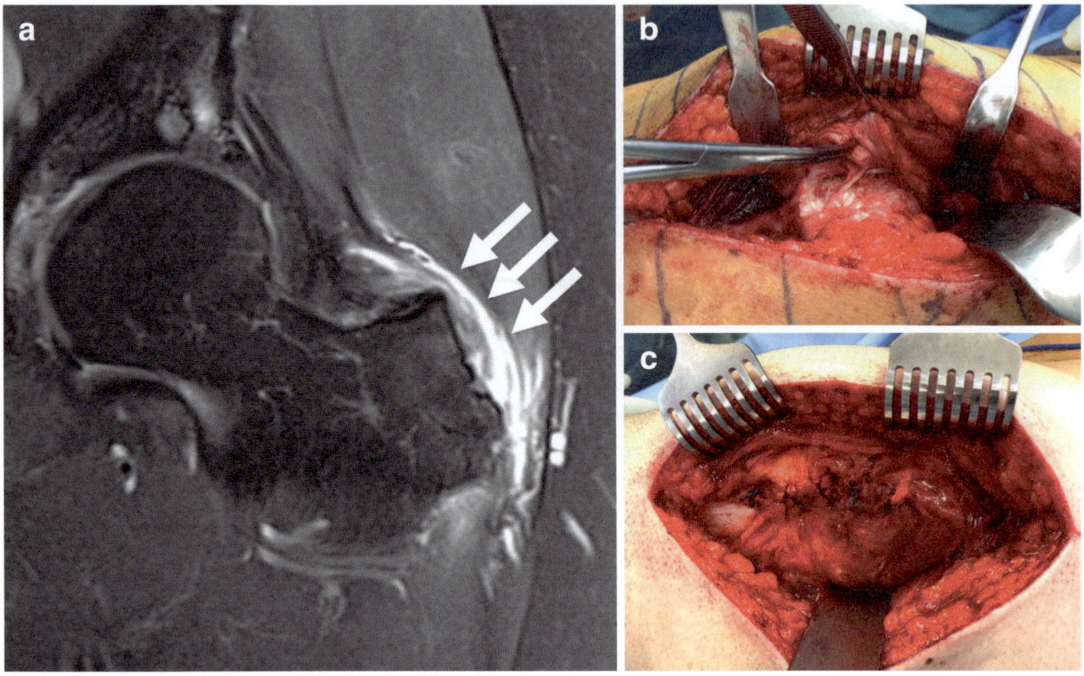

Fig. 6.12 Preoperative MRI with hyperdense infiltration and signs of interruption of the M. gluteus minimus and medius tendon insertions (**a**). Intraoperative image showing degenerative changes of the tendons (**b**) and after tendon repair (**c**) through a lateral approach

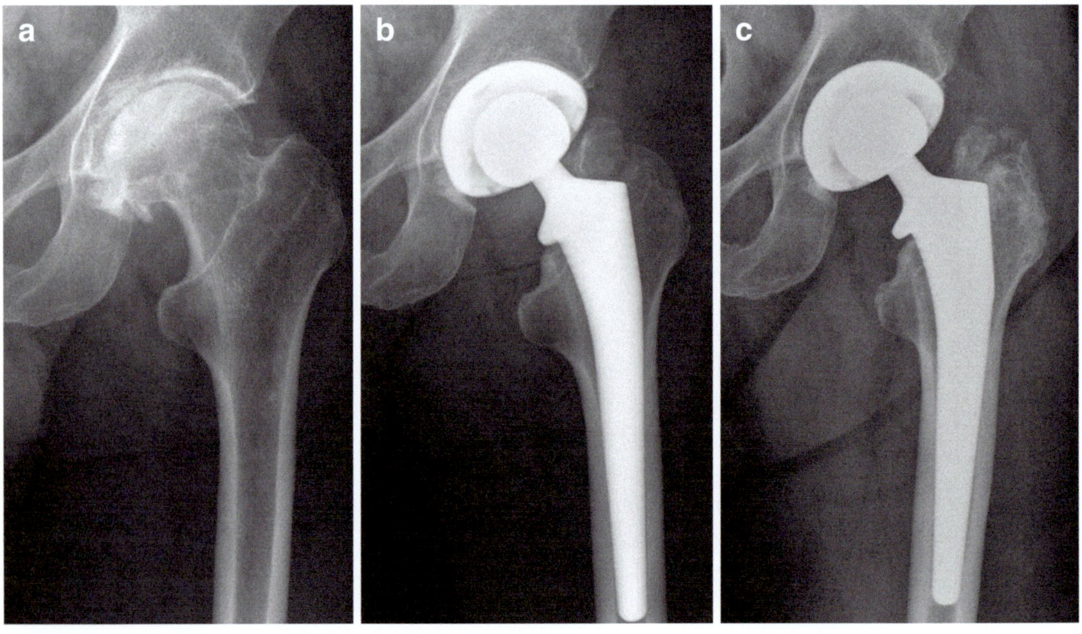

Fig. 6.13 Example of a trochanteric avulsion fracture. Preoperative radiograph (**a**), postoperative avulsion fracture (**b**), and radiograph following treatment with osteo sutures (**c**)

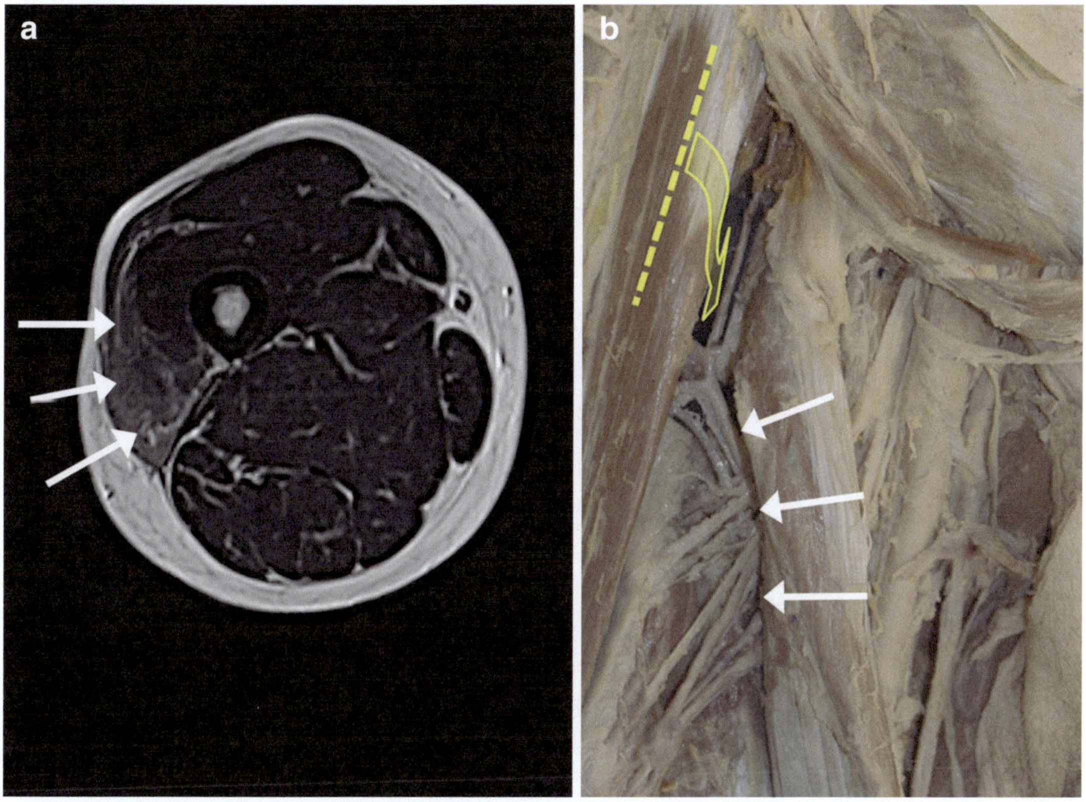

Fig. 6.14 Atrophy and fatty infiltration of the M. vastus lateralis (**a**) in the MRI. Probably based on an iatrogenic lesion of femoral nerves branches (**b**, white arrows) during the anterior approach (yellow arrow). (Adapted from Grob et al. [19])

DAA and complained about subjective atrophy of his thigh muscles on the first operated side. The MRI showed atrophy and fatty infiltration of the M. vastus lateralis. We attributed this pathology to an iatrogenic lesion of femoral nerve branches (Fig. 6.14).

Cup Orientation

We evaluated the accuracy and precision of cup orientation, as noted on postoperative radiographs, between the last 67 cases performed with our previous technique (transgluteal approach in lateral decubitus position) and the first 127 cases performed with DAA. We used previously described software that calculates cup orientation with respect to the anterior pelvic plane (Fig. 6.16). Our evaluation revealed that, even in the learning curve, our precision for cup orientation was better for DAA than the established routine at that time (Fig. 6.17).

Length of Stay

Over a three-year period, we reduced the in-hospital length of stay by 29%.

DAA in Switzerland

DAA has become, by far, the most commonly used approach in Switzerland. Since the initiation of the Swiss Implant Registry in 2015, the use of DAA has gradually increased, while the classic lateral and posterior approaches have declined (Fig. 6.18).

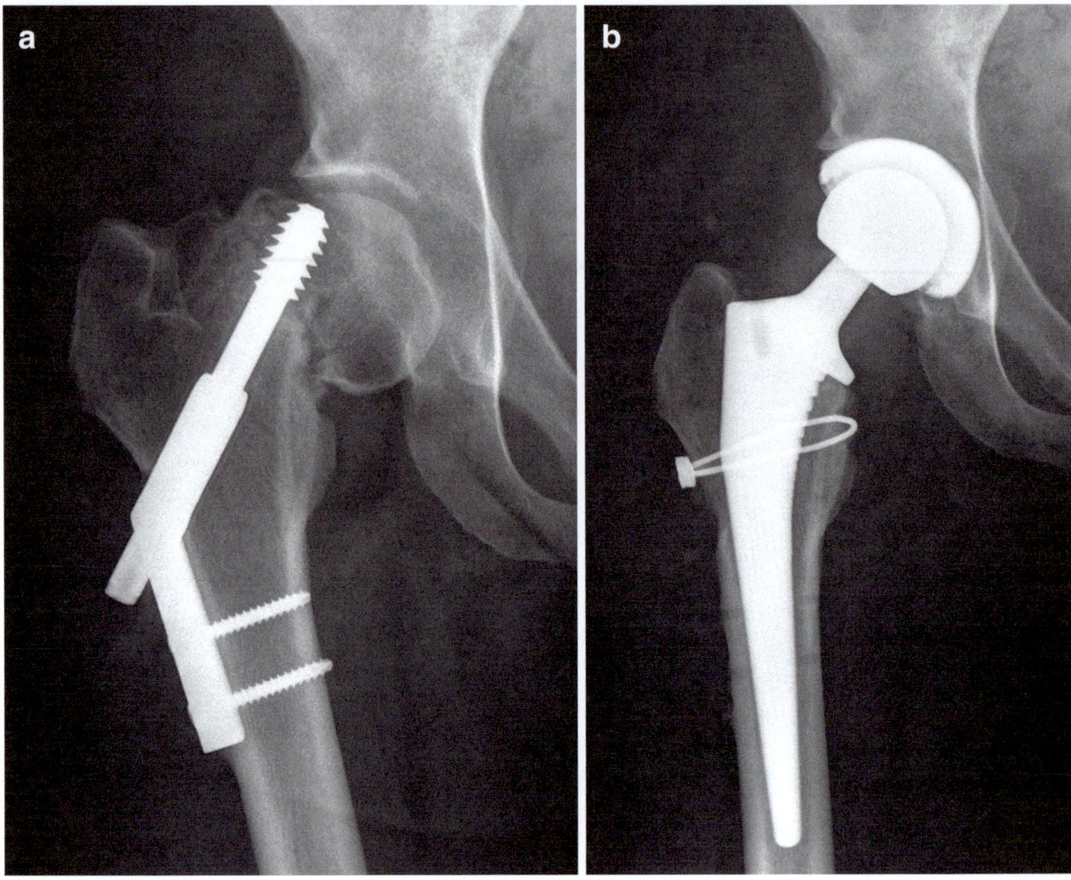

Fig. 6.15 Patient with a cut-out of a dynamic hip screw (**a**) with an intraoperative fracture of the calcar during implantation of the total hip arthroplasty (**b**)

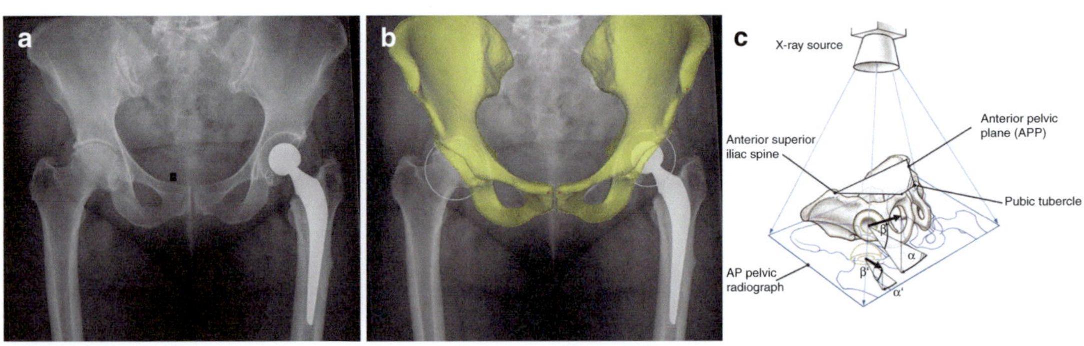

Fig. 6.16 Anterior-posterior pelvic radiograph with the radiolucent polyethylene cup (RM Pressfit or RM Pressfit vitamys cup, Mathys AG, Bettlach, Switzerland). (**b**) The three-dimensional cup orientation was calculated using a postoperative anterior-posterior pelvic radiograph and 2D/3D-matching software with a statistical shape model of the pelvis. (**c**) Cup inclination and anteversion are measured according to the anatomy of the pelvis with reference to the anterior pelvic plane (defined by the anterior superior iliac spines and pubic tubercles)

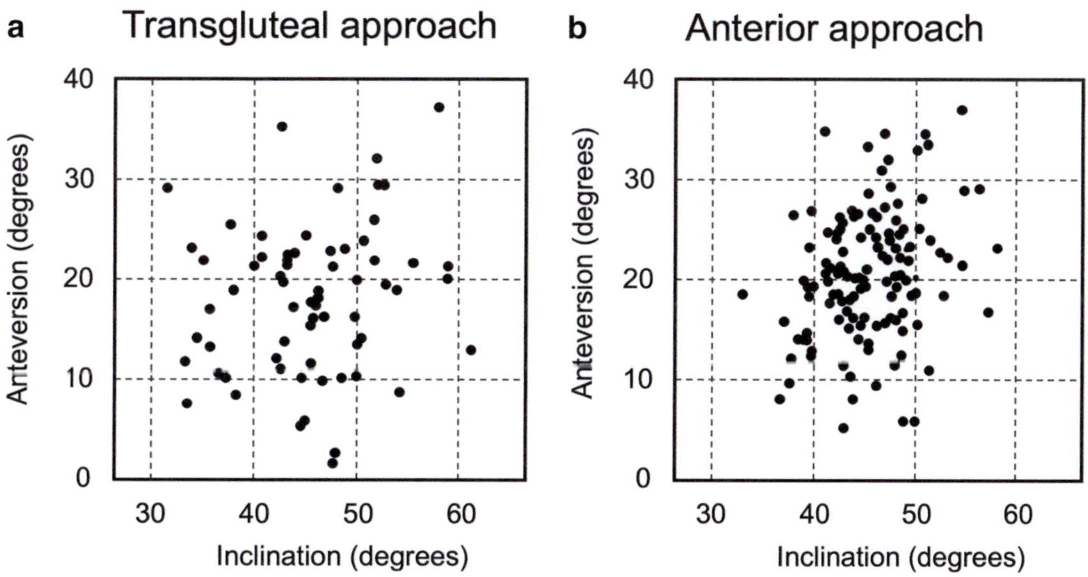

Fig. 6.17 The transgluteal approach (**a**) is compared to DAA (**b**), which shows higher postoperative precision of cup version and inclination. The target values for inclination (40°) and for anteversion (15°) were used based on Lewinnek's safe zone

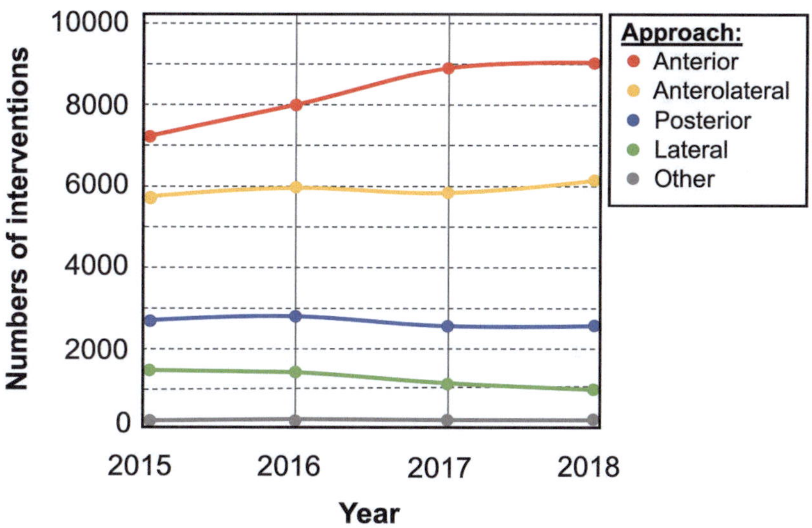

Fig. 6.18 Evolution of the different approaches to the hip joint for total hip replacement in Switzerland from 2015 through 2018

Literature

1. Barrett WP, Turner SE, Leopold JP. Prospective randomized study of direct anterior vs postero-lateral approach for total hip arthroplasty. J Arthroplast. 2013;28(9):1634–8.
2. Wang Z, Hou JZ, Wu CZ, Zhou JY, Gu XM, Wang H-H, et al. A systematic review and meta-analysis of direct anterior approach versus posterior approach in total hip arthroplasty. J Orthop Surg. 2018;13(1):229.
3. de Steiger RN, Lorimer M, Solomon M. What is the learning curve for the anterior approach for total hip arthroplasty? Clin Orthop. 2015;473(12):3860–6.
4. Rudin D, Manestar M, Ullrich O, Erhardt J, Grob K. The anatomical course of the lateral femoral cutaneous nerve with special attention to the anterior approach to the hip joint. J Bone Jt Surg. 2016;98(7):561–7.

5. Kong X, Grau L, Ong A, Yang C, Chai W. Adopting the direct anterior approach: experience and learning curve in a Chinese patient population. J Orthop Surg. 2019;14(1):218.
6. Lamb JN, Baetz J, Messer-Hannemann P, Adekanmbi I, van Duren BH, Redmond A, et al. A calcar collar is protective against early periprosthetic femoral fracture around cementless femoral components in primary total hip arthroplasty: a registry study with biomechanical validation. Bone Jt J. 2019;101-B(7):779–86.
7. Demey G, Fary C, Lustig S, Neyret P, si Selmi T. Does a collar improve the immediate stability of uncemented femoral hip stems in total hip arthroplasty? A bilateral comparative cadaver study. J Arthroplast. 2011;26(8):1549–55.
8. Ström H, Nilsson O, Milbrink J, Mallmin H, Larsson S. The effect of early weight bearing on migration pattern of the uncemented CLS stem in total hip arthroplasty. J Arthroplast. 2007;22(8):1122–9.
9. Dorr LD, Faugere MC, Mackel AM, Gruen TA, Bognar B, Malluche H. Structural and cellular assessment of bone quality of proximal femur. Bone. 1993;14(3):231–42.
10. Wilkerson J, Fernando ND. Classifications in brief: the Dorr classification of femoral bone. Clin Orthop. 2020;478(8):1939–44.
11. Lewinnek GE, Lewis JL, Tarr R, Compere CL, Zimmerman JR. Dislocations after total hip-replacement arthroplasties. J Bone Joint Surg Am. 1978;60(2):217–20.
12. Rüdiger HA, Fritz B, Impellizzeri FM, Leunig M, Pfirrmann C, Sutter R. The external obturator footprint as a landmark in total hip arthroplasty through a direct anterior approach: a CT-based analysis. Hip Int. 2019;29(1):96–101.
13. Beamer BS, Morgan JH, Barr C, Weaver MJ, Vrahas MS. Does fluoroscopy improve acetabular component placement in total hip arthroplasty? Clin Orthop. 2014;472(12):3953–62.
14. Navarro SM, Frey C, Blackwell T, Voges SB, Del Schutte H. Clinical results of direct anterior approach THA with minimal fluoroscopic exposure optimization techniques. Surg Technol Int. 2018;33:277–80.
15. Homma Y, Baba T, Kobayashi H, Desroches A, Ozaki Y, Ochi H, et al. Safety in early experience with a direct anterior approach using fluoroscopic guidance with manual leg control for primary total hip arthroplasty: a consecutive one hundred and twenty case series. Int Orthop. 2016;40(12):2487–94.
16. James JR, Peterson BE, Crim JR, Cook JL, Crist BDBD. The use of fluoroscopy during direct anterior hip arthroplasty: powerful or misleading? J Arthroplast. 2018;33(6):1775–9.
17. Pomeroy C, Mason JB, Fehring T, Masonis JL, Curtin BM. Radiation exposure during Fluoro-assisted direct anterior total hip arthroplasty. J Arthroplast. 2016;31(8):1742–5.
18. Chughtai M, Samuel LT, Acuña AJ, Kamath AF. Algorithmic soft tissue femoral release in anterior approach total hip arthroplasty. Arthroplasty Today. 2019;5(4):471–6.
19. Grob K, Monahan R, Gilbey H, Yap F, Filgueira L, Kuster M. Distal extension of the direct anterior approach to the hip poses risk to neurovascular structures: an anatomical study. J Bone Joint Surg Am. 2015;97(2):126–32.

Challenges in Anterior Approach Education

7

William G. Hamilton and Jonathan R. Dattilo

Introduction

The direct anterior approach (DAA) to total hip arthroplasty (THA) is becoming an increasingly popular technique, with many purported benefits, including faster earlier recovery, reduced dislocation risk, and less postoperative pain [1–4]. The DAA may be a more technically demanding operation to both perform and consequently teach. While the history of DAA has been extensively covered elsewhere in this text, a brief review is helpful to explain the framework of education with respect to the evolution of DAA.

The initial description of the anterior approach is most commonly attributed to German surgeon Carl Hueter in his *Der Grundriss der Chirurgie (The Compendium of Surgery)* published in 1881, and in many descriptions, this approach was termed the "Hueter interval" [5, 6]. Norwegian-born American surgeon Marius Smith-Petersen is credited with spreading the use of the anterior approach in the English-speaking world, and hence the Heuter interval became more commonly known as the "Smith-Petersen approach" in the United States [6]. While original applications for the DAA were described for pediatric hip dysplasia, the mid-1900s witnessed its gradual application to arthroplasty. This began with hemiarthroplasty for fracture management in France in 1950 [7] and subsequently in the United States in 1955 [5], followed by implementation for THA in the United States in 1980 [8]. However, it was not until the turn of the century, fueled by emerging interest in minimally-invasive hip replacement [9], that the DAA subsequently gained more widespread notoriety for elective THA in the United States [10, 11].

The past two decades have played witness to a slow, early adoption of the DAA followed by an exponential rise in recent years. Practice patterns of the American Association of Hip and Knee Surgeons (AAHKS) demonstrate that only 12% of members utilized the DAA in 2009, but by 2019, 56.2% of members had incorporated it into their practices [12, 13].

This pattern of evolution and adoption of the DAA in the United States has resulted in a bimodal distribution of learning. In the first generation, early adopters consisting of established, practicing surgeons challenged themselves to master the technique. However, as Malcom Gladwell's commonly quoted "10,000-hour rule" describes, mastery of a new task requires a tremendous amount of time and dedication [14]. There was therefore an inherent and necessary lag before this knowledge could be effectively incorporated into residency and fellowship training. However, early adopters are now capable of teaching the current generation of trainees. It is becoming more commonplace for residents and

W. G. Hamilton (✉) · J. R. Dattilo
Anderson Orthopaedic Research Institute,
Alexandria, VA, USA

J. M. Matta, A. P. Sah (eds.), *Anterior Hip Replacement*,
https://doi.org/10.1007/978-3-030-91896-5_7

fellows to learn the DAA. In fact, a survey of AAHKS members in 2019 demonstrated that DAA surgeons had been in practice for a shorter duration than surgeons using other approaches, suggesting that these trainees who had the opportunity to receive formal instruction are transitioning into practice [13].

As surgeons began using the DAA in THA, several reports were published demonstrating an early learning curve associated with increased complications, many of which attempted to quantify the number of cases constituting the learning period [15–18]. A systematic review demonstrated enormous variation in the reported volume of cases that constituted the learning curve, ranging from 10 to 200 [19]. Because there exists no standard definition for the learning curve, much of this variation is likely due to heterogeneity in how each study calculated its endpoint. In particular, because some early adopters of the DAA were more experienced surgeons, one must be mindful when interpreting these publications, as they may not be generalizable to the average surgeon. For example, one single-surgeon study utilized procedure time as an endpoint. The authors noted that 400 cases were required for a surgeon who was an expert in the posterior approach to achieve equivalent operative time with the DAA, which may not be a fair assessment of a true learning curve, but more closely mimic the time required to achieve equivalent mastery of the technique [20]. Furthermore, there is also substantial variation in the amount of formal training novice DAA surgeons receive prior to implementing it in practice, which has directly correlated with complication rates. A study of community surgeons with little or no formal training demonstrated a 9% complication rate [21], while another study found that those who had received formal instruction had no evidence of increased complications [22]. A learning curve is intuitively inherent to any surgeon performing an unfamiliar procedure and indeed has been demonstrated with other THA approaches [23]. Therefore, the burden of complications may reflect the amount of preoperative education and preparation for any new technique rather represent a phenomenon unique to the DAA.

We will utilize the remainder of this chapter to explore the various challenges to DAA education, first from the perspective of the educator and subsequently from two trainee perspectives. We will conclude with suggestions for both educators and trainee surgeons to safely and effectively learn to incorporate DAA THA into clinical practice.

Challenges for the Educator

Surgical education in the United States has historically relied on the apprenticeship model popularized by William Stewart Halsted [24]. However, compared to Halsted's era, contemporary educators and students now have increased access to cadaver labs, high-quality multimedia, and most recently surgical simulations designed specifically for arthroplasty procedures [25, 26]. Despite a wider armamentarium of educational tools, there remain challenges inherent to any apprenticeship model and the dissemination of information from teacher to apprentice.

A master surgeon may not be a master educator, as these represent two entirely separate skill sets. In fact, the majority of surgeons receive no formal pedagogical training [27]. Furthermore, it is an inherent challenge for someone who is a master of their trade to remember the basics and appeal to a novice learner. This phenomenon, described as "the more you know, the less you can clearly explain," has been dubbed the *knowledge paradox* [27]. The difficulties a master surgeon faces in communicating what they perceive to be basic concepts is a form of cognitive bias in which experts often overestimate the abilities of novices [28]. In other words, we assume that things we take for granted as fundamental are already mastered by the novice, which is often untrue. This is further manifested in what is known as the *threshold concept*, which means that once the boundary of understanding has been crossed, it is challenging to remember a time when the concept was not understood [27]. Therefore, the first step in educating a trainee is first one of self-reflection and a concerted effort to recall and relate to their perspectives.

A second tenet crucial to Halsted's model of surgical education was graduated autonomy [24]. The educator is tasked with not only imparting the knowledge of the procedure, but also guiding the trainee in the transition from supervised to independent practice. Surgical learning is a whole-task curriculum in which the trainee learns a summation of steps to complete the task from beginning to end. There are two processes that are fundamental to this model [29]. First, tasks increase from simple to complex, beginning with relatively straightforward principles such as anatomy and graduating to complex concepts and maneuvers. Second, as trainees progress, there is a concurrent decrease in support and guidance. This process of gradually diminishing support is known as *scaffolding* and continues until trainees are able to independently perform the task in its entirety [29].

This process of graduated autonomy is crucial to instilling confidence in the trainee and lessening the abruptness of transitioning to independent practice, but it may be challenging for the educating surgeon. Most importantly, this needs to be done in a manner that prioritizes patient care. Initially, the educator must evaluate the trainee's baseline skill. Equally important is for the educator to gain an understanding of the trainee's self-assessment of their skills. Trainees who understand their own strengths, and more importantly, their weaknesses, are ideal. A cavalier surgeon who has a poor assessment of his or her own skill or has a low threshold to take risk can pose a danger. Once it has been demonstrated that the trainee can be allowed unsupervised autonomy, the educator must decide how this can be accomplished. It can be helpful to have the trainee operate independently of the surgeon but with an assistant familiar with the procedure. In fact, for surgeons learning the DAA, operating with an assistant who had performed more than 100 cases may help mitigate complications [30].

Proper education of DAA THA presents multiple challenges. The approach has been adopted with a focus on minimally-invasive surgery, as well as having influence from industry and patient marketing [31]. In 2019 among AAHKS members who performed the DAA, 76% reported increased market share, while 66% of nonperformers lost market share [13]. This emphasis on minimally-invasive surgery leads to smaller incisions that may be less conducive for visualization and trainee education. Furthermore, variations in technique, such as the "bikini incision" [32], while perhaps more attractive to patients, may make it even harder for a novice surgeon to learn the fundamentals.

A prerequisite to trainee education is for the instructing surgeon to be proficient in preventing and managing complications that may arise. While an extensile exposure has been described for the DAA [33], many surgeons may not be comfortable managing complications through this approach. One study reported that of surgeons who normally perform the DAA, 79.3% cite revision status as a reason for preferential use of a posterior approach [13]. While many contemporary educators have mastered the primary DAA THA technique, they may remain in their learning period for revisions. This limited experience in utilizing an extensile DAA exposure poses a barrier for education, as surgeons may be reticent to allow trainees hands-on participation if they are not confident that they can address complications themselves.

In summary, mastery of the DAA technique is but the first step in the journey of becoming a proficient educator. There are multiple challenges that those educating novices in the DAA technique must master, including an appreciation of the foundation of knowledge and technical skills of their apprentice, as well as inherent challenges of minimally invasive surgery and identification of their comfort level in managing complications.

Challenges for the Trainee

In this section, we will examine the challenges of DAA education from two uniquely different perspectives. First, we will explore the challenges from the traditional perspective of a resident or fellow who has not yet completed training. We will then explore the different challenges that a practicing surgeon must face when transitioning to the DAA from another surgical approach.

Resident and Fellow Challenges

The resident or fellow learning the DAA in training can be considered a blank slate. They are devoid of the biases of a practicing surgeon who has mastered another approach. Conversely, they also enter with less foundational knowledge of hip arthroplasty and lack the mastery of basic surgical skills. Nevertheless, there is increasing demand for exposure to the DAA in residency and fellowship training, both because of community demand and employment opportunities that appear to be enhanced by prior training with DAA [31, 34].

Introduction to DAA THA for the resident or fellow begins with the core elements of whole-task curricula [29]. The first step is to understand the theory or the foundational knowledge of hip arthroplasty. The modern digital age affords trainees an endless array of textbooks, websites, and multimedia. The second step is the acquisition of procedural skills. These have historically been practiced in a cadaver lab, though modern technology now offers surgical simulations for dedicated learning in a controlled environment. Indeed, surgical simulations have demonstrated efficacy in teaching novices both in acetabular cup placement through a posterior approach [26] as well as improved performance in the DAA [25]. The transition to the operating room is not only desirable for the trainee and a necessity toward the transition to completing the whole-task curricula but also offers the opportunity for immediate individualized feedback. It appears that this personal feedback has been demonstrated to be more efficacious than self-study alone [35]. Additionally, compared to practicing surgeons who may only be able to attend single-day instructional courses, residents and fellows have the benefit of shorter individual teaching episodes, which are temporally distributed over a longer time period, a learning feature demonstrated to be more effective in surgical education [36].

There is a paucity of data specifically examining whether complication rates are reduced for trainees who have learned the approach in residency or fellowship. However, a learning curve has been demonstrated in other THA approaches [23], as well as a general learning curve for junior surgeons entering practice [37]. As the current generation of trainees matures, it will be interesting to see if their early complication rates differ from reports of practicing surgeons transitioning to the DAA, though it may be difficult to ascertain differences attributable specifically to the DAA as opposed to a product of transition to independent practice.

Several components of DAA may actually facilitate novice training. First, the patient is positioned supine, which may ease the burden of cognitive spatial orientation for the learner. Second, the supine positioning allows for the use of fluoroscopy, which many DAA surgeons choose to employ. The use of fluoroscopy in the DAA has been shown to eliminate severely malpositioned acetabular components [38] and benefits trainees by providing real-time feedback for component placement.

There are factors inherent to DAA THA that may pose challenges for the trainee. First, identification of the correct intermuscular interval may be challenging. Other surgical approaches utilized for THA use key muscular attachments to identify the correct interval, for instance, the junction of the vastus lateralis and gluteus medius in a direct lateral approach or the split of the easily identifiable gluteus maximus in a posterior approach. However, the anterior approach generally relies on blunt dissection to find the interval between the tensor fascia lata laterally and the sartorius medially [39], and it can be easy to inadvertently dissect too far medially and end up in the inappropriate, and dangerous, interval containing the femoral artery and nerve. The emphasis on small incisions associated with minimally invasive surgery may be an additional challenging factor, and we have provided a safety checklist for identifying the correct interval in Table 7.1. Second, while fluoroscopic guidance may provide immediate feedback, correct interpretation must be mastered for safe use. Without a thorough understanding of pelvic positioning, fluoroscopic views may be misleading [40]. Furthermore, while the patient is almost universally positioned supine during DAA THA, there

Table 7.1 Checklist to identify the correct interval in DAA THA

1. Feel through the wound for the anterior superior iliac spine (ASIS). Note the orientation of the muscle fibers of the tensor fascia lata (TFL), which should be originating from and extending laterally from the ASIS.
2. The fascia of the iliotibial band will become thicker posteriorly overlaying the TFL, and there are several perforating arteries that will enter the thickened portion of the fascia. The fascial incision should be made anterior to these perforating arteries.
3. The surgeon's finger should be able to slide over the muscle belly of the TFL, and orientation of the finger proximal and posteriorly should allow the finger to slide easily over the superior femoral neck.
4. If the medial muscle in the interval has white striations, this is the rectus femoris and serves to verify that the surgeon has achieved the correct interval.
5. The lateral circumflex artery and two venous comitans should be running in a medial-to-lateral orientation at the midpoint of the interval. If more than three vascular structures are visualized, particularly if they are traveling in a cranial-caudal direction, surgeons should be wary that they may be medial to the rectus muscle and encountering the femoral artery and its divisions.

are choices of orthopedic table utilized. Some surgeons use a standard operating room table, while others make use of specialized orthopedic tables, which must also be learned by the trainee. Femoral exposure and broaching may also be uniquely challenging in the DAA. A stepwise exposure of posterior capsule, conjoined tendon, and piriformis has been described to facilitate femoral access [41]. Failure to obtain adequate femoral exposure may result in perforation during broaching, which typically occurs due to inadequate femoral exposure or patient body habitus, and most commonly results in a posterior or lateral perforation [41].

As the educator strives to foster the trainee's sense of autonomy, the trainee is preparing for independent practice. This includes self-assessment and subsequent dedication to addressing areas of perceived deficiency. Time should be spent learning how to prepare for cases, as templating prior to THA has been shown to improve the accuracy of component sizing and help the surgeon anticipate complications [42]. Additionally, preoperative preparation and appropriate patient selection can help avoid intraoperative difficulties during the transition period. Among practicing DAA surgeons, 65% cited complex anatomy and 53% cited body habitus as a reason to abandon DAA in favor of a posterior approach [13].

In preparation for practice, the trainee should recognize that they will likely experience a high rate of personnel variability in the operating room. This requires they learn not only their own role as a surgeon in performing the operation but also the role of everyone in the operating room. This includes the actions of the surgical assistant, surgical technician, the radiology technician, and the circulating nurse who may be operating the orthopedic table. In an ideal setting, the surgeon would teach the surgeon, the radiology technician would teach that surgeon's radiology technician, and so on. Therefore, it may be valuable for the trainees to shadow the members of the team beyond the surgeon to help teach their new teams how to safely and effectively perform these roles.

Challenges for the Transitioning Surgeon

Concern for the learning curve has been cited as one of the top barriers for practicing surgeons to transition to the DAA [13]. Despite marketing pressures to perform the DAA [31, 34], they may already obtain favorable outcomes with an alternative approach and may not have the opportunity to pursue formal training once they have started practice. Furthermore, without unequivocal data supporting the superiority of the DAA over alternative approaches, they may feel that the risk to their patients during their learning curve is not justifiable. As previously discussed, the reported learning curve can range between 10 [19] and even 400 cases [20] depending on the outcome measured, but the most commonly quoted numbers appear to be 50 or 100 cases [16–18].

Devoting adequate time to learning a new technique can be a challenge for the practicing surgeon, both logistically and financially. Educational time often means time spent away from the practice. While the surgeon may forego some personal income to learn a new skill set and marketability, overhead, staff wages, and other practice costs may pose a challenge. While it is well accepted that inadequate preparation results in poor outcomes, the amount of educational time required to mitigate early complications has not been clearly defined. Woolson et al. reported five community surgeons whose only training was surgeon observation, and none practiced in a cadaver lab prior to starting the DAA. The authors noted a sixfold increase in major complication rate and nearly twofold increase in operating time and blood loss [21]. In contrast, multiple other studies have shown that surgeons who engage in formal education and cadaver training did not experience increased complications during their initial cases utilizing the DAA [22, 34, 43].

There are several technical aspects of the DAA that may pose unique challenges to transitioning surgeons. First, the DAA uses the supine position, while most approaches are performed in the lateral decubitus position. This requires a cognitive conversion in spatial orientation. Second, the surgeon must learn unfamiliar anatomy and the steps of a new procedure, and also new instrumentation and workflow. Many DAA surgeons employ specific tools designed for the approach, such as offset broach handles or lighted retractors designed for minimally-invasive surgery, which may be unfamiliar to the practicing surgeon. Additionally, there are a number of tables offered for the DAA, including a standard operating table, Hana (Mizuho OSI, Union City, CA), Arch (Innovative Orthopedic Technologies LLC, Houston, TX), and Medacta (Medacta International, Frauenfeld, Switzerland). The surgeon must choose which of these tables is most beneficial for their practice and then learn to operate the table. Because the intraoperative range of motion testing is more challenging when using a specialized table, many surgeons evolve into limiting their intraoperative range testing. This can be a challenging mental hurdle to overcome and requires accurate use of templating and/or intraoperative fluoroscopic measurements to ensure restoration of length and offset. Preoperative templating has been advocated as beneficial to estimate implant sizes and identify potential difficulties preoperatively [42]. Many surgeons who have mastered THA through other approaches may rely less on preoperative templating in favor of intraoperative decision-making based on hip stability and must necessarily adjust their preoperative preparation and workflow.

Mitigating the Challenges of DAA Education

The Dunning–Kruger affect is a term of cognitive bias described as "the less you know, the less you are able to recognize how little you know and your limitations" [44]. In their original article, Dunning and Kruger further argue that the skills that engender competence in a particular domain are often the very same skills necessary to evaluate competence in that domain" [45]. This phenomenon may plague the trainee, whether they are a resident, fellow, or practicing surgeon. This is exemplified when a trainee, who is early in their learning curve and lacks the full breadth of knowledge of a master surgeon, gains a boost of confidence through deliberate practice of one specific task that represents only a fraction of the entire procedure. Confidence then becomes artificially inflated, leading to a discrepancy between perceived ability and objective ability. This is precisely the period where complications can occur, and trainees may only become aware of this discrepancy when they encounter failure. This paradox highlights the importance of self-reflection coupled with education. Trainees must make an effort to identify their own limitations, but also be cognizant that, at that point in their learning curves, they may not have the skills necessary to identify their own areas of weakness and require the feedback of someone who has mastered the DAA.

In a case series of 120 DAA THA performed by three surgeons, Homma and colleagues have proposed four countermeasures to limit complications for inexperienced DAA surgeons [30]. First, they established defined patient exclusion criteria, specifically history of any hip osteotomy, dysplasia with Crowe three or four deformity, short neck secondary to Perthes disease, and a severe hip flexion contracture. Second, the authors argued in favor of a standard operating table rather than a specialized orthopedic table due to a perceived fear of potential complications from the specialized table. Third, they advocate for the use of unlimited fluoroscopy. Finally, and perhaps most importantly, they advocated for having an experienced surgical assistant, defined as someone who had performed greater than 100 DAA cases. The authors demonstrated no intraoperative complications or reoperations for any reason. Unfortunately, they did not detail the preoperative educational process of the three surgeons in this study, which significantly limits the interpretation and generalizability of these countermeasures.

In perhaps what is the most insightful publication on the transition to the DAA available, Pirruccio and colleagues detail an algorithmic approach employed by the senior author, an experienced posterior hip surgeon [34]. In this article, the authors outline a stepwise approach to learning the DAA that mimics the whole-task curricula and simultaneously exemplifies the circumvention of the Dunning–Kruger effect. Their algorithm begins with a period of self-study to learn the fundamentals of DAA anatomy and literature review. The senior author then observed an experienced DAA surgeon and took extensive notes. The final phases included a cadaver course in which he first assisted and subsequently performed a case with personalized, immediate feedback. When transitioning to the operating room, the initial operations performed by the senior author were proctored with an experienced DAA surgeon in the room. They also engaged the entire surgical team, including the physician assistant, resident, fellow, and surgical technician in preoperative preparation and postoperative debrief to identify areas of weakness. Lastly, the study emphasized a visit to the DAA mentor after 30 cases for additional training. The authors analyzed their first 100 DAA operations compared to the senior author's last 100 posterior THA and found an understandable 7-min increase in operating time but significantly shorter hospital length of stay for the DAA. No difference was found in blood loss, and most importantly, no differences in surgical complication rates were identified. This study shows that while learning a new technique can require a substantial investment, a dedicated, algorithmic approach can allow a surgeon to safely transition to the DAA and mitigate early complications.

Summary

The decision to employ the DAA is first and foremost a personal one. It should not be influenced by practice or industry marketing but rather should be made because the surgeon believes it is beneficial to patient care. Once the decision is made to learn the DAA, it is crucial to dedicate time and resources to this education. Identifying a mentor and establishing a relationship is paramount. It is unreasonable to expect that a single observership or weekend course will provide sufficient fundamental knowledge and procedural skills to succeed. Rather, learning occurs on a spectrum with continued self-evaluation and longitudinal mentorship. In summation, THA is an extremely successful operation, and the DAA offers many proposed benefits to augment this success, and with proper devotion to education, it can be safely adopted.

References

1. Barrett WP, Turner SE, Leopold JP. Prospective randomized study of direct anterior vs postero-lateral approach for total hip arthroplasty. J Arthroplast. 2013;28:1634–8.
2. Cheng TE, Wallis JA, Taylor NF, Holden CT, Marks P, Smith CL, Armstrong MS, Singh PJ. A prospective randomized clinical trial in total hip arthroplasty-comparing early results between the direct anterior approach and the posterior approach. J Arthroplast. 2017;32:883–90.
3. Miller LE, Kamath AF, Boettner F, Bhattacharyya SK. In-hospital outcomes with anterior versus posterior approaches in total hip arthroplasty: meta-analysis of randomized controlled trials. J Pain Res. 2018;11:1327–34.
4. Mirza AJ, Lombardi AV Jr, Morris MJ, Berend KR. A mini-anterior approach to the hip for total joint replacement: optimising results: improving hip joint replacement outcomes. Bone Joint J. 2014;96-b:32–5.

5. O'Brien RM. The technic for insertion of femoral head prosthesis by the straight anterior or Hueter approach. Clin Orthop. 1955;6:22–6.
6. Rachbauer F, Kain MS, Leunig M. The history of the anterior approach to the hip. Orthop Clin North Am. 2009;40:311–20.
7. Judet J, Judet R. The use of an artificial femoral head for arthroplasty of the hip joint. J Bone Joint Surg Br. 1950;32-b:166–73.
8. Light TR, Keggi KJ. Anterior approach to hip arthroplasty. Clin Orthop Relat Res. 1980;152:255–60.
9. Berger RA. Total hip arthroplasty using the minimally invasive two-incision approach. Clin Orthop Relat Res. 2003;417:232–41.
10. Matta JM, Shahrdar C, Ferguson T. Single-incision anterior approach for total hip arthroplasty on an orthopaedic table. Clin Orthop Relat Res. 2005;441:115–24.
11. Siguier T, Siguier M, Brumpt B. Mini-incision anterior approach does not increase dislocation rate: a study of 1037 total hip replacements. Clin Orthop Relat Res. 2004;426:164–73.
12. Abdel MP, Berry DJ. Current practice trends in primary hip and knee arthroplasties among members of the American Association of Hip and Knee Surgeons: a long-term update. J Arthroplast. 2019;34:S24–s7.
13. Patel NN, Shah JA, Erens GA. Current trends in clinical practice for the direct anterior approach total hip arthroplasty. J Arthroplast. 2019;34:1987–93.e3.
14. Gladwell M. Outliers: the story of success. New York: Back Bay Books; 2011.
15. Barnett SL, Peters DJ, Hamilton WG, Ziran NM, Gorab RS, Matta JM. Is the anterior approach safe? Early complication rate associated with 5090 consecutive primary Total hip arthroplasty procedures performed using the anterior approach. J Arthroplast. 2016;31:2291–4.
16. de Steiger RN, Lorimer M, Solomon M. What is the learning curve for the anterior approach for total hip arthroplasty? Clin Orthop Relat Res. 2015;473:3860–6.
17. Hartford JM, Bellino MJ. The learning curve for the direct anterior approach for total hip arthroplasty: a single surgeon's first 500 cases. Hip Int. 2017;27:483–8.
18. Kong X, Grau L, Ong A, Yang C, Chai W. Adopting the direct anterior approach: experience and learning curve in a Chinese patient population. J Orthop Surg Res. 2019;14:218.
19. den Hartog YM, Mathijssen NM, Vehmeijer SB. The less invasive anterior approach for total hip arthroplasty: a comparison to other approaches and an evaluation of the learning curve – a systematic review. Hip Int. 2016;26:105–20.
20. Stone AH, Sibia US, Atkinson R, Turner TR, King PJ. Evaluation of the learning curve when transitioning from posterolateral to direct anterior hip arthroplasty: a consecutive series of 1000 cases. J Arthroplast. 2018;33:2530–4.
21. Woolson ST, Pouliot MA, Huddleston JI. Primary total hip arthroplasty using an anterior approach and a fracture table: short-term results from a community hospital. J Arthroplast. 2009;24:999–1005.
22. Spaans AJ, van den Hout JA, Bolder SB. High complication rate in the early experience of minimally invasive total hip arthroplasty by the direct anterior approach. Acta Orthop. 2012;83:342–6.
23. Salai M, Mintz Y, Giveon U, Chechik A, Horoszowski H. The "learning curve" of total hip arthroplasty. Arch Orthop Trauma Surg. 1997;116:420–2.
24. Cameron JL. William Stewart Halsted. Our surgical heritage. Ann Surg. 1997;225:445–58.
25. Logishetty K, Rudran B, Cobb JP. Virtual reality training improves trainee performance in total hip arthroplasty: a randomized controlled trial. Bone Joint J. 2019;101-b:1585–92.
26. Logishetty K, Western L, Morgan R, Iranpour F, Cobb JP, Auvinet E. Can an augmented reality headset improve accuracy of acetabular cup orientation in simulated THA? A randomized trial. Clin Orthop Relat Res. 2019;477:1190–9.
27. Goldberg H, Hanlon C. When I say... the knowledge paradox: the more I know, the less I can clearly explain. Med Educ. 2019;53:13–4.
28. Burson KA, Larrick RP, Klayman J. Skilled or unskilled, but still unaware of it: how perceptions of difficulty drive miscalibration in relative comparisons. J Pers Soc Psychol. 2006;90:60–77.
29. Dolmans DH, Wolfhagen IH, Van Merrienboer JJ. Twelve tips for implementing whole-task curricula: how to make it work. Med Teach. 2013;35:801–5.
30. Homma Y, Baba T, Kobayashi H, Desroches A, Ozaki Y, Ochi H, Matsumoto M, Yuasa T, Kaneko K. Safety in early experience with a direct anterior approach using fluoroscopic guidance with manual leg control for primary total hip arthroplasty: a consecutive one hundred and twenty case series. Int Orthop. 2016;40:2487–94.
31. Churchill L, Pollock M, Lebedeva Y, Pasic N, Bryant D, Howard J, Lanting B, Laliberte Rudman D. Optimizing outpatient total hip arthroplasty: perspectives of key stakeholders. Can J Surg. 2018;61:370–6.
32. Leunig M, Faas M, von Knoch F, Naal FD. Skin crease 'bikini' incision for anterior approach total hip arthroplasty: surgical technique and preliminary results. Clin Orthop Relat Res. 2013;471:2245–52.
33. Ghijselings SGM, Driesen R, Simon JP, Corten K. Distal extension of the anterior approach to the hip using the femoral Interbundle technique: surgical technique and case series. J Arthroplast. 2017;32:2186–90.
34. Pirruccio K, Evangelista PJ, Haw J, Goldberg T, Sheth NP. Safely implementing the direct anterior total hip arthroplasty: a methodological approach to minimizing the learning curve. J Am Acad Orthop Surg. 2020;28(22):930–6.
35. Vogel D, Harendza S. Basic practical skills teaching and learning in undergraduate medical education –

a review on methodological evidence. GMS J Med Educ. 2016;33:Doc64.
36. Moulton CA, Dubrowski A, Macrae H, Graham B, Grober E, Reznick R. Teaching surgical skills: what kind of practice makes perfect?: a randomized, controlled trial. Ann Surg. 2006;244:400–9.
37. Unwin AJ, Thomas M. Dislocation after hemiarthroplasty of the hip: a comparison of the dislocation rate after posterior and lateral approaches to the hip. Ann R Coll Surg Engl. 1994;76:327–9.
38. Hamilton WG, Parks NL, Huynh C. Comparison of cup alignment, jump distance, and complications in consecutive series of anterior approach and posterior approach total hip arthroplasty. J Arthroplast. 2015;30:1959–62.
39. Cadossi M, Sambri A, Tedesco G, Mazzotti A, Terrando S, Faldini C. Anterior approach in total hip replacement. Orthopedics. 2017;40:e553–e6.
40. James CR, Peterson BE, Crim JR, Cook JL, Crist BD. The use of fluoroscopy during direct anterior hip arthroplasty: powerful or misleading? J Arthroplast. 2018;33:1775–9.
41. Gonzales FB, Ongwijitwat S, Hamilton WG. In: Cashman J, Goyal N, editors. The hip: preservation, replacement, and revision. Brooklandville: Data Trace Publishing Company; 2015. pp 61:1–19.
42. Della Valle AG, Padgett DE, Salvati EA. Preoperative planning for primary total hip arthroplasty. J Am Acad Orthop Surg. 2005;13:455–62.
43. Free MD, Owen DH, Agius PA, Pascoe EM, Harvie P. Direct anterior approach Total hip arthroplasty: an adjunct to an enhanced recovery pathway: outcomes and learning curve effects in surgeons transitioning from other surgical approaches. J Arthroplast. 2018;33:3490–5.
44. Pafitanis G, Nikkhah D, Myers S. The Dunning-Kruger effect: revisiting "the valley of despair" in the evolution of competency and proficiency in reconstructive microsurgery. J Plast Reconstr Aesthet Surg. 2020;73:783–808.
45. Kruger J, Dunning D. Unskilled and unaware of it: how difficulties in recognizing one's own incompetence lead to inflated self-assessments. J Pers Soc Psychol. 1999;77:1121–34.

Why I Favor a Standard Incision and Keys to Exposure for the Anterior Approach

8

Robert P. Runner and Steven L. Barnett

Since it was first described by Charles Hueter [1], the anterior approach has slowly increased in popularity for the treatment of many hip pathologies with a resurgence in use for total hip arthroplasty over recent years [2]. It has the benefits of supine positioning, can be done under neuraxial anesthesia, and is a truly internervous approach to the hip. This evolution is likely multifactorial and includes possible improved early outcomes [3–6], reduced pain and length of stay, and relative ease of intraoperative fluoroscopy [7]. Recent reviews of anterior vs posterior approach show improved length of stay and dislocation rate, though there is no clear superiority for one approach over the other [5, 8]. Multiple conclusions recommend the choice of approach be tailored to surgeon experience, patient factors, and patient anatomy/deformity [3, 4, 7, 8].

When choosing the anterior approach, there are two common skin incisions: the standard (vertical, proximal to distal) and the bikini (proximal/lateral to distal/medial oblique) incisions. This chapter will focus on the benefits of the standard incision.

R. P. Runner
Department of Orthopedic Surgery, Rancho Los Amigos National Rehabilitation Center, Downey, CA, USA

S. L. Barnett (✉)
Hoag Orthopedic Institute, Irvine, CA, USA

Proximal and Distal Extension

One of the major benefits of standard incisions is the ability to extend the incision. This extension may be needed intraoperatively at the index procedure to address surgical complexities (intraoperative femur fracture, difficult femoral exposure, acetabular bone grafting or augmentation, etc.) or during revision procedures (acetabular cage reconstruction, both femoral and acetabular fracture plating and augmentation, extended femoral osteotomies, etc.) We continue to use the standard incision for the majority of patients and strongly recommend it for surgeons who are just starting out on their journey with the anterior approach.

When extending the anterior incision, there have been several articles that describe a safe technique for access to the femur without endangering the nerve supply to the quadriceps muscles [9]. The main distal skin extension takes the incision distal and posterior to become essentially a lateral approach to the femur. The deep dissection will split the IT band to allow access to the posterior border of the vastus lateralis to maintain its innervation anteriorly from the branches of the femoral nerve [9]. In a cadaveric study of 20 hips, two distinguishable neurovascular bundles were found supplying the vastus lateralis. The first bundle is located an average of 12.3 cm from the ASIS, 3.2 cm from the gluteus minimus insertion, and 1.6 cm from the lesser

J. M. Matta, A. P. Sah (eds.), *Anterior Hip Replacement*,
https://doi.org/10.1007/978-3-030-91896-5_8

trochanter [10]. The average distance from the first and second bundle was 3.3 cm (range 1.8–6.1 cm) [10]. These extensions allow for more distal access of the femoral metadiaphysis for placement of cerclage wires or cables if an intraoperative proximal femoral fracture occurs [11] or for use in femoral revision for periprosthetic fracture [12]. Please see the chapters in the Revision Surgery section for further details on extending the anterior approach.

Soft Tissue Management

A concern following hip arthroplasty is superficial wound dehiscence/infection, and the anterior approach is not immune to these complications. One early retrospective case-control study of 651 DAA hips found that 11.5% sustain wound complications requiring intervention, with 1.9% requiring reoperation [13]. Obesity and diabetes mellitus were significantly associated with these complications in DAA patients, and the "optimal" cutoff for BMI was around 28 kg/m^2 [13]. Comparison of DAA and mini-anterolateral approach found similar results with a higher rate of wound healing complications following DAA at 8% vs 4% ($P = 0.036$) [14]. One retrospective study comparing DAA to a mini-posterior approach even found more wound complications in the mini-posterior group [15]. However, the same group's prospective randomized study of anterior vs mini-posterior THA found only slight differences in early functional recovery in favor of the DAA with no difference in complications between DAA and mini-posterior patients [16].

Previous studies have found obesity as an independent risk factor for complications in all patients undergoing THA regardless of approach. A 2016 retrospective series of 1621 DAA THA patients reported that obesity (BMI > 35 kg/m^2) was associated with higher rates of deep infection (2.5% vs 0.35%, $P = 0.0044$), all-cause reoperation (3.43% vs 0.92%, $P = 0.008$), and all studied complications (4.41% vs 1.27%, $P = 0.0040$, relative risk 3.5) [17]. One of the critiques of the anterior approach is the differential quality of the skin and subcutaneous tissues overlying the proximal/anterior thigh as compared to the lateral/posterior thigh, which may be accentuated in obese patients. The combination of immune dysfunction and malnutrition in obesity with the proximity of the skin incision to the inguinal fold, genitalia, and abdominal pannus may put patients undergoing DAA THA at risk [17].

This difference in soft tissue and retraction during the case can lead to wound complication issues. A large retrospective series comparing obese (BMI > 35 kg/m^2) and nonobese patients for THA done via anterior or posterior approaches found that there was no statistical difference in deep infection rates between the two approaches; however, patients who underwent the anterior approach had higher rates of superficial wound complications across all BMIs [18]. A smaller series did not find a difference in wound complications leading to reoperation between approaches; however, it may be underpowered to detect such a difference [19].

One 2017 cadaveric study of 18 hips showed similar amounts of muscle damage to the tensor fasciae latae muscle belly and lateral femoral cutaneous nerve for standard incision vs bikini incision [20].

In an attempt to reduce wound complications, alternative approaches such as the bikini oblique/horizontal skin incision have been studied. A 2019 case-control retrospective study for 3:1 matched standard vs bikini DAA patients found that the bikini incision patients had lower rates of delayed wound healing at 2.3% vs 6.1% ($P = 0.087$) [21]. Subgroup analysis of obese patients with a BMI of >30 kg/m^2 found statistically significant lower rates of wound complications, 0% vs 16.6% ($P < 0.05$) [21]. Additionally, there was no difference in incision cosmesis scores at 6 months for Patient Scar Assessment Scale or Vancouver Scar Assessment Scale [21].

In our opinion, both the standard vertical and horizontal/oblique bikini skin incisions are applicable to DAA THA, and the bikini incision may offer reduced rates of delayed wound healing, especially in obese patients. However, we would recommend mastery of the DAA via the standard incision first as it allows extension to address possible complications before routine utilization of the bikini incision.

Orthopedic Table

Use of an orthopedic table as an operative adjunct is not required for DAA THA but can be helpful. Since Dr. Matta's initial description [22] of his case series using a single incision anterior approach for THA, many surgeons have adopted the use of an orthopedic table when performing DAA THA. Although use of the table will be described in more detail elsewhere in this book, we provide tips to help ensure success to follow.

When positioning the patient on the table, ensure the pelvis sits level prior to draping as gluteal soft tissue can rotate the pelvis relative to the table and lead to errors in imaging. If you are using extensions to the orthopedic table for self-retractor placement, ensure they are clear of sheets/blankets or other obstructions that would impede the attachment of retractor arms and posts. Ensure you have appropriate padding and protection of the perineal soft tissues to avoid damage [23, 24]. Slight Trendelenburg positioning can help reduce perineal pressure and aid in appropriate pelvic positioning to match the standing pre-op film for cup insertion [24].

Draping

As previously discussed, obesity is an independent risk factor for wound complications following DAA THA. When treating patients with a redundant pannus, the first step in the clinic is to examine the patient supine to establish that the pannus is mobile enough to move away from the incision during the case and ensure there are no fungal infections in the groin crease that should be treated prior to surgery. After the patient is positioned on the table, the pannus can be retracted superiorly and held with silk tape or other soft tissue retraction systems draped over the contralateral shoulder to the side bar. Excessive traction on the abdominal skin at this point may result in superficial skin tears.

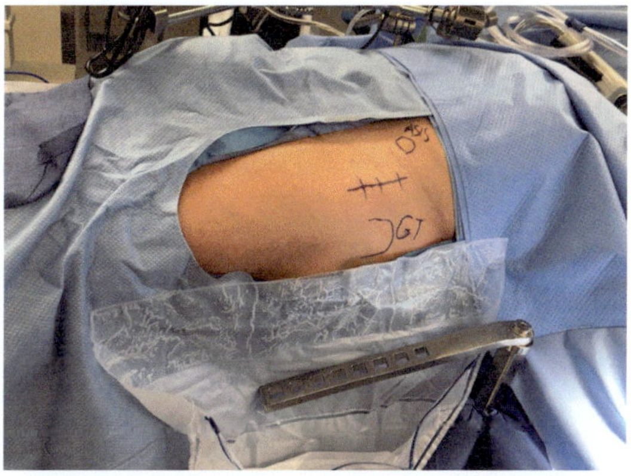

Fig. 8.1 Left hip draping demonstrating the location of anterior-superior iliac spine, incision, greater trochanter, and the femoral lift bar

Be cognizant of anatomic landmarks and future incision location during sterile draping. Necessary landmarks in the sterile surgical field include the anterior superior iliac spine (ASIS), iliac crest, greater trochanter, and proximal thigh. Keeping these four landmarks in the field allows for proper incision localization as well as the ability to extend the incision proximally or distally as needed (Fig. 8.1). The medial extent of draping should be just medial to the ASIS. Extending the surgical field more medial to this increases the risk of groin contamination in certain patients.

We utilize a second alcohol-based skin prep after draping immediately prior to application of an iodine impregnated adhesive drape over the incision site as a final precaution. Use of a "shower curtain" type drape has also been described in a similar technique to ORIF of femoral neck fractures. Though this varies based on surgeon preference, there is no clear superior draping technique.

Standing Low vs Standing High

Both the surgeon and first assist position themselves on the operative side of the patient. We utilize a self-retaining retractor system attached to the opposite side of the table, although a second assist can perform this function as well

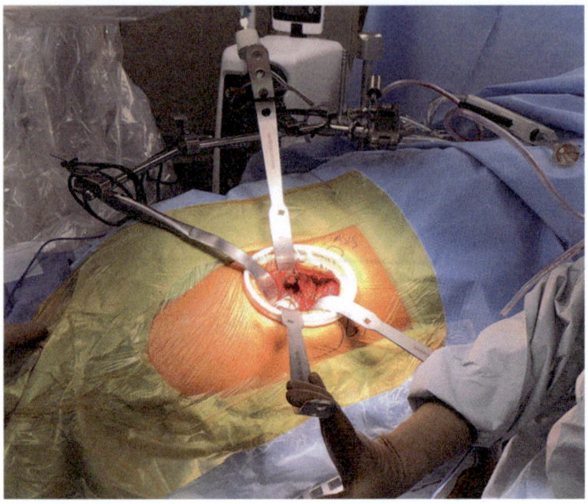

Fig. 8.2 Self-retaining retractor arm on the opposite side of operative table

(Fig. 8.2). It is personal preference whether the first assist stands toward the head (high) or toward the foot (low) during the procedure. Efforts are made to place the scrub tech on the opposite side of the table such that the surgeon and tech are face to face when passing instruments, which minimize the potential for contamination.

Fluoroscopic imaging can be placed on either side of the table and usually is positioned opposite of the scrub tech and instrument tables. Fluoroscopic aided acetabular reaming and component placement are facilitated if the C-arm is brought in from the opposite side of the table.

Superficial Dissection

Throughout the evolution of the anterior approach, many incisions have been described [1]. Although incision length, proximity to the ASIS, and obliquity vary by surgeon, the vertical nature of this incision lends it to be categorized as a "standard" approach.

The ASIS is the key landmark during soft tissue dissection, and localization throughout both superficial and deep dissection will prevent one from wandering into the wrong intermuscular interval as well as the femoral neurovascular bundle. The incision starts 1–2 fingerbreadths distal and lateral to the ASIS. Efforts are made to prevent crossing the groin crease at a right angle. In rare cases where proximal extension is necessary because of body habitus, the incision is curved posteriorly along the crease. The incision is approximately 10 cm and runs toward the lateral epicondyle of the femur. This should be in line with the muscles fibers of the tensor fasciae latae that runs deep originating postero-lateral to the ASIS. In general, the more lateral your skin incision, the lower the risk of irritation and neuropraxia to the branches of the lateral femoral cutaneous nerve (LFCN).

In a prospective randomized clinical trial comparing early results of anterior vs posterior THA, there was an 83% incidence of LFCN neuropraxia at the 12-week mark for DA with no neuropraxia in the posterior group [4]. In a separate review of long-term effects of LFCN neuropraxia, 1871 DAA THA patients found that the most commonly experienced symptom was "numbness" occurring in 37% of patients and only 11% of patients having some symptom at 6–8 years postoperatively [25]. In that large study of DAA patients, neuropathic symptoms continued to improve with time and were not correlated with hip functional outcome scores [25], which corroborated previous studies with similar findings [26, 27].

Full-thickness skin flaps are developed deep to the subcutaneous fat layer, and an elastic, circumferential soft-tissue protector is placed exposing the fascia overlying the tensor fascia muscle (Fig. 8.3). At closure, tacking down the subcutaneous tissue to the underlying fascia with

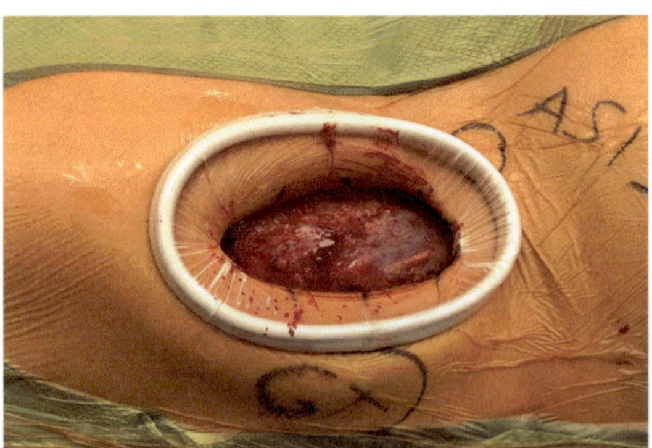

Fig. 8.3 Elastic incisional soft tissue protector

absorbable suture prevents postoperative seroma formation.

Deep Dissection

Once the fascia overlying the tensor muscle is exposed, sharp dissection is utilized to make a fascial incision lateral to the ASIS, extending distal and parallel to the skin incision. Staying lateral to the ASIS protects one from exposing the hip medial to the rectus femoris muscle in the vicinity of the femoral nerve and artery. These structures should not be routinely encountered in primary DAA THA.

Allis clamps are placed on the medial fascial edge, and blunt finger dissection is utilized to retract the tensor muscle laterally, exposing the intermuscular interval lateral to the rectus femoris. Expose this interval throughout the length of the incision.

Finger dissection is usually sufficient to develop the interval deep to the tensor muscle proximally over the femoral neck. A cobra or bent Hohmann retractor is then placed extracapsular deep to the tensor muscle and gluteus minimus. Efforts are made to keep this retractor immediately extraarticular in order to avoid damaging adjacent muscle fibers. The remaining posterior fascia is then split just lateral to the rectus muscle for circumflex vessel exposure.

Lateral Femoral Circumflex Artery

The ascending branches of the lateral circumflex vessels are identified with the use of a Weitlaner self-retainer or two Hibbs retractors in the intermuscular interval between the rectus femoris and tensor muscles. These vessels run proximo-lateral to disto-medial in the mid to distal third of the incision [29] (Fig. 8.4). If not immediately visualized, they can be found more distal in the incision and are rarely, if ever, not present. It is important to not confuse any transversely running perforating branches to the tensor with the ascending branch of the lateral femoral circumflex coming off the profunda femoris artery [28].

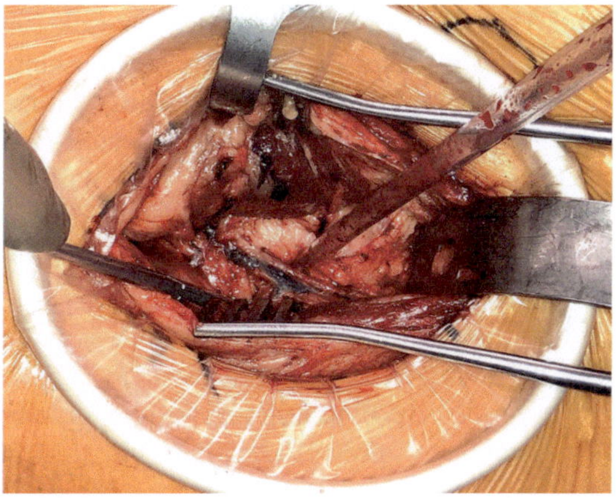

Fig. 8.4 Lateral circumflex vessels extending from infer-olateral to proximo-medial across the exposure field

Once visualized, the vessels are exposed and cauterized with the use of DeBakey forceps. Other options include use of silk ties as well as bipolar electro-cautery. Care is taken at this step to ensure coagulation of the transected vessel ends to prevent future bleeding later in the case, which can be more difficult to control.

Anterior Capsule Exposure

A Cobb elevator is utilized to sweep under the rectus femoris and iliocapsularis [30] muscle from distal to proximal along the inferior hip capsule up to the anterolateral acetabular rim. The iliocapsularis has some fibers that originate from the inferior border of the anterior-inferior iliac spine (AIIS), with an elongated attachment to the anteromedial hip capsule and inserts just distal to the lesser trochanter [30]. The indirect head of the rectus will be draped over the anterior capsule and inserted proximal/laterally. A second Cobra retractor is placed around the inferior femoral neck, and a bent Hohmann retractor is then placed over the anterior-lateral rim of the acetabulum just medial to the terminal insertion of the reflected head of the rectus muscle. It is important to direct this retractor perpendicular to the inguinal crease toward the contralateral shoulder to prevent placement infero-medial in the vicinity of the femoral nerve as it courses over the pelvic brim. The reflected head of the rectus muscle can be released to aid in exposure but is not usually necessary. It is also important to ensure that the anterior retractor is deep to all of the rectus muscle fibers. Intramuscular as well as medial placement of this retractor can lead to impingement of the femoral nerve against the pelvis leading to postoperative palsy (Fig. 8.5).

Femoral neuropathy following DAA is a rare (0.1–2.4%) but serious complication [31, 32]. In one large series of 1756 patients, the rate for femoral neuropathy after DAA THA was 0.34%, with all recovering motor function between 6 weeks and 1 year post-op [33]. Prior anatomic studies show that with more inferior/distal progression of retractor placement along the anterior wall, the distance to the femoral neurovascular bundle decreases [34] and recommend more superior placement at the 12-o-clock position to avoid damage [35]. One Japanese cadaveric study specifically identified the proximity of the femoral nerve in the supine position with respect to the acetabular rim during DAA THA [36]. They found the femoral nerve to be immediately adjacent within 16.6 to 33.2 mm of the acetabular rim at points from 0° to 150° of a line drawn from the ASIS, with the nerve being closest (16.6 mm) at the medial point of 90° [36]. Additionally, the femoral artery is nearby and not immune to damage and thrombosis [37].

Capsular Management

Visualization of the anterior hip capsule is now complete. In patients with larger tensor muscles, a Hibbs or Hohmann retractor can be positioned to retract the tensor muscle laterally for further exposure. An inverted T-shaped capsulotomy is performed by making a longitudinal incision from the anterior acetabular rim distal to the inter-trochanteric line. This is then extended in "T" fashion, both medial and lateral attempting to preserve as much capsular length as possible for later closure. The superior and inferior femoral neck retractors are then re-positioned intraarticularly in preparation for the femoral neck osteotomy (Fig. 8.6). Additional capsular incisions along the superior acetabular rim can also be undertaken to assist in exposure after femoral head removal. Tag stitches placed in the inferior edges of the capsular flaps can be useful in retraction during acetabular preparation as well as re-approximation at the end of the case.

Both capsulectomy and capsulotomy techniques have been described. A future randomized controlled double-blinded trial to assess differ-

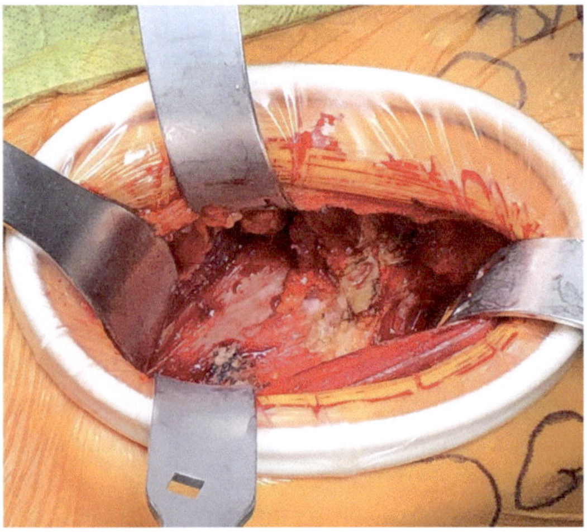

Fig. 8.5 Left hip anterior capsular exposure with Hohmann retractor deep to the reflected head of rectus m. over the anterolateral acetabular rim

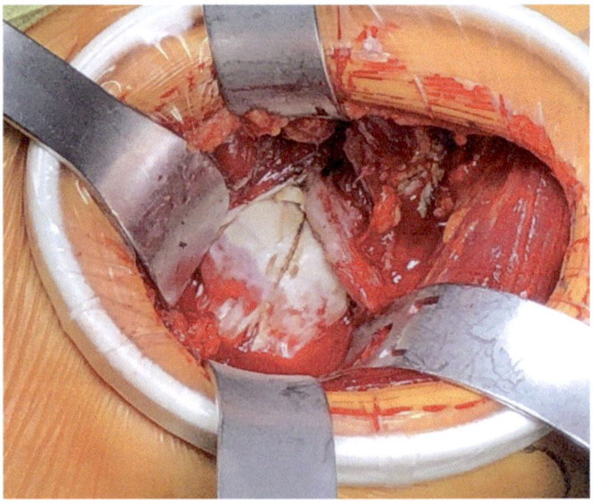

Fig. 8.6 Femoral neck exposure after inverted "T" capsulotomy with the intra-articular placement of superior and inferior neck retractors

ences between capsulectomy and capsulotomy is underway [38] to assess true differences between techniques. Both chapter authors agree that the proprioceptive fibers of the native capsule may contribute to improved results, and the retained capsule can help in soft tissue retraction during the case to protect the anterior rectus muscle fibers during dislocation/reduction and help confirm leg length and offset restoration during trialing.

Femoral Neck Osteotomy

In preparation for the femoral neck osteotomy, the leg is positioned in 20 degrees of external rotation, and gross traction is applied to partially subluxate the femoral head. The femoral neck cut is localized relative to the superior saddle where the femoral neck transitions into the greater trochanter. Current practice is to identify the shoulder or saddle of the trochanter and make the osteotomy approximately 45° inferomedial from that point. Unlike the posterior approach, the lesser trochanter is not easily visualized and therefore cannot routinely be used as a landmark. The osteotomy is then made in situ taking care to completely incise the medial calcar region in order to prevent inadvertent fracture around the lesser trochanter. This should be perpendicular to the angle of the neck in the AP plane; otherwise, the perceived neck version may be different from the shaft and can lead to issues during femoral broaching. Further traction is applied to the operative leg to create space at the osteotomy site, which allows for insertion of a corkscrew up the neck into the femoral head for retrieval (Fig. 8.7). Care is taken not to damage the tensor muscle fibers during femoral head removal utilizing a T-handle on the previously placed corkscrew. Surgeon preference is for an in situ cut rather than dislocation followed by osteotomy, though both are acceptable techniques. Fluoroscopy can be utilized prior to performing the osteotomy if landmark visualization is difficult. . Additionally, a small napkin ring of femoral neck can be removed if needed to assist in head extraction.

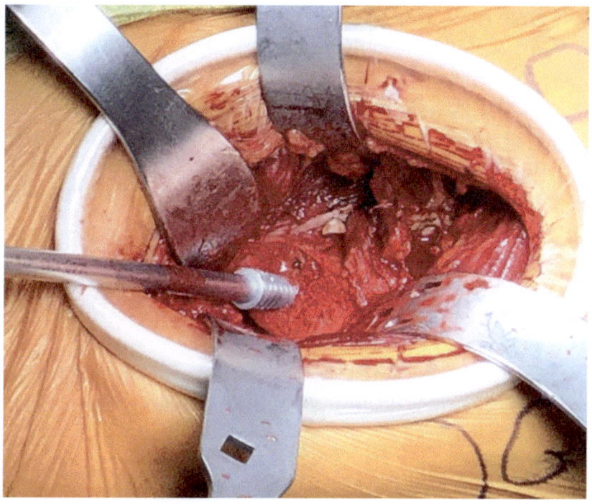

Fig. 8.7 Femoral head removal after osteotomy using corkscrew inserted up the cut surface of the femoral neck

Current Practice
Pearls

1. When starting out, use a standard incision and understand how to extend it as necessary in the case of intraop complications.
2. Patients with easier exposures for initial cases include: coxa valga, female, nonmuscular, no pannus, routine osteoarthritis.
3. Go sequentially with the exposure and ensure you can see what you need before moving on.
4. The femoral release is titrated to the patient, so only release as needed.
5. Sources of bleeding are commonly the lateral femoral circumflex, obturator branches, and the posterior capsule.
6. Be cognizant of the femoral nerve with retractors anteriorly and time in extension.
7. Be cognizant of the peroneal post with excessive traction.

Bibliography

1. Rachbauer F, Kain MS, Leunig M. The history of the anterior approach to the hip. Orthop Clin North Am. 2009;40(3):311–20.
2. Light TR, Keggi KJ. Anterior approach to hip arthroplasty. Clin Orthop Relat Res. 1980;152:255–60.
3. Miller LE, Gondusky JS, Bhattacharyya S, Kamath AF, Boettner F, Wright J. Does surgical approach affect outcomes in total hip arthroplasty through 90

days of follow-up? A systematic review with meta-analysis. J Arthroplast. 2018;33(4):1296–302.
4. Cheng TE, Wallis JA, Taylor NF, Holden CT, Marks P, Smith CL, et al. A prospective randomized clinical trial in total hip arthroplasty-comparing early results between the direct anterior approach and the posterior approach. J Arthroplast. 2017;32(3):883–90.
5. Barrett WP, Turner SE, Leopold JP. Prospective randomized study of direct anterior vs postero-lateral approach for total hip arthroplasty. J Arthroplast. 2013;28(9):1634–8.
6. Hozack WJ, Heller S. Direct anterior hip exposure for total hip arthroplasty. JBJS Essent Surg Tech. 2015;5(4):e22.
7. Kyriakopoulos G, Poultsides L, Christofilopoulos P. Total hip arthroplasty through an anterior approach: the pros and cons. EFORT Open Rev. 2018;3(11):574–83.
8. Higgins BT, Barlow DR, Heagerty NE, Lin TJ. Anterior vs. posterior approach for total hip arthroplasty, a systematic review and meta-analysis. J Arthroplast. 2015;30(3):419–34.
9. Nogler MM, Thaler MR. The direct anterior approach for hip revision: accessing the entire femoral diaphysis without endangering the nerve supply. J Arthroplast. 2017;32(2):510–4.
10. Ghijselings SG, Driesen R, Simon JP, Corten K. Distal extension of the direct anterior approach to the hip: a cadaveric feasibility study. J Arthroplast. 2017;32(1):300–3.
11. Ghijselings SGM, Driesen R, Simon JP, Corten K. Distal extension of the anterior approach to the hip using the femoral Interbundle technique: surgical technique and case series. J Arthroplast. 2017;32(7):2186–90.
12. Thaler M, Dammerer D, Krismer M, Ban M, Lechner R, Nogler M. Extension of the direct anterior approach for the treatment of Periprosthetic femoral fractures. J Arthroplast. 2019;34(10):2449–53.
13. Jahng KH, Bas MA, Rodriguez JA, Cooper HJ. Risk factors for wound complications after direct anterior approach hip arthroplasty. J Arthroplast. 2016;31(11):2583–7.
14. Herndon CL, Drummond N, Sarpong NO, Cooper HJ, Shah RP, Geller JA. Direct anterior versus mini-anterolateral approach for primary total hip arthroplasty: early postoperative outcomes and complications. Arthroplast Today. 2020;6(2):257–61.
15. Poehling-Monaghan KL, Kamath AF, Taunton MJ, Pagnano MW. Direct anterior versus miniposterior THA with the same advanced perioperative protocols: surprising early clinical results. Clin Orthop Relat Res. 2015;473(2):623–31.
16. Taunton MJ, Trousdale RT, Sierra RJ, Kaufman K, Pagnano MW. John Charnley award: randomized clinical trial of direct anterior and Miniposterior approach THA: which provides better functional recovery? Clin Orthop Relat Res. 2018;476(2):216–29.
17. Purcell RL, Parks NL, Gargiulo JM, Hamilton WG. Severely obese patients have a higher risk of infection after direct anterior approach total hip arthroplasty. J Arthroplast. 2016;31(9 Suppl):162–5.
18. Purcell RL, Parks NL, Cody JP, Hamilton WG. Comparison of wound complications and deep infections with direct anterior and posterior approaches in obese hip arthroplasty patients. J Arthroplast. 2018;33(1):220–3.
19. Tissot C, Vautrin M, Luyet A, Borens O. Are there more wound complications or infections with direct anterior approach total hip arthroplasty? Hip Int. 2018;28(6):591–8.
20. Lanting BA, Hartley KC, Raffoul AJ, Burkhart TA, Sommerville L, Martin GR, et al. Bikini versus traditional incision direct anterior approach: is there any difference in soft tissue damage? Hip Int. 2017;27(4):397–400.
21. Manrique J, Paskey T, Tarabichi M, Restrepo C, Foltz C, Hozack WJ. Total hip arthroplasty through the direct anterior approach using a bikini incision can be safely performed in obese patients. J Arthroplast. 2019;34(8):1723–30.
22. Matta JM, Shahrdar C, Ferguson T. Single-incision anterior approach for total hip arthroplasty on an orthopaedic table. Clin Orthop Relat Res. 2005;441:115–24.
23. Flierl MA, Stahel PF, Hak DJ, Morgan SJ, Smith WR. Traction table-related complications in orthopaedic surgery. J Am Acad Orthop Surg. 2010;18(11):668–75.
24. Lall AC, Saadat AA, Battaglia MR, Maldonado DR, Perets I, Domb BG. Perineal pressure during hip arthroscopy is reduced by use of Trendelenburg: a prospective study with randomized order of positioning. Clin Orthop Relat Res. 2019;477(8):1851–7.
25. Patton RS, Runner RP, Lyons RJ, Bradbury TL. Clinical outcomes of patients with lateral femoral cutaneous nerve injury after direct anterior total hip arthroplasty. J Arthroplast. 2018;33(9):2919–26 e1.
26. Goulding K, Beaule PE, Kim PR, Fazekas A. Incidence of lateral femoral cutaneous nerve neuropraxia after anterior approach hip arthroplasty. Clin Orthop Relat Res. 2010;468(9):2397–404.
27. Bhargava T, Goytia RN, Jones LC, Hungerford MW. Lateral femoral cutaneous nerve impairment after direct anterior approach for total hip arthroplasty. Orthopedics. 2010;33(7):472.
28. Zlotorowicz M, Czubak-Wrzosek M, Wrzosek P, Czubak J. The origin of the medial femoral circumflex artery, lateral femoral circumflex artery and obturator artery. Surg Radiol Anat. 2018;40(5):515–20.
29. Lakhiani C, Lee MR, Saint-Cyr M. Vascular anatomy of the anterolateral thigh flap: a systematic review. Plast Reconstr Surg. 2012;130(6):1254–68.
30. Ward WT, Fleisch ID, Ganz R. Anatomy of the iliocapsularis muscle. Relevance to surgery of the hip. Clin Orthop Relat Res. 2000;374:278–85.
31. Fox AJ, Bedi A, Wanivenhaus@ F, Sculco TP, Fox JS. Femoral neuropathy following total hip arthroplasty: review and management guidelines. Acta Orthop Belg. 2012;78(2):145–51.

32. Farrell CM, Springer BD, Haidukewych GJ, Morrey BF. Motor nerve palsy following primary total hip arthroplasty. J Bone Joint Surg Am. 2005;87(12):2619–25.
33. Patton RS, Runner RP, Lazarus D, Bradbury TL. Femoral neuropathy following direct anterior total hip arthroplasty: an anatomic review and case series(dagger). J Surg Case Rep. 2018;2018(9):rjy171.
34. Shubert D, Madoff S, Milillo R, Nandi S. Neurovascular structure proximity to acetabular retractors in total hip arthroplasty. J Arthroplast. 2015;30(1):145–8.
35. Sullivan CW, Banerjee S, Desai K, Smith M, Roberts JT. Safe zones for anterior acetabular retractor placement in direct anterior total hip arthroplasty: a cadaveric study. J Am Acad Orthop Surg. 2019;27(21):e969–e76.
36. Yoshino K, Nakamura J, Hagiwara S, Suzuki T, Kawasaki Y, Ohtori S. Anatomical implications regarding femoral nerve palsy during a direct anterior approach to total hip arthroplasty: a cadaveric study. J Bone Joint Surg Am. 2020;102(2):137–42.
37. Mortazavi SMJ, Kazemi M, Noaparast M. Femoral artery intimal injury following total hip arthroplasty through the direct anterior approach: a rare but potential complication. Arthroplast Today. 2019;5(3):288–91.
38. Ometti M, Brambilla L, Gatti R, Tettamanti A, La Cava T, Pironti P, et al. Capsulectomy vs capsulotomy in total hip arthroplasty. Clinical outcomes and proprioception evaluation: study protocol for a randomized, controlled, double blinded trial. J Orthop. 2019;16(6):526–33.

9 Anterior Approach to the Hip Through the Oblique "Bikini" Incision

Brandon H. Naylor, Jeremy Statton, and Charles A. DeCook

Introduction

Total hip arthroplasty (THA) has rapidly become one of the most successful orthopedic surgical procedures performed, considered by many the surgery of the century [1]. Multiple techniques to facilitate the procedure have emerged to facilitate the procedure, including the anterior THA (ATHA) as originally described by Hueter in 1881, introduced as a minimally invasive intermuscular and internervous interval approach [2]. The orthopedic community has witnessed a resurgence in the ATHA over recent decades following multiple reported advantages compared to other traditional approaches including improved dislocation risk, patient satisfaction, and functional recovery [3–6]. Multiple techniques have been described to facilitate the procedure, largely based on surgeon preference, where the choice of table, implants, instruments, and the use of fluoroscopy have continued to provide fodder for discourse. Numerous authors have also noted a higher incidence of wound-related complications when comparing the ATHA to alternative approaches, particularly in those with obesity and diabetes mellitus (DM) [7, 8]. Particularly along the proximal aspect of the incision, skin thickness and vascularity declines maceration and stretching can be seen, often resulting from difficult exposure and errant broaching or retractor placement. These findings have led to the latest technique divergence, regarding where to place the incision, with the introduction of the "bikini" approach to ATHA.

Proponents of the bikini approach note that the incision is made in line with the body's natural Langer lines, resulting in reduced scar formation without compromising exposure, and importantly, avoiding traversing the natural skin crease in a perpendicular fashion. Langer lines, also known as skin cleavage or tension lines, were described by Karl Langer in 1861 [9] (Fig. 9.1). Langer studied the mechanical properties of the skin and how tension lines differed depending on the regional orientation of the underlying collagen fibers. Specifically, he noted a consistent oblique direction of the line about the anterior surface of the thigh in the orientation of the hip crease and unchanged by hip position. Since then, numerous guidelines have been developed to determine the ideal placement of reduced tension incisions, including a focus on lines perpendicular to the action of the underlying muscle and relaxed skin tension lines [10, 11]. Borges [12], for example, described relaxed skin tension lines as a means of reducing scar formation. These lines are produced from furrows formed from the pinching and relaxing of skin surfaces.

B. H. Naylor · J. Statton · C. A. DeCook (✉)
Northside Hospital, Arthritis and Total Joint Specialists, Cumming, GA, USA
e-mail: brandon.naylor@northside.com

J. M. Matta, A. P. Sah (eds.), *Anterior Hip Replacement*,
https://doi.org/10.1007/978-3-030-91896-5_9

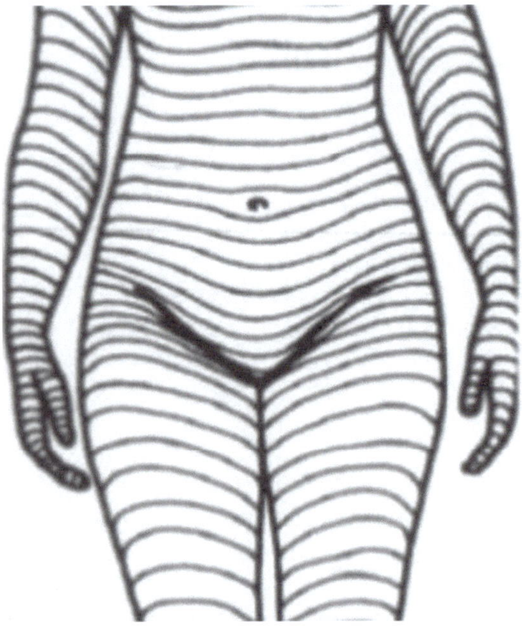

Fig. 9.1 Natural skin tension lines

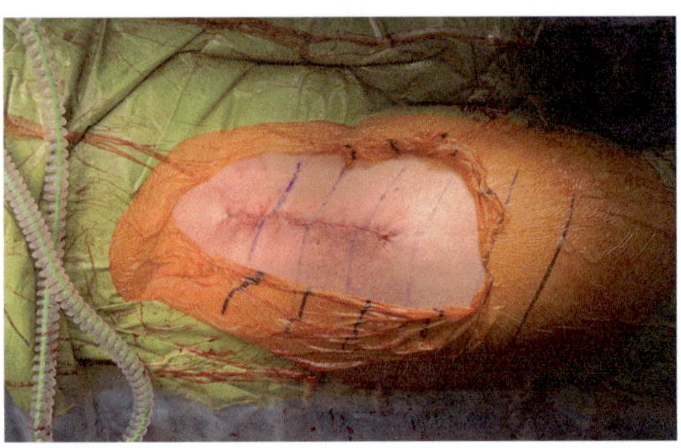

Fig. 9.2 Tradition longitudinal anterior hip incision following closure

Arthroplasty surgeons have continued to seek the optimal incision for the ATHA. Traditionally the incision for anterior hip arthroplasty begins approximately 2 cm distal and 2 cm lateral to the anterior superior iliac spine (ASIS). The incision is typically extended approximately 8 cm along the trajectory of the tensor fascial lata (TFL) muscle belly toward the lateral femoral condyle (Fig. 9.2). Unfortunately, the classic longitudinal incision does not follow the natural skin tension lines, which often leads to scar widening and poor cosmesis. To improve cosmesis, the use of the short oblique skin incision is increasing, an approach that follows the anatomic skin creases previously described in hip preservation and vascular surgery [13, 14].

The approach follows a short oblique incision in line with the skin crease of the groin. With deeper dissection, the superficial window can be mobilized superior or inferior as needed for implant preparation with no change in the deep dissection between "bikini" and traditional approaches. The increased mobility of the superficial window results from the trajectory of the underlying collagen fibers, which illustrates the anisotropy of skin, where tissue tension depends on the trajectory of the external pulling force. In fact, it is our experience that femoral exposure and instrumentation have improved while becoming more in line with the femur. Here, we describe our technique for ATHA as it relates to the "bikini" incision, followed by a discussion of the reported outcomes and applicability. Further technical descriptions of the ATHA procedure are found elsewhere throughout this text and beyond the scope of this chapter.

Technique

Positioning and Draping

Following appropriate anesthesia, the patient's feet are secured in adequately sized boots prior to transferring the patient to the HANA table (Mizuho, Union City, CA). The ipsilateral hip is preliminarily flexed to identify the natural flexion crease and marked using a nonsterile marker. Nonsterile U drapes are then used to demarcate the operative area, from the level of the umbilicus superiorly to the distal thigh inferiorly, and from the exposed buttock posteriorly to the medial groin centrally. After skin prep, drapes are placed superior and inferior to the surgical field followed by adhesive drapes placed along the superior, inferior, medial, and lateral aspects of the surgical field. Multiple hash marks across the hip flexion crease are created using a sterile marking pen. An iodine impregnated adhesive "shower curtain" drape is placed, ensuring adequate seal of the perineal region. A hook bracket is then

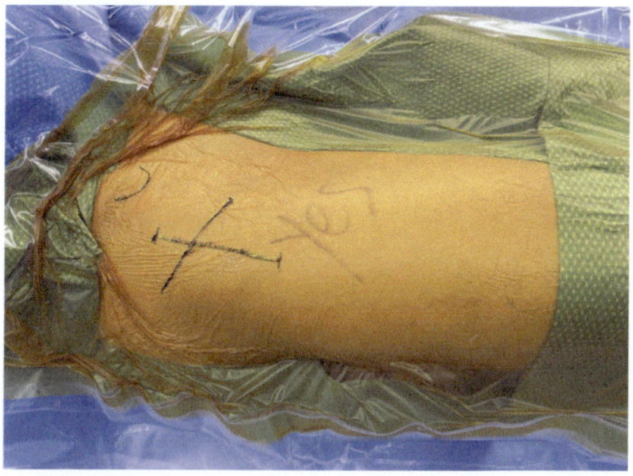

Fig. 9.3 "Bikini" incision marked compared to traditional incision

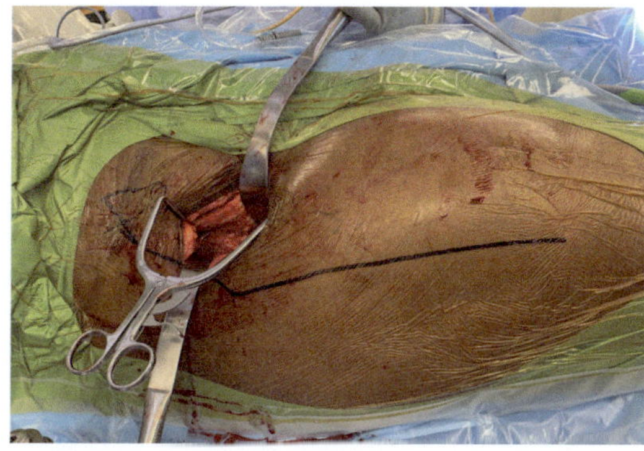

Fig. 9.4 Anterior total hip arthroplasty capsular exposure following the "bikini" incision

secured in place, and a towel and clip are used to drape the junction.

Incision and Approach

The anterior superior iliac spine (ASIS) is identified and marked. The incision is then marked in line with the previous flexion crease mark, approximately 6–8 cm, with two-thirds of the incision lateral to the ASIS and one-third medial (Fig. 9.3). The skin is incised to the level of the subcutaneous fat at which point traditional longdituinal dissection can proceed in line with the fibers of the TFL muscle belly. The TFL fascia is incised, typically between the anterior two-thirds and posterior one-third of the TFL muscle, thus exposing the underlying muscle belly. The obliquity and location of this fascial incision are thought to reduce the occurrence of LFCN injury. An Allis clamp is then placed along the medial limb to assist with blunt digital development of the interval between the TFL muscle and medial investing fascia. Angled retractors are then used to retract the TFL lateral and the rectus medial. A cobra retractor is then placed along the superior neck over the capsule to retract gluteal structures where the lateral circumflex vessels are identified and cauterized or ligated. In some cases, the "bikini" approach may allow complete avoidance of the lateral circumflex vessels. An additional cobra retractor is then placed between the capsule and iliopsoas tendon along the medial neck (Fig. 9.4). Gluteus medius, minimus, and TFL are retracted laterally while the iliocapsularis and rectus femoris are retracted medially to fully expose the hip capsule. A cobb elevator is used to gently elevate the iliocapsularis from the capsule for further exposure and interval identification, followed by a T-type capsulotomy beginning at the anterior superior acetabular rim, traversing obliquely along the neck to the inferior aspect of the intertrochanteric line. The superior capsular limb is carried along the shoulder of the superior neck, or saddle, staying medial to the greater trochanter. The inferior limb is carried around the calcar to the level of the lesser trochanter, effectively releasing the pubofemoral ligament complex. The two capsule limbs are tagged using a heavy vicryl suture, used for manipulation during both implant preparations and capsulotomy closure. The respective cobra retractors are then placed intracapsular, exposing the femoral neck from the "saddle" to the calcar. An oscillating saw is used to cut the neck at a predetermined level based on templated leg length and offset. The saw is angled in a slightly medial direction so as to avoid contact with the greater trochanter. Gross traction is applied, and a corkscrew is inserted through the base of the head, which is then used to rotate and lever the head and bring it forth from the wound.

Implant Preparation and Evaluation

A blunt tip angle retractor is placed anteriorly between the labrum and capsule, ensuring protection from the adjacent neurovascular structures. A sharp cobra is placed along the posterior rim of the acetabulum. With these retractors in place, the "bikini" window will naturally mobilize inferiorly, revealing adequate exposure and direct access for cup preparation. The labrum and pulvinar are sharply excised, and appropriately sized sequential reamers are applied to the bone using fluoroscopic evaluation to achieve adequate circumferential bleeding subchondral bone achieving the planned cup position. The final cup and liner are then placed.

A blunt bone hook is then placed around the femur just distal to the vastus ridge with the leg in neutral rotation. The femur is then externally rotated to 90 degrees without traction. Ensure full release of the pubofemoral ligament to the level of the lesser trochanter. Superior release is then performed to allow further femoral external rotation. This is achieved with the safe and strategic placement of a medial calcar retractor or Muller, followed by the gentle placement of a trochanteric retractor directly lateral to the greater trochanter while staying medial to the abductor musculature. At this point, the remaining superolateral capsule should be visualized and is releases from the superior neck, typically at the 1 o'clock position for a right hip, to the piriformis fossa and short of the piriformis tendon. Adequate femoral exposure typically requires a 270-degree capsular release, preserving structures posterior to the femoral neck, including the obturator externus, which holds important anti-dislocation properties. At this point, the bone hooked can be used to pull the femur anterolateral for further mobility, ensuring the greater trochanter does not lever on the posterior rim of the acetabulum, which may result in fracture. Further external to 115–125 degrees is then achieved, often "flipping" the piriformis posterior to the greater trochanter, where the leg is then brought to the floor, both extending and adducting the hip. Again, with the retractors in place, the bikini incision should naturally mobilize superior to afford excellent access to the canal (Figs. 9.5 and 9.6).

A box osteotome is then used to remove proximal bone in the posterolateral neck region followed by a canal finder or rat-tail. Sequential broaching is performed, ensuring the broach is parallel to the posterior cortex of the femoral neck following the patient's natural anatomic version. Once the appropriate broach is identified based on preoperative templating, a trial reduc-

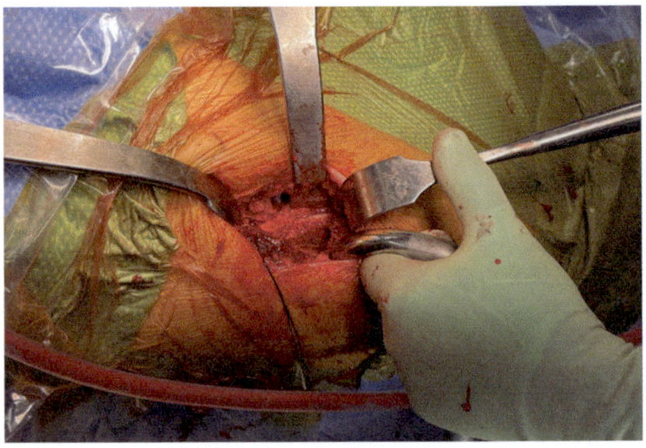

Fig. 9.5 Femoral exposure using the "bikini" incision

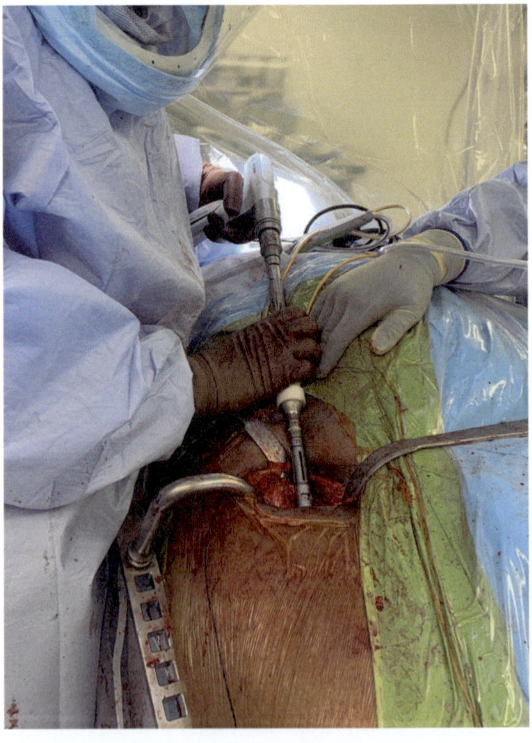

Fig. 9.6 Femoral instrumentation following the "bikini" incision, demonstrating adequate exposure to perform in-line reaming, if needed

tion is performed. Stability is critically assessed as is appropriate position, leg length, and offset using fluoroscopy. Final implants are then placed.

Closure and Wound Care

Thorough irrigation is achieved along with a periarticular injection, careful to avoid surrounding neurovascular structures, including the LFCN. A running barbed suture is used to close the TFL fascial, followed by the subdermal tissue. A running monofilament barbed suture is used for subcuticular skin closure, followed by the application of a topical skin adhesive and sterile silver-impregnated island dressing. The dressing is maintained for 5 days prior to removal, with the wound then left open to air if dry.

Outcomes

Cosmesis, wound healing, exposure compromise, and functional outcomes are essential metrics to assess the efficacy of the "bikini" approach. As such, multiple studies have compared the results of the new incision to the traditional longitudinal incision for ATHA [14–19]. Leunig et al. [14] sought to retrospectively compare the scar formation, functional and pain scores, and the efficacy with regard to complications, blood loss, implant position, and lateral femoral cutaneous nerve (LFCN) symptoms at 6 months post-procedure. The authors found significantly shorter and narrower scar formation along with a greater patient cosmetic satisfaction. Importantly, no difference in function and pain scores, complications, and LFCN injury were identified. Recently, Wang et al. [17] performed a prospective randomized control trial among 100 patients undergoing the ATHA with either the traditional or "bikini" incision. Outcomes included a scar cosmesis assessment at 6 months, visual analog score for pain, Oxford hip score, UCLA activity-level rating, serum markers for muscle damage, LFCN damage, component positioning, and wound healing. The authors identified a significantly improved scar cosmesis assessment and rating scores among those with the "bikini" incision when compared to the traditional longitudinal approach at 6 months, with no statistical difference in functional outcomes or complications at any time point. A trend was also noted toward a lower incidence of delayed wound healing among the bikini group (1 case vs 6 cases). It is important to note patients with a BMI of over 30 kg/m^2 were excluded from the study. Menzies-Wilson et al. [16] retrospectively compared the two incisions by a single surgeon with respect to functional outcomes and complications at a minimum 6 months postoperatively. The authors found a significantly larger improvement from baseline EQ-5D among those with the "bikini" incision. However, slightly less improvement in Oxford hip scores was identified among those with the "bikini" incision but failed to reach a clinically significant difference. Importantly, among the 214 patients included (90 bikini, 124 traditional), only one patient in each group developed a superficial wound infection. Leunig et al. [18] recently assessed a large cohort for functional and cosmesis outcomes and complications at a minimum 2 years following ATHA through the "bikini" versus the traditional approach. Those undergoing the bikini approach demonstrated higher cosmetic satisfaction with decreased scar numbness. No difference was noted between Oxford hip scores, component positioning, LFCN dysesthesias, or heterotopic ossification formation.

Those using the traditional incision may consider the smaller orthogonal bikini incision a nidus for further soft tissue damage in already limited exposure. To investigate this concern, Lanting et al. [15] performed a bilateral comparative cadaveric analysis between the exposures, with the bikini approach performed on one side, and the traditional approach on the other. Blinded anatomists assessed muscle and LFCN damage between the two sides. The authors noted no increase in muscle or LFCN damage between the two approaches.

The "bikini" incision has been purported as advantageous for young female patients with encouraging results; however, concern remains regarding the safety of the approach in those with obesity, where the incision can be partially or completed covered by an abdominal pannus [7, 8, 20].

Manrique et al. [19] performed a case-control retrospective study comparing the "bikini" ($n = 86$) and traditional incision ($n = 230$). Wound complications, acute periprosthetic joint infection, length of surgery, and dysesthesia were assessed with subgroup analysis in those with BMI greater than 30 kg/m^2(16 bikini and 48 conventional). Obese patients had a statistically significant lower rate of delayed wound healing when the "bikini" approach was utilized (0% vs 16.6%, $P < 0.05$). Among the obese population, the "bikini" approach also demonstrated reduced LFCN dysesthesia (0% vs 6.3%), shorter operative time, and reduced length of stay. This is in contrast to the entire cohort, where no statistical difference was identified in regard to delayed wound healing, dysesthesia, operative time, or intraoperative complications. Importantly, all wounds demonstrated healing by 3 months, and the majority of dysesthesia cases resolved, with the remaining patients reporting only mild peri-incisional numbness.

LFCN compromise manifesting as numbness is common following ATHA using the traditional longitudinal incision, with an incidence ranging from 15% to 88% [21–24]. Concerns regarding an increased risk when using the bikini incision draw on the medial extent of the skin incision and the conceivable increased retraction force required in the address potential limited exposure. The natural history of LFCN dysesthesia has been well documented, with most cases improving over time without functional limitations [21]. Patton et al. [22] noted a 16% rate of continued neuropathic symptoms at a mean of 3.9 years, with "numbness" the most commonly reported finding. However, before adopting the anterior approach, or the bikini incision for that matter, a comprehensive understanding of the anatomic course of the LFCN is paramount. Multiple studies have sought to evaluate the relevant anatomy regarding the LFCN as it relates to the anterior approach, each noting the highly variable branching patterns [25–27]. Sugano et al. [25] classified their findings as the anterior type (37%), which largely coursed along the medial aspect of the TFL, and the posterior type (63%), with branches equal to or thicker than the anterior division. Importantly, they noted that 42% of specimens had LFCN crossing the skin incision placed along the midline of the TFL muscle belly. The branching patterns were further classified by Rudin et al. [27] into three types. The sartorius-type was identified in 36% of specimens, with the dominant anterior nerve coursing along the lateral border of the sartorius, the posterior-type in 32%, and a fan-type in 32%, characterized by the nerve spreading in equal distributions. Interestingly, the authors also described an 11% occurrence of the nerve entering the thigh lateral to the ASIS. Importantly, the nerve was found to consistently traverse the deep layer of the subcutaneous fat tissue. Finally, Thaler et al. [26] evaluated several incisions for the anterior approach with regard to the LFCN, including the bikini incision. In their specimens, they identified a 70.5% prevalence of the sartorius type, 13.6% posterior-type, and 15.9% fan-type. Notably, the authors found the bikini incision to cross the main branch of the LFCN in 100% of cases. This finding illustrates the importance of transitioning the "bikini" approach to the longitudinal technique once subcutaneous fat is encountered so as to avoid the transection of the deep underlying LFCN branch or branches. Interestingly, when using the bikini incision, Leunig et al. [18] found a higher incidence of numbness within the scar in the longitudinal incision (14.5% vs 7.5%). Conversely, Wang et al. [17] noted a slight trend toward a higher incidence of LFCN dysesthesia with the "bikini" incision in their prospective RCT; however, this was not statistically significant. Ultimately, most reports comparing the two approaches identified no difference in the incidence of LFCN dysesthesia [14–16].

Considerations

Based on the available literature, we feel this approach is safe and effective for patients ranging from thin, young females to those with obesity and an overhanging pannus, with numerous advantages compared to the alternative longitudinal incision. We would, however, stress the

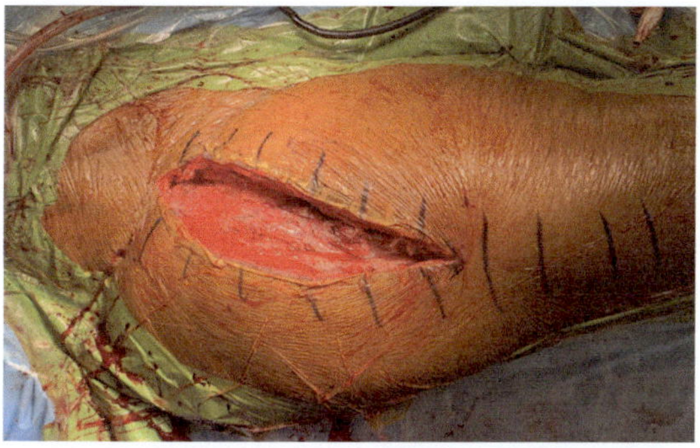

Fig. 9.7 Traditional distal longitudinal extension, which lies slightly medial to that of the extensile approach using the "bikini" incision

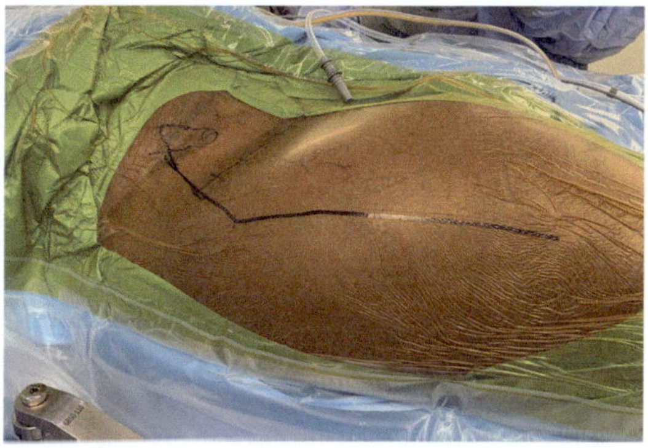

Fig. 9.8 Proposed "bikini" incision extensile approach marked

importance of appropriate skill development and relative comfort performing the ATHA, with mastery of the technique prior to adopting the "bikini" incision.

Additionally, while the extensile nature of the longitudinal incision is well described, scant literature exists regarding the extensile options with the bikini incision should further exposure or revision be required [28, 29] (Fig. 9.7). Our extensile approach to the bikini incision is predicated on previous literature describing the blood supply to the thigh as it relates to fasciocutaneous flap elevation [30, 31]. With more robust blood flow and soft tissue along the lateral aspect of the bikini incision, we typically extend the incision both proximal and distal 60–90 degrees perpendicular to the previous incision beginning at the lateral edge (Fig. 9.8). Furthermore, if only femoral revision is required, a separate standard lateral incision can be utilized. However, further research will be needed to best determine the appropriate extensile approach with the "bikini" incision.

Summary

The "bikini" incision is a safe and effective modification to the highly successful ATHA. While patients report improved cosmesis, surgeons utilizing the approach can realize reduced wound complications with often improved exposure. Importantly, no difference in functional recovery or LFCN dysesthesia is seen between approaches. Surgeons within the learning curve should become proficient with the ATHA using the traditional longitudinal incision prior to adopting the "bikini" approach. Further research is needed to identify the ideal extensile nature of the "bikini" incision.

References

1. Learmonth ID, Young C, Rorabeck C. The operation of the century: total hip replacement. Lancet. 2007;370(9597):1508–19.
2. Rachbauer F, Kain MSH, Leunig M. The history of the anterior approach to the hip. Orthop Clin North Am. 2009;40(3):311–20.
3. Berend KR, Lombardi AV, Seng BE, Adams JB. Enhanced early outcomes with the anterior supine intermuscular approach in primary total hip arthroplasty. J Bone Jt Surg. 2009;91 Suppl 6:107–20.
4. Ponzio DY, Poultsides LA, Salvatore A, Yu LY, Memtsoudis SG, Alexiades MM. In-hospital morbidity and postoperative revisions after direct anterior vs posterior total hip arthroplasty. J Arthroplast. 2018;33(5):1421–5.
5. Zhao HY, De KP, Xia YY, Shi XJ, Nie Y, Pei FX. Comparison of early functional recovery after total hip arthroplasty using a direct anterior or posterolateral approach: a randomized controlled trial. J Arthroplast. 2017;32(11):3421–8.
6. Kaufman K, Taunton M. Direct anterior approach for total hip arthroplasty results in quicker functional recovery compared to the mini-posterior approach. J Orthop Res. 2017:35.
7. Christensen CP, Karthikeyan T, Jacobs CA. Greater prevalence of wound complications requiring reop-

eration with direct anterior approach total hip arthroplasty. J Arthroplast. 2014;29(9):1839–41.
8. Jahng KH, Bas MA, Rodriguez JA, Cooper HJ. Risk factors for wound complications after direct anterior approach hip arthroplasty. J Arthroplast. 2016;31(11):2583–7.
9. Abyaneh MAY, Griffith R, Falto-Aizpurua L, Nouri K. Famous lines in history: Langer lines. JAMA Dermatol. 2014;150(10):1087.
10. Wilhelmi BJ, Blackwell SJ, Phillips LG. Langer's lines: to use or not to use. Plast Reconstr Surg. 1999;104(1):208–14.
11. Maranda EL, Heifetz R, Cortizo J, Hafeez F, Nouri K. Kraissl lines – a map. JAMA Dermatol. 2016;152(9):1014.
12. Borges AF. Relaxed skin tension lines. Dermatol Clin. 1989;7(1):169–77.
13. Swinnen J, Chao A, Tiwari A, Crozier J, Vicaretti M, Fletcher J. Vertical or transverse incisions for access to the femoral artery: a randomized control study. Ann Vasc Surg. 2010;24(3):336–41.
14. Leunig M, Faas M, Von Knoch F, Naal FD. Skin crease "bikini" incision for anterior approach total hip arthroplasty: surgical technique and preliminary results hip. Clin Orthop Relat Res. 2013;471(7):2245–52.
15. Lanting BA, Hartley KC, Raffoul AJ, Burkhart TA, Sommerville L, Martin GR, Howard JL, Johnson M. Bikini versus traditional incision direct anterior approach: is there any difference in soft tissue damage? Hip Int. 2017;27(4):397–400.
16. Menzies-Wilson R, Marino IT, Mahalingham K, Field R. Functional outcomes of direct anterior approach hip arthroplasty: oblique 'bikini' versus longitudinal skin incision. J Orthop Trauma Rehabil. 2020;27(1):52–6.
17. Wang Q, Yue Y, Yang Z, Chen L, Li Q, Kang P. Comparison of postoperative outcomes between traditional longitudinal incision and bikini incision in total hip arthroplasty via direct anterior approach: a randomized controlled trial. J Arthroplast. 2020;36(1):222–30.
18. Leunig M, Hutmacher JE, Rüdiger HA, Naal FD, Ricciardi BF, Impellizzeri FM. Skin crease "bikini" incision for the direct anterior approach in total hip arthroplasty. Bone Jt J. 2018;100-B(7):853–61.
19. Manrique J, Paskey T, Tarabichi M, Restrepo C, Foltz C, Hozack WJ. Total hip arthroplasty through the direct anterior approach using a bikini incision can be safely performed in obese patients. J Arthroplast. 2019;34(8):1723–30.
20. Faldini C, Mazzotti A, Perna F, Stefanini N, Panciera A, Pilla F, Ruffilli A, Neonakis EM, Traina F. Modified minimally invasive direct anterior approach through a bikini incision for total hip arthroplasty: technique and results in young female patients. J Biol Regul Homeost Agents. 2017;31(4 suppl 1):83–9.
21. Gala L, Kim PR, Beaulé PE. Natural history of lateral femoral cutaneous nerve neuropraxia after anterior approach total hip arthroplasty. Hip Int. 2019;29(2):161–5.
22. Patton RS, Runner RP, Lyons RJ, Bradbury TL. Clinical outcomes of patients with lateral femoral cutaneous nerve injury after direct anterior total hip arthroplasty. J Arthroplast. 2018;33(9):2919–26.
23. Goulding K, Beaulé PE, Kim PR, Fazekas A. Incidence of lateral femoral cutaneous nerve neuropraxia after anterior approach hip arthroplasty. Clin Orthop Relat Res. 2010;468(9):2397–404.
24. Ropars M, Morandi X, Huten D, Thomazeau H, Berton E, Darnault P. Anatomical study of the lateral femoral cutaneous nerve with special reference to minimally invasive anterior approach for total hip replacement. Surg Radiol Anat. 2009;31(3):199–204.
25. Sugano M, Nakamura J, Hagiwara S, Suzuki T, Nakajima T, Orita S, Akazawa T, Eguchi Y, Kawasaki Y, Ohtori S. Anatomical course of the lateral femoral cutaneous nerve with special reference to the direct anterior approach to total hip arthroplasty. Mod Rheumatol. 2020;30(4):752–7.
26. Thaler M, Dammerer D, Hechenberger F, Hörmann R, Van Beeck A, Stofferin H. The anatomical course of the lateral femoral cutaneous nerve in relation to various skin incisions used for primary and revision total hip arthroplasty with the direct anterior approach. J Arthroplast. 2020;36(1):368–73.
27. Rudin D, Manestar M, Ullrich O, Erhardt J, Grob K. The anatomical course of the lateral femoral cutaneous nerve with special attention to the anterior approach to the hip joint. J Bone Jt Surg Am. 2016;98(7):561–7.
28. Manrique J, Chen AF, Heller S, Hozack WJ. Direct anterior approach for revision total hip arthroplasty. Ann Transl Med. 2014;2(10):100.
29. Molenaers B, Driesen R, Molenaers G, Corten K. The direct anterior approach for complex primary total hip arthroplasty: the extensile acetabular approach on a regular operating room table. J Arthroplast. 2017;32(5):1553–9.
30. Cormack GC, Lamberty BGH. The blood supply of thigh skin. Plast Reconstr Surg. 1985;75(3):342–54.
31. Kimata Y, Uchiyama K, Ebihara S, Nakatsuka T, Harii K. Anatomic variations and technical problems of the anterolateral thigh flap: a report of 74 cases. Plast Reconstr Surg. 1998;102(5):1517–23.

10 My Keys to Getting the Acetabulum Right with the Anterior Approach: Exposure, Preparation, Sizing, Position, Stability

Nicholas H. Mast

The innominate bone and its confluence of sweeping arches and buttresses make for interesting orthopedic work. The various corridors between the tables of cortical bone, the proximity to major neurovascular structures, and the variability of surgical landmarks throughout the range of pathology we encounter as surgeons must all be respected. But for the student of the anatomy of the hip, I don't know of a more satisfying problem to solve than the problem of the acetabulum.

Casual introduction to surgical osteology cannot overlook the contributions of Judet and Letournel to our modern understanding of the innominate bone. The acetabulum is thought to be contained within the "open arms of an inverted Y" (Fig. 10.1). It is from this understanding of the osseous support to the native acetabulum that we learn how to gain stability of the prosthetic acetabular cup. Achieving a stable acetabular construct is no different in the anterior approach to the hip than any other approach. Advantages related to patient positioning, exposure, and the ability to use fluoroscopy make the anterior approach preferable for addressing acetabular problems as they relate to arthroplasty of the hip.

N. H. Mast (✉)
The Hip and Pelvis Institute, San Francisco, CA, USA
e-mail: doctormast@sfhips.com

Exposure

The exposure of the acetabulum is one of the advantages of the anterior approach. The Smith-Petersen or Heuter approach is a truly inter-nervous and inter-muscular plane that allows extension to both the intrapelvic and extrapelvic surfaces of the innominate bone. Using the standard (Heuter) approach, we find a very straightforward and nearly unparalleled exposure to the acetabulum. While most surgeons adept at the anterior approach for arthroplasty of the hip are very familiar with this exposure, understanding how the Heuter relates to the larger approaches such as the Smith-Petersen approach, the Levine approach, and the extended iliofemoral approach give the surgeon a broader understanding of how to optimize the approach for some of the surgical problems encountered in prosthetic surgery of the acetabulum [1].

The standard surgical approach is well described in the literature as well as elsewhere in this manual [2, 3]. However, a brief review is discussed as it relates specifically to exposure of the acetabulum that is discussed below.

For maximal exposure of the acetabulum, this author routinely utilizes the orthopedic table or table extension [3–5]. Advantages of the orthopedic table include near circumferential access to the acetabulum and pelvis and ability to hold the position of the extremity out of the way with traction or other maneuvers without the need for a scrubbed assistant. It is acknowledged however

J. M. Matta, A. P. Sah (eds.), *Anterior Hip Replacement*,
https://doi.org/10.1007/978-3-030-91896-5_10

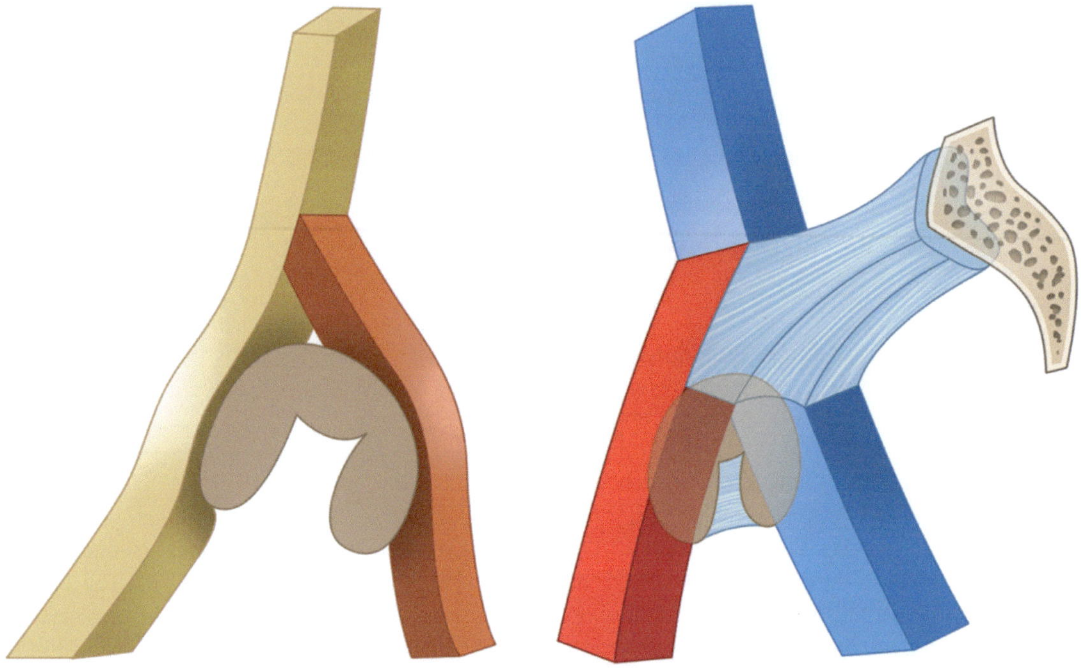

Fig. 10.1 Schematic of the two columns of bone that support the native acetabulum. The anterior (blue) and posterior column (red) are linked to the sacral bone by the "sciatic buttress." The structural support for the prosthetic acetabulum is guided by placing the cup underneath this arch of bone. When either the anterior or posterior column is deficient, the cup has a tendency to fail through that column. Structural support to a deficient column can be accomplished by buttressing, spanning, or other techniques

that many surgeons prefer to operate on the standard operating table, and this is typically without detriment to the access [6–10].

A standard 8–10-cm surgical incision is utilized for most patients. Skin incisions may vary in terms of orientation. A bikini incision may be utilized for cosmesis or wound-healing concerns [9, 11, 12]. A more direct linear incision placed in line with the muscle belly of the tensor may be selected due to advantages of the extensile nature of this approach. The deep exposure however remains consistent.

The fascia of the tensor fasciae latae is split and the tensor fasciae latae muscle is mobilized from within its sheath in an effort to protect the lateral femoral cutaneous nerve [13, 14]. In cases in which a previous anterior approach was used, the medial border of the tensor is a good landmark to follow around the muscle belly to find the interval. Once the tensor fasciae latae muscle is mobilized, the surgeon continues through the floor of the tensor sheath. Typically elevating the rectus and the underlying iliocapsularis off of the anterior capsule of the hip is performed to improve the exposure of the anterior capsule. Identification of the anterior border of the gluteus minimus allows for exposure of the more superior capsule. Distally, the lateral femoral circumflex vessels are ligated in order to extend the approach and improve the access along the intertrochanteric line and capsular insertion along the femur.

A typical "L" shaped capsulotomy is performed to achieve access to the joint. The capsule is incised from just lateral to the anterior inferior iliac spine and down to the anterolateral femur. Commonly, a small tubercle representing the most proximal and lateral origin of the vastus lateralis is a good landmark for the capsulotomy. The distal limb of the "L" releases the iliofemoral ligament medially from the anterior surface of the femoral neck along the intertrochanteric line toward the lesser trochanter. Having the hip in slight external rotation and flexion relaxes the capsule and facilitates exposure to the acetabulum. Many times, if the anterior capsule is incompletely released off of the femur, there is difficulty getting exposure to the acetabulum. Spending extra time to make sure the iliofemoral and pubofemoral ligaments are fully released off of the femur all the way down to the lesser trochanter is worth the time invested. This can be performed either before sectioning of the femoral neck using the "dislocation first" method or after the neck osteotomy.

In the setting of primary total hip arthroplasty, the most common reasons for poor exposure of the acetabulum are the following: (1) inadequate release of the anterior capsule (iliofemoral and pubofemoral ligaments), (2) leaving too long a neck resection with femur impeding the exposure of the acetabulum, (3) anterior osteophytes with the encroachment of the working space to the acetabulum and resultant difficulties with ingress or egress of instruments, and (4) poor positioning of the femur, either with too much traction tightening the soft tissues, or too much internal or external rotation that brings the trochanter or femoral neck into the field of view.

In cases of acetabular protrusion, post-traumatic deformity or complex hip arthroplasty, there is value in performing all capsular releases prior to addressing the acetabulum. In these cases, a femur first approach to the hip may offer some value for later acetabular preparation, as completing these releases first unlocks the femur from the acetabulum and allows access around the proximal femur.

If challenges are anticipated in the exposure of the acetabulum, one can further develop the Heuter exposure. The superficial interval can be developed proximally by dissecting between Tensor and Sartorius all the way up to the level of the anterior superior iliac spine (ASIS). Distally the tensor can be mobilized to the level of the aponeurotic insertion of the tensor fascia latae upon the iliotibial tract. This latter move improves mobilization of the tensor muscle belly and allows more direct in-line access to the acetabulum.

The deep dissection may be enhanced by sectioning of the indirect head of the rectus allowing the rectus muscle belly to roll medially. This is frequently helpful in muscular males. Laterally, the gluteus minimus can be elevated sharply off of capsule and ilium to allow more superior and posterior exposure of the acetabular rim. One should recognize however that these maneuvers carry with them the risk of development of heterotopic ossification. One should handle such deep tissues with care.

Converting the typical L-shaped capsulotomy to a "Z" or "H" type capsulotomy may offer even a wider exposure of the acetabulum. While not typically required for routine cases, taking the proximal capsule posterior along the acetabular rim to create a "Z" will give a posterior superior access to the rim, while going medial underneath the rectus, or even performing a rectus tenotomy to take the capsule medial in an "H" will allow for improved exposure of the anterior superior rim (Fig. 10.2). Additional release of the inferior

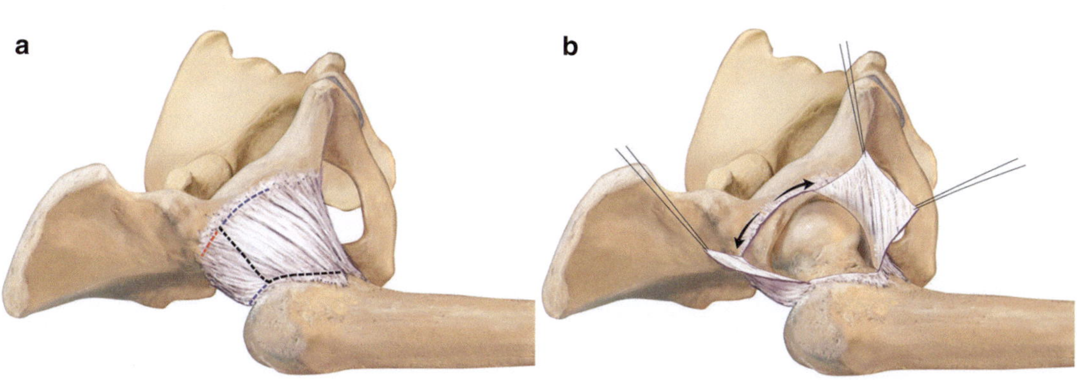

Fig. 10.2 Diagram of capsular management. (**a**) The standard "L"-shaped capsulotomy (black) can be extended to a "Z" by releasing capsule off of the posterior wall (red), which can provide more exposure to superior acetabular wall. Extension to more of an "H" (blue) by releasing off the anterior wall and lateral shoulder depicted in (**b**) can also be considered if additional mobilization is required (e.g., resurfacing arthroplasty, revision)

capsule just above the transverse acetabular ligament will aid in the anterior to posterior excursion of retraction to improve visualization. In cases of severe contracture or revision surgery, a capsulectomy can be performed with no obvious detriment to function. However, there may be a protective role of the anterior capsule from psoas irritation in the setting of primary hip surgery.

In cases such as revision surgery or resurfacing arthroplasty where the femoral head and neck are to be retained while acetabular preparation is to be completed, flexing and externally rotating the femur allows one to work overtop the femoral neck by subluxating the femoral neck or trunion posteriorly and superiorly (Fig. 10.3).

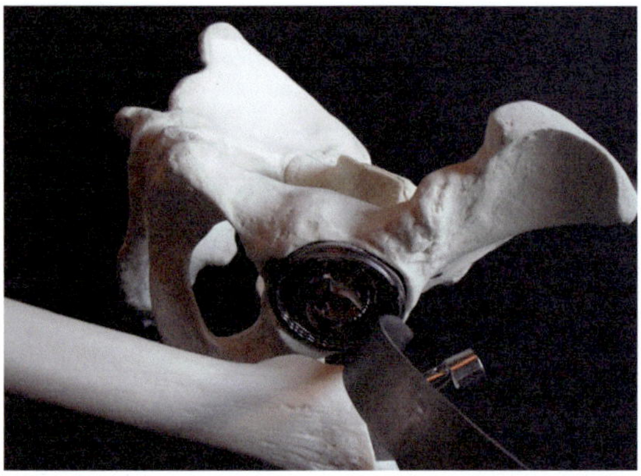

Fig. 10.3 Diagramming a technique of working "overtop" the femoral neck by bringing the extremity into slight flexion and external rotation, one can leave the femoral neck in place and access the acetabulum. Be mindful, however, of the psoas tendon in the distal portion of the surgical field. (From Mast and Laude [10], Fig. 10.1)

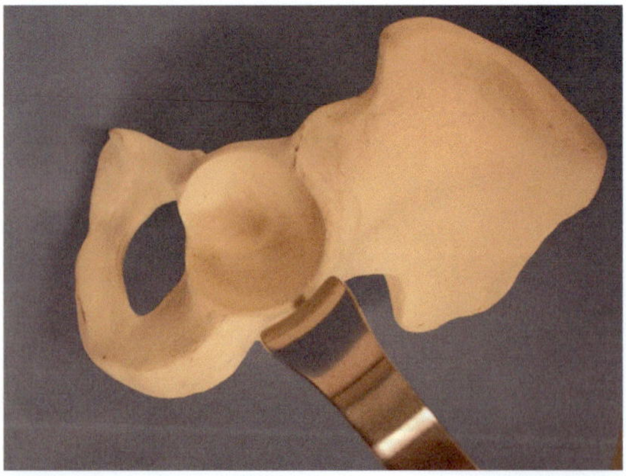

Fig. 10.4 Posterior acetabular retractor and its placement along the posterior wall. Typically a smooth tipped cobra retractor is used for this purpose

During primary total hip arthroplasty utilizing the anterior approach, there are typically three locations for retractor placement that are useful in acetabular exposure. The posterior superior retractor may be placed along the acetabular rim or along the posterior column; typically a broad smooth cobra retractor is helpful in this application (Fig. 10.4). This retractor commonly holds the tensor posteriorly, so it must be placed being mindful of the tension on the tensor as this can be easily ruptured. A retractor may also be placed into the obturator foramen just distal to the transverse acetabular ligament (Fig. 10.5). The obturator retractor is useful for exposure or visualization, especially in revision settings, but may deflect reaming or cup placement proximally. The anterior retractor requires specific mention as it is placed just distal to the pectineal eminence (Fig. 10.6). Care must be utilized to place this intracapsularly and directly onto the bone, as it sits immediately adjacent to the femoral nerve and vascular structures [15, 16].

The extensile exposure of the Anterior Approach has its roots in acetabular fracture surgery [17]. The Levine approach or intrapelvic Smith-Petersen is still commonly utilized as a portion of an anterior intrapelvic approach for acetabular fractures, periacetabular osteotomy, or hip arthrodesis [18–20]. It improves upon the standard Heuter exposure by providing excellent

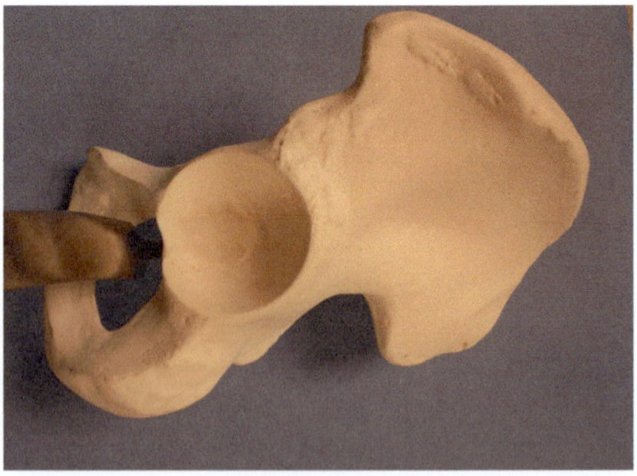

Fig. 10.5 Obturator retractor and its placement just distal to the transverse acetabular ligament (TAL). This retractor gives excellent exposure to the inferior acetabulum; however, this must be balanced against the tendency of this retractor to deflect reamers and cup inserters during cup implantation

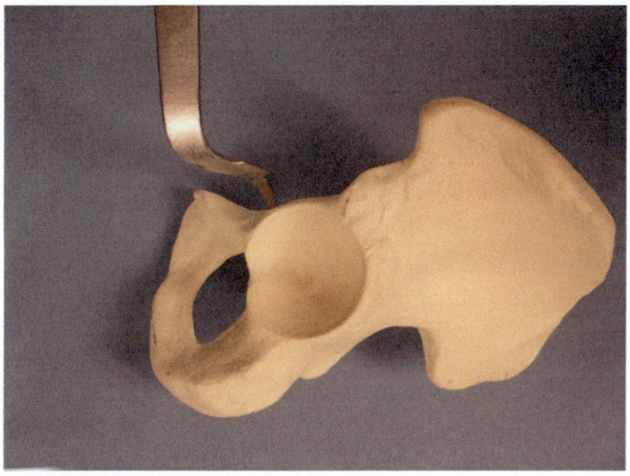

Fig. 10.6 The anterior retractor and its placement just distal to the pectineal eminence. Care must be taken to place this retractor intracapsularly and directly onto bone due to this location being immediately adjacent to the femoral neurovascular bundle

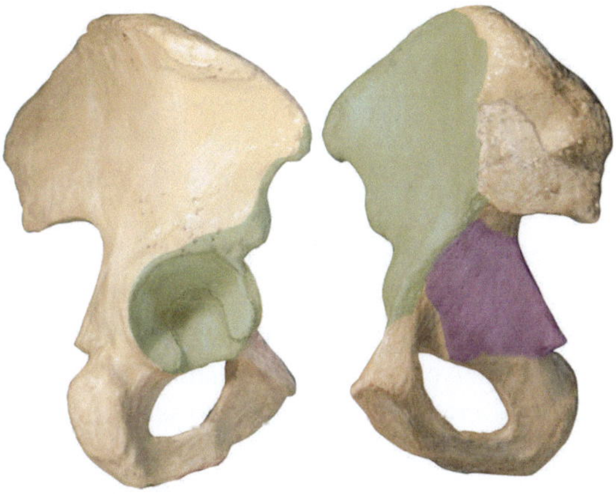

Fig. 10.7 Schematic of the visible (green) and palpable (red) osseous landmarks through the intrapelvic extension of the Smith-Petersen approach

exposure to the intrapelvic anterior column, sciatic buttress, and quadrilateral surface.

The intrapelvic exposure begins by exposing the fascia of the tensor fasciae latae to the anterior superior iliac spine. The fascia is divided until the ASIS is reached. Care is taken at the anterior superior iliac spine to protect the lateral femoral cutaneous nerve. The skin incision commonly curves along the palpable landmarks of the iliac crest, and subcutaneous exposure proceeds to expose the external oblique aponeurosis as it inserts on the iliac crest. Sharp dissection or electrocautery is used to elevate the abdominal muscles off the iliac crest, and the iliacus muscle is elevated in a subperiosteal manner off the inner table of the iliac wing. A laparotomy sponge is placed on the inner table of the pelvis. Finally, the inguinal ligament with the attachments of the sartorius and direct head of the rectus femoris muscle is released to connect the two exposures. Care is taken to stay within the tensor fasciae latae sheath distally to maintain this structure so as to protect the lateral femoral cutaneous nerve. The exposure is then extended medially, following the inner surface of the anterior column, as the psoas muscle is elevated in a subperiosteal manner. At this point, the entirety of the inner table of the pelvis and much of the anterior column and anterior wall of the acetabulum are visible (Fig. 10.7). With flexion of the hip, the quadrilateral surface can be palpated. Additional exposure can be afforded distally by tagging and releasing the rectus tendon off of the anterior inferior iliac spine.

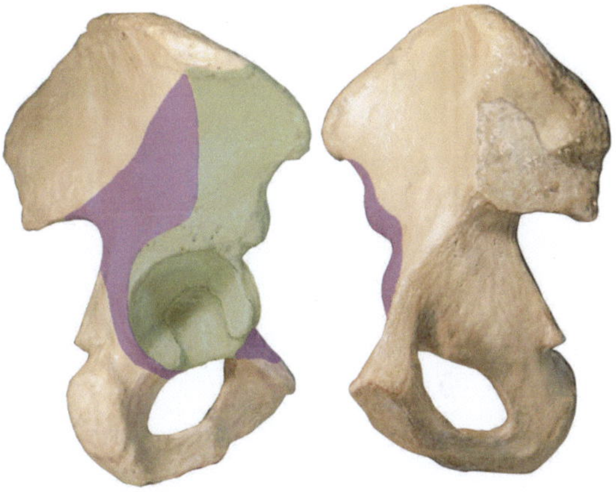

Fig. 10.8 Schematic of the visible (green) and palpable (red) osseous landmarks through the extrapelvic extension of the Smith-Petersen approach

Proximal extension of the exposure can proceed in an extrapelvic fashion. This gives visual access to the external surface of the anterior column anterior to the medius pillar but can afford palpable access as far back as the sciatic notch (Fig. 10.8). In this case, the exposure follows the classic Smith-Petersen approach. The approach is again directed proximally along the palpable landmarks of the iliac crest. The skin incision courses proximally and along the iliac crest at the anterior superior iliac spine. The incision of the tensor fasciae latae fascia extends to the anterior superior iliac spine. The tensor fasciae latae muscle may then be mobilized proximally but not divided from its origin at this point. Once the tensor fasciae latae is mobilized, the anterior column of the ilium can be palpated. Subperiosteal dissection then proceeds underneath the gluteus minimus muscle and along the outer surface of the ilium from anterior to posterior. This creates a pocket underneath the gluteus minimus and tensor fasciae latae where implants or instruments can be placed. Care should be taken at the proximal aspect of the greater sciatic notch to not injure the neurovascular pedicle to the superior gluteal artery. If bleeding is encountered, packing is recommended, as blind cauterization or clamping may injure the superior gluteal nerve and affect hip abductor muscle function. If additional exposure is required posteriorly, the tensor fasciae latae must be mobilized from the ilium. To mobilize the tensor fasciae latae from its origin, an osteotomy of the anterior superior iliac spine, including the anterior third of the crest, can be performed (Fig. 10.9). Alternatively, reinforcing the tendinous origin with suture prior to sharply elevating the fibers off the crest can minimize fraying of the tensor and facilitate its closure. This latter technique can be helpful if only a few centimeters of excursion of the tensor fasciae latae is required by the exposure.

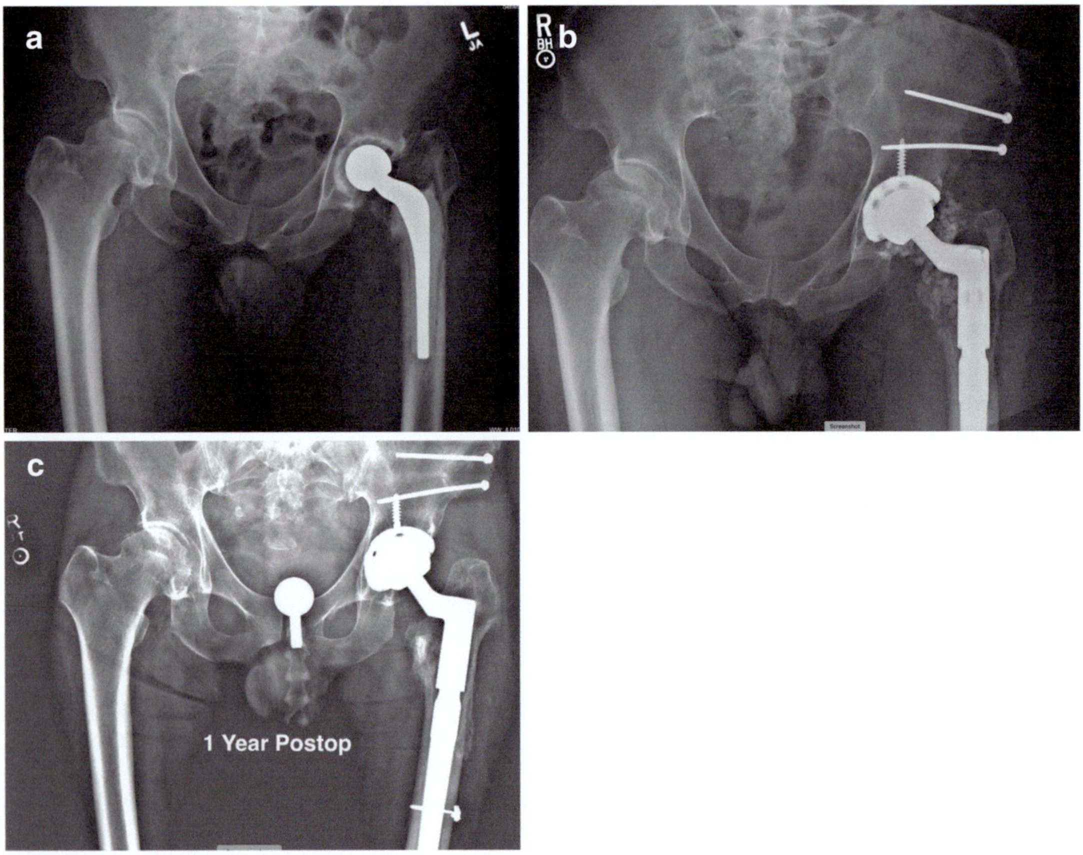

Fig. 10.9 Case demonstrating the utility of ASIS osteotomy. A PMMA spacer subsided within the femoral canal (**a**) making "in-line" femoral access difficult. An osteotomy was required of the ASIS, which made preparation for a straight stem more straightforward (**b**). Postoperative x-ray demonstrating screw fixation of the ASIS after the resulting osteotomy (**c**)

Sizing and Preparation

Preparation of the acetabulum for acetabular component placement proceeds as it does in any other approach. The principles of acetabular reconstruction are the same, namely, (1) reestablish hip center to restore normal biomechanics of the hip, (2) achieve bony coverage of the implant to provide stable early fixation and to allow for long-term fixation of the implant, and (3) achieve implant position that balances coverage and impingement and optimizes wear of the biomaterials.

At the time of the writing of this chapter, titanium shells with high friction porous coatings are available from most manufacturers. They offer advantages in early fixation of uncemented acetabular components and have been the preferred implants in the hands of this author; however, excellent results can be achieved with standard uncemented designs and even with cemented fixation. Fixation techniques and implants will be selected prior to the procedure based upon the technical demands of the procedure. Preoperative templating proceeds either using analog overlays or digital templating software and gives guidance to implant choice, size, and position.

One of the major advantages of the supine positioning afforded by the anterior approach is the ability to use fluoroscopy to guide reaming and implant placement. Upon completion of acetabular exposure, the reamer is introduced and reaming proceeds under fluoroscopy. Nearly all cases will proceed with fluoroscopy assist.

Acetabular preparation occurs after exposure obtained. Again, acetabular exposure with the Heuter approach should be excellent. If inadequate circumferential visualization of the acetabulum cannot be achieved, there is generally a problem with either inadequate release of the iliofemoral and pubofemoral ligaments, or too long a neck cut leading to the femoral neck being in the field of view of the acetabulum. One should consciously make sure that the release of the iliofemoral ligament has been performed so that the lesser trochanter of the femur can be visualized. This can be aided by external rotation of the femur. The neck cut can be checked using fluoroscopy. If excessive femoral neck is present, re-cutting of the neck may be required. In rare cases, anterior osteophytes may be present that impede ingress of reamers; these may require resection.

Typically, the extracted femoral head provides a good reference for the final cup size. The extracted femoral head generally measures about 4–6 mm smaller than the anticipated cup size. Therefore, the first reamer is selected to match the extracted head size with the goal of reaming line-to-line with the final shell diameter. The exceptions to this rule include cases of dysplasia and impingement. When dealing with dysplasia, a starting reamer should be 2–4 mm smaller than the extracted head size. This allows for adequate medialization and coverage without risking overthinning of the anterior and posterior columns in what is typically an ovoid or dish-shaped acetabulum. Similarly, in protrusion where the overhanging rim impedes preparation of the acetabulum, starting with a reamer 2–4 mm larger than the extracted head size will preferentially remove bone from the acetabular rim without further deepening the deformity. A general rule for dysplasia is "go small and medial," while "large and lateral" is reserved for protrusio.

Reaming is generally performed in the same anteversion of the cup. Be aware of the tendency of the femur to deflect the reamer anteriorly, leading to excessive reaming of the anterior wall/column. The direction of reaming should follow the final anticipated cup location. Because of medial osteophyte formation and subsequent lateralization of the hip in the typical patient with osteoarthritis, the first couple of reamers should be directed medially. The direction of reaming should reflect the location of the final hip center as opposed to the final cup position. For example, in the high dysplastic hip, it is not uncommon to be reaming distally to ensure the reproduction of a low hip center. The common mistake is to try to match the final cup position with the reamer, which commonly removes supracetabular bone and leads to a high hip center. Using a "pulsed" reaming technique coupled with intermittent fluoroscopy allows the surgeon to "fine tune" hip center position and make adjustments as necessary.

The goal of reaming is to prepare a hemispherical bed of bleeding bone that is well-covered and reproduces the normal center of rotation of the hip.

Surgeon preference will dictate whether under-reaming the acetabulum offers any advantage in the fixation of the acetabular component. Typically reaming under the final shell size by 1 or 2 mm is safe and may provide an additional "press-fit"; however, this has to be balanced by the risk of acetabular or pelvic fracture.

Positioning and Stability

Acetabular trials are not generally used in the experience of this author, as definitive acetabular shell insertion is typically done at this point. A curved or straight cup impactor may be used for this step. Accessory portals for the straight cup inserter may be utilized to ensure appropriate cup positioning (Fig. 10.10). Appropriate cup position is realized radiographically by judging the shape of the ellipse formed by the opening of the hemispherical shell. Inclination is judged by the relationship to the ilioischial and trans-teardrop or transischial line. Another good landmark is that the inserter should generally point toward the ipsilateral sacroiliac joint. Clinical checks for cup position would include the relationship of the shell to the rim of the anterior wall of the acetabulum. Ideal anteversion has the cup generally just underneath the anterior wall. Adequate acetabular inclination is seen by the amount of acetabular components left uncovered by the superolateral acetabulum. The TAL can also be seen and utilized for reference. For those new to the anterior approach, keep in mind that there is a tendency to place the cup with too much anteversion and inclination.

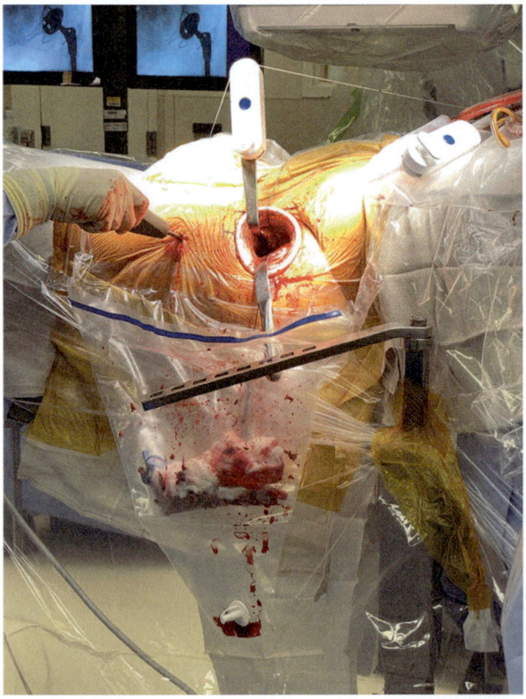

Fig. 10.10 Accessory portals are sometimes necessary to place acetabular components, deal with locking mechanisms (pictured), or remove impeding hardware. Fluoroscopy can be helpful in guiding these accessory incisions

Acetabular screw fixation proceeds with placement into the posterior superior quadrant of the acetabulum for adjunctive fixation. Liberal use of oblique (Judet) views of the hip can give immediate feedback guiding screw placement, length, and orientation (Fig. 10.11). Powerful long screw fixation can be obtained in the sciatic buttress just proximal to the sciatic notch. These long screws are typically placed between the tables of the flat bones of the pelvis and can get cortical bite along large stretches of bone. During insertion of these long screws into the buttress, be aware of the tendency of the screw to shift the position of the cup as it is tightened. In revision cases, placing one or more "position" screws prior to placing the long "power" screw can be helpful in maintaining the cup position while the screws are applied.

A common strategy to deal with superolateral deficiency associated with wear or dysplasia has been to use an autologous graft from the patient's femoral head. When acetabular dysplasia or wear creates superolateral deficiency, a strategy that we have employed takes advantage of newer, higher friction surfaces on modern acetabular shells to place the cup in the anatomic hip center getting provisional fixation between the anterior and posterior columns, placing screws to get definitive cup fixation but then buttressing the construct by placing a wedge of the autologous

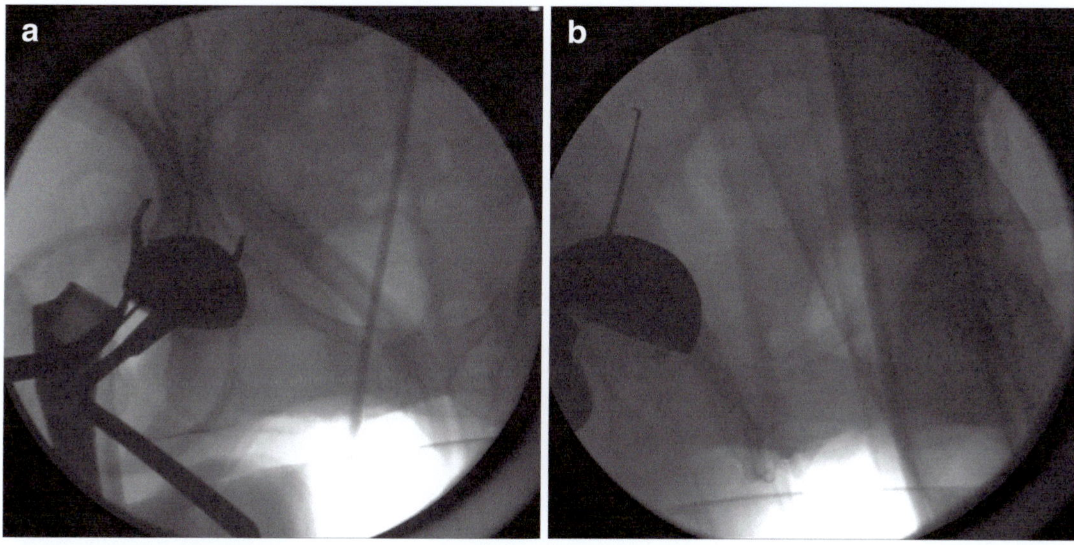

Fig. 10.11 Intraoperative oblique (Judet) views of the innominate bone (**a**, **b**) confirming the use of intraosseous corridors for screw placement

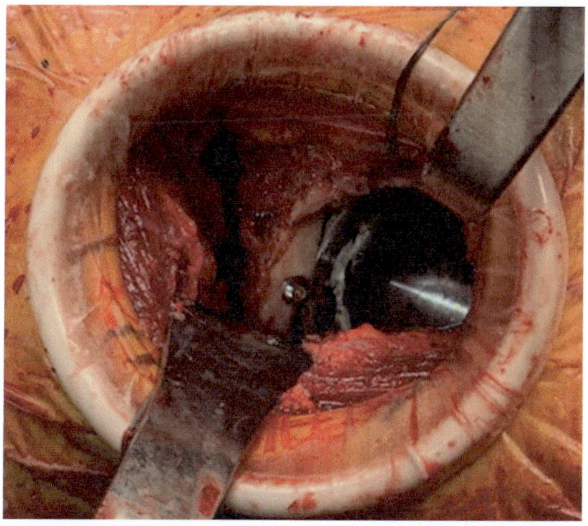

Fig. 10.12 Case demonstration of a superolateral deficiency due to wear. Placement of the cup at the anatomic hip center and use of femoral head autograft as an augment for structural support can be accomplished easily through the anterior approach. Typically, the use of a high friction cup with provisional fixation between the columns followed by grafting is the sequence employed by this author

femoral head into the superolateral defect. This avoids problems associated with using a high hip center and more accurately reproduces the biomechanics of the hip while offering a simpler approach to fashioning the superolateral graft construct (Fig. 10.12).

Conclusion

With proficiency with the anterior approach, many will find the acetabulum to be ideally addressed through this interval. Except in cases where access to the posterior column is required (such as posterior wall defects requiring grafting and/or buttressing, or posterior column deficiencies requiring spanning with an implant), the anterior approach is the preferred approach to address the acetabulum. The extensile nature of the approach respects muscular and neurologic contributions to hip function. This is important in the primary setting but can be even more valuable in the tenuous and compromised tissues of revision hip surgery. Spending time understanding how to maximize the exposure will facilitate the complex case and extend the applicability of the approach to even more complex pathology.

References

1. Mast NH, Laude F. Revision total hip arthroplasty performed through the Hueter interval. J Bone Joint Surg. 2011;93 Suppl 2:143–8.
2. Matta JM, Shahrdar C, Ferguson T. Single-incision anterior approach for total hip arthroplasty on

an orthopaedic table. Clin Orthop Relat Res. 2005;30(441):115–24.
3. Matta JM, Ferguson TA. The anterior approach for hip replacement. Orthopedics. 2005;28(9):927–8.
4. Laude F. Total hip arthroplasty through an anterior Hueter minimally invasive approach. Interactive. Surgery. 2006;
5. Anterior Total Hip Arthroplasty Collaborative Investigators, Bhandari M, Matta JM, Dodgin D, Clark C, Kregor P, et al. Outcomes following the single-incision anterior approach to total hip arthroplasty: a multicenter observational study. Orthop Clin North Am. 2009;40(3):329–42.
6. Molenaers B, Driesen R, Molenaers G, Corten K. The direct anterior approach for complex primary total hip arthroplasty: the extensile acetabular approach on a regular operating room table. J Arthroplast. 2017;32(5):1553–9.
7. Hozack WJ, Heller S. Direct anterior hip exposure for Total hip arthroplasty. JBJS Essent Surg Tech. 2015;5(4):e22.
8. Seng BE, Berend KR, Ajluni AF, Lombardi AV. Anterior-supine minimally invasive total hip arthroplasty: defining the learning curve. Orthop Clin North Am. 2009;40(3):343–50.
9. Connolly KP, Kamath AF. Direct anterior total hip arthroplasty: Literature review of variations in surgical technique. World J Orthop. Baishideng Publishing Group Inc;. 2016;7(1):38–43.
10. Kennon R, Keggi J, Zatorski LE, Keggi KJ. Anterior approach for total hip arthroplasty: beyond the minimally invasive technique. J Bone Joint Surg Am. 2004;86-A Suppl 2:91–7.
11. Leunig M, Faas M, Knoch von F, Naal FD. Skin crease "bikini" incision for anterior approach total hip arthroplasty: surgical technique and preliminary results. Clin Orthop Relat Res. Springer-Verlag;. 2013;471(7):2245–52.
12. Lanting BA, Hartley KC, Raffoul AJ, Burkhart TA, Sommerville L, Martin GR, et al. Bikini versus traditional incision direct anterior approach: is there any difference in soft tissue damage? Hip Int. 2017;27(4):397–400.
13. Goulding K, Beaulé PE, Kim PR, Fazekas A. Incidence of lateral femoral cutaneous nerve neuropraxia after anterior approach hip arthroplasty. Clin Orthop Relat Res. 2010;468(9):2397–404.
14. Sugano M, Nakamura J, Hagiwara S, Suzuki T, Nakajima T, Orita S, et al. Anatomical course of the lateral femoral cutaneous nerve with special reference to the direct anterior approach to total hip arthroplasty. Mod Rheumatol. 2019;33(7):1–6.
15. Short AJ, Barnett JJG, Gofeld M, Baig E, Lam K, Agur AMR, et al. Anatomic study of innervation of the anterior hip capsule: implication for image-guided intervention. Reg Anesth Pain Med. 2018;43(2):186–92.
16. Stubbs T, Moon AS, Dahlgren N, Patel HA, Jha AJ, Shah A, et al. Anterior acetabular retractors and the femoral neurovascular bundle in anterior total hip arthroplasty: a cadaveric study. Eur J Orthop Surg Traumatol. Springer Paris;. 2020;30(4):617–20.
17. Levine M. A treatment of central fractures of the acetabulum: a case report. J Bone Joint Surg; 1943.
18. Beaulé PE, Griffin DB, Matta JM. The Levine anterior approach for total hip replacement as the treatment for an acute acetabular fracture. J Orthop Trauma. 2004;18(9):623–9.
19. Matta JM. Hip joint arthrodesis utilizing anterior compression plate fixation. J Arthroplast. 1994;9(6):665.
20. Leunig M, Ganz R. (iii) Bernese periacetabular osteotomy. Curr Orthop. 2007;21(2):100–8.

11 My Keys to Getting the Femur Right: Exposure, Preparation, Sizing, Depth of Insertion of Stem, Ball Head, Stability

Anthony T. Carter

The keys to success in exposing the femur via the DAA include the following:

- A firm understanding of the anatomy of the proximal femur, including the neurovascular anatomy, to minimize blood loss and avoid nerve injury.
- Consistent sequential releases are required to maximize femoral exposure titrated to only what is necessary to safely prepare the femur. Be patient and reassess femoral mobility after each and every release. Never settle for "it is good enough."
- Anticipate required releases based on preoperative radiographic assessment and body habitus.
- Predictable proper retractor placement.
- Lower extremity positioning.
- Proper instrumentation for femoral preparation.

Difficulty with exposure and manipulation of the femur for proper canal preparation has been reported, including fractures of the greater trochanter, calcar fractures, and femoral canal perforation. Based on current literature, these rates range from 0% to 5.3% [1–10]. The majority of these fractures can be managed intraoperatively and do not require further intervention. The majority of studies comparing intraoperative fracture rates between anterior, posterior, and lateral approaches do not demonstrate a statistical difference [11–16]. However, Malek et al. [17] found a significantly higher fracture rate in the DAA group compared to the posterior approach group. There does not appear to be a significant difference of intraoperative femoral fracture rate whether performed on a specialized fracture or regular operating room table [18]. Most studies suggest that these complications are related to surgeon experience with a steep learning curve effect. The number of cases varies widely from 25 to 100 cases [19–21]. There is a lower incidence of these fractures with larger volume centers and higher volume surgeons [22, 23].

Additionally, improper femoral canal preparation due to poor exposure has been suggested as a cause of early stem loosening requiring early revision [22, 24–26]. In a multicenter study of 1277 DAA cases, the Anterior Total Hip Collaborative found an early revision rate of 2.7%, 1.3% of which was attributed to femoral loosening [5]. In this study, there was a significant correlation between surgeon and early revision rates. Interestingly, Ponzi et al. [27] found a reduced rate of early revision compared to the posterior approach including the learning curve

Supplementary Information The online version contains supplementary material available at [https://doi.org/10.1007/978-3-030-91896-5_11].

A. T. Carter (✉)
Hampton Roads Orthopaedics & Sports Medicine, Newport News, VA, USA

J. M. Matta, A. P. Sah (eds.), *Anterior Hip Replacement*, https://doi.org/10.1007/978-3-030-91896-5_11

in the anterior approach cohort. Varus positioning and undersizing of the femoral component have been reported as high as 7.5% of cases, especially during the learning curve [28]. However, there does not appear to be a significant difference when compared to posterior or lateral approaches [14, 29]. In fact, some studies report significantly better stem positioning with the anterior approach, possibly due to the intraoperative use of fluoroscopy [30].

These complications are not approach specific but inherent with any surgical procedure about the hip. These complications can be minimized with a firm understanding of the anatomy of the hip and a consistent stepwise approach to soft tissue management. Consistent predictable retractor placement is also a key to success. Whether performed on a specialized table or on a standard operating room table, the anatomy of the hip does not change. Consistent landmarks are utilized. The true tissue sparing intermuscular/internervous interval developed to reach the hip capsule has been extensively detailed previously in this book and will not be covered here. Ensure that all fascial bands tethering the TFL to the iliac crest have been released to release tension on the TFL. Understanding the capsular anatomy and tendinous insertions of the proximal femur and their functional significance is critical to proper management of the proximal femur. In the vast majority of cases, appropriate capsular release is all that is required to obtain adequate exposure of the femur. The capsule is made up of several ligaments, which are often indistinguishable, including the pubofemoral, iliofemoral, and ischiofemoral ligaments (Fig. 11.1a, b).

The capsule is the primary static stabilizer of the hip joint and is often thickened and contracted secondary to chronic inflammation. This also enhances its robust vascularity. The initial release of the femur begins with initial capsulotomy. I prefer the inverted T method as classically described by Dr. Matta beginning at the lateral acetabular rim, following parallel to the femoral neck, down to the palpable femoral tubercle (Fig. 11.2). The limbs are then completed laterally and medially along the intertrochanteric line and tagged with different colored sutures, and cobra retractors are placed intracapsulary (Fig. 11.3; Video 11.1).

Some authors propose a sail-type capsular flap, while others may prefer a capsulectomy, which has demonstrated equal outcomes to capsulotomy and repair at 1 year after surgery. Caution should be taken to achieve meticulous hemostasis during this part of the procedure as the capsule itself has a robust blood supply and branches of the medial femoral circumflex vessel course along the intertrochanteric ridge. It is important to extend the lateral or superior limb of the capsulotomy past the saddle of the femur as far toward the greater trochanter as possible without damaging the gluteus minimus tendon or muscle (Fig. 11.4).

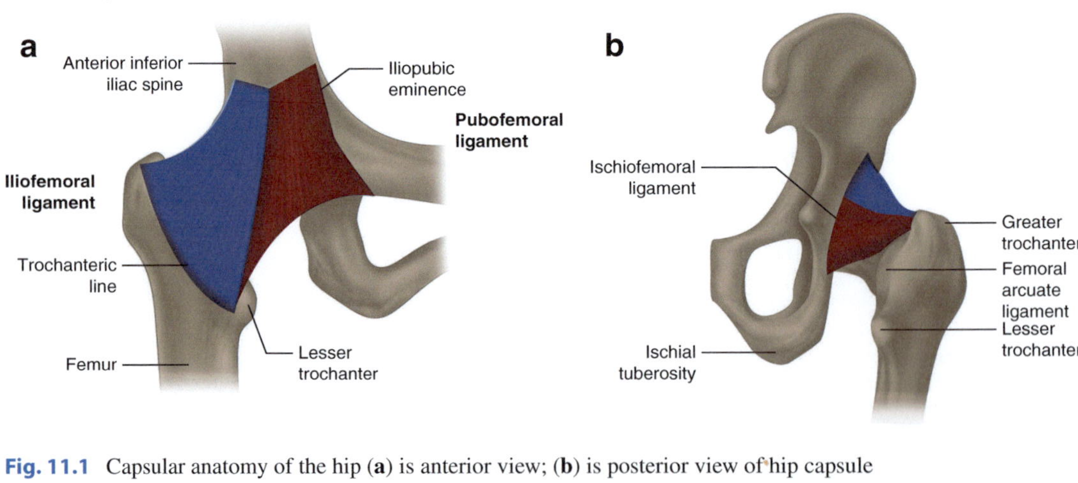

Fig. 11.1 Capsular anatomy of the hip (**a**) is anterior view; (**b**) is posterior view of hip capsule

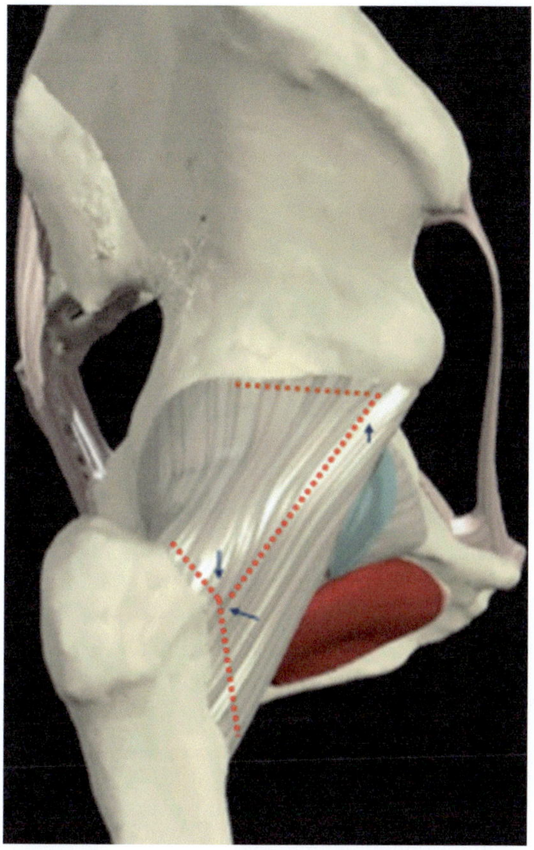

Fig. 11.2 Classic inverted "T" capsulotomy. The superior aspect can also be converted to an "H" to aid in exposure

In the classical description of the technique, the hip is now dislocated prior to the neck cut, which strips the capsule from the femur, further completing the capsular release both medially and posteriorly. In a contracted hip, coxa breva, Perthes disease, prior trauma, or protrusio, this dislocation maneuver can be challenging. If this step is skipped and a neck cut in situ was planned, it is extremely helpful to complete the pubofemoral ligament release (Fig. 11.5) by externally rotating the femur maximally at this point (at least 80 degrees to 90 degrees), tilting the medial Cobra retractor toward the head to place the pubofemoral ligament under tension, while lifting up on the tagline of the suture. The release can then be completed along the medial border of the femur, down to the lesser trochanter (Fig. 11.6; Video 11.2).

This important maneuver, performed early in the case, allows the femur to relax posteriorly and laterally to assist in acetabular exposure as well as later with femoral exposure. This release also aids in retractor placement around the posterior medial calcar later in the procedure. Once again, caution should be exercised during this release as bleeding may be encountered from the medial circumflex vessels. In addition, care should be taken to avoid the neurovascular bundles entering

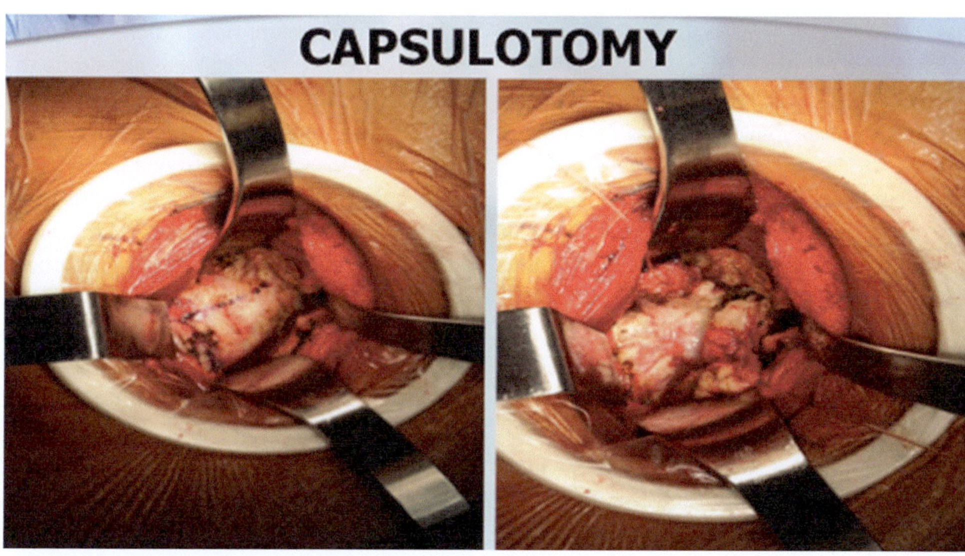

Fig. 11.3 Be sure to extend the distal limb of the capsulotomy completely to the intertrochanteric ridge. The vastus lateralis can be retracted with a Homan retractor to allow better visualization. The cobras are placed intracapsularly at this point

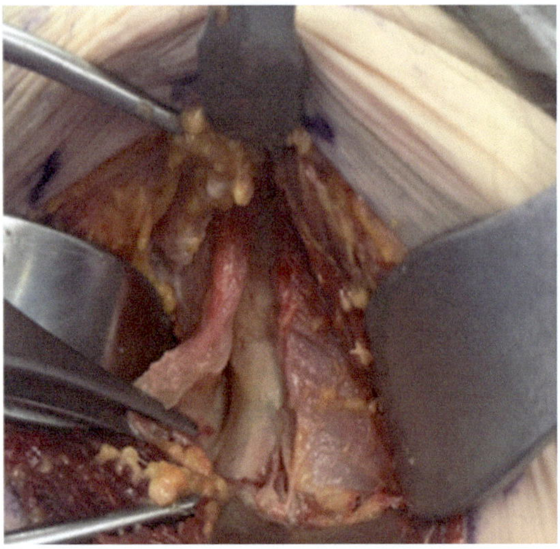

Fig. 11.4 Visualization of the saddle of the femur

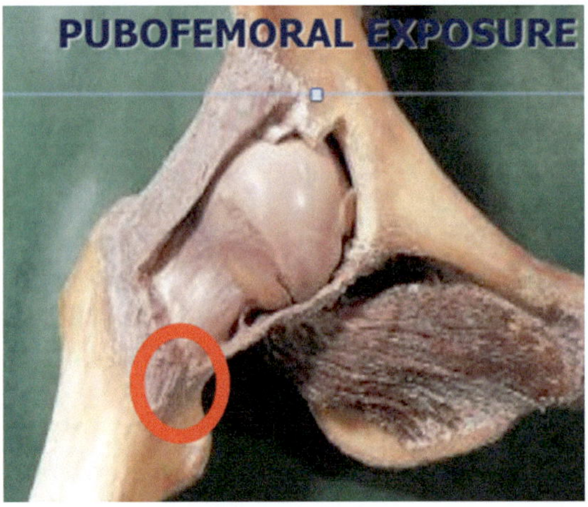

Fig. 11.5 The inferior extent of the pubofemoral ligament (stout inferomedial capsule) to the lesser trochanter

the medial border of the vastus. The neck cut is typically made with the femur in neutral rotation and slight traction to allow easy evaluation of the completed osteotomy. Either a single cut or a napkin ring technique can be employed (Fig. 11.7a–d). Since the posterior capsule may be tensioned against the posterior neck, care must be taken not to plunge with the saw blade and inadvertently damage the posterior retinacular vessels. A corkscrew is drilled into the cut neck in a retrograde fashion with the femur externally rotated approximately 60 degrees, and the head and neck fragments are removed by lifting the

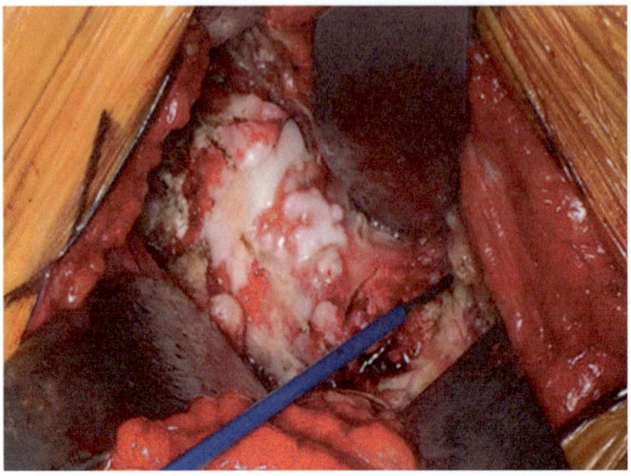

Fig. 11.6 Release of the pubofemoral ligament

handle of the corkscrew superiorly toward the patient's opposite shoulder. Twisting the corkscrew during this maneuver can be helpful to strip the capsule off of the neck (Fig. 11.8). Anterior osteophytes of the acetabular rim may impede head removal. The level of the neck cut is based on preoperative templating and chosen stem design. This important step is often overlooked and underappreciated. A neck cut that is too long can impede acetabular exposure from bony impingement and extensive retained capsular tethering. Too low a neck cut, while aiding with acetabular exposure, can risk fracture of the greater trochanter and potentially affect proximal stem fixation (Fig. 11.9).

Without sufficient bone stock, a low neck cut can also affect retractor placement along the posteromedial calcar. The Mueller can slip off the bone during femoral preparation, and often a retractor with a long wide paddle placed along the remaining posterior neck provides better and more stable retraction. Adequate release of the inframedial capsule (pubofemoral ligament) can also be reassessed after the in situ neck cut. If inadequate, the femur may impede acetabular preparation, especially if traction is applied to the anterior capsule from retractors placed around the acetabulum. This release is complete when the lesser trochanter can be easily palpated manually. Any residual bands of the pubofemoral ligament can be easily released from the femur manually by sliding the finger down to the lesser trochanter, which again allows the femur

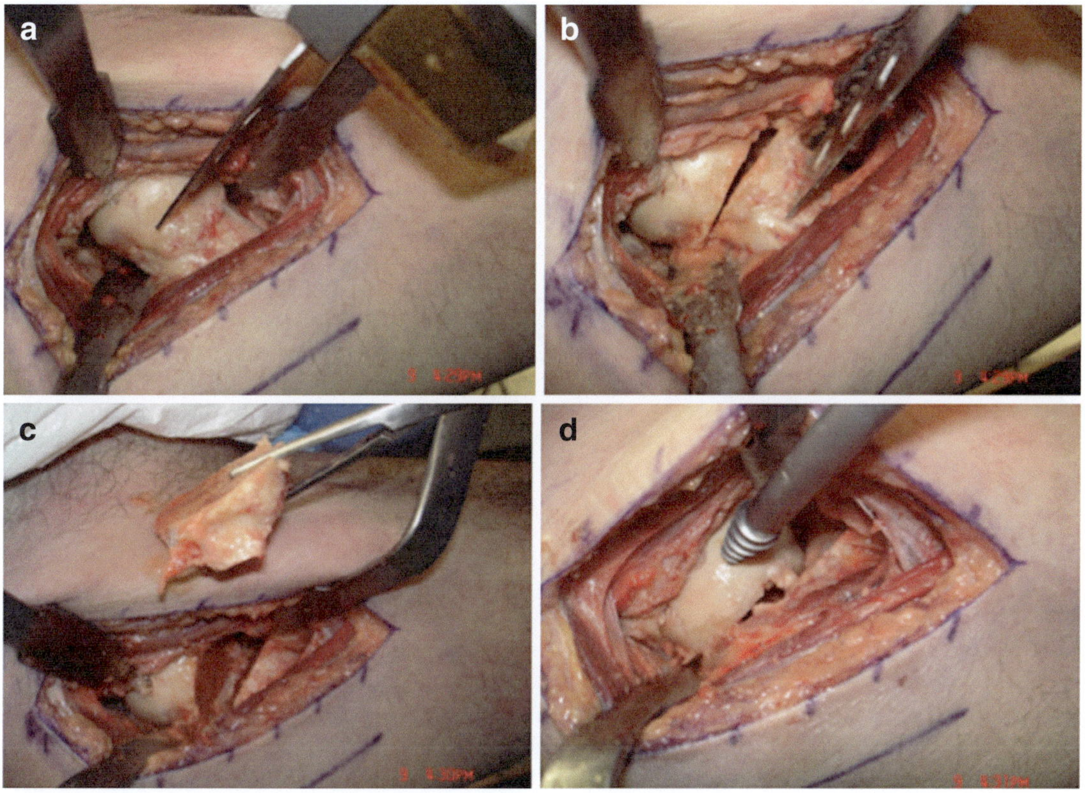

Fig. 11.7 Napkin ring neck cut. (**a**) initial subcapital neck cut. (**b**) secondary neck cut to remove approx 1cm of neck. (**c**) removal of napkin ring with a kocher or tenaculum. (**d**) removal of head with corkscrew

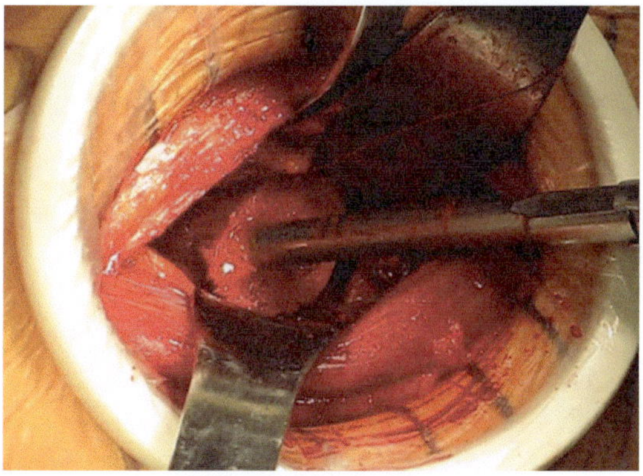

Fig. 11.8 Rotation of the head with the corkscrew can release capsular attachments to neck

to assume a relaxed position laterally and posteriorly (Fig. 11.10). Once the acetabulum has been prepared, the femur, which is typically held at about 45 degrees of external rotation and slight traction during acetabular preparation, is placed in neutral rotation and traction removed. The femoral hook for the femur lift (if being used) is typically placed at the base of the greater trochanter in the interval between the gluteus maximus tendon and the vastus lateralis (Fig. 11.11a, b).

It is important to note that the hook does not go against the bone but outside or deep to the vastus lateralis. If resistance is encountered during placement, redirect the hook in the proper plane. Another trick for finding the correct interval is to palpate the cut calcar medially and run your finger laterally to the edge of the femur and around the vastus lateralis. Your finger will fall into the correct interval. Do not place the hook into the lift until after the leg has been externally rotated and extended, as inadvertent tension applied to the proximal femur prior to capsular release could result in fracture of the greater trochanter (Fig. 11.12).

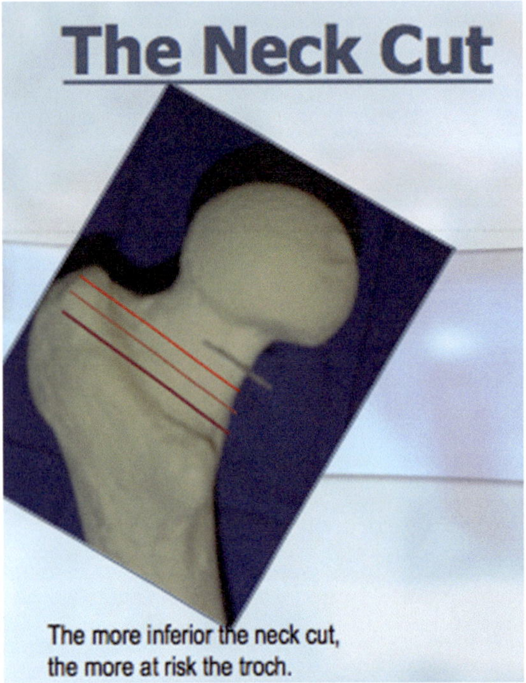

Fig. 11.9 A low neck cut risks fracture of the greater trochanter. The greater trochanter is at risk if the saw blade penetrates too far posterior. The metaphysis at this level is very patulent, and proper filling of the canal with rotational stability may be difficult to maintain

Alternatively, if performed on a regular table, a bone hook can be placed around the femur or carefully into the cut neck, and the femur can be lifted manually superiorly and laterally as the leg is externally rotated and extended. I like to try to achieve at least 90 degrees to 120 degrees of external rotation prior to extending the leg. Another helpful trick is while externally rotating the femur, slight traction can be applied to the leg as it is externally rotated by grasping the distal femur about the knee and manually externally rotating the leg (Video 11.3). This can often "unlock" the greater trochanter from the posterior rim of the acetabulum and allow greater external rotation (Fig. 11.13a, b).

A Mueller retractor is placed along the posterior medial calcar, with either limb of the Mueller around the lesser trochanter (Fig. 11.14), which should be easy to accomplish if the pubofemoral capsular release was sufficient, as described earlier.

Alternatively, a Cobra retractor can be placed along the posterior neck of the femur. This can be especially helpful if a low neck cut was performed and the Mueller may slip off the posterior

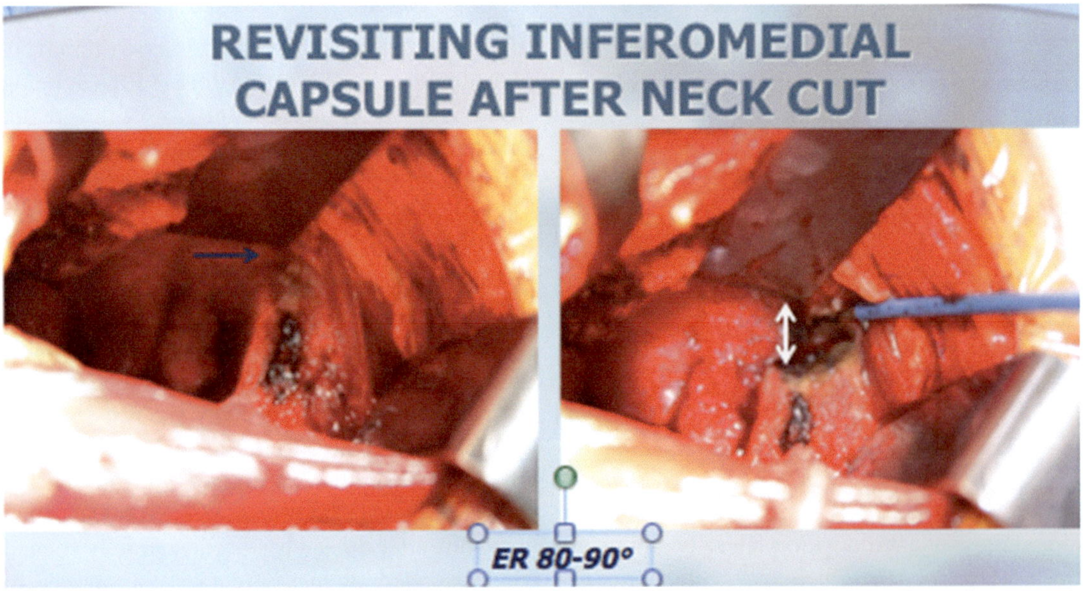

Fig. 11.10 Note the relative posterior movement of the femur after completion of the pubofemoral ligament release

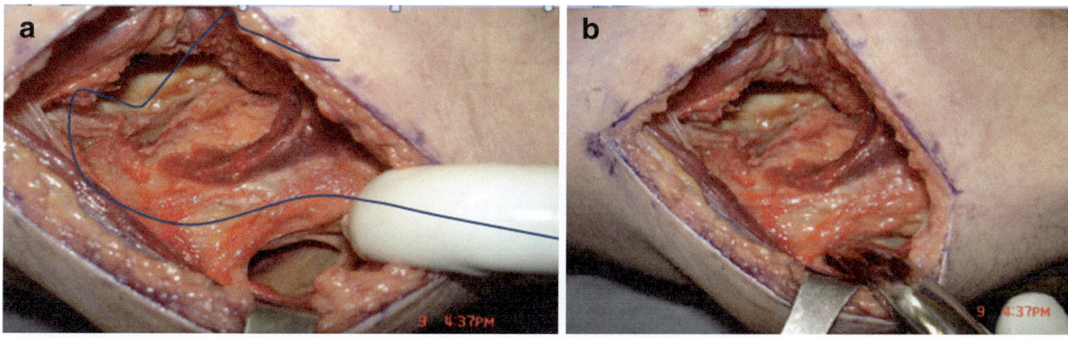

Fig. 11.11 Correct interval for placement of Hana hook (**a**) is demonstrating proper interval; (**b**) is with hook in place

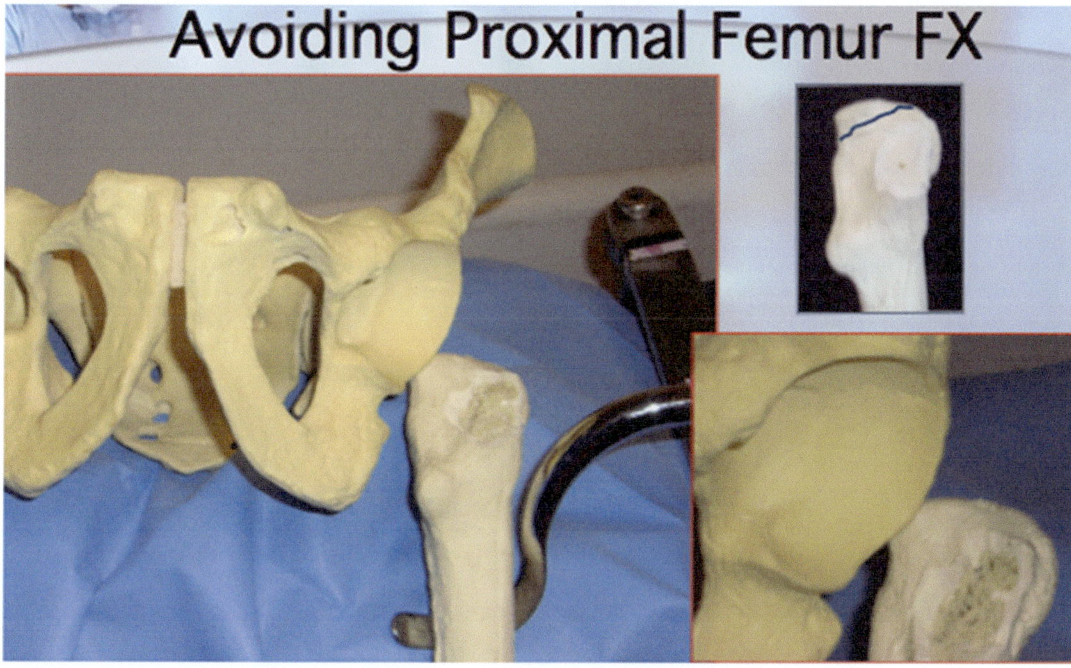

Fig. 11.12 Excessive anterior force can inadvertently be applied to the femur as the leg is externally rotated and extended prior to capsular release. The posteriorly tethered greater trochanter can be avulsed or fractured

neck. A long Homan is then carefully placed extracapsularly (Video 11.3), and the superolateral capsule (iliofemoral and ischiofemoral ligaments) release is completed exposing the underlying external rotators (Fig. 11.15a, b). The tagged capsule can be released from the leading edge of the greater trochanter circumferentially around the trochanter to its posterolateral edge (Fig. 11.16a, b; Video 11.4). Care must be taken to not cut the abductor muscles, which may be between the retractor and the capsule. Frequent repositioning of the Homan, moving it from extracapsular to intracapsular, can be helpful to define the correct plane. Alternatively, a Chevron-type opening in the superolateral capsule over the trochanter can be performed with a vertical episiotomy extending superiorly from the apex of the trochanter and the Homan placed through this capsular perforation (Fig. 11.17).

The capsule can then be peeled off on either side of the trochanter. After each release of the capsule, mobility of the femur both superiorly and laterally should be reassessed manually. In the vast majority of cases, only capsular release

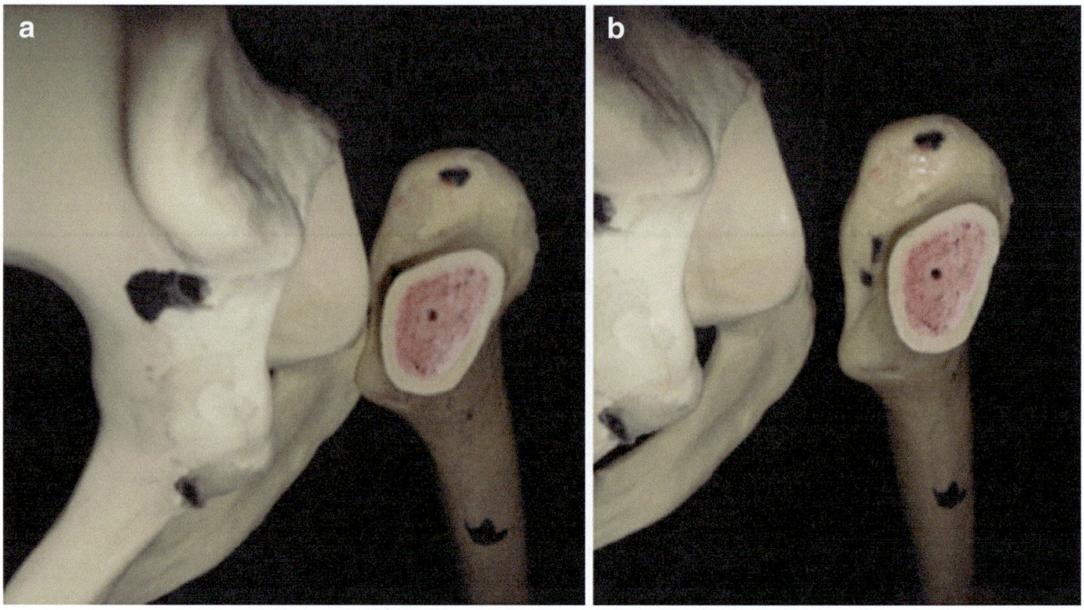

Fig. 11.13 Prior to capsular releases, the greater trochanter can be trapped medially against the pelvis, limiting elevation and lateralization. This also increases the risk of avulsion of the greater trochanter if forceful extension is applied to the femur during manipulation of the leg (**a**) inadequate lateralization of proximal femur. note that trochanter is locked behind acetabulum; (**b**) demonstrates appropriate lateralization of proximal femur away from pelvis to allow adequate exposure

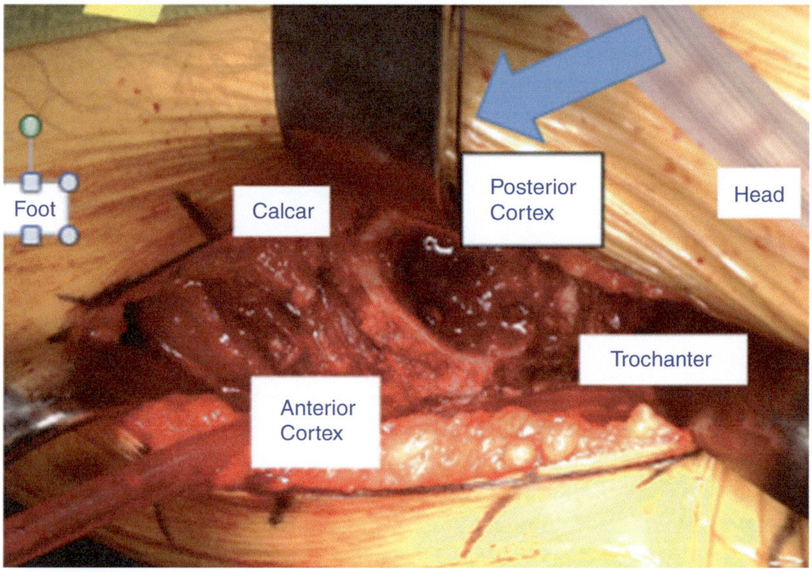

Fig. 11.14 Placement of the Mueller retractor along posterior cortex femur. Forced exposure with this retractor could fracture the femur in thin osteoporotic bone

of the femur is necessary to properly prepare the femur. Patience and persistence are key here, and repositioning of the large Homan and repeated manual checks of femoral mobility are necessary. A Cobb or Key elevator can be used as well to peel the capsule off the trochanter. A thin fat pad typically exists between the capsule and the short external rotators, which will appear as shiny tendons beneath the capsule (Video 11.5). A common error is to mistake any residual lateral cortex of the femur for the greater trochanter, especially if a longer neck cut was made initially (Fig. 11.18). In this case, the superior capsule is adequately released around the rim of the greater

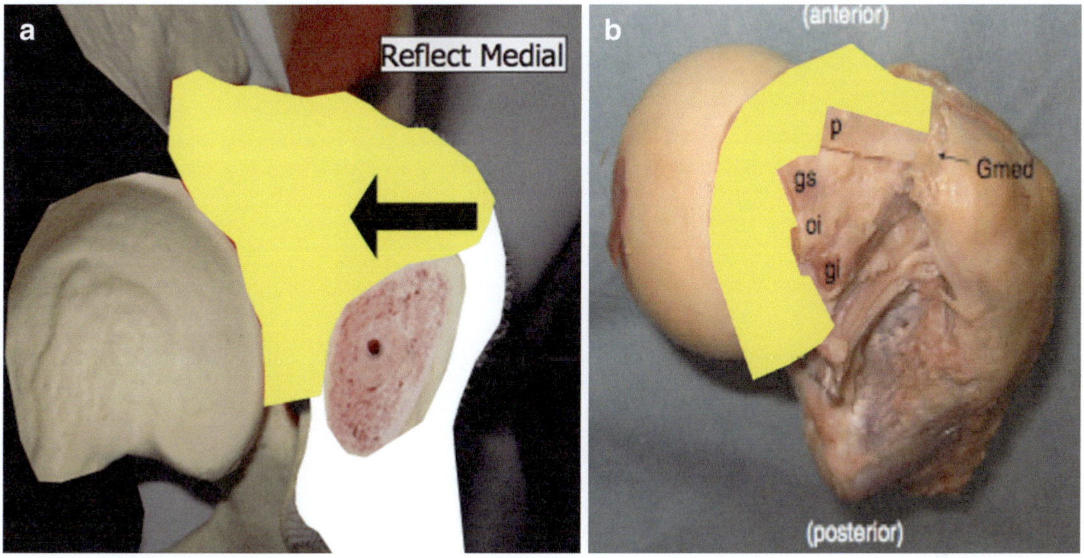

Fig. 11.15 (**a**, **b**) Schematic illustration of mobilization of the superior capsule (iliofemoral and ilioischial ligaments). The external rotators can then be visualized

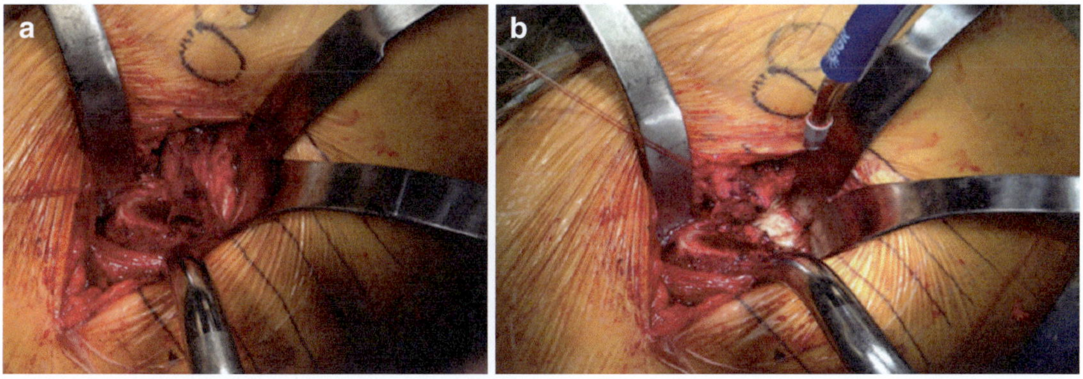

Fig. 11.16 (**a**, **b**) Intraoperative photo demonstrating reflection of the tagged superolateral capsule. This is essentially working from "inside-out" relative to the posterior approach

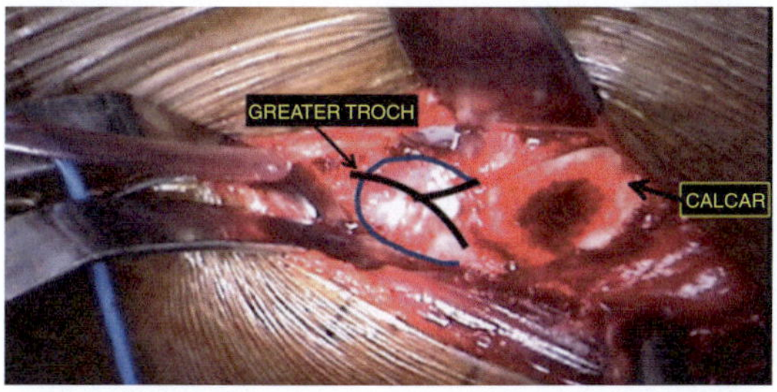

Fig. 11.17 The black line illustrates an alternative to peeling the entire capsule off the greater trochanter; a chevron type episiotomy can be made, perforated with the pointed Homan, and the capsule dissected off the trochanter in either direction

trochanter, which should be easily visible and palpable, as should the piriformis fossa. Of note, the tip of the trochanter is almost always more posterior medial in this externally rotated extended position and again should be easily palpated and identified to ensure adequate capsular release. If further releases are necessary, they are usually done in a sequential manner, identifying the short external rotators, which will appear beneath the capsule on the inner or medial aspect of the greater trochanter (Fig. 11.19).

Any dissection that remains on the medial border of the greater trochanter within the fossa

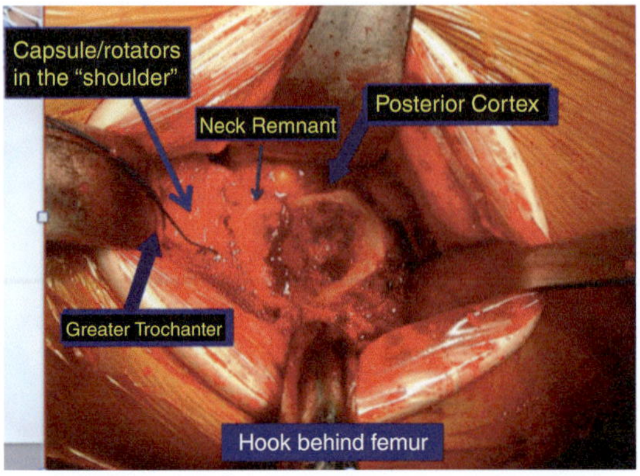

Fig. 11.18 Residual neck remnant. notice that the greater trochanter is completely covered by residual capsule and the external rotators are not visualized beneath the capsule

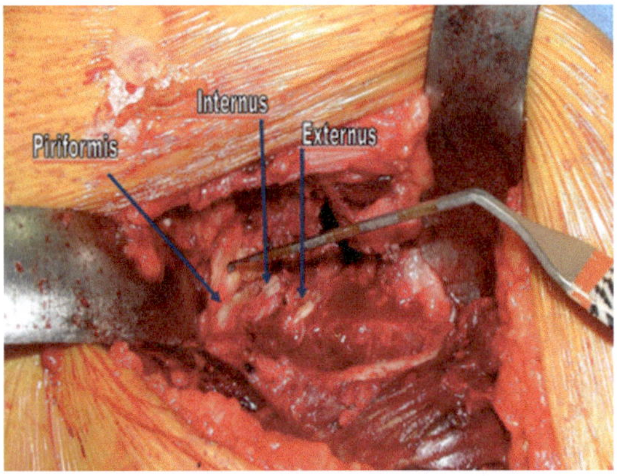

Fig. 11.19 Insertion of the external rotator of the right hip. The piriformis insertion is superior and anterior on the greater trochanter; the conjoined tendon inserts just below the piriformis and slightly more posteriorly. The obturator externus inserts low and posterior at the greater trochanter/neck junction

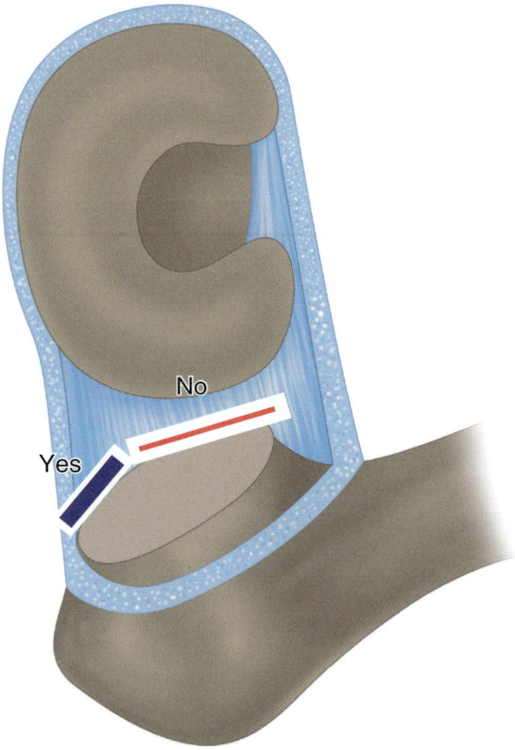

Fig. 11.20 Obturator internus release. (Courtesy of F. Boetner, MD)

is safe. The piriformis tendon inserts very superior and anterior on the trochanter, while the conjoined tendon inserts lower and more posterior, and finally the obturator internus, which has the most direct medial pull of the femur to prevent posterior dislocation, inserts very low and posterior on the neck of the femur. Release of the obturator externus is never necessary and provides little, if any, additional exposure. The posterior capsule should also be spared, as no additional exposure is provided [31] with an increased risk of posterior dislocation (Fig. 11.20). Typically, the conjoined tendon is released first by running the Bovie tip from the base of the trochanter directed superiorly toward the tip, and care should be taken not to release the piriformis (Fig. 11.21; Video 11.5).

Again, manual traction is applied after any release to assess any incrementally increased mobility of the femur. If this release is inadequate, prior to releasing the piriformis, it is often helpful to hit the "reset button." Remove all retractors, return the leg to a neutral position with regard to extension and rotation, and repeat the entire maneuver of external rotation and extension of the leg while manually lifting the femur superior and lateral. The retractors are then reinserted. This "up and down" maneuver often provides enough additional elevation and lateralization of the femur to allow the preparation of the femur. If still tight, a release of the piriformis can be performed after re-evaluating the previous capsular releases. Release of the piriformis is typically required in less than 10% of cases. There are certain clinical and radiographic signs that more extensive releases may be required and should be part of the

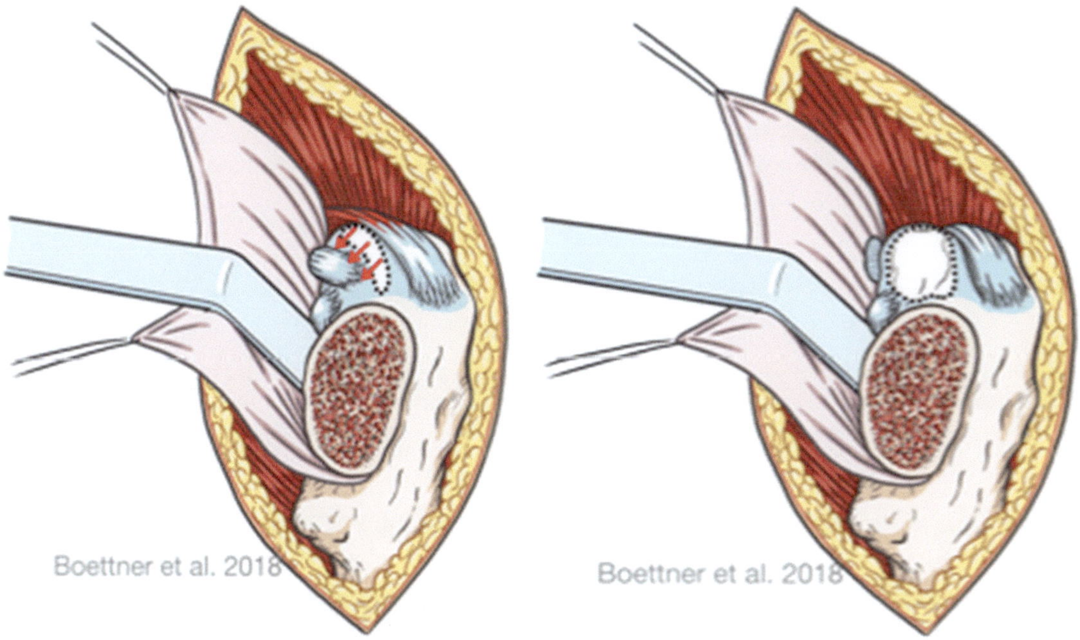

Fig. 11.21 Initial isolated release of the obturator internus tendon from the greater trochanter with preservation of the piriformis and obturator externus

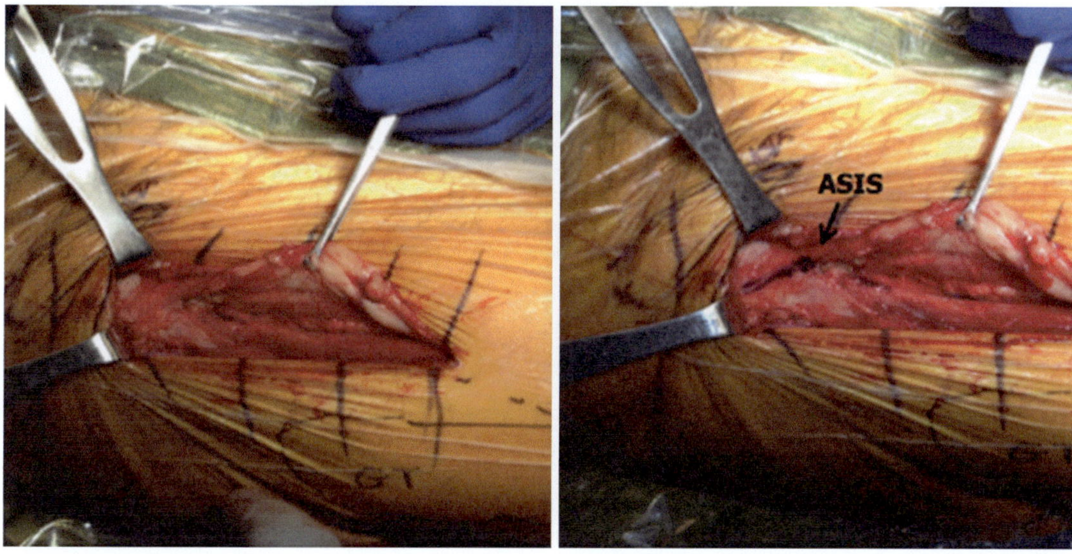

Fig. 11.22 With slight proximal extension of the incision, the leading edge of the TFL can be identified at the ASIS and carefully released for approximately 1–2 cm. Ensure a cuff of tendon for later repair

preoperative assessment. Radiographic signs that a more extensive release will be required include those factors where the femur starts closer to the pelvis, such as a short neck, protrusio, a wide pelvic flare with wide iliac crest, and relatively narrow ischium. In addition, body habitus traits such as obesity, large muscular young males, or previous trauma may require more extensive releases, although each case should be performed in a stepwise consistent manner. In rare cases, again especially in young muscular males or where there has been previous injury or scarring, one can consider

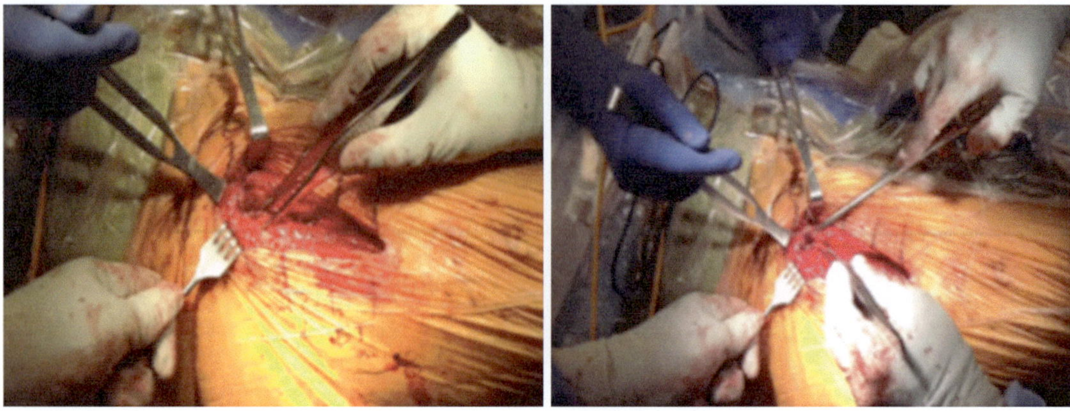

Fig. 11.23 The tendinous cuff of the reflected TFL can be repaired directly or through drill holes in the crest

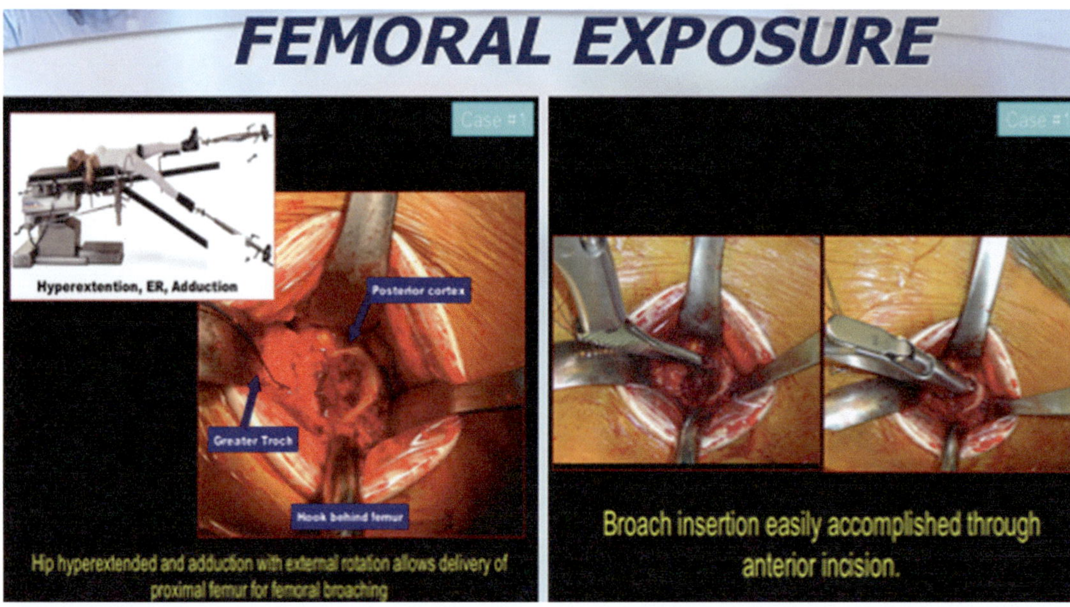

Fig. 11.24 Proper exposure of the femur for preparation. No attempts at broaching the canal should be attempted prior to adequate exposure

a release of the TFL from its origin on the iliac crest. This maneuver can also be useful in revision surgery. This release is performed using electrocautery, peeling the tendonous leading edge of the TFL off the iliac crest 1 cm to 2 cm posteriorly, leaving a cuff of the tendon for repair (Figs. 11.22 and 11.23, Videos 11.6, 11.7, and 11.8). Alternatively, the cuff can be repaired through drill holes in the crest.

Broaching of the femur should only begin when adequate exposure has been obtained (Fig. 11.24).

The proximal femur should be lateralized away from the pelvis, elevated into the wound beyond the acetabulum, and rotated such that the calcar should be pointing to the ceiling (Fig. 11.25).

At this point, the femur can be prepared. A canal sounder can be placed manually to define canal orientation to avoid canal perforation or varus placement of the broaches with potential fracture of the calcar (Fig. 11.26a, b).

A box osteotome can also be used to open the proximal canal typically directed along the poste-

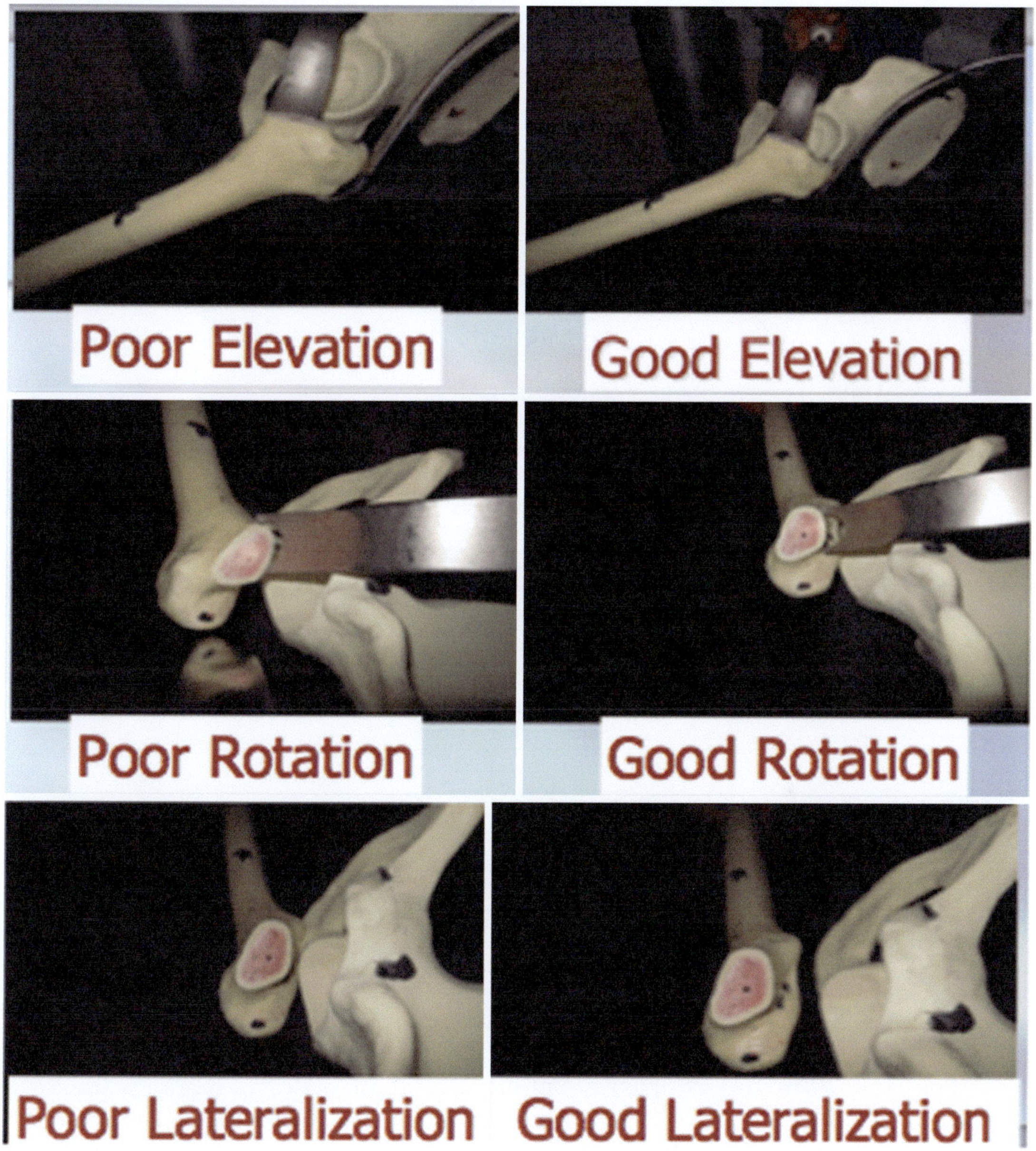

Fig. 11.25 Schematic of correct femoral positioning relative to the pelvis

rior border of the calcar and toward the apex of the calcar (Fig. 11.27). Care should be taken to account for the normal anteversion and anterior position of the neck relative to the shaft of the femur to prevent inadvertent removal of anterior metaphyseal bone by starting the broach too anteriorly initially (Fig. 11.28).

A Rongeur or rasp can be employed to remove any remaining lateral neck remnant to prevent varus positioning of the broaches and stem (Fig. 11.29).

Dual offset type handles in an attempt to compensate for poor exposure can lead to wallowing out of the proximal femur (Fig. 11.31a–c) or

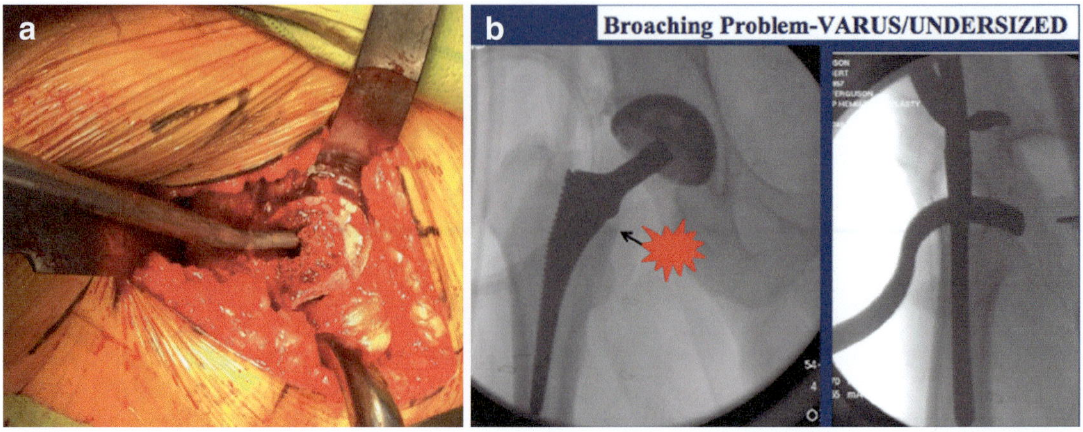

Fig. 11.26 (**a**, **b**) The correct plane of the femoral canal must be identified. Forced broaching with inadequate femoral exposure, or in obese patients with a protuberant abdomen, out-of-plane broaching can result in perforation or fracture

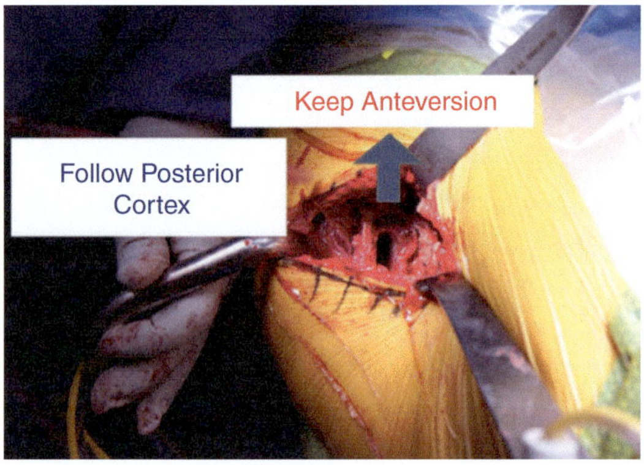

Fig. 11.27 Maintain proper version by following the posterior cortex and directed toward the apex of the calcar

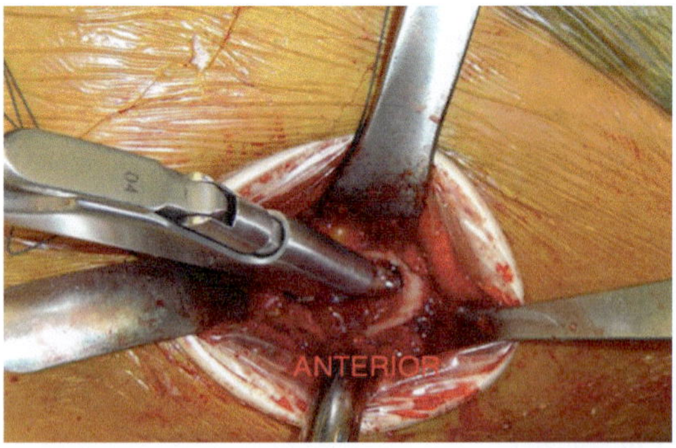

Fig. 11.28 The broach should be started in a relative posterior position along the posterior cortex to ensure placement down the canal

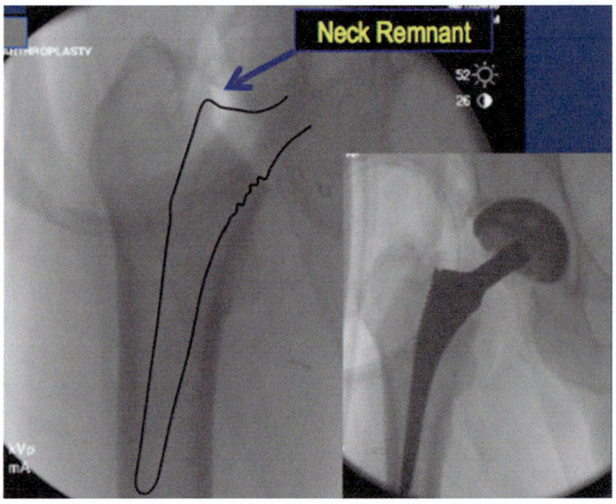

Fig. 11.29 Ensure proper lateralization by removing any lateral neck remnant. Broaching then begins to the templated size, typically plus or minus one size. It is very important to template preoperatively to determine approximate stem size, as well as the appropriate stem choice, based on the patient's anatomy. While most surgeons are comfortable using a particular stem for most of their cases, there is not one stem that can always be used 100% of the time. Broach-only stems are most commonly used, but in door type A canals, distal reaming may be required to prevent distal potting with unintended lengthening or inadvertent fracture. Broaching must not be forced, and I advocate the use of straight broach handles in order to perform consistent high fidelity broaching with force imparted in a single plane (Fig. 11.30)

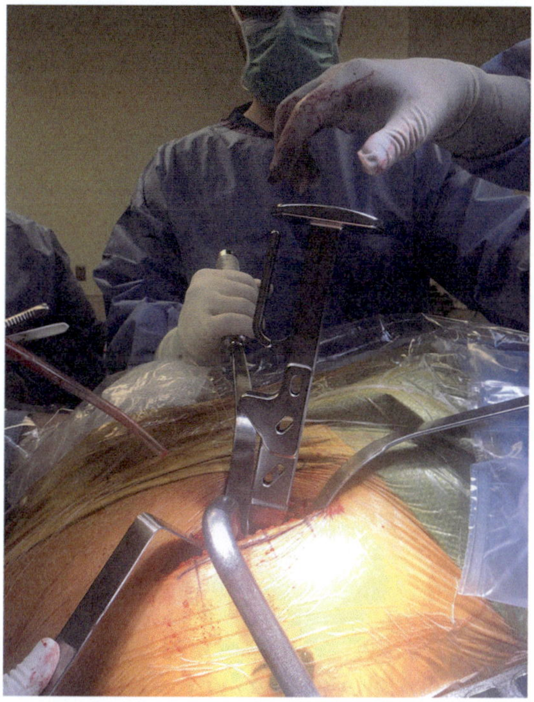

Fig. 11.30 Straight broach handle

rasping away the anterior metaphysis, especially when offset forces are applied to the broach handle with broach removal.

In addition, to avoid varus alignment or posterior perforation, the broach handle should always be directed with a slightly downward force to the floor and a medial force directed toward the patient's body. Once again, this should not be forced to avoid fracture of the greater trochanter. If canal perforation occurs, it is typically very proximal and posterior (Fig. 11.32).

By simply placing the broach in the correct plane, the defect can be bypassed, and no additional fixation is usually required as long as the rotational stability of the stem can be obtained. I typically try to sink the broach so that the lateral shoulder of the broach is sitting at the depth of the confluence of the lateral neck and base of the trochanter (saddle) and broach up until rotational stability is obtained (Fig. 11.33).

I try to not over counter-sync the broach and try to once again be consistent with high fidelity broaching. There are newer technologies, such

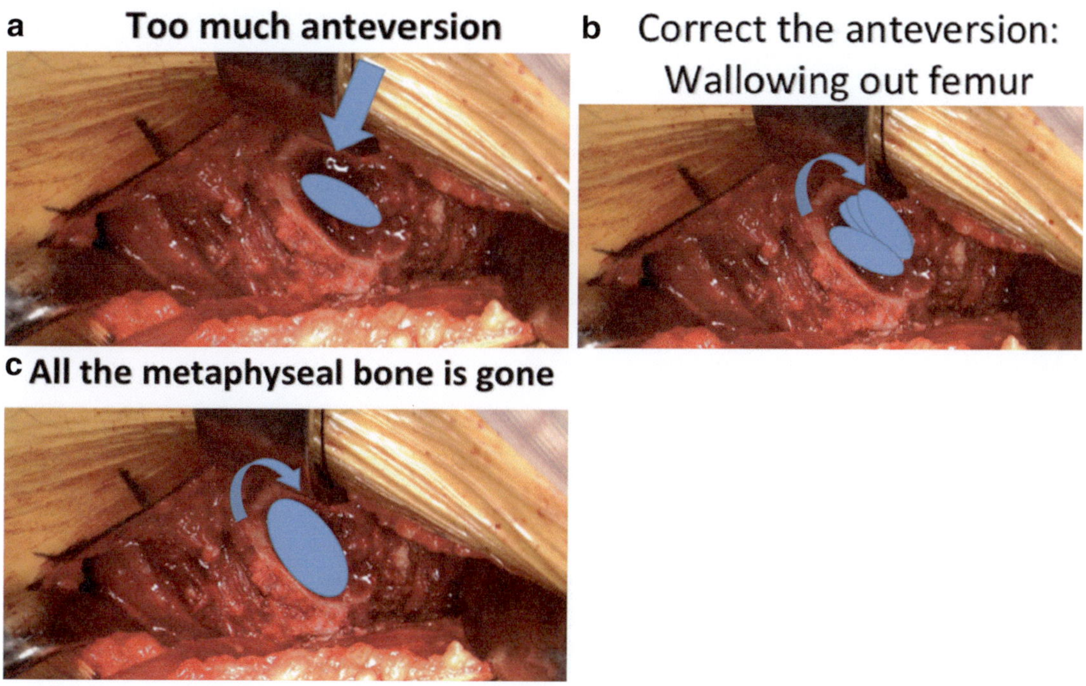

Fig. 11.31 (**a–c**) Inadvertent excessive removal of cancellous metaphyseal bone

as the Kincise, that may help in achieving more consistent broaching. I refrain from calcar planing until after trial reduction and fluoroscopic evaluation of stem positioning, fill, and leg length and offset. If I have not planed the femur, I can always adjust the stem up or down by up or downsizing the broach, as long as rotational stability and good fill of the metaphysis is obtained in a medial to lateral direction. Comparing the cut head/neck to the proposed trial head and neck can also be used as a check of appropriate trial size if the neck has not been planed (Fig. 11.34).

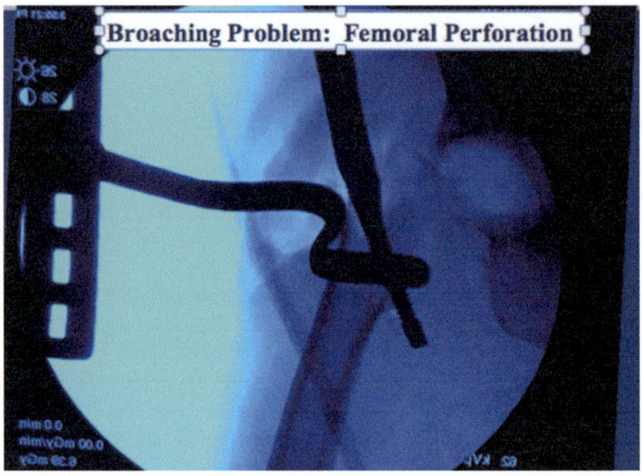

Fig. 11.32 Fluoroscopic image of typical proximal posterolateral perforation

If the final broach is difficult to remove and requires somewhat excessive blows to remove it from the stem, I would consider downsizing the stem or consider reaming distally to distal prevent potting of the stem or inadvertently having the stem sit high and adding additional leg length. After trialing, and prior to removal of the final broach, a twist test of the broach handle is performed to ensure rotational stability (Video 11.9). If rotation occurs, either broach larger if there is still room distally without diaphyseal impingement or consider using a different stem with a broader metaphyseal fill. Care should be taken during final stem insertion to avoid varus align-

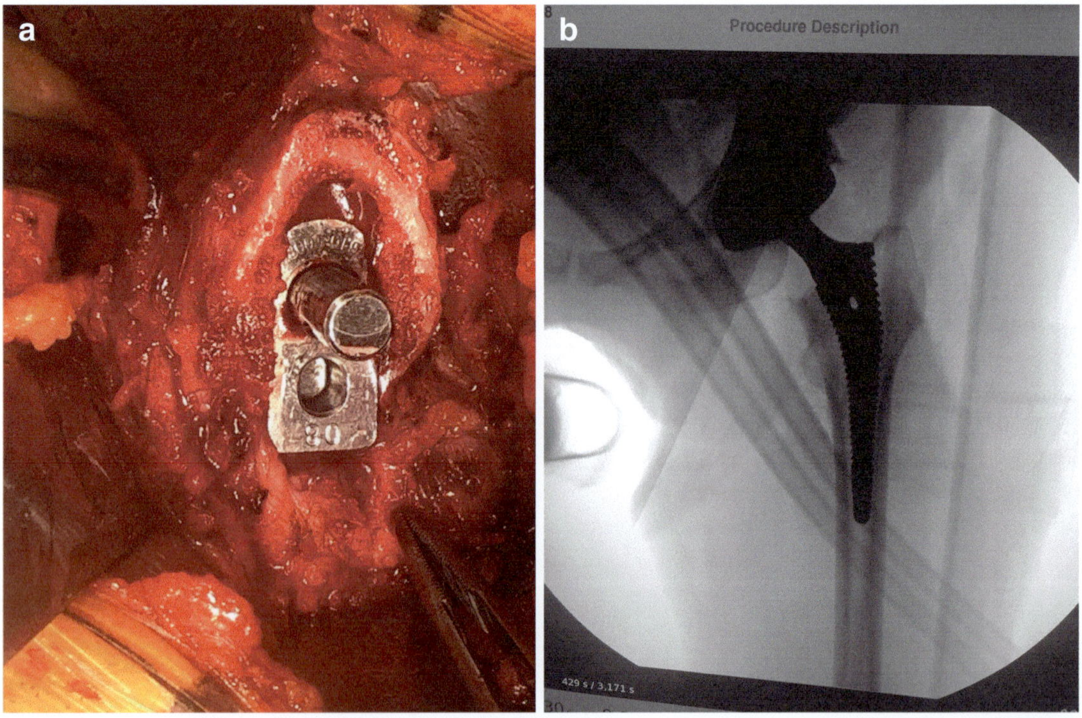

Fig. 11.33 Lateral edge of broach sitting flush with a saddle of the femur. This is a good starting point for trialing allowing up or downsizing easily as long as rotational stability is maintained. Note fill of canal and height of broach on AP x-ray (**a**) note lateral shoulder of broach is seated at the level of the saddle of the proximal femur; (**b**) placement of broach at this level typically results in appropriate neck length as evidenced by intraoperative fluoroscopic image

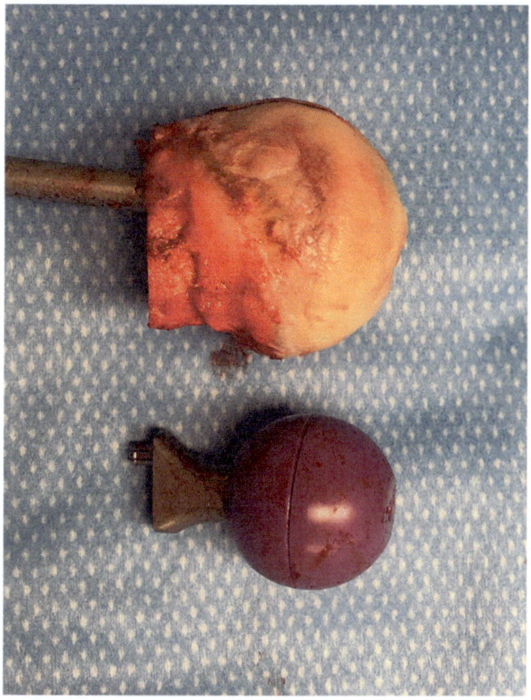

Fig. 11.34 Comparing the cut head neck height to the trial head and neck can give a good approximation of restored leg length and can be used as an additional check to the radiographic or navigational findings

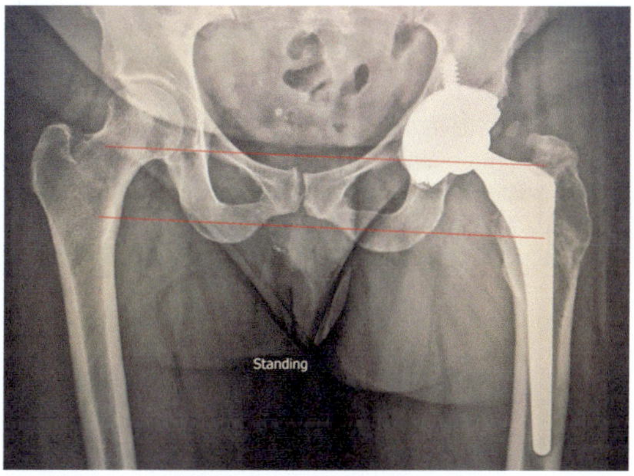

Fig. 11.35 Radiograph demonstrating marked lengthening due to poor stem positioning. The varus placement of the undersized stem resulted in the stem sitting too proud

ment or change in version prior to impaction to prevent fracture with forced impaction or the stem sitting proud with inadvertent lengthening (Fig. 11.35).

The reduction maneuver should be gentle, the retractors removed, and the leg is elevated to a neutral to a slightly flexed position.

The leg is then internally rotated to approximately 60–70 degrees to position the head beneath the rectus and prevent impingement. Gentle longitudinal traction is applied, and the femoral head is manually guided digitally into the socket as the leg is internally rotated to zero. The reduction should be gentle with perhaps a slight bump as the ball enters the acetabulum (Video 11.9). If a head pusher is required to force reduction or excessive traction is required, the hip is typically either too long or there is too much offset. Typically 32 mm and 36 mm head balls are used, and my preference is to try to achieve as much poly as possible, especially in younger active patients, than compromise poly thickness in order to upsize the head. Stability is typically not an issue. If leg length and offset have been restored radiographically during the trial maneuver, the hip should be stable. Conventional stability testing, such as the shuck test, is unnecessary during the DAA. With the leg in neutral extension, I typically will externally rotate the leg maximally to assess for posterior impingement. If the hip is unstable without achieving at least 90 degrees of external rotation, or if there is evidence of subluxation of the head at less than 90 degrees of external rotation, check for posterior osteophytes and reassess cup position with regard to anteversion and/or vertical placement, and anteversion of the stem. Also, critically reassess offset. Some advocate hyperextending the leg 20 degrees to 30 degrees and performing the same maneuver of external rotation to at least 90 degrees to once again assess stability. If there is instability with this maneuver, I would not artificially increase leg length or offset if they were restored radiographically. Find and fix the underlying etiology for the instability.

In summary, with patience and experience, essentially all cases of all total hip replacement cases can be done safely through an anterior approach. A solid understanding of the anatomy of the proximal femur with meticulous capsular management and serial sequential releases as necessary will greatly aid in accomplishing this goal.

References

1. Berend KR, Lombardi AV, Seng BE, Adams JB. Enhanced early outcomes with the anterior supine intermuscular approach in primary total hip arthroplasty. J Bone Joint Surg (Am). 2009;91(suppl 6):107–20.
2. Seng BE, Berend KR, Ajluni AF, Lombardi AV. Anterior-supine minimally invasive total hip arthroplasty: defining the learning curve. Orthop Clin North Am. 2009;40:343–50.
3. Schwartz BE, Sisko ZW, Mayekar EM, Wang OJ, Gordon AC. Transitioning to the direct anterior approach in total hip arthroplasty: is it safe in the current health care climate? J Arthroplast. 2016;31:2819–24.
4. Barnett SL, Peters DJ, Hamilton WG, Ziran NM, Gorab RS, Matta JM. Is the anterior approach safe? Early complication rate associated with 5090 consecutive primary total hip arthroplasty procedures performed using gthe anterior approach. J Arthroplast. 2016;31:2291–4.
5. Anterior Total Hip Arthroplasty Collaborative Investigators, Bhandari M, Matta J, et al. Outcomes following the single-incision anterior approach to total hip arthroplasty: a multicenter observational study. Orthop Clin North Am. 2009;40:329–42.
6. Cidambi KR, Barnett SL, Malette PR, Patel JJ, Na N, Gorab RS. Impact of femoral stem design on failure after anterior approach total hip arthroplasty. J Arthroplast. 2018;33:800–4.
7. Mirza AJ, Lombardi AV, Morris MJ, Berend KR. A mini-anterior approach to the hip for total joint replacement: optimizing results: improving hip joint replacement outcomes. Bone Joint J. 2014;96B:32–5.
8. Tamaki T, Jonishi K, Miura Y, Oinuma K, Shiratsuchi H. Cementless tapered-wedge length affects the risk of periprosthetic femoral fractures in direct anterior total hip arthroplasty. J Arthroplast. 2018;33:805–9.
9. Dietrich M, Kabelitz M, Dora C, Zingg PO. Perioperative fractures in cementless total hip arthroplasty using the direct anterior minimally invasive approach: reduced risk with short stems. J Arthroplast. 2018;33:548–54.
10. Lanting BA, Sm O, Cope RP, Patterson AH, Masonis JL. Incidence of perioperative events in single setting bilateral direct anterior approach total hip arthroplasty. J Arthroplast. 2015;30:465–7.
11. Zhoa HY, DeKang P, Xia YY, Shi XJ, Nie Y, Pei FX. Comparison of early functional recovery after total hip arthroplasty using a direct anterior or posterolateral approach: a randomized controlled trial. J Arthroplast. 2017;32:3421–8.
12. Alecci V, Valente M, Crucil M, Minerva M, Pellegrino CM, Sabbadini DD. Comparison of primary total hip replacements performed with a direct anterior approach versus the standard lateral approach: perioperative findings. J Orthop Traumatol. 2011;12:123–9.
13. Rodriguez JA, Deshmukh AJ, Rathod PA, et al. Does the direct anterior approach in THA offer faster rehabilitation and comparable safety to the posterior approach? Clin Orthop Relat Res. 2014;472:455–63.
14. Spaans AJ, Van Den Hout JAAM, Boldr SBT. High complication rate in the early experience of minimally invasive total hip arthroplasty by the direct anterior approach. Acta Orthop. 2012;83:342–6.
15. Nakata K, Nishikawa M, Yamamoto K, Hirota S, Yoshikawa H. A clinical comparative study of the direct anterior with mini-posterior approach: two consecutive series. J Arthroplast. 2009;24:698–704.
16. Sendtner E, Borowiak K, Schuster T, Woerner M, Grifka J, Renkawitz T. Tackling the learning curve: comparison between the anterior, minimally invasive (micro-hip) and the lateral, transgluteal(Bauer) approach for primary total hip replacement. Arch Orthop Trauma Surg. 2011;131:597–602.
17. Malek IA, Royce G, Bhatti SU, et al. A comparison between the direct anterior and posterior approaches for total hip arthroplasty: the role of an "enhanced recovery" pathway. Bone Joint J. 2016;98-B:754–60.
18. Cohen EM, Vaughn JJ, Ritterman SA, et al. Intraoperative femur fracture risk during primary direct anterior approach cementless total hip arthroplasty with and without a fracture table. J Artthroplasty. 2017;32:2847–51.
19. York PJ, Logterman SL, Hak DJ, Mavrogenis A, Mauffrey C. Orthopaedic trauma surgeons and direct anterior total hip arthroplasty: evaluation of learning curve at a level I academic institution. Eur J Orthop Surg Traumatol. 2017;27:421–4.
20. Zawadsky MW, Paulus MC, Murray PJ, Johansen MA. Early outcome comparison between the direct anterior approach and the mini-incision posterior approach for primary total hip arthroplasy: 150 consecutive cases. J Arthroplast. 2014;29:1256–60.
21. deSteiger RN, Lorimer M, Solomon M. What is the learning curve for the anterior approach for total hip arthroplasty? Clin Orthop Relat Res. 2015;473:3860–6.
22. Degeest T, Fennema P, Lenaerts G, DeLoore G. Adverse effects associated with the direct anterior approach for total hip arthroplasty: a Bayesian meta-analysis. Arch Orthop Trauma Surg. 2015;135:1183–92.
23. Lee GC, Marconi D. Complications following direct anterior hip procedures: costs to both patients and surgeons. J Arthroplast. 2015;30:98–101.
24. Eto S, Hwang K, Huddleston JI, Amanatullah DF, Maloney WJ, Goodman SB. The direct anterior approach is associated with early revision total hip arthroplasty. J Arthroplast. 2017;32:1001–5.
25. Brun O-CL, Mansson L, Nordsletten L. The direct anterior minimal invasive approach in total hip replacement: a prospective departmental study on the learning curve. Hip Int. 2018;28:156–60.
26. Meneghini RM, et al. Direct anterior approach: risk factor for early femoral failure of cementless total hip

arthroplasty: a multicenter study. J Bone Joint Surg. 2017;99:99–105.
27. Ponzio DY, Poulsides LA, Salvatore A, Lee YY, Memtsoudis SG, Alexiades MM. In-hospital morbidity and postoperative revisions after direct anterior vs posterior total hip arthroplasty. J Arthroplast. 2018;33:1421–5.
28. Homma Y, Baba T, Kobayashi H, et al. Safety in early experience with a direct anterior approach using fluoroscopic guidance with manual leg control for primary total hip arthroplasty: a consecutive one hundred and twenty case series. Int Orthop. 2016;40:2487–94.
29. Kobayashi H, Homma Y, Baba T, et al. Surgeons changing the approach for total hip arthroplasty from posterior to direct anterior with fluoroscopy should consider potential excessive cup anteversion and flexion implantation of the stem in their early experience. Int Orthop. 2016;40:1813–9.
30. Barrett WP, Turner SE, Leopold JP. Prospective randomized study of direct anterior vs postero-lateral approach for total hip arthroplasty. J Arthroplast. 2013;28:1634–8.
31. Matsuura M, Ohashi H, Okamoto Y, Inori F, Okijima Y. Elevation of the femur in THA through a direct anterior approach: cadaver and clinical studies. Clin Orthop Relat Res. 2010;468:3201–6.

Diagnosing and Managing Complications from the Anterior Approach

12

Samuel W. Carlson and Michael J. Taunton

Introduction

Each surgical approach employed for THA is associated with unique risks and complications in addition to the general risks of THA. The popularity of THA through the direct anterior approach (DATHA) is increasing due to several purported advantages, including shorter hospital stays, quicker recovery, reduced narcotic consumption, and reduced dislocation rates [1–4]. While the advantages of DATHA are numerous, it is not without risk, and there are several complications unique to the DATHA.

For surgeons experienced with DATHA, overall rates of complications associated with the approach are similar to complication rates for all THA surgical approaches [5]. Multiple studies have attempted to investigate the learning curve associated with DATHA, with studies reporting various case numbers, ranging from 10 to 100, representing the learning curve [4, 6–9]. In a multicenter observational study of DATHA, Bhandahari et al. demonstrate a two-fold increase in complication rates associated with surgeons who had performed less than 100 cases compared to surgeons who performed 100 or more DATHAs [6]. The overall rate of reoperation in this study was 2.7%, which is comparable to published complication rates for other THA approaches. Seng et al. studied a surgeon's initial experience with DATHA and reported a learning curve of 6 months and 37 cases, after which blood loss, operating room time, and approach-related complications decreased [7]. The complication rate over the entirety of this study period was no different for the implementation of the DATHA than it was for the surgeon's traditional surgical approach. Hart et al. studied 30-day major and minor complications following total hip arthroplasty performed through direct anterior, lateral, and posterior approaches [2]. Following multivariable regression analysis, no significant differences in 30-day major and minor complications existed between the three different THA approaches.

The purpose of this chapter is to examine the intraoperative and postoperative complications associated with DATHA, how they are diagnosed, and how they are managed.

S. W. Carlson
Mayo Clinic, Rochester, MN, USA

M. J. Taunton (✉)
Hip & Knee Reconstructive Surgery, Mayo Clinic, Rochester, MN, USA
e-mail: taunton.michael@mayo.edu

J. M. Matta, A. P. Sah (eds.), *Anterior Hip Replacement*,
https://doi.org/10.1007/978-3-030-91896-5_12

Intraoperative Complications

Neurologic Complications

Lateral Femoral Cutaneous Nerve Injury

The most common and frequently discussed neurologic complication associated with DATHA is injury to the lateral femoral cutaneous nerve (LFCN). The LFCN is a purely sensory nerve that emerges from the lumbar plexus and travels along the lateral border of the psoas, superficial to the iliacus, and emerges superficial to the deep inguinal ligament, traveling between the sartorius and the tensor fascia lata (TFL) in the thigh. Injury to the LFCN typically occurs during the approach, as it is encountered in the interval between the sartorius and the TFL. The true incidence of injury to the LFCN is unknown, but reports in the literature can range from 2% to 81% depending on the study [6, 10, 11]. Injury to the LFCN is usually in the form of neurapraxia resulting from compression with retractor placement or scar tissue formation, as well as the stretch from patient positioning. It is important to know that the branching pattern of the nerve is variable [12]. Injury to the nerve can also result from laceration to the main branch of the LFCN or to its subsidiary branches. Symptoms of LFCN injury include numbness or paresthesias of the anterolateral thigh, and, in the worst-case scenario, dysesthesias.

Diagnosis of LFCN injury can be difficult for surgeons as there is significant variability in symptoms among patients. Certain questionnaires, such as the DN4 questionnaire, exist to examine the severity of peripheral nerve injury [10]. However, one can diagnose LFCN injury simply by asking patients if they have symptoms consistent with LFCN injury as described above. Preoperative counseling to explain the symptoms as a known—and common—complication of DATHA is important to ensure patients aren't surprised by the symptoms postoperatively.

Treatment of LFCN injury is observation and symptomatic management. Goulding et al. reported that 67% of 55 patients who underwent primary DATHA demonstrated symptoms consistent with LFCN injury with no effect on functional outcomes [11]. In this study, only three of the patients reported complete resolution of their symptoms at the final follow-up [11]. Gala et al. described 77 patients who underwent primary DATHA or hip resurfacing through a direct anterior approach [10]. Fifty-five patients still reported some anterolateral thigh symptoms at a mean 5.5-year follow-up, and 22 patients (27%) demonstrated complete resolution of symptoms. Regardless of whether a patient still expressed anterolateral thigh symptoms, patients still had a statistically significant improvement in their preoperative pain scores and a significant improvement in their postoperative function. Patton et al. described 768 hips that underwent DATHA, with 24% reporting neuropathic pain before a minimum 2-year follow-up and only 11% reporting neuropathic symptoms at 6–8-year follow-up, demonstrating a statistically significant reduction [13]. Neuropathic symptoms had no effect on clinical outcomes following DATHA. This study further demonstrated limited improvement in symptoms at 1 year postoperatively but continued improvement over time [13]. While the majority of the literature demonstrates low rates of LFCN following DATHA and low rates of functional impairment or decreases in quality of life, Homma et al. and Ozaki et al. described reduced quality of life in patients with persistent neuropathic pain following DATHA [14, 15].

Femoral Nerve Injury

Femoral nerve (FN) injury following THA is rare, with various studies in the literature reporting rates ranging from 0.01% to 2.27% [16–23]. Multiple studies have demonstrated increased rates of FN injury with DATHA. Fleischman et al. demonstrated an incidence of 0.21% among all patients undergoing THA at their institution from 2011 to 2016 and an incidence of 0.4% for patients undergoing DATHA and 0.64% for patients undergoing anterolateral THA [23]. The authors also note an increase in the incidence of femoral nerve injury in DATHA over time, with an incidence of 0.29% from 2011 to 2013 and 0.57% from 2014 to 2016. Ishimatsu et al. reported the intraoperative status of the femoral nerve in patients undergoing DATHA and 77% of patients experienced a reduction of femoral nerve conduction amplitude after placement of the anterior acetabular retractor, but the femoral nerve conduction amplitude improved by the end of the procedure [24]. None of the patients in the Ishimatsu study experienced neurologic impairment postoperatively.

With DATHA, injury to the FN can occur due to compression or direct injury from retractors, stretch injury with hip extension and anterior femoral retraction, postoperative hematoma, or laceration. Cadaveric studies have shown the shortest distance from the acetabulum to the femoral nerve is 16.6 mm from the anterior rim of the acetabulum [24]. Symptoms following FN injury include reduced quadriceps strength and anteromedial thigh numbness or paresthesias. Initial evaluation may be cross-sectional imaging to identify a compressing lesion such as a hematoma or a laceration. If femoral nerve function does not return in the absence of other findings, electromyography or nerve conduction studies may be helpful to confirm the diagnosis after a few weeks. Consultation with a neurologist or peripheral nerve surgeon may be helpful in these situations.

FN palsy is typically treated with observation and symptomatic treatment. Physical therapy, gait aids, and braces such as a knee-ankle-foot orthosis can be used to assist with motor and functional deficits. Gait aids and gait training are important for these patients as they are at increased risk for falling, which could result in subsequent complications such as dislocations or periprosthetic fractures. In specific cases, such as FN palsy from a postoperative hematoma, surgical management may be required to decompress the FN. FN palsy is associated with a better prognosis than other nerve palsies, such as sciatic nerve palsy, which is a complication associated with posterior approaches to the hip and avoided by DATHA. Simmons et al. reported an incidence of femoral nerve palsy of 2.3% during 440 consecutive THAs over a 1-year period [25]. All patients in this series recovered fully within 1 year postoperatively [25]. Fleischman et al. reported that motor weakness had resolved in 75% of 36 patients with femoral nerve palsies by 33.3 months and recovery did not occur for a majority of patients until at least 6 months postoperatively [23]. At final follow-up, 40% required the use of an assisted device and sensory symptoms had not resolved in more than 80% of patients with femoral nerve palsy. Therefore, while it is a rare complication, it is a complication that can produce devastating consequences for patients.

Pudendal Nerve Injury

Pudendal nerve (PN) injury in DATHA can occur when providers utilize a traction Table. PN injury results from stretch due to excessive and prolonged traction on the operative leg or due to compression against an inadequately padded perineal post. Diagnosis of PN injury is a clinical diagnosis with signs and symptoms consisting of numbness and paresthesias in the perineum and sexual dysfunction. Sexual dysfunction following DATHA with a traction table has been reported in the literature and has been shown to resolve within weeks to months [26, 27]. Treatment of PN injury is with observation and symptomatic management.

Intraoperative Femur Fracture

Intraoperative femur fracture (IFF) is a well-described complication of all THA—regardless of the surgical approach [28–32]. IFF is more common in uncemented THA than in cemented THA, with the incidence for uncemented THA ranging from 2.95% to 27.8% compared to 0.3% to 1.2% for cemented THA [30–32]. An increased rate of IFFs has been reported as a common complication associated with DATHA [33, 34]. Reasons for the increased rate of IFFs include some surgeons' preference to utilize fracture tables during DATHA and learning the necessary techniques for femoral preparation and femoral stem insertion unique to DATHA. The frequency of IFFs in DATHA reported in the literature varies from 0.8% to 7%, with most reports demonstrating a decrease in frequency with increasing surgeon experience [4, 35–39].

Intraoperative femur fractures occur in various forms ranging from nondisplaced fractures of the calcar that are common with cementless THA regardless of approach, to displaced femoral shaft fractures requiring open reduction and internal fixation. As with all THA, the femur must be adequately exposed to allow for safe femoral preparation and stem insertion. For the DATHA, this can be one of the most challenging aspects of the exposure. One technique to assist with this aspect of the approach is to use a fracture table that allows the surgeon to extend the operative leg and place an instrument under the femur to elevate the femur, providing sufficient exposure for the surgeon [40]. The original paper discussing DATHA with the use of a fracture table reported a fracture rate of 1.8% in 494 consecutive DATHAs [40]. Among the IFFs, 3 were greater trochanter fractures, 2 femoral shaft fractures, and 4 calcar fractures. The literature reports the incidence of IFF with the use of a fracture table to range from 0.8% to 6.5%, while the incidence of IFF with a standard OR table ranges from 1% to 7% [4, 35–39]. Cohen et al. performed a retrospective review of 472 consecutive patients who underwent DATHA over a 1-year period by two experienced DATHA surgeons—one of whom utilizes a fracture table while the other surgeons utilize a standard OR table [41]. There were 12 intraoperative femur fractures: 6 fractures occurred using the fracture table and 6 occurred with the standard OR table for a rate of 2.2% and 2.8%, respectively. No statistically significant difference was observed. Hartford et al. performed a retrospective review of 500 primary DATHAs performed by a single surgeon with a fracture table in all cases [38]. There were 13 IFFs (2.6%), and the rate of IFF decreased after the first 100 patients [38]. Masonis et al. reviewed complications of the first 300 DATHAs and reported IFFs in the first 62 cases and none in the remaining 238 [35]. Jewett and Collis reviewed complications of the first 800 DATHAs and found the majority of their intraoperative fractures were in the first 200 cases [36]. For all THA, the rate of IFF increases with uncemented THA, stem design, and certain patient factors such as osteoporosis. Some studies have demonstrated increased rates of IFF with DATHA compared to other hip approaches, but most of the DATHA complications data examine a surgeon's initial experience with DATHA and include the learning curve. However, with experience, the incidence of IFF in DATHA decreases to rates comparable to other surgical approaches.

Diagnosis of an IFF requires the surgeon to maintain vigilance and a high degree of suspicion during femoral preparation and stem insertion. With the positioning of the femur during DATHA, increased stress is placed on the greater trochanter, which can result in an IFF. Furthermore, delivering the femur with or without the use of a fracture table can result in proximal femur fractures that can extend distally. Lastly, as with all other surgical hip approaches, when inserting an uncemented stem, calcar fractures can occur due to increased hoop stresses at the level of the calcar during broaching or stem insertion. If one is suspicious for an IFF, extending one's exposure to better examine the femur and obtaining an intraoperative radiograph to check for fracture lines is essential. The DA approach can be extended distally, and it can be used to treat both IFFs and postoperative periprosthetic fractures [42, 43]. If adequate exposure with the extensile DA approach cannot be obtained, converting to a standard lateral approach to the femur can be performed. Treatment options for the above-listed fractures are the same through the DA approach as they are for any other surgical approach. Greater trochanter fractures can either be treated nonoperatively or with open reduction and internal fixation with plates and screws or various forms of wires or heavy suture. Calcar fractures are treated as they would be with any other surgical approach: cerclage wires or cables with or without modified weight-bearing postoperatively. Proximal femur fractures that extend distally are treated with open reduction and internal fixation following routine fracture treatment principles.

Component Malposition

Instability following THA remains one of the predominant causes of early failure and revision.

One of the concerns with DATHA is the ability to obtain adequate acetabular exposure and the possibility for component malposition leading to an increased risk of instability and dislocation [33, 36, 37]. However, one of the advantages of DATHA is performing the procedure in the supine position and the ease with which intraoperative fluoroscopy can be utilized. Lin et al. compared radiographic outcomes between DATHA and THA performed from a posterior approach with intraoperative fluoroscopy and found that there was a lower percentage of patients in the posterior group with acceptable acetabular inclination angles [44]. There was no difference between the two groups in terms of acetabular anteversion, leg length, or offset. Brun et al. performed a randomized controlled trial comparing radiographic outcomes of component placement through the direct lateral approach compared to the DATHA [45]. The degrees of both cup inclination and anteversion were significantly higher in the DATHA group; however, the differences in the means between the two groups are unlikely to be clinically significant as both means fall within the acceptable range of anteversion. There was no difference in leg length, femoral stem position, or offset between the two groups. There were no dislocations in either group at 2-year follow-up [45].

While fluoroscopy has been shown to improve component position in THA, successful results with DATHA can still be achieved without fluoroscopy [46]. Bingham et al. investigated whether the use of intraoperative fluoroscopy significantly improved acetabular cup position and leg length discrepancy by retrospectively comparing radiographic outcomes of DATHA performed by one surgeon who employs intraoperative fluoroscopy and another surgeon who does not use intraoperative fluoroscopy [47]. The authors found no statistically significant difference with regard to postoperative leg length discrepancy and differences in component anteversion or inclination. Both surgeons included in this analysis are fellowship trained, high-volume arthroplasty surgeons at academic institutions, and therefore the results may not be generalizable. As a result, and due to the ease with which intraoperative fluoroscopy can be utilized with the DATHA, it is recommended that a surgeon either learning the DATHA or early in one's practice utilizes intraoperative fluoroscopy to minimize the risk of component malpositioning.

Postoperative Complications

Instability and Dislocation

One of the purported advantages of DATHA is a decreased risk of postoperative instability and dislocation [1]. This advantage is the result of leaving the posterior capsule and short external rotators intact during the surgical approach. With modern posterior approaches (PA) that involve meticulous soft tissue repair, dislocation rates are oftentimes quoted to range from 1% to 2% at one-year follow-up [48–50]. The consequences of instability can be devastating to patients, potentially resulting in revision surgery. Therefore, by reducing the risk of postoperative instability and dislocations, DATHA can provide a substantial benefit to patients.

The reported dislocation rates following DATHA typically range from 0.6% to 3.0% [6, 51–53]. In a large meta-analysis incorporating 38 studies with 11,810 DATHAs with an average follow-up of 18 months, the overall dislocation rate was 1.2% [48]. In studies directly comparing the postoperative dislocation rates of DATHA versus other hip approaches, DATHA either compares favorably or demonstrates no difference compared to other approaches. Fleischman et al. compared the rates of mechanical complications following THA based on the surgical approach [54]. This study demonstrated a dislocation rate with DATHA of 0.6% at 90 days and 0.74% at 2 years, which compared favorably to the dislocation rate for PATHA of 1.4% and 1.7% at 90 days and 2 years, respectively [54]. Sheth et al. utilized a large insurance database to analyze the dislocation rates of 22,237 THAs stratified by the hip approach. THAs performed from a PA demonstrated a dislocation rate of 1.4% compared to 0.8% for DATHA, and there was no significant difference between the two groups with respect to the overall complication rate [55]. In a similar study employing a large insurance database to compare dislocation rates between DATHA and PATHA at 2-year follow-up, DATHA demonstrated a significantly lower dislocation rate of 0.84% compared to 2% for PATHA [56]. Few studies have examined the long-term dislocation rates following DATHA. Berry et al. reported the cumulative risk of first-time dislocation for patients who underwent primary Charnley THA at a single institution from 1969 to 1984 and reported a risk of 1% at 1 month, 1.9% at 1 year, and a 1% increase in cumulative risk every 5 years to 7% at 25 years [50]. Tamaki et al. investigated the cumulative mid-term risk of dislocation following DATHA in 871 hips and reported a dislocation rate of 0.69% at 1 month, 0.80% at 1 year, and 0.93% at 5 years [51].

While the approach employed by a surgeon certainly influences the risk of postoperative instability and dislocation, there are many other variables that affect postoperative instability. One such variable that influences postoperative stability is component positioning. As discussed earlier, one of the initial concerns with DATHA was the risk for component malposition due to limited exposure. However, as the previous section highlighted, there is no difference in rates of component malpositioning between the DATHA and other surgical approaches. Furthermore, DATHA facilitates the use of intraoperative fluoroscopy, allowing one to check one's positioning and make whatever necessary adjustments are required. In a double-blinded randomized controlled trial, Brun et al. found no significant differences in component positioning between patients who underwent DATHA and those who underwent direct lateral THA, and no dislocations occurred at 2-year follow-up in either group [45]. Tripuranemi et al. performed a retrospective matched cohort analysis comparing acetabular abduction and anteversion angles and dislocation rates between patients who underwent PATHA and DATHA. There was no statistically significant difference between the two groups with respect to abduction or anteversion angles [57]. The dislocation rate in the PATHA group was 1.5% and 3.0% for the DATHA group [57].

Dislocations following DATHA are typically anterior dislocations, but dislocations can still occur in any direction [3]. Diagnosis of periprosthetic dislocation is with physical exam and orthogonal radiographs. Treatment of a dislocated DATHA is the same as for any periprosthetic dislocation. First-time dislocations can be treated with closed versus open reduction. As with all other THAs, recurrent instability deserves further work-up for an underlying cause of the instability. Recurrent instability could be the result of many variables, including patient and surgical factors. A more thorough review of recurrent instability is outside the scope of this chapter. Revision surgery to correct the majority of underlying causes of recurrent instability can be treated through the DA approach.

Wound Complications

Due to the location of the incision, DATHA is associated with an increased risk of postoperative wound complications requiring reoperation [36]. The skin over the anterior thigh is thinner, which decreases its healing potential. Furthermore, the skin in this area is susceptible to more shear stresses, increasing the risk of dehiscence and decreasing the healing potential. The incision is frequently close to—or through—the inguinal crease, a moist environment that lends itself to bacterial growth and a difficult healing environment. In obese patients, skin folds from the abdomen frequently overlap with the skin incision, further complicating the healing environment [58]. Christensen et al. compared 1288 primary PATHAs to 505 DATHAs and demonstrated a statistically significant greater number of wound complications requiring reoperation with the DATHA (0.2% vs. 1.4%) [59]. Jewett and Collis reported a rate of wound complications requiring reoperation with DATHA of 1.6% [36]. Statz et al. retrospectively reviewed 1573 DATHAs performed at a single institution and reported a wound complication rate of 1.1% [58]. Fortunately, none of the patients with wound complications were found to have a deep infection, and none required head and liner exchanges.

The authors also demonstrate a statistically significant increased rate of wound complications in females and obese patients [58]. An increased risk of wound complications in obese patients undergoing DATHA is well established [60–63]. Watts et al. reported a 1.7% rate of wound complications in 716 DATHAs compared to 1.9% for PATHAs performed at a single institution, and obesity was found to be a stronger risk factor for wound complications in DATHA than for PATHA [61]. Purcell et al. reviewed 4651 primary THAs performed by the PA and the DA at a single institution [62]. The rate of wound complications in nonobese DATHA compared to nonobese PATHA was significantly increased at 1.7% compared to 0.3%, respectively [62]. There was no statistically significant difference in the rate of wound complications between obese DATHA compared to obese PATHA, and there was no difference in reoperations due to wound complications between DATHA and PATHA regardless of BMI [62].

Diagnosis of wound complications is a clinical diagnosis. One can reduce the risk of wound complications following DATHA with meticulous surgical technique, respect for skin and soft tissues, meticulous wound closure, and protecting the incision from shear forces during the first several weeks postoperatively. It is important to plan the surgical incision away from skin folds to the best of one's ability. If one cannot perform DATHA without placing the incision in a tenuous area, or if the incision will be compromised by abdominal skin folds, then we recommend utilizing a different surgical approach. If a wound complication is significant enough to warrant a reoperation and irrigation and debridement, one must interrogate the fascia to determine if the infection is a deep infection. If it is determined to be a deep infection, the fascia must be opened, cultures obtained, and a head and liner exchange performed. We utilize 24 hours of perioperative antibiotics with weight-based Cefazolin preferred. We typically keep patients on oral antibiotics for prophylaxis, usually cefadroxil or cephalexin, for 14 days until cultures result. If cultures turn positive, we recommend coordinating with an infectious disease team in order to ensure proper antibiotic coverage.

Aseptic Loosening

Data from large registry studies reveal that aseptic loosening remains one of the primary reasons for revision THA—regardless of surgical approach [64–67]. In a study examining reasons for revision after 4555 primary THAs performed at single institution, aseptic loosening was the second most common cause of implant revision [68]. Eto et al. reviewed 483 revision THAs performed at their institution and compared the rea sons for revision for THAs performed via a DA and those performed by all other THA approaches [69]. The authors found that aseptic loosening was a more common reason for revision in patients who underwent DATHA compared to all other THA approaches [69]. Meneghini et al. performed a retrospective review of 342 THAs who underwent revision THA and found an increased rate of aseptic loosening and revision for early femoral failure in patients who underwent DATHA compared to PATHA [34]. In contrast, Cidambi et al. reviewed 1120 THAs at a minimum 2-year follow-up who underwent primary DATHA at their institution [70]. There were 9 revisions in their cohort, 5 of which were for aseptic loosening of the femoral component, yielding a rate of femoral component loosening of only 0.5% in this cohort. Sheth et al. utilized a large Kaiser-Permanente database and found no statistically significant difference in rates of aseptic femoral loosening between DATHA (1.1%) and PATHA (1.9%) [55]. While the data comparing rates of aseptic loosening for DATHA compared to other THA approaches is inconclusive, aseptic loosening is a common cause of revision THA regardless of the surgical approach. Diagnosis of aseptic loosening is accomplished by serial radiographs. Patients oftentimes present with new and increased pain that is typically worse with weight-bearing activities. In patients who present with signs and symptoms consistent with aseptic loosening, it is imperative to rule out infection with an ESR and CRP and aspiration if clinically indicated. When infection has been ruled out, treatment of aseptic loosening in symptomatic patients consists of revision THA.

Postoperative Periprosthetic Femur Fracture

Postoperative periprosthetic femur fractures are common causes of THA failure regardless of surgical approach, with the incidence reported in the literature ranging from 0.47% to 7.1% and the Swedish National register reporting an annual incidence of 0.1% [32]. Periprosthetic femur fractures are devastating complications associated with increased mortality at 30 days and 1 year [71, 72]. Common risk factors for periprosthetic femur fracture include age, gender, and uncemented femoral components [73]. We previously described the risk of intraoperative femur fracture associated with DATHA. Several studies have reported early periprosthetic femur fracture as a common complication following DATHA [39]. Berend et al. reported 26 (0.9%) periprosthetic femur fractures in 2869 DATHAs at a mean of 35 days postoperatively and found increasing age was a significant risk factor [39]. Twenty-three of these fractures required revision THA, two required open reduction and internal fixation, and one was treated nonoperatively [39]. In a consecutive series of 500 DATHAs, Hartford reported a postoperative periprosthetic femur fracture incidence of 2% [38]. Meneghini et al. examined reasons for early femoral component failure and subsequent revision in 342 THAs performed at several academic centers [34]. The authors found the prevalence of periprosthetic femur fractures among the entire cohort was 11.7%. The incidence of periprosthetic femur fractures in patients who underwent DATHA was 17.8% compared to 6.2% for patients who underwent direct lateral THA and 10.8% for those who underwent PATHA. There was no statistically significant relationship between approach and incidence of periprosthetic femur fracture [34]. In a retrospective review comparing complications after DATHA versus anterolateral THA, there was no difference in rates of postoperative periprosthetic femur fractures [74]. In another retrospective review of 1967 primary THAs of various surgical approaches performed at a single institution, there was no difference in postoperative fractures at 30 days postoperatively between different surgical approaches [2].

Postoperative femur fractures result from trauma and are subsequently diagnosed with radiographs. Treatment of postoperative femur fractures depends on the fracture type, location, stability of the stem, and host bone stock remaining. Treatment can range from nonoperative management to proximal femoral replacement.

Conclusion

As with any surgical approach for THA, there are risks and benefits to performing DATHA. The benefits of DATHA are numerous and include shorter hospital stays, quicker functional recovery, and the potential for improved stability. The risks are also numerous and decrease as the surgeon's familiarity with the approach improves, at which point the risks of DATHA are different but equal to the risks of other approaches. When selecting an approach to utilize for THA, it is thus up to the surgeon to determine which risk profile one is most comfortable with and will provide patients with the best possible outcome.

References

1. Higgins BT, et al. Anterior vs. posterior approach for total hip arthroplasty, a systematic review and meta-analysis. J Arthroplast. 2015;30(3):419–34.
2. Hart A, et al. Thirty-day major and minor complications following total hip arthroplasty-a comparison of the direct anterior, lateral, and posterior approaches. J Arthroplast. 2019;34(11):2681–5.
3. Barton C, Kim PR. Complications of the direct anterior approach for total hip arthroplasty. Orthop Clin North Am. 2009;40(3):371–5.
4. Barnett SL, et al. Is the anterior approach safe? Early complication rate associated with 5090 consecutive primary total hip arthroplasty procedures performed using the anterior approach. J Arthroplast. 2016;31(10):2291–4.
5. Mjaaland KE, et al. Implant survival after minimally invasive anterior or anterolateral vs. conventional posterior or direct lateral approach: an analysis of 21,860 total hip arthroplasties from the Norwegian Arthroplasty Register (2008 to 2013). J Bone Joint Surg Am. 2017;99(10):840–7.

6. Bhandari M, et al. Outcomes following the single-incision anterior approach to total hip arthroplasty: a multicenter observational study. Orthop Clin North Am. 2009;40(3):329–42.
7. Seng BE, et al. Anterior-supine minimally invasive total hip arthroplasty: defining the learning curve. Orthop Clin North Am. 2009;40(3):343–50.
8. Stone AH, et al. Evaluation of the learning curve when transitioning from posterolateral to direct anterior hip arthroplasty: a consecutive series of 1000 cases. J Arthroplast. 2018;33(8):2530–4.
9. de Steiger RN, Lorimer M, Solomon M. What is the learning curve for the anterior approach for total hip arthroplasty? Clin Orthop Relat Res. 2015;473(12):3860–6.
10. Gala L, Kim PR, Beaule PE. Natural history of lateral femoral cutaneous nerve neuropraxia after anterior approach total hip arthroplasty. Hip Int. 2019;29(2):161–5.
11. Goulding K, et al. Incidence of lateral femoral cutaneous nerve neuropraxia after anterior approach hip arthroplasty. Clin Orthop Relat Res. 2010;468(9):2397–404.
12. Rudin D, et al. The anatomical course of the lateral femoral cutaneous nerve with special attention to the anterior approach to the hip joint. J Bone Joint Surg Am. 2016;98(7):561–7.
13. Patton RS, et al. Clinical outcomes of patients with lateral femoral cutaneous nerve injury after direct anterior total hip arthroplasty. J Arthroplast. 2018;33(9):2919–2926 e1.
14. Homma Y, et al. Lateral femoral cutaneous nerve injury with the direct anterior approach for total hip arthroplasty. Int Orthop. 2016;40(8):1587–93.
15. Ozaki Y, et al. Spontaneous healing of lateral femoral cutaneous nerve injury and improved quality of life after total hip arthroplasty via a direct anterior approach. J Orthop Surg (Hong Kong). 2017;25(1):2309499016684750.
16. Farrell CM, et al. Motor nerve palsy following primary total hip arthroplasty. J Bone Joint Surg Am. 2005;87(12):2619–25.
17. Eggli S, Hankemayer S, Muller ME. Nerve palsy after leg lengthening in total replacement arthroplasty for developmental dysplasia of the hip. J Bone Joint Surg Br. 1999;81(5):843–5.
18. Oldenburg M, Muller RT. The frequency, prognosis and significance of nerve injuries in total hip arthroplasty. Int Orthop. 1997;21(1):1–3.
19. van der Linde MJ, Tonino AJ. Nerve injury after hip arthroplasty. 5/600 cases after uncemented hip replacement, anterolateral approach versus direct lateral approach. Acta Orthop Scand. 1997;68(6):521–3.
20. Navarro RA, et al. Surgical approach and nerve palsy in total hip arthroplasty. J Arthroplast. 1995;10(1):1–5.
21. Nercessian OA, Macaulay W, Stinchfield FE. Peripheral neuropathies following total hip arthroplasty. J Arthroplast. 1994;9(6):645–51.
22. Schmalzried TP, Amstutz HC, Dorey FJ. Nerve palsy associated with total hip replacement. Risk factors and prognosis. J Bone Joint Surg Am. 1991;73(7):1074–80.
23. Fleischman AN, Rothman RH, Parvizi J. Femoral nerve palsy following total hip arthroplasty: incidence and course of recovery. J Arthroplast. 2018;33(4):1194–9.
24. Ishimatsu T, et al. Motor-evoked potential analysis of femoral nerve status during the direct anterior approach for total hip arthroplasty. J Bone Joint Surg Am. 2018;100(7):572–7.
25. Simmons C Jr, et al. Femoral neuropathy following total hip arthroplasty. Anatomic study, case reports, and literature review. J Arthroplast. 1991;6 Suppl:S57–66.
26. Vajapey SP, et al. Nerve injuries with the direct anterior approach to total hip arthroplasty. JBJS Rev. 2020;8(2):e0109.
27. Pailhe R, et al. Pudendal nerve neuralgia after hip arthroscopy: retrospective study and literature review. Orthop Traumatol Surg Res. 2013;99(7):785–90.
28. Scott RD, et al. Femoral fractures in conjunction with total hip replacement. J Bone Joint Surg Am. 1975;57(4):494–501.
29. Davidson D, et al. Intraoperative periprosthetic fractures during total hip arthroplasty. Evaluation and management. J Bone Joint Surg Am. 2008;90(9):2000–12.
30. Young PS, Patil S, Meek RMD. Intraoperative femoral fractures: prevention is better than cure. Bone Joint Res. 2018;7(1):103–4.
31. Schwartz JT Jr, Mayer JG, Engh CA. Femoral fracture during non-cemented total hip arthroplasty. J Bone Joint Surg Am. 1989;71(8):1135–42.
32. Berry DJ. Epidemiology: hip and knee. Orthop Clin North Am. 1999;30(2):183–90.
33. Flevas DA, Tsantes AG, Mavrogenis AF. Direct anterior approach total hip arthroplasty revisited. JBJS Rev. 2020;8(4):e0144.
34. Meneghini RM, et al. Direct anterior approach: risk factor for early femoral failure of cementless total hip arthroplasty: a multicenter study. J Bone Joint Surg Am. 2017;99(2):99–105.
35. Masonis J, Thompson C, Odum S. Safe and accurate: learning the direct anterior total hip arthroplasty. Orthopedics. 2008;31(12 Suppl 2)
36. Jewett BA, Collis DK. High complication rate with anterior total hip arthroplasties on a fracture table. Clin Orthop Relat Res. 2011;469(2):503–7.
37. Woolson ST, Pouliot MA, Huddleston JI. Primary total hip arthroplasty using an anterior approach and a fracture table: short-term results from a community hospital. J Arthroplast. 2009;24(7):999–1005.
38. Hartford JM, Knowles SB. Risk factors for perioperative femoral fractures: cementless femoral implants and the direct anterior approach using a fracture table. J Arthroplast. 2016;31(9):2013–8.
39. Berend KR, et al. Risk of periprosthetic fractures with direct anterior primary total hip arthroplasty. J Arthroplast. 2016;31(10):2295–8.
40. Matta JM, Shahrdar C, Ferguson T. Single-incision anterior approach for total hip arthroplasty on

an orthopaedic table. Clin Orthop Relat Res. 2005;441:115–24.
41. Cohen EM, et al. Intraoperative femur fracture risk during primary direct anterior approach cementless total hip arthroplasty with and without a fracture table. J Arthroplast. 2017;32(9):2847–51.
42. Thaler M, et al. Extension of the direct anterior approach for the treatment of periprosthetic femoral fractures. J Arthroplast. 2019;34(10):2449–53.
43. Nogler MM, Thaler MR. The direct anterior approach for hip revision: accessing the entire femoral diaphysis without endangering the nerve supply. J Arthroplast. 2017;32(2):510–4.
44. Lin TJ, et al. A comparison of radiographic outcomes after total hip arthroplasty between the posterior approach and direct anterior approach with intraoperative fluoroscopy. J Arthroplast. 2017;32(2):616–23.
45. Brun OL, et al. Component placement in direct lateral vs minimally invasive anterior approach in total hip arthroplasty: radiographic outcomes from a prospective randomized controlled trial. J Arthroplast. 2019;34(8):1718–22.
46. Beamer BS, et al. Does fluoroscopy improve acetabular component placement in total hip arthroplasty? Clin Orthop Relat Res. 2014;472(12):3953–62.
47. Bingham JS, et al. Does intraoperative fluoroscopy improve limb-length discrepancy and acetabular component positioning during direct anterior total hip arthroplasty? J Arthroplast. 2018;33(9):2927–31.
48. Lee GC, Marconi D. Complications following direct anterior hip procedures: costs to both patients and surgeons. J Arthroplast. 2015;30(9 Suppl):98–101.
49. Leichtle UG, et al. Dislocation after total hip arthroplasty: risk factors and treatment options. Acta Orthop Traumatol Turc. 2013;47(2):96–103.
50. Berry DJ, et al. The cumulative long-term risk of dislocation after primary Charnley total hip arthroplasty. J Bone Joint Surg Am. 2004;86(1):9–14.
51. Tamaki T, et al. Epidemiology of dislocation following direct anterior total hip arthroplasty: a minimum 5-year follow-up study. J Arthroplast. 2016;31(12):2886–8.
52. Sariali E, Leonard P, Mamoudy P. Dislocation after total hip arthroplasty using Hueter anterior approach. J Arthroplast. 2008;23(2):266–72.
53. Siguier T, Siguier M, Brumpt B. Mini-incision anterior approach does not increase dislocation rate: a study of 1037 total hip replacements. Clin Orthop Relat Res. 2004;426:164–73.
54. Fleischman AN, et al. Mechanical complications following Total hip arthroplasty based on surgical approach: a large, Single-Institution Cohort Study. J Arthroplasty. 2019;34(6):1255–60.
55. Sheth D, et al. Anterior and anterolateral approaches for THA are associated with lower dislocation risk without higher revision risk. Clin Orthop Relat Res. 2015;473(11):3401–8.
56. Charney M, et al. A comparison of risk of dislocation and cause-specific revision between direct anterior and posterior approach following elective cementless total hip arthroplasty. J Arthroplast. 2020;35(6):1651–7.
57. Tripuraneni KR, et al. Acetabular abduction and dislocations in direct anterior vs posterior total hip arthroplasty: a retrospective, Matched Cohort Study. J Arthroplasty. 2016;31(10):2299–302.
58. Statz JM, et al. Outcome of direct anterior total hip arthroplasty complicated by superficial wound dehiscence requiring irrigation and debridement. J Arthroplast. 2019;34(7):1492–7.
59. Christensen CP, Karthikeyan T, Jacobs CA. Greater prevalence of wound complications requiring reoperation with direct anterior approach total hip arthroplasty. J Arthroplast. 2014;29(9):1839–41.
60. Jahng KH, et al. Risk factors for wound complications after direct anterior approach hip arthroplasty. J Arthroplast. 2016;31(11):2583–7.
61. Watts CD, et al. High risk of wound complications following direct anterior total hip arthroplasty in obese patients. J Arthroplast. 2015;30(12):2296–8.
62. Purcell RL, et al. Comparison of wound complications and deep infections with direct anterior and posterior approaches in obese hip arthroplasty patients. J Arthroplast. 2018;33(1):220–3.
63. Purcell RL, et al. Severely obese patients have a higher risk of infection after direct anterior approach total hip arthroplasty. J Arthroplast. 2016;31(9 Suppl):162–5.
64. Puolakka TJ, et al. The Finnish Arthroplasty Register: report of the hip register. Acta Orthop Scand. 2001;72(5):433–41.
65. Malchau H, et al. The Swedish total hip replacement register. J Bone Joint Surg Am. 2002;84-A Suppl 2:2–20.
66. Bozic KJ, et al. The epidemiology of revision total hip arthroplasty in the United States. J Bone Joint Surg Am. 2009;91(1):128–33.
67. Haynes JA, et al. Contemporary surgical indications and referral trends in revision total hip arthroplasty: a 10-year review. J Arthroplast. 2016;31(3):622–5.
68. Ledford CK, et al. What are the contemporary etiologies for revision surgery and revision after primary, noncemented total hip arthroplasty? J Am Acad Orthop Surg. 2019;27(24):933–8.
69. Eto S, et al. The direct anterior approach is associated with early revision total hip arthroplasty. J Arthroplast. 2017;32(3):1001–5.
70. Cidambi KR, et al. Impact of femoral stem design on failure after anterior approach total hip arthroplasty. J Arthroplast. 2018;33(3):800–4.
71. Parvizi J, Ereth MH, Lewallen DG. Thirty-day mortality following hip arthroplasty for acute fracture. J Bone Joint Surg Am. 2004;86(9):1983–8.
72. Bhattacharyya T, et al. Mortality after periprosthetic fracture of the femur. J Bone Joint Surg Am. 2007;89(12):2658–62.
73. Singh JA, et al. Are gender, comorbidity, and obesity risk factors for postoperative periprosthetic fractures after primary total hip arthroplasty? J Arthroplast. 2013;28(1):126–31 e1–2.
74. Klasan A, et al. Complications after direct anterior versus Watson-Jones approach in total hip arthroplasty: results from a matched pair analysis on 1408 patients. BMC Musculoskelet Disord. 2019;20(1):77.

13 Tips and Tricks for Your First Anterior Hip Replacement

Friedrich Boettner

Switching to an approach that you do not know or that you did not learn during training is always challenging. You have the responsibility toward your patients to not increase complication risk and, on the other hand, take the benefits of this new approach into consideration. No surgeon, that starts with the anterior approach, should take it lightly, and one has to make sure to be fully prepared for this transition. This chapter focuses on the steps you can take to minimize the chance of getting into complications and to make the transition as easy as possible.

Anterior Training Courses

Today, many companies offer training courses for anterior hip replacement (Fig. 13.1). These courses usually offer a very succinct way to obtain all of the information that you need to start implementing this new approach into your clinical practice. They usually combine educational sessions and presentations by experienced hip replacement surgeons, as well as a hands on instructions. In addition, there usually is the opportunity to practice how to deal with some of the possible complications like placing a cerclage wire around the femur.

Some courses also offer a mentoring option that connects the student surgeon to one of the instructors and later on might even offer the mentor to join the surgeon for their first cases. In addition it can be helpful to review the first cases with an experienced surgeon to avoid selecting a patient with a likely more challenging intra-operative exposure or component placement.

Getting Comfortable with the Implants

Often we use slightly different implants from what we are used to in our traditional approach. When I switched approaches, I initially spent 6

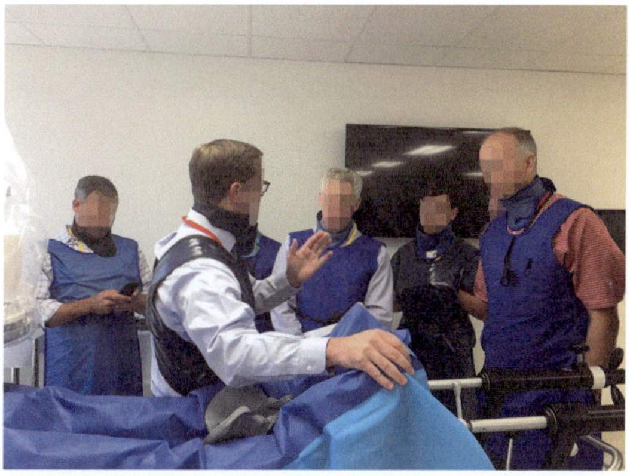

Fig. 13.1 During a Joel Matta DePuy anterior training course reviewing visualization of components on the C-arm

F. Boettner (✉)
Hospital for Special Surgery, New York, NY, USA
e-mail: boettnerf@hss.edu

J. M. Matta, A. P. Sah (eds.), *Anterior Hip Replacement*,
https://doi.org/10.1007/978-3-030-91896-5_13

months using the implants I wanted to use for the anterior approach through my old posterior approach. I wanted to make myself comfortable with how to insert these implants and comfortable with how the it feels to broach for the implant. In addition, I wanted to have my traditional approach to deal with any complications I might encounter like intraoperative calcar fractures or potential loosening. You want to minimize the stress that you have when you start a new approach, being familiar with the implants, having a feel for how the broach should sit, and understanding the head and liner options decreases stress at the time of surgery and allows you to focus on the approach itself.

Technology Can Help!

Familiarize yourself with the available technology. This ranges from tools to minimize blood loss (Aquamantys©, Medtronic, Dublin, Ireland) to software to interpret C-arm images (JointPoint©, DePuy Orthopedics, Warsaw IN, Radlink Inc., OrthoGrid Salt Lake City, UT), navigation systems (Brainlab AG, Munich, Germany), or robotic tools (Mako©, Stryker, Kalamazoo MI). The latter all can help you with positioning of the components. Switching to a new approach also means that you are less familiar with how to use anatomic landmarks to position your components. The biggest benefit of the anterior approach is that it allows you to take intraoperative C-arm images and therefore gives you an opportunity to control your component position in the operating room. There are now a number of software tools available that can help you better understand the image and allow you to accommodate for artifacts or parallax that is still an issue with many of our current fluroscopy units. Other technology tools that are now available include insertion devices that help you adjust the cup position easily or facilitate broaching of compression broaches (Kincise©, DePuy Orthopaedics, Warsaw IN).

Today there are many tools available, and it makes sense to review them and try them before you start switching to an anterior approach.

Patient Position and Familiarizing Yourself with the Table

The patient is usually placed in a supine position, and the surgery can be performed on either a special table or on a standard operating room table. One way or the other, you need to make sure that the table accommodates taking a C-arm image of the pelvis. If you have access to a special table like the Hana table, you need to familiarize yourself with the table and train a team member to manage the table and its leg extensions during surgery. There are reports of complications that are the result of inadequate use of the table, and it is very important to adjust traction and control the leg extensions appropriately. In my experience, it helps to write down the successive steps of the surgery and table handling so you can make sure not to miss a step during surgery and your assistant can anticipate the next change in table position. It also gives you time to think about the most efficient order of steps for each part of the surgery. In the beginning, we taped a list of the steps onto the wall of the operating room for everybody to see. When you start operating, you might run into difficult situations, that occupy your mind, and it is beneficial that every member of the team knows the next step so they can remind you in case you forget. I also recommend a dry run through the steps of the surgery and desired table positions without a patient so that everybody knows how the leg extensions are handled before an actual patient is positioned on the table.

The table is a powerful tool, and the leg extensions have some weight, and they ultimately could cause fractures if moved uncontrolled. In addition, I have observed in some very thin females that too much traction can result in temporary irritation of the pudendal nerve. Usually aim for enough traction on the legs to stabilize the pelvis and allow for insertion of the components without the pelvis shifting, but on the other hand I do not want to have so much traction that the hip already subluxes like we see in hip arthroscopies (Fig. 13.2).

Also, we assure the appropriate position of the arms. Usually, we favor crossing the arms over

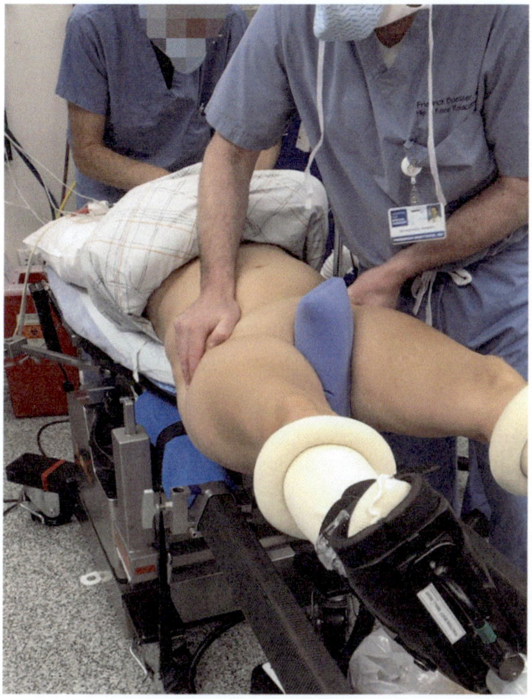

Fig. 13.2 Enough traction to stabilize the pelvis

the chest but make sure they do not slide too far down since that could impact on the angle that the broach takes into the femur. Also, we discuss with the anesthesiologist whether they need access to one of the arms for the IV line. We do recommend applying a support under the unoperated leg so that it does not hang unsupported throughout the surgery. Finally, it is important to stress that if you extend and externally rotate the hip for insertion of the femoral component, traction needs to be released to avoid excessive soft tissue tension and potential injury. Finally make sure that the boots are tightly screwed onto the leg extension, since they can slide out of its holding during positioning of the femur resulting in the leg falling to the ground.

Anesthesia and Perioperative Management

I recommend a standardized approach for your anterior hip replacement surgeries. For me, that means using spinal anesthesia. The main benefit of spinal anesthesia besides accommodating outpatient surgery is that it results in very predictable muscle relaxation. This helps to judge soft tissue tension as one factor indicating adequate leg length, but, even more importantly, makes sure that the patient is fully relaxed for exposure of the femur.

Patient Selection

Probably, the most important step is to select the right patient for the first cases. There are a number of things that I look for in an ideal patient. The perfect patient is female, has a normal BMI of less than 30 kg/m2, does not have excessive abdominal tissue overhanging the anterior hip (Fig. 13.3), and is not excessively muscular. Stay away from muscular patients, with short femoral necks and varus alignment or coxa profunda (Fig. 13.4). Also, male patients with a very narrow pelvis or significant flexion contractures are usually not ideal candidates for the first surgeries. On radiographs, I prefer patients with primary osteoarthritis, a door B femur, and slight valgus neck alignment with the center of the hip at the level or above the tip of the greater trochanter (Fig. 13.5). The longer the neck the easier it will be to get exposure to the acetabulum. While with more experience you can absolutely consider doing anterior approaches for any hip pathology, I don't recommend patients with osteoarthritis secondary to pediatric hip disorders since broaching of a very sclerotic neck (Fig. 13.6) and metaphysis or acetabular fixation in more dysplastic hips can be challenging when you are not used to operating through an anterior approach. As you get more comfortable, you will realize that you will extend your indications to ultimately include most of your patients.

Preoperative Templating

Preoperative templating is an important step to anticipate any difficulties during surgery. In my practice, I still use two different stems to accommodate a more valgus femur or a type A femur with

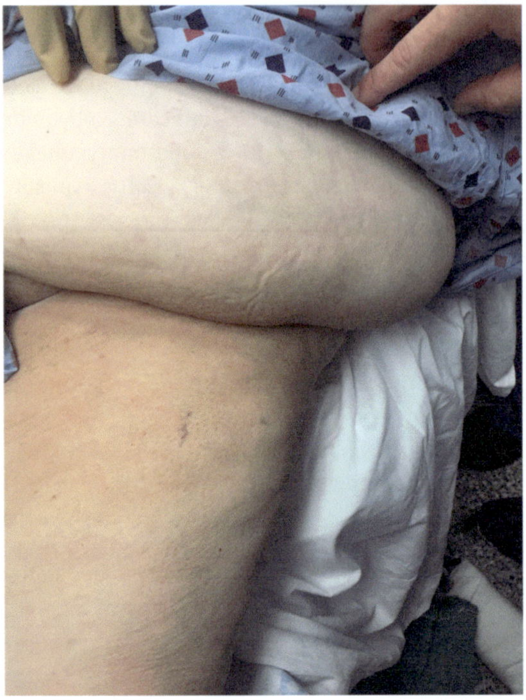

Fig. 13.3 Morbidly obese patient with a skin fold in the area of the anterior approach. Careful skin closure using staples or interrupted nylon stitches and a vacuum dressing are recommended to avoid wound complications

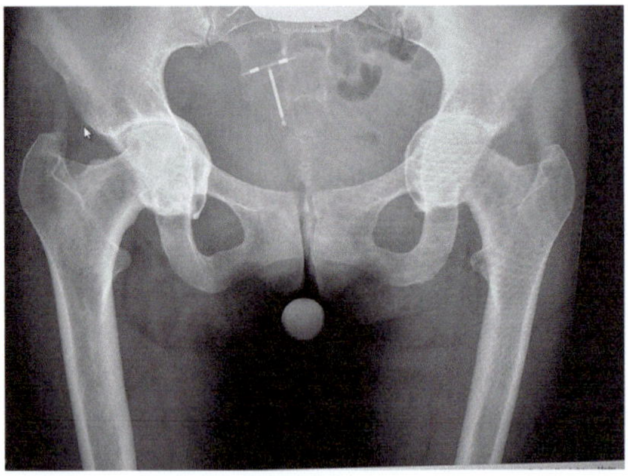

Fig. 13.4 Coxa profunda with a short, varus neck and a center of the femoral head below the tip of the trochanter. Not the ideal patient for an anterior approach

a more varus neck alignment. Be aware of patients with very small bones that might challenge the femoral component placement (Fig. 13.7). Special care should be taken to anticipate the amount of neck resection and the size of the stem and length

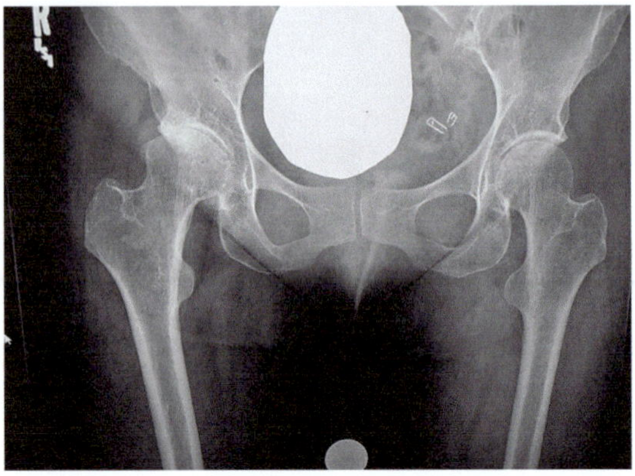

Fig. 13.5 Ideal patient, DORR type B femur, long femoral neck, and slight valgus neck orientation

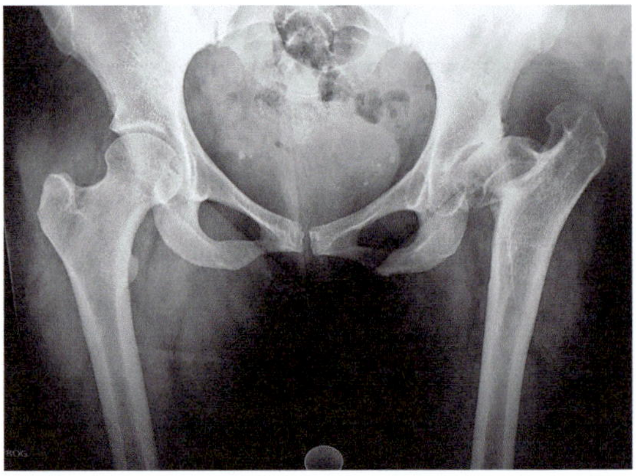

Fig. 13.6 Shortened neck status post prior surgeries for Perthes disease. A more difficult exposure and broaching of the femoral canal should be anticipated in this case

of the head to restore leg length. If I can reproduce the preoperative plan at the time of surgery, I can usually achieve adequate leg length during trial reductions, which avoids repetitive reductions and intraoperative C-arm imaging. Finally, templating for me especially in the beginning was the last check to make sure that this is a relatively straightforward surgery and I do not have to expect any unusual difficulties. I also pay attention to the overall pelvic position. I might increase my anteversion for patients with excessive forward flexion of the pelvis resulting in an inlet view and decrease acetabular anteversion in patients with a significant outlet view. If you use a C-arm you will not have to worry about this as long as the pelvis position on the table resembles the standing AP pelvis image

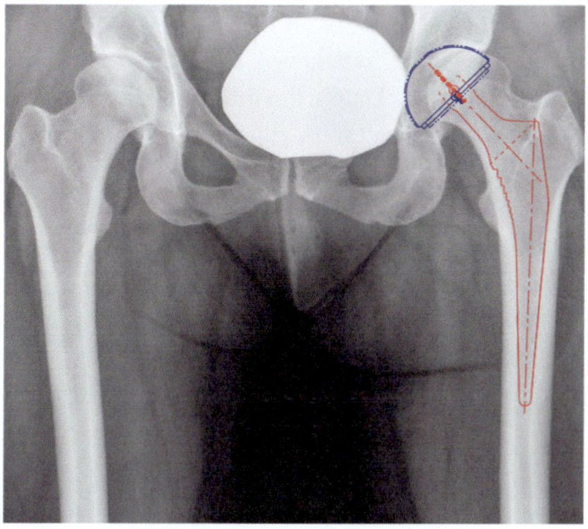

Fig. 13.7 Smallest template available for the femoral component in a small patient with a narrow canal. Broaching for the femoral component will be a challenge during surgery

you automatically adjust the anteversion to the individual pelvic tilt. A definite plus for using a c-arm intraoperatively.

The Incision

There are many ways to identify the appropriate position of the incision. I usually angle my incision a little bit more to the side to avoid the branches of the lateral femoral cutaneous nerve (Fig. 13.8). I confirm alignment of the fibers of the tensor fascia lata muscle running toward the side of the hip to avoid placing my incision accidentally over the more medially oriented sartorius muscle. If I have a tough time to identify the tensor, I might feel with my index finger subcutaneously the anterior superior iliac spine, which is a good landmark to identify the insertion of the tensor. I also prefer to mark my incision in the holding area. If I have difficulties finding the tensor muscle, I ask the patient to elevate the extended leg, which will usually tension the tensor muscle and make it easy to palpate it through the skin. It is wise to remind the patient that there is a chance of numbness on the side of the incision after surgery. Marking the incision in the holding area, while the patient is still awake, makes the patient realize that you do everything possible to avoid the nerve.

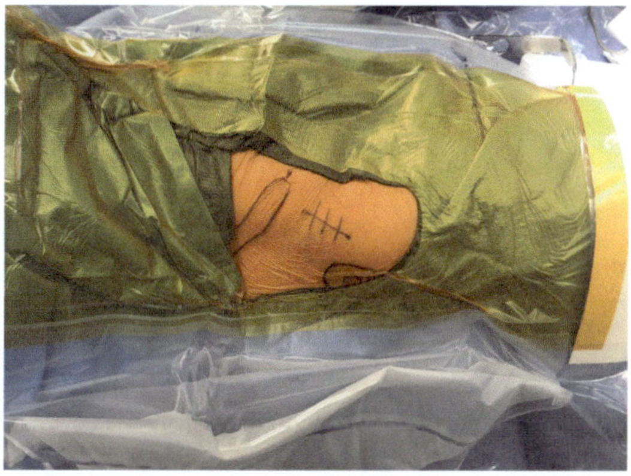

Fig. 13.8 Incision for an MIS anterior total hip replacement

Femoral Exposure

While we usually get quite comfortable exposing the acetabulum, we are most concerned with getting adequate femoral exposure. An increased risk of femoral fractures has been reported in the literature with the anterior approach, which highlights the importance of adequate soft tissue releases to expose the femur. Without question, patient selection is crucial in the beginning. More flexible female patients might not require any releases, while more muscular patients, with a dominant tensor muscle and narrow pelvis, can make it more difficult to mobilize the femur. I routinely release the insertion of the conjoined tendon over the tip of the greater. It is in my mind the main resistance to anterior elevation of the femur and if not released can result in fractures of the tip of the greater trochanter. I virtually never release the piriformis or obturator externus muscle. Both are in my mind important posterior stabilizers of the hip. As you start to extend the hip and elevate the femur, make sure to pull the femur slightly lateral to allow the tip of the trochanter to clear the posterior rim of the acetabulum. If you are unable to elevate the femur, then check your release one more time, and make sure the tip of the trochanter is not caught behind the acetabular component or blocked by overlying tissue and repeat the maneuver. Sometimes, just bringing the leg back into extension and repeating the maneuver can be all that is needed to facilitate better elevation of the femur. Once exposure is achieved, make sure you use a canal finder and confirm that you are in the canal. I also check anteversion by feeling the position of the knee and using the posterior cortex of the neck resection for orientation. Using a saw bone model with a femoral component and placing it in different positions helps to fully understand what it means to increase or decrease anteversion in an externally rotated femur (Fig. 13.9).

Cemented Versus Uncemented

I am almost always able to use uncemented fixation. Compression broaches together with a collar today accommodate uncemented fixation in more severely osteoporotic femurs. However, occasionally you might have to cement a femoral component through an anterior approach (Fig. 13.9). Despite rumors that cementing is not possible from the front, I actually find it quite straightforward. Plan your neck resection. It has been helpful for me to place the templates of my cemented stem of choice over my uncemented stem templates to get an idea if I need to resect additional neck whenever I switch over to a cemented stem. Use a flexible insertion tool for the cement restrictor. A rigid metal insert might not be able to seat the cement restrictor all the way down in the canal. When cementing the femoral component, I also pay attention to the position of the collar in relation to the medial calcar to avoid excessive varus or valgus component alignment. Once you have done the first few cemented stems, you will realize that it is possible to achieve a good cement mantle through an anterior approach.

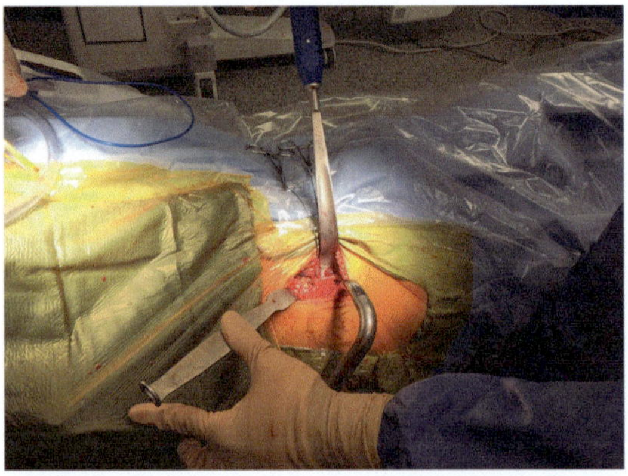

Fig. 13.9 Excellent exposure of the femur to accommodate cementless or cemented femoral component fixation

Restoring Leg Length

One of the benefits of the anterior approach is that it is usually easier and more accurate in restoring leg length. This is probably the biggest benefit of operating on a standard operating table without leg extensions since both legs are sterilely prepped and the surgeon can easily assess the leg lengths. If a HANA table is used, leg length is usually judged by the radiographic appearance of the hip or by the soft tissue tension. The later is examined by putting the index and middle finger around the neck of the femoral component and pulling the ball out of the socket after it was reduced. One should be able to pull out the head 2–3 mm. If you are unable to pull the head out of the socket at all, that usually means that the hip is over lengthened, and if it is easy to sublux the head, that usually means that you left the leg too short. Spinal anesthesia should result in comparable relaxion, but general anesthesia might be less predictable in regard to the amount of relaxation achieved at the time of trial reduction. The ultimate confirmation of the leg length discrepancy is always done radiographically.

Especially in the beginning, it can be difficult to get the leg length within range at the time of trial reduction. Under-resecting the femoral neck makes it more difficult to broach and reduce the femoral component. Care therefore should be taken to template and plan the amount of neck resection. I make an effort to check the neck resection prior to positioning the femur for broaching. Once I have confirmed that the neck resection is at the appropriate level, all I have to do is to sink the templated femoral implant to that level and usually my leg length will be within an acceptable range for the trial reduction. Since I preserve the capsule my final check is to make sure the distal capsule can be closed without too much tension.

Closure

The skin over the anterior hip is more sensitive to wound complications than the lateral skin over the greater trochanter. In my experience, we have struggled with more frequent stitch abscesses secondary to vicryl sutures. Additional care should be taken for patients with a skin fold in the front of the hip from excessive abdominal tissue overhanging the hip area. Try not to extend the incision into the skin fold itself since wound problems are more likely to occur. We recommend the use of vacuum-assisted closure dressings (Provena©, Acelity, San Antonio TX) for morbidly obese patients or patients with risk factors for poor wound healing, including smoking or diabetes (Fig. 13.10). Whenever we use a vacuum-assisted wound dressing, we usually close the skin with staples or interrupted nylon sutures. All other patients receive subcutaneous sutures with skin glue to accommodate showering once the dressing comes off. More recently, we have started to use monofilament suture material that is now easily available as barbed wire sutures (V-Lock©, Medtronic, Dublin, Ireland; Quill©, Surgical Specialties Inc., Wyomissing, PA; STRATAFIX©, Ethicon, Johnson & Johnson, New Brunswick NJ). These monofilament sutures are less likely to cause stitch abscesses. In addition, we advise our patients not to wear underwear that irritates the incision. Any form of massage or manual irritation of the incision should be avoided for the first 3 months after surgery.

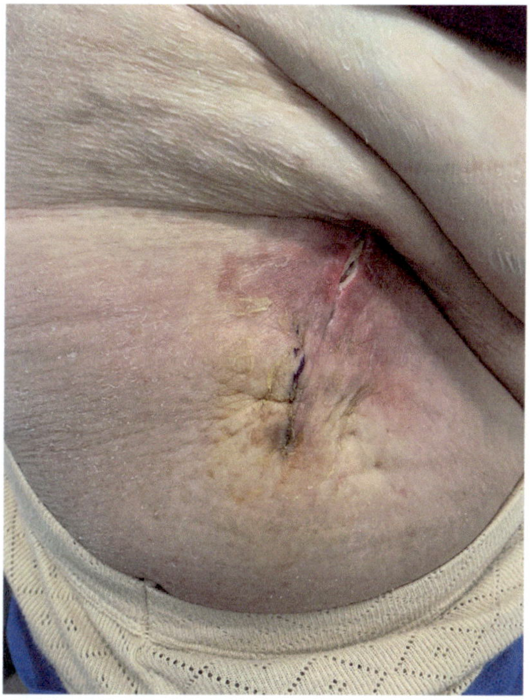

Fig. 13.10 Stitch abscess in the skin fold of a more obese patient after anterior approach total hip replacement

Getting the Patient Off the Table

Care should be taken when moving the patient off the table. We usually use a rolling board. Avoid excessive external rotation of the hip, since the hip during spinal anesthesia might be more vulnerable to anterior subluxation. In my experience, the anterior approach is extremely stable and dislocation has not been an issue in my practice.

Rehabilitation

Initially, I have been quite impressed with the amount of control patients exhibit immediately after surgery and the ability to be mobile early on. Now, this has pros and cons. It facilitates outpatient surgery and also allows the patient to be independent early on; however, it also increases the risk that a physical therapist not familiar with the approach starts excessive exercises too early and aggravates the hip. Since I have little control over home and outpatient physical therapy, I have stopped doing postoperative physical therapy. In my experience, patients recover fine without it.

I recommend never to put a pillow or anything under the knee and avoid resting the leg in hip flexion at night. I also encourage my patients to walk upright and to avoid hunching over the hip and keeping the hip flexed while walking. Once patients get to the 3- or 4-week time point, we usually start implementing quadriceps stretching exercises to increase the flexibility of the anterior hip tissue. I routinely close the anterior capsule and repair the reflected head of rectus femoris muscle. The latter, in my mind, is an important anterior stabilizer, and with the repair, I feel comfortable not to enforce hip precautions after surgery. If you do not repair the anterior capsule, it might be beneficial to enforce standard anterior precautions for the first 4 weeks. I do encourage my patients to use a toilet seat elevation for comfort in the first 4 weeks. To avoid strenuous activities, I give them some guidance on how far to walk in the first 4 weeks and encourage the use of a cane in the first 2 weeks. Usually, the goal is to walk one mile in the fourth week and less walking early on. I let patients return to driving after left hip replacement within 2 weeks and delay driving after right hip replacement until comfort and leg control accommodate driving after 3–5 weeks. I strongly discourage any hip flexion exercises in the first 3 months, which include straight leg raises and work with weights on the legs or thera-bands. It is my belief that strength training is in general not required for the hip and if you restore the anatomy including leg length and offset most anterior hip replacement patients will have a normal gait and activity level for everyday activities by 6 weeks after surgery. I let patients return to low-impact sports like golf or biking as early as 4–6 weeks after surgery, but discourage any higher-impact sports including tennis in the first 2–3 months. The main benefit of the anterior approach in my mind is that I am much less hesitant to allow my female patients to return to yoga or pilates. I have felt that restrictions that I usually apply to patients after posterior hip replacement do not need to be enforced in patients with an anterior approach. There is no doubt in my mind that the anterior approach is more stable than a posterior approach. In my first 1000 anterior hip replacements, I have not had a dislocation that required close reduction. This is a successful story I cannot reproduce with the posterior approach.

A Few Final Words

I am a high-volume hip surgeon, performing close to 300 hip replacements every year. I visited many surgeons that allowed me to benefit from their experience and helped me get comfortable with the overall setup for the surgery. While back then there was not an established way of doing the surgery, today, thanks to pioneers like Joel Matta, we have achieved major progress in standardizing the surgery. After I made up my mind it took me 2 years to ultimately do my first anterior hip placement surgery. I just did not want to leave my comfort zone. It took me 100 surgeries to feel somewhat comfortable and probably close to 400 surgeries to feel that I was cruising along as I was used to with a posterior approach. Today, I cannot envision a practice without the anterior approach. It has allowed my patients to return to activities that I would not have allowed them after posterior approach hip replacement. In addition, it has minimized the need for dual mobility articulations and I no longer feel the pressure to chase maximum head sizes. Take the first step and do not get discouraged from any difficulties that you will face in the beginning. Ask for help, visit one of the excellent training courses, and then be brave enough to do the first case. If you were trained on the anterior approach in residency or fellowship, you have a major advantage. I always will be greateful to the surgeons that pioneered this approach and trained me on it. We have come a long way and it is difficult for me today to envision an arthroplasty practice without the option of an anterior approach.

OR Efficiency: Radical Time Transparency and Operational Excellence

14

Jeremy Statton and Charles A. DeCook

Introduction: Why Efficiency Is Needed?

How is the efficiency of your operating room? Ask any orthopedic surgeon and the response will be some combination of disgust, disappointment, and disillusionment. Left to wait in surgeon lounges and complain about wasted time, we often spend more of our operative day waiting than operating. Most joint surgeons are left to do on average of 3–4 cases per day [1] and wonder why they cannot do more. Our decision to become surgeons was based on our love of operating, and our job satisfaction is directly related to our ability to operate more [2]. Unfortunately, there are few surgeons that are satisfied with their level of efficiency and the number of cases they perform. During a time of increased healthcare cost that is driving the US GDP, we must develop new technologies, ideas, and techniques that will disrupt our healthcare industry. This disruption must provide care that offers improved outcome, at lower cost, in a more convenient form. While most other industries have undergone this type of disruption, health care continues to lag. One of the greatest disruptions to health care will occur in the operating room.

Disrupting the current operating room productivity and efficiency will be a major step toward true disruption in the healthcare industry. The authors have utilized a simple formula of radical time transparency coupled with operational excellence to fundamentally change the productivity and efficiency of our hospital and ASC. Presently, we are routinely doing 12 primary total joint cases by 12:00 pm in two operating rooms. This production and efficiency have brought true value to our healthcare system, and we believe this is a simple and reproducible process that can disrupt today's operating room and bring true value to all parties.

Insights From Other Industries

Disruption has occurred in most of the industries from media, food and beverage, travel, automotive, travel, commerce, and manufacturing. In general, this disruption involves new technology and ideas that deliver goods or services faster, cheaper, and better than the status quo. The last two major industry holdouts to disruption have been education and health care. Gaining insights into how other industries were disrupted can help us understand how we improve the overall value we bring to the operating room and health care.

Walmart and Amazon have been the most recent disruptors of the commerce industry, driving down prices and delivering products in an

J. Statton · C. A. DeCook (✉)
Northside Hospital, Arthritis and Total Joint Specialists, Cumming, GA, USA

J. M. Matta, A. P. Sah (eds.), *Anterior Hip Replacement*,
https://doi.org/10.1007/978-3-030-91896-5_14

incredibly simple manner. One of Amazon's four core principles since its inception has been operational excellence. Bezos described this principle as "Delivering continuous improvement in customer experience and driving productivity, margin, efficiency, and asset velocity across all our businesses" [3]. No truer words have been used to describe every orthopedic surgeon's desire for operational excellence in his/her operating room.

Of course, the concept of operational excellence has been around long before Amazon and it was the cornerstone of the industrial revolution. Henry Ford was the biggest disruptor of the automobile industry and brought reliability and reproducibility to a new industry that was competing with the horse and carriage. One of Ford's most famous quotes was "you can have any color as long as its black" [4]. It has been suggested that Ford knew that black paint dried much faster than the other colors because he knew down to the second how long each step of the process took. From frame assembly times to paint drying times, Ford's stopwatch helped him keep track of not only how long the entire process would take but how each individual component contributed to the overall time. The genius of his moving assembly line was that one step in the process would automatically lead to the next step and avoid the long wait times between different steps of the manufacturing process. The Japanese manufacturer Toyota, much later, described this type of time waste as Mura, meaning lack of uniformity [5, 6].

From Ford to Toyota, time transparency allows manufacturers to determine where waste is occurring, make changes to the process and improve. This improvement not only improves time but the overall product quality. Time transparency and operational excellence are a critical component of every manufacturing process and to date have not been incorporated into operating rooms in order to enact change, disruption, and true improvements to operational efficiency. We have found that having an obsession with time, cost, and efficiency in the operating room brings about true disruption to the operating room and improving quality of care.

The goods and services of healthcare are actual human beings, making our job ever so critical. The drive to improve patient outcomes and reduce complications and readmissions will continue to be the number one driving force with our precious products. But as cost rise and overall healthcare spending increase, we must consider new ways to drive better outcomes. The great lessons learned from other industries are that time is a critical metric to obtain increases in quality and cost. Although it would seem ridiculous to any other industry to not measure time, our industry has been plagued by ignoring it. We have sought to distinguish ourselves from assembly lines of cars and have been mortified to treat our patients like cars on a conveyor belt. The great irony is that the quicker we realize our industry is no different than any other our patients will benefit from improved outcomes.

Time is a critical success metric that can no longer be ignored in our industry. Having radical time transparency allows for more efficiency, less cost, and a better end product. As total joint surgeons, much of our surgeries are similar and repeatable placing us in a unique opportunity to apply these principles to achieve true efficiency.

Part I: The Problem

The OR Inefficiency "Culture"

The causes of operating room inefficiency are always multifactorial, with each institution having its own unique set of challenges and deficiencies that lead to time delays, lost revenue, and poorer outcomes. While blame is often placed on turnover, anesthesia, inexperienced staff, miscommunication, instrument/implant readiness, and patient readiness, each individual problem never strikes at the fundamental causes. What caused the OR delay today is often a different cause tomorrow. Almost universally, it becomes difficult to assign fault to one individual or one process. When a particular individual or process is identified as mediocre and partially contributing to operating room inefficiency, there are often insufficient data to enact process changes. Most surgeons and OR administrators are left to simply summarize their institution as having a "culture" problem because they can't identify the root causes of their inefficiency. The OR "culture" proves insurmountable, and the status quo remains unaffected.

Core Problem: Time Transparency

Every operating room in the country measures time. Surgeons schedule cases at a particular time. Nurses are required to document several timestamps during a surgery including surgery start and end times, incision times, timeout times, etc. Yet, with all these time measurements, no one really knows where the time goes. Despite measurements being performed, these metrics are not easily accessible and are not actionable. These institutions lack time transparency.

For those rare institutions that make time measurements available to their teams and staff, it is often accessed days or weeks later and is not accessed real time when intervention is still possible. Time is locked away in an EMR or tracking system, never to be seen or used again. Ask the manager of your surgery department what your average turnover time was last month. Ask your partner what their average time to close their total hip or how long it takes to expose and prepare the acetabulum. Ask yourself what is the actual time it takes you to do a total hip? Almost no one has access to their own time metrics. Why is that? Lack of time transparency.

We submit that the core problem of any inefficient institution is a lack of time transparency. Every step of the patient journey must not only be measured, but readily displayed so that it can be utilized to effect change. When time transparency becomes ingrained in the culture of an operating room and when those time metrics lead to fundamental changes in operation, we call this "Radical Time Transparency." Time transparency becomes radical when fundamental operational changes occur.

As Mother Theresa said, "Honesty and transparency make you vulnerable. Be honest and transparent anyway." If your institution wants to improve patient care, cut down on waste, and become more efficient, they must achieve radical time transparency. It will show the true faults of any organization and can lead to real operational change.

Why Surgical Time Matters

Surgical Times

The average surgical time for a total hip arthroplasty is 95 min from incision to closed [7]. Despite advances in implants and technology, dramatic reductions in length of stay, improved recovery times, and reduction in complications, operative times have not changed over the last two decades [7]. Total knee arthroplasty average times are quite similar at 96 min and have also been equally stable over time [8]. Hospital volume has had an inverse effect on surgical time, with higher volume centers actually having longer surgical times [9]. In European countries where there is a large distinction between public and private hospitals, no significant difference in operative time exits [10].

Outcomes have been clearly associated with length of time required to complete the surgical procedure. Readmissions, reoperations, surgical site infections, and wound complications all rise with longer operative times [11]. Stearns et al. determined for TKA that operative times less than 80 min resulted in significantly fewer complications [11]. Della Valle et al. found similar results with prolonged operative times over 15 min resulted in higher: transfusion rates, wound dehiscence, renal insufficiency, sepsis, SSI, UTI, readmissions, and LOS [12]. Similar findings also occur in partial knee replacements that average 85 min per case. Gerlinger et al. found that re-operation, SSI, transfusion, and prolonged length of stay all related to longer operative times [13].

Infection has been a well-accepted complication of prolonged operative times in both hip and knee arthroplasty populations. Parvizi et al. in 2019 reviewed close to twenty thousand joint arthroplasties and found that for every 20 min of operative time the risk of 1 year PJI increased 25% [14]. They further demonstrated that operative times over 90 min demonstrated a twofold increase in SSI than those whose operations took 60 min [14]. Iorio et al. also proved that the only modifiable risk factors that could decrease infection risk included lower BMI, DM, and lower operative times [15]. With the average hip arthroplasty case taking over 90 min, there is clear incentive to significantly decrease operative times. Stearns et al. suggested that operative times less than 80 min could significantly reduce complications including infection [11].

Part II: Radical Time Transparency

True Time Transparency

- Measured
- Live
- Visible
- Valued
- Personal
- Radical

Measure Time

The first step toward true OR efficiency is measuring time. While some time metrics are measured in operating rooms today, there remain many time metrics that remain unmeasured. Having a complete and complimentary set of time measurements is key to understand the true efficiency problems in your operating room. Many institutions measure room turnover but do not measure the individual components of that turnover. Simply stating that the room turnover is 45 min will not help unless you know what your in room to prepped and draped time is. If your turnover continues to be high, it may be that your closed to out of room time is excessive. Do you know that your closed to out of the room time is? Have you ever known? What are your scrub techs opening time for a total hip? What is your instrument time out of room? Having detailed time metrics is key to better understanding broad metrics like turnover time. It is important to be aware of basic time metrics (see Table 14.1).

Live Time

Looking at time in retrospect can be helpful. Reviewing past time metrics can provide a benchmark for improvement in the future. Live time metrics carry the advantage of allowing on-demand staff changes to continue the flow in the OR. Live metrics demonstrate where bottlenecks and delays are occurring in real time. Your live time is actionable and can help reduce time that would have otherwise been excessively long.

Visible Time

Time must be visible. "What was incision time?" In-room time? How many times have you heard team members attempt to find out what time an event occurred? Having time visible brings more value to the metric and it helps everyone stay focused on the common goal. With so many potential pitfalls, bottlenecks, and delays, it is impossible to determine the fundamental sources of inefficiency in your institution without having this time transparency. By placing time more prominently in the OR, staff are more aware of their current progress. Imagine if each OR room has their turnover time prominently displayed for all to see. Each team member that contributes to turnover has a personal vested interest in the time

Table 14.1 Basic time metrics

Important Time Metrics:
First case start time
In-room to prepped/draped
In-room to cut time
Cut to closing time
Cut to closed time
Closing time
Closed to out time
Breakdown time
Cleaning time
Opening time
Room ready to in-room time
Nonsurgical patient OR time

displayed. Imagine if you could see how ahead or behind you are in your OR room.

Valued Time

Time must be valued. It is obvious which teams have embraced time metrics as one measure of team effectiveness. Those teams who value time recognize when they are running behind and know how to get help. Those who value time make efforts to improve processes that improve efficiency. Those teams who do not value time are unaware of time around them and do not recognize when delays are occurring. Teams that do not value time do not have meaningful ways to improve their process.

$$\text{Time} = \text{Value}$$

We have always considered health care different from any other industries. Quality patient care cannot be rushed, or mass-produced. Some even take a moral stand against measuring time in an OR. If a surgeon is thinking about time, or how many cases they need to do in a day, they cannot have excellent outcomes for their patients. From a place of good intention, health care has been slow to transition from thinking solely about patient outcomes to thinking of overall Value.

$$\text{Value} = \frac{\text{Outcomes} + \text{Patient Satisfaction}}{\text{Cost}}$$

As we become more accepting of value in health care [16], we must also embrace that time plays a major role in delivering value. If surgeon A performs three total hips with the same outcomes as surgeon B who performs seven in the same amount of time, it is no doubt that surgeon B's performance provides more value to the system. Interestingly, regardless of time, the higher the volume the better the outcome [17, 18]. This phenomenon has been seen across total joints and across specialties [19]. What has also proven out, just like other industries, is that as efficiency improves, so does patient outcomes. Delphin et al. found that OR efficiency had no negative impact on patient safety and quality of care [20].

Personal Time

Time must be personal. Hospitals typically do not capture time based on individuals, teams, or OR rooms. Instead, they report overall, generalized time measurements about turnover or start times. If the data are not personalized, the change cannot be personalized. Just because a nurse noted when a patient entered a room does not mean that this helps your team become better. For some teams, the problem may be start times, for others it may be slow turnover, and for yet others it may be that there is not enough staff to open trays. When used properly, personalized time serves as one of our most effective tools to track our improvement and compare ourselves to our peers. This means that the surgeon is not telling the anesthesiologist he is slow, rather the anesthesiologist recognizes it and makes a change in his or her process. Personalized data draw out the native competitiveness in most people and give them a goal to work toward [21] (see Table 14.2).

Radical Time

Time must be radical. To become radical, time must be used to improve the operation of the OR. Those transparent times need to be embraced and used by all parties of your organization from SPD to the administrator. Every staff member uses their metric to change their process. Whether that is turnover of trays or the duration of spinals, radical time transparency means that it changes the process of how we improve. Radical time transparency is the fuel for the second key ingredient to operating room efficiency and operational excellence.

Part III Operational Excellence: Practical Solutions

Operational Excellence

Time by itself is not enough. You must connect those time metrics to a system of process improvement to achieve operational excellence.

Table 14.2 Team member metrics

Circulator Efficiency
What is your average true turnover time (closed prior case to incision this case—how long does it take from the time the surgeon stops to when the surgeon starts again)?
What is your wheels-in to incision time?
What is your closed to wheels-out time?
How do your metrics compare to other circulators in the hospital/ASC and how do they compare across the country?
Scrub Tech Efficiency
What is your average case opening time (time from when the room is clean to all trays are open)?
What is your average turnover time?
How do your metrics compare to other techs in the hospital/ASC and how do they compare across the country?
Anesthesia Efficiency
What is the time from request to spinal complete?
What is the in-room time to anesthesia?
What is your closed to patient out time?
How do your metrics compare to other anesthesia in the hospital/ASC and how do they compare across the country?
Assistant Efficiency
What is your average surgical time?
What is your closing time for each procedure (time from when the surgeon has finished to full closure)?
How do your metrics compare to other assistants in the hospital/ASC and how do they compare across the country?

The time transparency is the fuel needed to run an efficient engine, but operational excellence is the real engine of efficiency. Remember the goal is never to be faster, but to be more efficient. In fact, the goal is never about time at all. The real goal is to improve the process. Time and efficiency are a delightful and natural byproduct of the process of measuring time and operational excellence.

Commitment by management and staff to improve operational control of the OR has shown true time savings in multiple studies. Ertl et al. looked at the application of six sigma program in the OR and noted on time starts improved from 32 to 73%, room utilization improved from 56% to 68%, and overall revenue increased 10% [22]. Similar interventions occurred at a children's hospital that led to a reduction of turnover time from 41 to 32 min [23]. Fundamentally "redesigning" OR operations with interventions like parallel process, minimizing nonoperative tasks, and reducing disruptions can have profound effects on OR efficiency [24]. Implementing operational changes can be particularly effective in the ASC, as Richter et al. described a 13-min reduction in turnover time resulting from these changes [25].

Certainly, the goal of efficiency and operational excellence is to increase the volume of cases being done by a single surgeon and/or the institution. If efficiency improves enough to increase the OR production, more cases can be performed, and more value brought to the process. Bolognesi demonstrated that by changing operations at an academic facility the number of total joint cases improved by 29% [26].

A. Waiting Room

Patients should be brought to pre-op based on OR and pre-op availability. Priority is based on the OR bottleneck, which is the operating room itself. Do not bring back the next patient of surgeon A if it is going to be another 4 h before the OR is ready. Instead, bring back the patient of surgeon B who is going to be ready in 30 min. Without transparency, a patient will be waiting in a pre-op room for an extended period of time, which wastes time and resources. The waiting room opens the funnel of patients, and if there are problems getting patients from their home to the waiting room or from the waiting room to the pre-op area, delays will occur.

B. Pre-op

Pre-op must know their average time from in the room to ready for surgery. They must also know how long each pre-op nurse average time to ready is. Dealing with a late patient is a common occurrence. Recognizing when a patient arrives late and recognizing the readiness of the OR and surgeon are critical to determine flexible additional staffing needs to ready that patient in time. Monitoring how many patients were not prepared when the OR was ready is a key metric to pre-op efficiency. The pre-op nurse has to be aware of the OR status and the OR needs to be aware of the pre-op status. Staffing must be flexible to meet the immediate needs of the OR. If pre-op administrators or charge nurses are unaware of how long the process takes, there will be times in which patients will not be ready for the OR. Ensuring an open line of communication between the waiting room and pre-op is critical to ensure patients are brought back in a timely manner. The communication also extends to the OR where the OR readiness takes precedents over other factors (see Table 14.3).

C. Anesthesia

Anesthesia plays a large part in the pre-op area. Anesthesia often performs regional blocks and spinals in pre-op. We have found spinals/blocks administered in the pre-op area to be a critical aspect of efficiency in the OR. The OR should be left for operating and not for time-consuming anesthesia procedures. The communication between the OR and anesthesia is absolutely critical. Anesthesia always needs to be alerted as to the appropriate time to start the block and or spinal or the appropriate time to go back to the OR. This often is complicated if a surgeon utilizes two rooms as the exact time to perform these tasks require a good awareness of surgical time. Too often, surgeons are unaware of how long it will take them to finish a case and wait until the very end of the procedure to initiate the next room. This often translates into lost time, waiting on the next patient to be prepped and draped. Surgeons need to know their surgical times and communicate clearly with anesthesia as to when to administer spinals and or general anesthesia. If general anesthesia is utilized, the anesthesia team needs to know how much time is left in the case so that the patient can be awakened at the same time the case is over. Prolonged extubations have been studied and result in on average of 12.5 min of time of patients in the OR [27]. In addition to other advantages, spinals can lead to improved efficiency as there is no wake-up time and no time putting the patient to sleep in the OR [28].

Table 14.3 Pre-op efficiency questions:

What is the average time required to prepare the patient for surgery?
Who are your fastest and slowest pre-op nurses?
What type of patient takes the longest to get ready?
How much faster is it if a tech or assistant helps the pre-op nurse?
When do you tell patients what their arrival time will be?
Who is responsible for alerting patients to arrive earlier or later? What cues are in place to call patients to change their arrival time?
Are you flexible enough to change patient arrival times the day before surgery?
How long are patients waiting from arrival to being brought back to pre-op?
How long after a patient is ready for surgery do they wait to be brought back?
How many pre-op rooms are being utilized at the beginning of the day versus the busiest time of day?

D. Operating

Room Overlapping of cases refers to the process of beginning the anesthesia on the next case prior to the completion of the case before. While this generally occurs with surgeons who have two or more operative rooms, it can also occur with surgeons who have a "flip" room or even one room. This is a critical component of any successful efficient OR and represents significant time savings. Szucs et al. randomized to overlapping vs sequential anesthesia and found significant reductions in turnover time by 13 min and more OR occupancy time of 1 h per day [29]. Often times, this also refers to initiating blocks and spinals in the pre-op area as opposed to the operating room. Significant reductions in turnover times can result from the use of induction rooms instead of OR rooms [30]. This concept of alternative sites for anesthesia was demonstrated in a Canadian study by Schwarz et al. who found a significant reduction in average turnover time from 54 min to 15 min [31]. This concept of parallel processing with anesthesia was validated by a recent meta-analysis that demonstrated improvement in all OR time metrics [32].

Drum-Buffer-Rope Theory

Drum-Buffer-Rope theory is a manufacturing concept that identifies and handles constraints in a process in order to improve efficiency [33]. The theory is that the slowest aspect of the process (constraint) is identified and then buffers are placed in order to keep the process moving at a steady pace in order to prevent bottlenecks. The operating room is the bottleneck of the OR assembly line. The Drum-Buffer-Rope theory tells us that there need to be cues (rope) in place to continue to feed patients (the buffer) into the OR. Creating a system in which patients are ready to go back to the OR at the perfect time is where true efficiency lies.

A truly efficient OR consistently works to improve this metric, which we call true turnover time. A thorough understanding of the Drum-Buffer-Rope theory is needed to accomplish this. Pre-op's role is to continue to feed the buffer (the patient) to the operating room. Patients need to be ready and waiting to enter the operating room. If the OR is empty, then the system has failed. A successful operating room is operating. Even if a patient is in the OR but surgery is not occurring, it is still not producing. To keep the buffer ready, there must be cues and communication between the OR and pre-op so that patients are ready for surgery. In a perfect setting, the wound is closed, and the next patient is incised immediately with no time between. Appreciating the contributing parts of the operating room is critical to efficiency.

E. Parallel vs Sequential Tasks

The typical approach to room turnover is to perform each necessary task in a particular sequence. A typical example of sequential tasks in the OR is as follows. The wound is closed. Nursing removes the drapes. Anesthesia then extubates patients. Transfer help is then called for. Patient is transferred to the stretcher. Patient, circulator, and anesthesia move the patient to PACU. The trays from surgery are broken down by the scrub tech. The trays are then moved out of the room. Cleaning help is then called for. The room is then moped, wiped, and cleaned. The OR staff is then alerted that the OR is clean. The scrub tech brings in the next cart of instruments. The circulator is then called to help open trays, and the circulating nurse then moves to pre-op to get the next patient. Sequential tasks are often assigned to particular team members, and this process often relies on the next person in the sequence to be alerted that their tasks are ready to be performed.

An alternative approach is to perform the same tasks simultaneously or in parallel. Instead of waiting for each necessary task to finish before proceeding with the next, multiple steps occur in parallel. Often these task duties can be performed by multiple members of the team. Patient and instrument turnover are prime examples of parallel tasks. Anesthesia, scrub techs, orderlies, circulators, and surgeons can all be working in parallel to reduce total turnover time. An efficient scrub tech will know when the surgeon is done with a specific instrument and begins to clean it and pack it for removal. In a highly efficient room, the instruments can be removed before the patient leaves. Team members responsible for cleaning can also help remove trays and can help assist in patient transfer.

Opening trays and preparing instruments for the next case are the longest aspect of turnover. This task can be quite onerous with total joint cases and in our institute averaging 19 min. While traditionally this process is done by one scrub tech and one circulator, improving time metrics means evaluating different ways to improve times. Having additional staff to open, reduced number of trays, and even disposable instruments has been shown to be effective at reducing opening times [34]. Reducing instrument variability from surgeon to surgeon has also been effective in opening times. Running parallel tasks means having the right number of staff available at the right time. Effective communication and flexible staffing allow these parallel processes to occur.

F. Dedicated Staff

Surgeons understand the importance of working with the same staff on a consistent basis. The general public would be aghast if they knew that often surgeons and staff who have never worked together before start doing cases together for the first time. Dedicated teams have clearly demonstrated reductions in surgical times.

Dedicated staff can also affect turnover times as well. A study by Matullo et al. looked at turnover times comparing cases that were done with orthopedic staff vs nonorthopedic staff. Dedicated and familiar orthopedic staff on average had turnover times of 20 min compared to 31 min for nonorthopedic staff [35]. Heiji et al. found similar results when using "fixed" staff that worked with the same surgeon every day and found lower turnover times and lower operative times by over 10 min [36].

G. Fist Case Start Times

The importance of starting the day on time could not be understated. Most surgeons experience delays in start times, and in the study by Onyebum et al., they found 99% of first cases started late [37]. Defining what an on time start time actually means is also important. We have chosen to define start time as incision time. The rationale is that there is a large amount of variability between in-room and incision time. Mazzei reviewed their in-room to incision time and found between 21 and 49 min prior to incision [38]. Tardiness has a tendency to build over the course of the day, and starting late for the first case of the day makes this phenomenon worse [39].

H. Two Room Models

Clearly, two room models can improve overall efficiency. A study by Namdari et al. looking at high volume total shoulder surgeons found significantly more efficiency [40]. In fact, one room over a 10-h period resulted in 3 total shoulder cases vs 4 total shoulder cases in two rooms over a shorter 9-h period [40].

Part IV: Surgeons

We operate throughout our careers in a relative vacuum. It is rare for other surgeons to observe or critique our own performance. As such, there often becomes a stagnation in our technique and overall efficiency. Too many of us do the same things over and over because this is how we learned to do it in training. Attempts to learn new techniques or even new instruments can be difficult to learn. The application of any new technique means a learning curve and a period of uncertainty and prolonged OR times. Change is difficult, and it is a normal human response to resist it.

In order to improve efficiency, we must be willing to see the world, or at least how we perform surgery, in a different light. Constantly analyze your surgical flow. "Operative efficiency is a critical ingredient to surgical success" [41]. Our surgical skills and behaviors are formed early in our career but are "rarely consciously analyzed or critically evaluated thereafter" [41]. Far too often we perform steps that are not necessary simply because that is the way we have always done it. Be willing to question each step and make beneficial changes.

Perform the surgery the same way every time. Consistency from the surgeon allows the opportunity for everyone around you to also be consistent. If you are constantly changing how you do a particular step or the order you do the steps in, there is no way for your assistant and scrub tech to anticipate your next move.

Limit the surgical tools that are required for every case. Instead of having everything possible for each case, be critical about what you need and create a tray that meets your needs in 95% of your cases. Plan for the norm not the exception. Any extra tools can be placed in peel packages that can be opened in unique circumstances.

Be a leader. Surgeons that lead the process of efficiency and process improvement see improved results. A study by Hendahewa et al. found a 58% reduction in turnover times with teams led by the surgeon themselves [42]. Often times surgeons go to the lounge and wait for the next case. The most productive surgeons are part of the team, they pick up the mop, they assist with opening cases, and they are an active participant in the process. Hitchin et al. determined that turnover time improved significantly when the surgeon was present in the room [43].

Lastly, adopt technology that makes you more efficient. Like every other industry, new technology for anterior hip arthroplasty is constantly being developed and introduced. Carefully evaluate these technologies and then do not hesitate to introduce any that will make it easier for you to perform the surgery. Do not adopt all technologies. Some devices or techniques complicate the surgery and add steps that make it take longer (see Table 14.4).

Table 14.4 Surgeon efficiency metrics

OR Room Metrics
1st Case Cut Time
What is your average first case cut time last month?
What are the latest you have started and the earliest you have started this year?
Time to Incision—How many minutes does it take for you to cut after the patient enters the room?
Time to Out—When the wound is closed, how long does it take for your patient to leave the room?
True Turnover—Time from closure prior case to incision next case.
Which teams have the fastest turnover?
Surgery Times
Skin to skin, what is your average time for a total hip this year?
What is the longest step in a total hip replacement for you?
What was your fastest and slowest total hip case this year?
How was your surgical time changed over the last 3 years? Are you getting faster, slower, or are you stagnant?
How long does it take for you to expose a total hip?
When you have two rooms, at what point in a total joint do you send the patient back to the other room?
How often is your waiting on the second room?
How do these times compare to your peers at the hospital and around the country?
Closure Times
How long does it actually take for your first assist to close a total knee?
What percent of the total surgical time is spent closing?
Which of your assistants close the fastest?
How much time do you save by assisting with closing?
How do these times compare with your peers?

Part V: Does Location Affect Efficiency? Hospital Versus ASC

Total joint arthroplasty is currently in a transition state from hospitals to ambulatory surgery centers. We have traditionally only performed total joints in the hospital setting due to concerns about pain control, the patient's ability to ambulate, and the desire to monitor and treat complications.

The Hospital Efficiency Dilemma

Hospital organizational and incentive structure can be a major challenge to efficiency. By nature of the multiple layers of nursing leadership, change can be slow and sometimes nonexistent. ASCs are often physician-run and have few if any bureaucratic layers that allow change to occur quickly. The stakeholder structure is often at odds in hospital settings where the hospital profits go solely to the hospital. ASCs have the benefit of multiple owners that incentivize efficiency and cost reduction.

Operating room staffing in hospitals vs. ASCs can be quite different. Typically, hospitals rotate different nurses and scrub techs through many different types of surgery, and as a result, the experience level can be quite different. Staff often rotates, and it can be difficult to predict who will be helping on a given day. Because of the sheer volume of cases and varied types of procedures, hospitals have on average much lower experienced staff compared to ASCs. ASCs also attract high-level performers as a result of the draw of smaller facilities, less variability, and less call responsibility.

Anesthesia and staff also suffer from similar stresses in the hospital setting that is not required in an ASC. The sheer volume and call associated with hospitals often mean that there is great variability of numbers and talent of its team members. ASCs have the luxury of a significantly reduced number of anesthesia providers, which can lead to less variability in care. The sheer reduction in space also is beneficial for the anesthesiologist who is a step away from pre-op, OR, and PACU.

Turnover time, a surrogate for overall efficiency, is on average remarkably different between an ASC and hospital. A study by Phelan et al. found a significant difference in mean turnover time, ancillary time, procedural time, exit time, and nonoperative in the ASC setting vs the hospital [44]. Sippel et al. also found significant reductions in turnover time by over 18 min in the ASC setting [45].

ASC Efficiency Advantage

Over the last 5–10 years, we have seen a shift of total joint cases moving from the hospital to the ASC. There are multiple reasons for this including patient outcomes, experience, and surgeon preference. Improved efficiency is also one of the major drivers of this change.

ASC's footprints are smaller. Smaller footprints lend to more efficiency at multiple levels including the transportation of patients, anesthesia movement from pre-op to PACU, and for surgeons to move from pre-op to OR to family consultation and back to pre-op multimodes times a day.

ASC's Organizational Structure Lends Well to Adaption

ASC staffing has several advantages. They can incentivize staff in different and unique ways to keep them motivated. The staff at the ASC should feel like part of a team that is accomplishing something worthwhile adding a sense of a fulfillment to their work.

ASC stakeholder incentive structure is geared toward cost reduction and overall production. Surgeons often have ownership in ASCs and as such are a motivated shareholder to bring true value. From implant costs to staff hours, surgeons have visibility into the true cost of joint replacement and are financial motivated to limit those costs.

Not only does the ASC provide an easier environment to make the changes needed to become more efficient, but the ASC also thrives on improved efficiency. When staff sees that it is possible to finish 12 cases by 12 pm, they develop a sense of pride that carries on to the next day. Patient experience improves with improved efficiency as well. When patients leave a facility mere hours after undergoing total hip replacement and can ambulate with adequate pain controls, they tell everyone they know.

Physician burnout is a problem, especially among orthopedic surgeons [46]. Physician burnout has been found to be twice that of the average occupation and leads to twice the normal number of medical errors, a decrease in quality of care, and a decrease in patient satisfaction [47]. When operating in an ASC with improved efficiency, surgeons thrive on this felt sense of knowing that they will have a good day. They arrive to the ASC confident that they will have everything they need. Each staff member will know their job and will get it done. Delays and obstacles are rare.

Part VI: Efficiency and the Anterior Approach

Intra-Operative Times Versus Other Approaches

There are numerous clinical studies that address surgical times with anterior approach. Most studies often compare anterior approach to other approaches. In comparison with posterior approach, Benoit et al. performed a randomized clinical trial and found the average time for anterior approach to be 69 min vs 45 min for posterior approach [48]. Pagnano found similar results in their single-institution study with anterior approach averaging 114 min vs 60 min for the mini-posterior approach [49]. Singh et al. performed a prospective randomized study of anterior to posterior and found similar results of 125 min vs 100 min [50]. The single-surgeon randomized trial by Barrett found anterior approach average time of 84 min vs his standard posterior approach of 60 min [51]. Comparison to anterolateral approach also exists. Gellar et al. found no difference between the two approaches, [52] whereas Lindgren et al. found significantly longer operative time with anterior approach averaging 101 min vs 80 min for anterolateral approach [53].

While single institutions generally demonstrated significantly longer operative times for anterior approach, meta-analysis generally shows a different story. Haddad et al. in 2017 did a systemic review and noted a trend toward increased surgical time, and there were no differences that reached statistical significance [54]. Bao et all performed a meta-analysis of all randomized clinical trials in 2018 comparing approaches and found no significant differences in operative times [55]. In 2020, Tian found similar findings of no differences [56].

Learning Curve

Certainly, the surgeon experience level affects surgical time in any operation including the anterior approach. Batailler et al. aimed to quantify the improvement of operative time as experience level increased [57]. They found that operative times were stabilized after 70 anterior approach cases. They also found that senior surgeons' operative times were lower during the learning curve, averaging 80 min vs junior surgeons at 93 min. Operative times can be a good surrogate for proficiency in a new approach, but complications can also be used as a surrogate. Chai et al. noted a learning curve of 88 cases before complications normalized [58]. Solomon in Australia reached similar conclusions with 50 cases as their threshold learning curve [59]. Nordsletten found a higher learning curve of 200 cases until proficiency was reached [60].

Case Difficulty

While operative experience, number of cases, and learning curve contribute to operative time, the difficulty of the particular case can also contribute. Shiratsuchi found that certain radiographic parameter could help predict the case duration. The most significant radiographic findings included proximal femoral migration and greater trochanter being higher than the femoral head. Other factors included younger age, male, higher BMI, height, previous hip surgery, and cement use.

Practical Implications

While not studied, preoperative timing may be improved with patients being left in a supine position. Often, a lateral position requires significant time and effort to level the pelvis. Often, the surgeon is required or prefers to be in the room, while this takes place in order to ensure accuracy. The anterior approach affords the surgeon less pelvis position time. Closing times between anterior and posterior approaches have not been specifically studied; however, it is generally acknowledged that anterior incisions are shorter, shallower, and take less time to close.

Part VII: Summary

The development of the low friction total hip arthroplasty by Sir John Charnley via a trans-trochanteric approach in a supine position revolutionized the treatment for osteoarthritis of the hip. Since its inception, the procedure has undergone further development through the improvement of implants, the development of alternative anatomical approaches, and the implementation of new technologies that amplify the skills of the surgeon. What has not improved significantly in total hip arthroplasty is operative efficiency. The average operative times over the last two decades have been stagnant with the average operative time being 95 min. Some would make a compelling case that the operative time has increased with the advent of the anterior approach although anterior advocates suggest this is likely due to the learning curve and the use of additional technologies to ensure more accurate cup position, leg length, and offset.

Certainly, the anterior approach and its broad adoption have been astounding and transformative in the modern era of hip arthroplasty. A recent survey of AAHKS members found a current anterior approach utilization of 56% of all US surgeons [61]. One area of improvement in the anterior approach should be operative efficiency. Reductions in operative times reduce many common complications and would improve the overall value of this operation.

To achieve true surgical efficiency, the application of radical time transparency and operational excellence must be performed at both the institutional and operating room levels. Applying the same general principles in other disrupted industries will help us in our quest to improve the value we bring to our healthcare industry.

References

1. https://www.aaos.org/quality/practice-management/aaos-orthopaedic-surgeon-census/orthopaedic-practice-in-the-u.s.-2018/
2. Holzer E, Tschan F, Kottwitz MU, Beldi G, Businger AP, Semmer NK. The workday of hospital surgeons: what they do, what makes them satisfied, and the role of core tasks and administrative tasks; a diary study. BMC Surg. 2019;19(1):112. https://doi.org/10.1186/s12893-019-0570-0. PMID: 31412843; PMCID: PMC6694625.
3. https://www.forbes.com/sites/carminegallo/2021/02/11/how-jeff-bezos-consistently-communicates-four-core-values-that-made-amazon-a-success/?sh=698466ab6e24
4. Ford H, Crowther S. My life and work. Doubleday; 1922. p. 92.
5. Masuda K. Kenkyusha's new Japanese-English dictionary. 5th ed. Tokyo: Kenkyusha; 2003. p. 2536.
6. Emiliani B, Stec D, Grasso L, Stodder J. Better thinking, better results: case study and analysis of an enterprise-wide lean transformation. 2nd ed. Kensington: Center for Lean Business Management; 2007. ISBN 978-0-9722591-2-5.
7. Cantrell WA, Samuel LT, Sultan AA, Acuña AJ, Kamath AF. Operative times have remained stable for total hip arthroplasty for >15 years. JBJS Open Access. 2019;4(4):e0047. https://doi.org/10.2106/JBJS.OA.19.00047.
8. Shah RP, Lauthen D, Geller JA, Cooper HJ. Average operative times for 1,313 primary total hip arthroplasty and 1,300 primary total knee arthroplasty over 39 months are roughly equal to medicare attributed operative times. J Arthroplast. 2019;34(8):1553–6. https://doi.org/10.1016/j.arth.2019.04.053. PMID: 31109757.
9. Anis HK, Mahmood BM, Klika AK, Mont MA, Barsoum WK, Molloy RM, Higuera CA. Hospital volume and postoperative infections in total knee arthroplasty. J Arthroplast. 2020;35(4):1079–83. https://doi.org/10.1016/j.arth.2019.10.044. PMID: 31759799.
10. Cowley RJ, Frampton C, Young SW. Operating time for total knee arthroplasty in public versus private sectors: where does the efficiency lie? ANZ J Surg. 2019;89(1–2):53–6. https://doi.org/10.1111/ans.14905. PMID: 30347508.
11. George J, Mahmood B, Sultan AA, Sodhi N, Mont MA, Higuera CA, Stearns KL. How fast should a total knee arthroplasty be performed? An analysis of 140,199 surgeries. J Arthroplast. 2018;33(8):2616–22. https://doi.org/10.1016/j.arth.2018.03.012. PMID: 29656973.
12. Bohl DD, Ondeck NT, Darrith B, Hannon CP, Fillingham YA, Della Valle CJ. Impact of operative time on adverse events following primary total joint arthroplasty. J Arthroplast. 2018;33(7):2256–2262.e4. https://doi.org/10.1016/j.arth.2018.02.037. PMID: 29551302.
13. Cregar WM, Goodloe JB, Lu Y, Gerlinger TL. Increased operative time impacts rates of short-term complications after unicompartmental knee arthroplasty. J Arthroplast. 2021;36(2):488–94. https://doi.org/10.1016/j.arth.2020.08.032. PMID: 32921548.
14. Wang Q, Goswami K, Shohat N, Aalirezaie A, Manrique J, Parvizi J. Longer operative time results in a higher rate of subsequent periprosthetic joint infection in patients undergoing primary joint arthroplasty. J Arthroplast. 2019;34(5):947–53. https://doi.org/10.1016/j.arth.2019.01.027. PMID: 30765229.
15. Maoz G, Phillips M, Bosco J, Slover J, Stachel A, Inneh I, Iorio R. The Otto Aufranc award: modifiable versus nonmodifiable risk factors for infection after hip arthroplasty. Clin Orthop Relat Res. 2015;473(2):453–9. https://doi.org/10.1007/s11999-014-3780-x. PMID: 25024028; PMCID: PMC4294894.
16. Porter ME. What is value in health care? N Engl J Med. 2010;363(26):2477–81. https://doi.org/10.1056/NEJMp1011024. PMID: 21142528.
17. Lau RL, Perruccio AV, Gandhi R, Mahomed NN. The role of surgeon volume on patient outcome in total knee arthroplasty: a systematic review of the literature. BMC Musculoskelet Disord. 2012;13:250. https://doi.org/10.1186/1471-2474-13-250.
18. Kreder HJ, Deyo RA, Koepsell T, et al. Relationship between the volume of total hip replacements performed by providers and the rates of postoperative complications in the state of Washington. J Bone Joint Surg Am. 1997;79:485–94. https://doi.org/10.2106/00004623-199704000-00003.
19. Birkmeyer JD, Stukel TA, Siewers AE, Goodney PP, Wennberg DE, Lucas FL. Surgeon volume and operative mortality in the United States. N Engl J Med. 2003;349(22):2117–27. https://doi.org/10.1056/NEJMsa035205. PMID: 14645640.
20. Chernov M, Vick A, Ramachandran S, Reddy S, Leyvi G, Delphin E. Perioperative efficiency vs. qual-

ity of care – do we always have to choose? J Investig Surg. 2020;33(3):265–70. https://doi.org/10.1080/08941939.2018.1492049. PMID: 30212251.
21. Gabriel RA, Gimlich R, Ehrenfeld JM, Urman RD. Operating room metrics score card-creating a prototype for individualized feedback. J Med Syst. 2014;38(11):144. https://doi.org/10.1007/s10916-014-0144-8. PMID: 25315824.
22. Bender JS, Nicolescu TO, Hollingsworth SB, Murer K, Wallace KR, Ertl WJ. Improving operating room efficiency via an interprofessional approach. Am J Surg. 2015;209(3):447–50. https://doi.org/10.1016/j.amjsurg.2014.12.007. PMID: 25770394.
23. Tagge EP, Thirumoorthi AS, Lenart J, Garberoglio C, Mitchell KW. Improving operating room efficiency in academic children's hospital using lean six sigma methodology. J Pediatr Surg. 2017;52(6):1040–4. https://doi.org/10.1016/j.jpedsurg.2017.03.035. PMID: 28389078.
24. Harders M, Malangoni MA, Weight S, Sidhu T. Improving operating room efficiency through process redesign. Surgery. 2006;140(4):509–14. https://doi.org/10.1016/j.surg.2006.06.018; discussion 514-6. PMID: 17011897.
25. Kubala M, Gardner JR, Criddle J, Nolder AR, Richter GT. Process improvement strategy to implement an outpatient surgery center efficiency model in an academic inpatient setting. Int J Pediatr Otorhinolaryngol. 2021;144:110650. https://doi.org/10.1016/j.ijporl.2021.110650. PMID: 33756390.
26. Attarian DE, Wahl JE, Wellman SS, Bolognesi MP. Developing a high-efficiency operating room for total joint arthroplasty in an academic setting. Clin Orthop Relat Res. 2013;471(6):1832–6. https://doi.org/10.1007/s11999-012-2718-4. PMID: 23208123; PMCID: PMC3706640.
27. Dexter F, Epstein RH. Increased mean time from end of surgery to operating room exit in a historical cohort of cases with prolonged time to extubation. Anesth Analg. 2013;117(6):1453–9. https://doi.org/10.1213/ANE.0b013e3182a44d86. PMID: 24257395.
28. Caggiano NM, Avery DM 3rd, Matullo KS. The effect of anesthesia type on nonsurgical operating room time. J Hand Surg Am. 2015;40(6):1202–9.e1. https://doi.org/10.1016/j.jhsa.2015.01.037. PMID: 25823623.
29. Sokolovic E, Biro P, Wyss P, Werthemann C, Haller U, Spahn D, Szucs T. Impact of the reduction of anaesthesia turnover time on operating room efficiency. Eur J Anaesthesiol. 2002;19(8):560–3. https://doi.org/10.1017/s026502150200090x. PMID: 12200944.
30. Friedman DM, Sokal SM, Chang Y, Berger DL. Increasing operating room efficiency through parallel processing. Ann Surg. 2006;243(1):10–4. https://doi.org/10.1097/01.sla.0000193600.97748.b1. PMID: 16371730; PMCID: PMC1449970
31. Head SJ, Seib R, Osborn JA, Schwarz SK. A "swing room" model based on regional anesthesia reduces turnover time and increases case throughput. Can J Anaesth. 2011;58(8):725–32. https://doi.org/10.1007/s12630-011-9518-2. PMID: 21638194.
32. El-Boghdadly K, Nair G, Pawa A, Onwochei DN. Impact of parallel processing of regional anesthesia with block rooms on resource utilization and clinical outcomes: a systematic review and meta-analysis. Reg Anesth Pain Med. 2020;45(9):720–6. https://doi.org/10.1136/rapm-2020-101397. PMID: 32699101.
33. Goldratt EM. 1947–2011. The goal: a process of ongoing improvement. Great Barrington: North River Press; 2004.
34. Marchand KB, Taylor KB, Salem HS, Mont MA, Marchand RC. Surgical tray optimization and efficiency: the impact of a novel sealed sterile container and instrument tray technology. Surg Technol Int. 2020;37:349–55. PMID: 33245139.
35. Avery DM 3rd, Matullo KS. The efficiency of a dedicated staff on operating room turnover time in hand surgery. J Hand Surg Am. 2014;39(1):108–10. https://doi.org/10.1016/j.jhsa.2013.09.039. PMID: 24268833.
36. Stepaniak PS, Vrijland WW, de Quelerij M, de Vries G, Heij C. Working with a fixed operating room team on consecutive similar cases and the effect on case duration and turnover time. Arch Surg. 2010;145(12):1165–70. https://doi.org/10.1001/archsurg.2010.255. PMID: 21173290.
37. Okeke CJ, Okorie CO, Ojewola RW, Omoke NI, Obi AO, Egwu AN, Onyebum OV. Delay of surgery start time: experience in a Nigerian teaching hospital. Niger J Surg. 2020;26(2):110–6. https://doi.org/10.4103/njs.NJS_61_19. PMID: 33223807; PMCID: PMC7659763.
38. Mazzei WJ. Operating room start times and turnover times in a university hospital. J Clin Anesth. 1994;6(5):405–8. https://doi.org/10.1016/s0952-8180(05)80011-x. PMID: 7986513.
39. Wachtel RE, Dexter F. Influence of the operating room schedule on tardiness from scheduled start times. Anesth Analg. 2009;108(6):1889–901. https://doi.org/10.1213/ane.0b013e31819f9f0c. PMID: 19448219.
40. Padegimas EM, Hendy BA, Lawrence C, Devasagayaraj R, Zmistowski BM, Abboud JA, Lazarus MD, Williams GR, Namdari S. An analysis of surgical and nonsurgical operating room times in high-volume shoulder arthroplasty. J Shoulder Elb Surg. 2017;26(6):1058–63. https://doi.org/10.1016/j.jse.2016.11.040. PMID: 28131689.
41. Booth RE. Keys to OR efficiencies. International society for tech in arthroplasty. In: Orthopaedic Proceedings, vol. 93-B. The British Editorial Society of Bone & Joint Surgery; 2011. p. 452.
42. Mizumoto R, Cristaudo AT, Hendahewa R. A surgeon-led model to improve operating theatre change-over time and overall efficiency: a randomised controlled trial. Int J Surg. 2016;30:83–9. https://doi.org/10.1016/j.ijsu.2016.04.033. PMID: 27109202.
43. Ricketts D, Hartley J, Patterson M, Harries W, Hitchin D. An orthopaedic theatre timings survey. Ann R Coll Surg Engl. 1994;76(3):200–4. PMID: 8017817; PMCID: PMC2502313.

44. Imran JB, Madni TD, Taveras LR, Cunningham HB, Clark AT, Cripps MW, GoldenMerry Y, Diwan W, Wolf SE, Mokdad AA, Phelan HA. Analysis of operating room efficiency between a hospital-owned ambulatory surgical center and hospital outpatient department. Am J Surg. 2019;218(5):809–12. https://doi.org/10.1016/j.amjsurg.2019.04.017. PMID: 31072593.
45. Clark N, Schneider DF, Vrabec S, Bauer PS, Chen H, Sippel RS. Increased efficiency of endocrine procedures performed in an ambulatory operating room. J Surg Res. 2013;184(1):200–3. https://doi.org/10.1016/j.jss.2013.04.038. PMID: 23702288; PMCID: PMC3759536.
46. Daniels AH, DePasse JM, Kamal RN. Orthopaedic surgeon burnout: diagnosis, treatment, and prevention. J Am Acad Orthop Surg. 2016;24(4):213–9. https://doi.org/10.5435/JAAOS-D-15-00148. PMID: 26885712.
47. Panagioti M, Geraghty K, Johnson J, Zhou A, Panagopoulou E, Chew-Graham C, Peters D, Hodkinson A, Riley R, Esmail A. Association between physician burnout and patient safety, professionalism, and patient satisfaction: a systematic review and meta-analysis. JAMA Intern Med. 2018;178(10):1317–31. https://doi.org/10.1001/jamainternmed.2018.3713. Retraction in: JAMA Intern Med. 2020;180(7):931. Erratum in: JAMA Intern Med. 2019;179(4):596. PMID: 30193239; PMCID: PMC6233757.
48. Moerenhout K, Derome P, Laflamme GY, Leduc S, Gaspard HS, Benoit B. Direct anterior versus posterior approach for total hip arthroplasty: a multicentre, prospective, randomized clinical trial. Can J Surg. 2020;63(5):E412–7. https://doi.org/10.1503/cjs.012019. PMID: 33009898; PMCID: PMC7608717.
49. Poehling-Monaghan KL, Kamath AF, Taunton MJ, Pagnano MW. Direct anterior versus miniposterior THA with the same advanced perioperative protocols: surprising early clinical results. Clin Orthop Relat Res. 2015;473(2):623–31. https://doi.org/10.1007/s11999-014-3827-z. PMID: 25082624; PMCID: PMC4294903.
50. Cheng TE, Wallis JA, Taylor NF, Holden CT, Marks P, Smith CL, Armstrong MS, Singh PJ. A prospective randomized clinical trial in total hip arthroplasty-comparing early results between the direct anterior approach and the posterior approach. J Arthroplast. 2017;32(3):883–90. https://doi.org/10.1016/j.arth.2016.08.027. PMID: 27687805.
51. Barrett WP, Turner SE, Leopold JP. Prospective randomized study of direct anterior vs postero-lateral approach for total hip arthroplasty. J Arthroplast. 2013;28(9):1634–8. https://doi.org/10.1016/j.arth.2013.01.034. PMID: 23523485.
52. Herndon CL, Drummond N, Sarpong NO, Cooper HJ, Shah RP, Geller JA. Direct anterior versus mini-anterolateral approach for primary total hip arthroplasty: early postoperative outcomes and complications. Arthroplast Today. 2020;6(2):257–61. https://doi.org/10.1016/j.artd.2020.02.009. PMID: 32577474; PMCID: PMC7303493. DA vs Mini AL similar OR times
53. Brismar BH, Hallert O, Tedhamre A, Lindgren JU. Early gain in pain reduction and hip function, but more complications following the direct anterior minimally invasive approach for total hip arthroplasty: a randomized trial of 100 patients with 5 years of follow up. Acta Orthop. 2018;89(5):484–9. https://doi.org/10.1080/17453674.2018.1504505. PMID: 30350758; PMCID: PMC6202757.
54. Meermans G, Konan S, Das R, Volpin A, Haddad FS. The direct anterior approach in total hip arthroplasty: a systematic review of the literature. Bone Joint J. 2017;99-B(6):732–40. https://doi.org/10.1302/0301-620X.99B6.38053. PMID: 28566391.
55. Wang Z, Hou JZ, Wu CH, Zhou YJ, Gu XM, Wang HH, Feng W, Cheng YX, Sheng X, Bao HW. A systematic review and meta-analysis of direct anterior approach versus posterior approach in total hip arthroplasty. J Orthop Surg Res. 2018;13(1):229. https://doi.org/10.1186/s13018-018-0929-4. PMID: 30189881; PMCID: PMC6127950.
56. Yang XT, Huang HF, Sun L, Yang Z, Deng CY, Tian XB. Direct anterior approach versus posterolateral approach in total hip arthroplasty: a systematic review and meta-analysis of randomized controlled studies. Orthop Surg. 2020;12(4):1065–73. https://doi.org/10.1111/os.12669. Erratum in: Orthop Surg. 2020;12(6):2048. PMID: 32558261; PMCID: PMC7454221.
57. Foissey C, Fauvernier M, Fary C, Servien E, Lustig S, Batailler C. Total hip arthroplasty performed by direct anterior approach – does experience influence the learning curve? SICOT J. 2020;6:15. https://doi.org/10.1051/sicotj/2020015. PMID: 32500856; PMCID: PMC7273835.
58. Kong X, Grau L, Ong A, Yang C, Chai W. Adopting the direct anterior approach: experience and learning curve in a Chinese patient population. J Orthop Surg Res. 2019;14(1):218. https://doi.org/10.1186/s13018-019-1272-0. PMID: 31311597; PMCID: PMC6636028.
59. de Steiger RN, Lorimer M, Solomon M. What is the learning curve for the anterior approach for total hip arthroplasty? Clin Orthop Relat Res. 2015;473(12):3860–6. https://doi.org/10.1007/s11999-015-4565-6. PMID: 26394641; PMCID: PMC4626490.
60. Tamaki T, Nakakita Y, Miura Y, Higashi H, Oinuma K, Shiratsuchi H. Radiographic factors to predict operation time of direct anterior total hip arthroplasty for dysplastic hips. Hip Int. 2021;31(1):90–6. https://doi.org/10.1177/1120700019873877. PMID: 31496293.
61. Patel NN, Shah JA, Erens GA. Current trends in clinical practice for the direct anterior approach total hip arthroplasty. J Arthroplast. 2019;34(9):1987–1993.e3. https://doi.org/10.1016/j.arth.2019.04.025. PMID: 31076194.

Results of the Direct Anterior Approach for Total Hip Arthroplasty

15

William P. Barrett

When reviewing the results of the direct anterior approach (DAA) for total hip arthroplasty (THA), it is important to recognize that THA has been a life-changing procedure for millions of patients over the last 50 years. As described by Ian Learmonth in 2007 as the operation of the century, it has continued to evolve and improve [1]. The global hip replacement device market will approach 6 billion dollars in 2020 [2]. Thus, from both a clinical and financial perspective it has a significant impact on our lives. I began performing DAA THA in 2008, and in many ways, my experience is an example of the changing paradigm for approaches to THA. Having performed posterior approach THA for 20 years, one could ask why change? In the early 2000s, the results of posterior approach THA were very good. When we contemplate introducing new technology, techniques, or materials into our clinical practice, it is useful to consider the recommendations of Malchau: identify the problem, what is the proposed solution (risks, complications, cost, and chances of success), how do you deal with what you think will happen versus what happens (universal dilemma), what compromises are justifiable in pursuit of the change, and what are the costs [3]. A confluence of factors over the last 10–15 years has helped identify some of the problems with our approaches to THA. Patients are seeking care at a younger age, wanting to return to active lifestyles, not wanting to follow postoperative precautions and expecting faster recoveries while having a short stay or outpatient procedure. In addition, the emphasis on value in joint replacement surgery (quality/cost) and bundled payments made us all consider alternatives. Modifiable factors in technique, patient optimization, and implant selection present opportunities to improve the value of THA.

The established paradigm for surgical approaches in the early 2000s was a posterior or direct lateral approach. As Thomas Kuhn noted in 1962, established paradigms can stifle progress and evolution of thought [4]. But as we will review in this chapter, surgeons from around the world began exploring the anterior approach and challenging established paradigms and building on the success of previous techniques. As results from multiple centers with various modifications of the technique began to emerge interest in DAA increased, this interest was influenced by surgeon curiosity, marketing by industry, hospitals, and patient demand. The methods for establishing the usefulness of new technology or techniques are not standardized and often left up to surgeons and industry to decide. A survey of American Academy of Hip and Knee Surgeons (AAHKS) in 2018 found that 56.2% of respondents perform DAA, while 43.8% did not [5]. The DAA performing surgeons felt that outcomes differed between DAA and PA with regard to length of

W. P. Barrett (✉)
Proliance Orthopedic Associates, Renton, WA, USA

J. M. Matta, A. P. Sah (eds.), *Anterior Hip Replacement*,
https://doi.org/10.1007/978-3-030-91896-5_15

stay, postoperative pain, dislocation rate, component accuracy, and short-term patient outcomes. Non-DAA surgeons cited increased complication rates, steep learning curve, and lack of clinical superiority as reasons for not switching to DAA. The purpose of this chapter is to understand how a surgical approach that was used by less than 5% of AAHKS members increased to more than 50% over a 15-year period. We will follow the results of DAA from early observational cohort studies, to current meta-analysis reports. We will track the evolution of results with the early emphasis on learning curves issues, DAA, and technique-specific complications and the impact of education and surgeon learning on results.

Early Results

As noted in the first chapter of this book, Judet and Judet had been using the Hueter approach since 1947 and evolved to use a similar approach for THA [6]. They described removing the insertion of the tensor fascia lata from the anterior iliac crest and cutting the piriformis tendon. Since that time, many surgeons have used a modification of this approach to perform THA. Many of the early publications emphasized the safety and lower dislocation rate of anterior approach as dislocation had evolved as the "problem" with posterior approach (PA) THA.

In 2003, Kennon described their experience with "A minimally invasive anterior surgical approach" [7]. Patients were positioned supine on a regular operating room table with a bump under the operative hip. The skin incision was similar to the distal portion of a Smith–Peterson approach, and the interval between the tensor fascia lata and sartorius muscle was utilized. Additional small stab incisions could be utilized to introduce acetabular reamers or femoral broaches/reamer/insertors (Fig. 15.1). Due to the limited femoral exposure, the authors often used a dual modular femoral design to facilitate placement of the femoral component. The authors had been using this approach for over 30 years at the time of publication. A ten-year review of 1281

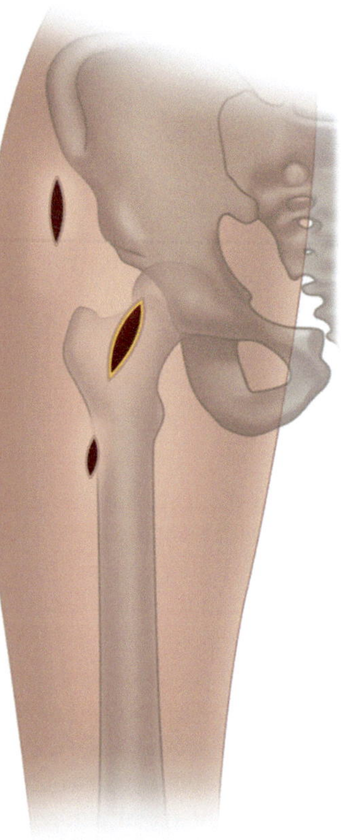

Fig. 15.1 Drawing of early anterior approach skin incision as described by Kennon et al. [7]

cemented stems and 851 cementless stems focusing on complications was reported. There were 25 (2%) fractures of the femur in the cemented group and 60 (7%) in the cementless group. They concluded that their review of 2132 consecutive cases revealed a low rate of intraoperative and postoperative complications, short operative times (50–60 min) for "noncomplex" cases, and a "low" blood loss. In their study, this approach led to faster postoperative mobilization and rehabilitation.

In 2004, Siguier reported the results of 1037 cemented THAs with a 22 mm femoral head using a modified Hueter approach [8]. They began using a mini-incision anterior approach for THA in 1993. Patients were positioned supine on a Judet fracture table. A 6–8 cm skin incision was utilized centered over the tensor fascia lata (TFL). The interval between the TFL and the sartorius was developed. Following surgery, patients were allowed to be weight-bearing as tolerated on postoperative day 1 or day 2. Ten of 1037 (0.96%) hips dislocated at 2 weeks to 8 months postoperatively. Two patients developed a femoral nerve palsy both resolved with time. At the time of their paper, the rate of dislocation with a 22 mm femoral head ranged from 1.78% to 2.59% using trans-trochanteric or posterior approaches. They concluded that the mini-incision anterior approach was a safe and reproducible technique with low morbidity and fast postoperative recovery due to preservation of the soft tissue.

Matta in 2005 reported a series of 494 THAs performed through a single anterior incision utilizing the interval previously described with the patient on a fracture-type table combined with intraoperative fluoroscopy to improve implant positioning [9]. This was a retrospective, single-surgeon, study of 437 consecutive patients who had 494 THAs performed between 1996 and 2004. Fifty-four stems were cemented and 442 were cementless. The surgical approach evolved during the course of the study. A classic Smith–Petersen approach was used from 1996 to 2002. In 2002, the author switched to a smaller incision starting just distal and lateral to the anterior superior iliac spine. In his 2005 paper, he described the step-by-step approach and use of intraoperative fluoroscopy to confirm implant position and leg length. The average cup inclination was 42 degrees with 96% in the range of 35–50 degrees. Following surgery, limb length discrepancy averaged 3 ± 2 mm. There were 3 (0.61%) post-op dislocations, 17 (3.4%) operative complications including 3 greater trochanter fractures, 2 femoral shaft fractures, 4 calcar fractures, and 3 ankle fractures from use of the fracture table. The average operative time was 75 min, and blood loss averaged 350 ml. The authors concluded that the use of a tissue-sparing anterior approach with fluoroscopic guidance allowed consistent implant positioning and leg length restoration.

These 3 papers demonstrated that this approach could be performed safely, reproducibly, and with a lower dislocation rate than previously reported with posterior approach THA in the hands of experienced anterior approach surgeons. However, the question remained that could this approach be used in a widespread manner by a significant number of orthopedic surgeons.

Learning Curve

A chapter of this book is dedicated to the learning curve for DAA; however, it is important to review how the literature responded to this evolving paradigm shift in approach to THA. Several articles highlighted the possible risks and learning curve associated with DAA. While authors noted that this approach could be performed by experienced surgeons, they questioned the assimilation of DAA into general use. Learning curve can be defined in a variety of ways but in essence is the number of cases a surgeon requires to obtain a steady state of outcomes. Many factors influence that number including surgeon experience, case volume, surgeon preparation with regard to independent learning, availability of courses, cadaver training, mentoring, and ease of assimilation of a new technique. Malcom Gladwell in his book Outliers published in 2008 examined factors that lead to high levels of success and states world-class expertise requires approximately 10,000 hours of practice to master a skill [10]. While learning the DAA does not require that time commitment, the role of practice and education in adopting the DAA will be explored using the following articles.

In 2009, the results of a multicenter observational cohort study were published to answer the question: Can the results of DAA be extrapolated to surgeons with less experience using DAA [11]. They reviewed 1277 DAA THAs from 9 sites with up to 3-year follow-up. Data were analyzed by an independent data center. The average operative time was 95 min, fluoroscopy time averaged 30 s, and average blood loss was 427 ml. Thirty-five patients (2.7%) required revision surgery. Seventeen patients (1.3%) developed loose implants, and dislocations occurred in 8 (0.6%) patients. Surgeons who performed less than 100 cases were twice as likely (20.2%) to have a complication versus those that performed more than

100 procedures (9.8%). They concluded that the procedure was associated with an acceptable complication rate, low dislocation rate, and early return to function that plateaued at 3 months postoperatively and noted that complications declined after 100 cases.

Woolson in 2009 reported on short-term results from 5 community orthopedic surgeons performing DAA starting in 2004 [12]. Of note, these 5 surgeons were all low-volume hip surgeons, with 4 out of 5 performing less than 1 THA per month. Four of the 5 visited a surgeon champion of the DAA; however, none of the surgeons did any cadaver training or had available mentoring opportunities. The study included 247 DAA THAs. The average operative time was 164 mins, average blood loss was 858 ml, and major complications occurred in 9% of patients. These included proximal femoral or greater trochanteric fractures in 16 (6.5%) patients, 2 peroneal nerve palsies, and 3 re-operations for limb length inequalities. There were no post-op dislocations. The authors noted that major complications decreased after 30–50 cases. This study raised awareness of the importance of preoperative preparation prior to adopting a new procedure or technique.

Jewett in 2011 reported his experience with DAA using a fracture table and technique outlined by Matta [13]. This retrospective study included 800 THAs performed between 2004 and 2009. They noted 26 (3.2%) intraoperative complications including 19 trochanteric fractures and 3 femoral canal perforations. The majority of these occurred in the first 200 cases in the series. They reported 91 (11.3%) postoperative complications. Seven (0.88%) dislocations, 37 (4.6%) wound complications, and 26 reoperations, the majority for wound complications requiring debridement. The authors noted the greater trochanteric fracture rate was primarily in the first 200 cases, and wound complications persisted throughout the series but were not associated with an increased infection rate. They stressed the importance of education and training for surgeons prior to adopting this technique.

In 2015, de Steiger published a study asking "What is the learning curve for the Anterior Approach for Total Hip Arthroplasty?" [14]. Using data from the Australian Orthopaedic Association National Joint Replacement Registry (AOANJRR), the authors evaluated 4138 DAA cases, using the same implant system, performed by 13 surgeons from 2007 to 2013. All of these surgeons had performed more than 100 cases. They divided the surgeon case volume into 5 groups: group 1 cases 1–15 cases to group 5 greater than 100 cases. The primary outcome measure was time to first revision and reason for revision. The cumulative revision rate for all surgeons at 4 years was 3%. For their first 15 cases, the revision rate was 6%, and for greater than 100 cases 2%. It was not until surgeons had performed 50 cases that the revision rate approached a steady state. The most common reason for revision was fracture, which occurred in 34 hips (29%) of all revisions followed by loosening, dislocation, and infection. They noted that surgeons with more experience had lower revision rates and they needed to perform 50 cases to reach a steady state, i.e., 50 case learning curve.

In 2016, Schwartz addressed the question "Is it safe to transition to Direct Anterior Approach in the current health care climate" [15]. They published a retrospective, single-surgeon cohort study of consecutive primary THAs over a transition period from PA to DAA. These included 201 PA and 211 DAA. Prior to switching, the surgeon completed 2 cadaveric courses and consulted with several surgeons using the DAA. During his first 25 DAA cases, he "cherry-picked" patients with lower BMI and more favorable anatomy. All cases were performed on a special table using fluoroscopy. They noted no difference in 30- or 90-day readmission rates, no difference in rates of complications, and no difference in revision rates. DAA patients had longer operative and overall procedure times. However, the DAA patients had half the rate of acetabular components placed outside the goal inclination range of 35–50 degrees. They concluded that transitioning from a PA to DAA can be done with appropriate surgeon preparation and patient selection without increased risks to patients.

Stone in 2018 reported on the learning curve when transitioning from a posterolateral to DA for THA [16]. This was a single-surgeon retrospective study of 1000 DAA consecutive cases. The surgeon was an experienced hip surgeon who had performed over 1500 PA THAs prior to starting the DAA. He participated in didactic training, surgeon mentorship, assisted another DAA surgeon, and did cadaver training before transitioning to the DAA. They compared the average operative time, total procedure time, and complications of the prior PA cases to 1000 consecutive DAA cases. There was an initial increase in both operative time and total procedure time of 34% and 30%, respectively, when compared to the PA. The operative time became statistically equivalent after the 400th DAA case and shorter than the PA time after 600 cases. The total procedure time was statistically equivalent after 900 cases. Thirty-six complications requiring reoperation occurred in the DAA group with a minimum of 2-year follow-up. Among these were 7 femoral component loosenings, 4 periprosthetic femur fractures, 12 infections, and 1 dislocation. They concluded that when transitioning from a PA to DAA THA, surgeons will experience decreased efficiency up to 500 cases, low complication rates with a particularly low dislocation rate.

In 2020, Pirruccio reported on a prospective, single-surgeon study comparing the first 100 DAA cases and comparing them to the surgeons last consecutive PA THAs [17]. The surgeon went through the following process prior to implementing the DAA: one-month period of anatomy and literature review followed by visitation to an experienced DAA surgeon to observe 3 cases. He then created a 30-page annotated technique guide. He then attended a cadaver course and then performed 2 DAA cases with a surgeon mentor. From case 3 to 30, the surgeon would meet the night before surgery with his joint replacement fellow, PA, resident, and scrub tech to watch a surgical technique video and review the annotated technique guide. After each case, the team would meet to debrief and update their technique guide. After case #30, the surgeon and PA revisited the experienced DAA surgeon. The authors noted the DAA cases took 7 min longer, were associated with a 0.7 shorter length of stay, and no significant difference in estimated blood loss or surgical complications. They attributed the no significant difference in THA complication rate when transitioning from PA to DAA to a fully engaged learning methodology prior to transitioning.

Gofton in 2020 published results of a retrospective review of prospectively collected data for an observational cohort of patients undergoing DAA THA between 2006 and 2017 by 4 surgeons at a single tertiary care center [18]. Between 2006 and 2016, DAA THA rose from 1.5% to 53.2% of annual THAs at their institution. The overall adverse event rate was 6.4%. The adverse event rate was higher in the surgeon's first 15 cases (11.7%) compared to the remaining cases (4.1%) The dislocation rate was 0.7% (8/1078), and there was a canal perforation/femoral shaft fracture rate of 0.5%. The authors recommended a stepwise approach by introducing a new implant and then new approach and mentoring for the first 20 cases to insure patient safety.

Review of these 8 different studies reveals that surgeon preparation and experience are directly related to the length of the learning curve and risk of complication when transitioning from another surgical approach to the DAA. These studies reflect the experience of surgeons who are already in practice following their training. In the following section, we will review some of the common complications associated with the DAA.

Complications

The most common complications following THA include infection, dislocation, periprosthetic fracture, and neurovascular injury. Along with the discussion of learning curve, examination of complication rates associated with the DAA is useful when considering its use in THA.

Wound complications can occur with any surgical approach for THA. There are some generally agreed-upon risk factors some of which are modifiable such as patient weight and smoking. Wound complications with the DAA have been thought to be related to the thinner skin anteriorly, increased shear forces due to the proximity of the inguinal crease, and overlying pannus in obese individuals. Christensen in 2014 reported on a retrospective, single-surgeon, registry data study from 2003 to 2014 comparing 1288 PA THA and 505 DAA THA [19]. They noted a significantly higher rate of reoperation for wound-related complications 1.4% in the DAA group versus 0.2% for the PA group. Reoperation for infection was not significantly different 0.6% versus 0.2%. They advocated counseling patients preoperatively regarding the risk of wound-related problems with the DAA.

In 2015, Watts reported on a single-center, single-surgeon, retrospective cohort analysis of 716 patients undergoing a DAA THA and compared them to a group of 3040 posterior approach patients during the same time interval (2010–2014) [20]. In the DAA group, 12 patients (1.7%) developed wound complications following surgery. Dehiscence or necrosis of a portion of the incision required a return to the OR for 9 (75%) of these patients. This was compared to 59 (1.9%) patients with wound complications in the PA group. Of these, 31 (53%) required reoperation for wound debridement. The authors found that obese (BMI > 40) females were at higher risk of wound complications in the DAA group. Wound complication rates were similar in both the DAA and PA groups.

Russo in 2015 performed a retrospective review of 210 consecutive patients who had a DAA THA and divided the patients into 3 categories: normal BMI, pre-obese, and obese (BMI > 30) [21]. The obese group had a longer surgery time, length of stay, and narcotic use all statistically significant. Complications and wound complications were also significantly higher in the obese group. They noted the obese group had an 8.8 higher risk of complications and 3.6 times higher risk of wound complications compared to patients with BMI < 30.

In 2016, Jahng reported on 651 DAA arthroplasties the majority of which were primary THAs [22]. The majority of patients had uneventful wound healing, but 75 (11.5%) had post-op wound complications that required additional treatment. Of this group of patients, 13 (1.9%) of the overall cohort required reoperation for the wound complications. Multivariate analysis showed that BMI > 30 and diabetes were significantly associated with the development of wound complications.

Dislocation after THA has been and remains one of the major causes for additional treatment and or surgery after THA. Early and subsequent studies have demonstrated a lower rate of dislocation following DAA THA. This is due to many factors including supine positioning, intraoperative use of fluoroscopy, and software programs to evaluate implant positioning, leg length, and offset.

In 2015, Sheth reported on a review of the Kaiser Permanente Total Joint Registry [23]. They identified primary THAs performed between 2001 and 2011. They evaluated septic revisions, aseptic revisions, and dislocations by surgical approach. 42,438 THAs were available for analysis of revision outcomes, and 22,237 were available for dislocation outcomes. They found no difference in the risk of revision (either septic or aseptic) between any of the approaches but noted the DAA and anterolateral approach had a lower risk of dislocation versus the PA.

In 2018, Fleischman reported on a single institution, retrospective study of 16,186 THAs performed between 2010 and 2016 [24]. This review revealed the risk of dislocation was 0.74% for DAA versus 1.74% for PA. The risk of femoral failure due to periprosthetic fracture or loosening was 1.2% for DAA versus 0.47% for PA. The authors noted this higher rate of femoral failure may be due to difficulty with femoral exposure and canal preparation particularly early on in a surgeon's experience. Preservation of the posterior soft tissue structures and more accurate component positioning were credited to the lower dislocation rate for DAA.

Charney in 2020 reported on a cohort study from the Kaiser Permanente's Total Joint Replacement Registry for primary THA [25]. There were 38,399 primary THAs, and 6428 (16.7%) were DAA THAs. They noted the DAA was associated with a lower risk of dislocation, revision for instability, revision for periprosthetic fracture, and 90-day unplanned readmission following THA when compared to PA THA. However, the DAA was associated with a higher risk of revision for aseptic loosening.

Periprosthetic fractures can occur with any surgical approach, and the majority occur during surgery and may or may not be recognized at the time of occurrence. Lee in 2015 reported a meta-analysis of complications following DAA THA [26]. They reviewed 38 studies with an aggregated total of 11,810 DAA THAs. Intraoperative femoral fractures occurred in 2.3% of cases with trochanteric, calcar fracture, and femoral perforations being the most common.

In 2016, Barnett presented a cohort study of 5090 primary DAA THAs performed between 2006 and 2013 [27]. Five surgeons from 3 sites contributed to study. The 90-day complication rate was 1.9%. There were 41 (0.8%) intraoperative femur fractures (29 calcar fractures, 9 greater trochanteric fractures, and 3 femoral shaft fractures). There were 7 postoperative fractures. The authors all of whom were experienced DAA THA surgeons concluded that the 90-day periprosthetic fracture rate demonstrated an acceptable risk profile.

In 2019, Hart reported on 1967 THAs performed at a single institution by multiple surgeons between 2010 and 2017 [28]. The data were a synthesis of the institution joint registry database and National Surgical Quality Improvement data. Three surgical approached were utilized PA 56%, direct lateral 29%, and DAA 15%. Thirty-day major and minor complications occurred in 3.9% and 9.4%, respectively, for all the approaches combined. The rates 30-day complications were similar between all 3 approaches.

While the DAA takes advantage of the internervous plane between the TFL and Sartorius muscles, there is a risk of injury to the lateral femoral cutaneous nerve (LFCN) because of its proximity to the skin incision and approach. Damage to this nerve does not result in functional impairment but it can cause numbness or neuralgia on the anterolateral thigh. In 2016, Rudin using cadaveric specimens described the variable branching patterns of the LFCN [29]. They noted 62% of the nerves entered the proximal thigh medial to the anterior superior iliac spine (ASIS), while 27% entered superior to the ASIS and 11% lateral to the ASIS. The nerve consistently coursed in the deep layer of the subcutaneous fat tissue. In 2015, Grob published "Potential Risk to the Superior Gluteal Nerve During the Anterior Approach" [30]. The hemipelvis from 19 cadaveric specimens were dissected to locate the innervation of the TFL muscle. In 17 of 19 cases, a branch from the inferior branch of the superior gluteal nerve entered the TFL muscle within 10 mm of the entry point of the ascending branch of the lateral circumflex femoral artery. The authors concluded that coagulation of the ascending branch of the lateral circumflex artery and placement of retractors carry the potential risk of injury to the motor branch of the TFL muscle. They recommended ligation/coagulation of the vascular leash slightly medial to the medial border of the TFL muscle to avoid damage to the motor branch. Lee in the previously referenced meta-analysis of complications following DAA THA noted that injury to the femoral nerve from the DAA is not higher than other approaches [26].

The most common complications following THA can also occur with the DAA THA. There is an increased risk of wound complications with obese, diabetic patients. In obese patients with a large pannus, we use a wound vac to minimize soft tissue problems and promote wound healing (Fig. 15.2). There is an increased risk of femoral fractures and implant loosening early in the learning curve due to challenges of femoral exposure without adequate releases. Dislocation rates are consistently lower with the DAA. Sensory nerve injuries are more common due to the location of the LFCN but typically do not cause functional impairment.

A unique risk of DAA THA with the use of fluoroscopic guidance is radiation exposure to the surgeon and patient. McArthur in 2015 reported on a consecutive series of 51 patients who underwent a DAA THA [31]. They found that the average radiation exposure to the surgeon was slightly higher than a hip injection but substantially less than placement of cannulated screws for a femoral neck fracture, guidance for

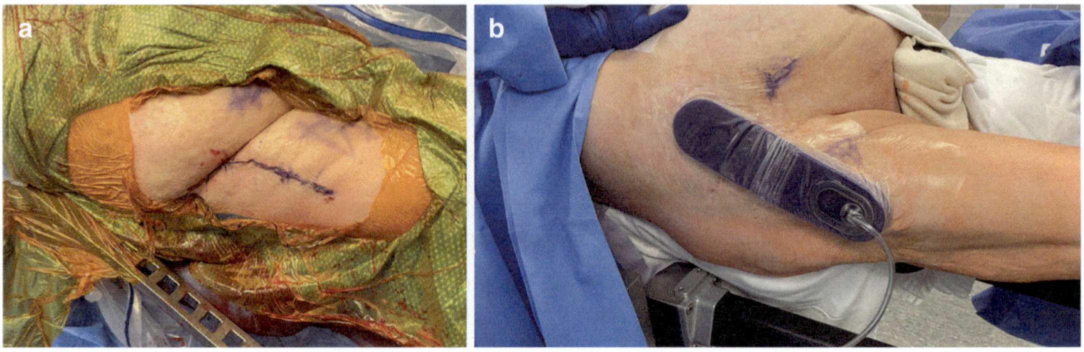

Fig. 15.2 (a) Intraoperative photograph of patient with right anterior approach THA with large pannus. (b) Same patient after application of negative pressure wound vac dressing

hip arthroscopy, or placement of an intramedullary nail for a femoral shaft fracture. Curtin in 2016 evaluated patient radiation exposure during fluoroscopically assisted DAA THA [32]. This was a retrospective review of 157 consecutive DAA THAs from 2 institutions. They evaluated total exposure time, radiation emittance, and peak kilovoltage. There was an association between radiation exposure and body mass index. The average exposure time per procedure was 23.74 s. The total radiation exposure was nearly identical with screening mammograms, and 4 times less than a standard chest CT scan. The authors concluded that the 1 time exposure to radiation for the patient during a DAA THA is negligible.

Advantages

As noted previously, the cause of dislocation is multifactorial. In 2015, Abdel published a study of 9784 hips from a single institution between 2003 and 2012 [33]. A group of 206 THAs that had a dislocation were identified. The acetabular implant position was evaluated with regard to inclination and anteversion. They found that 84% of the cups were in Lewinnek's "safe zone" of 40 degrees ± 10 degrees and 69% were in the safe zone for anteversion 15 degrees ± 10 degrees. They also noted that 65% of dislocated hips performed through a PA had an acetabular component in the combined safe zone versus 33% of dislocated hips performed through an anterolateral approach. They concluded that hip stability is dependent on multiple factors including cup position, patient anatomy, and implant design. More recently, the influence of spinopelvic issues has been associated with THA stability.

Hamilton in 2015 reported a retrospective 2 cohort review of 100 PA THAs, and the first 100 DAA THAs performed by the senior author [34]. The PA group had posterior capsular repair and 6 weeks of PA precautions. The DAA group utilized a fracture-type table, intraoperative fluoroscopy, and no post-op precautions. The authors noted more accurate cup position with the DAA (90% in safe zone versus 79% for PA) for abduction. The variance in cup abduction was greater in the PA group (44.4 degrees versus 24.9 degrees in the DAA group). There were 4 dislocations in the PA group vs. 2 in the DAA group. The study was underpowered to detect a statistical difference. The authors concluded that supine positioning and use of intraoperative fluoroscopy contributed to more accurate implant positioning.

McLawhorn in 2020 published an article titled "Prospective Evaluation of the Posterior Tissue Envelope and Anterior Capsule after Anterior Total Hip Arthroplasty" [35]. Thirty-two patients following a DAA THA had metal artifact reduction MRIs of their hips immediately postoperatively, 3 months postoperatively, and at 1-year follow-up. Fifteen of the hips had an anterior capsulotomy and repair versus 17 patients with capsulectomy. Immediately post-op, 75% of the piriformis tendons were intact. Of those not intact, the gap was 2–3 mm from bone. At 1-year follow-up, 97% of the piriformis tendons were intact. Immediately post-op, 35% of conjoined tendons were intact, 94% showed no sign of obturator internus atrophy. Of the released conjoined tendons, at 1 year 95% were intact with scar in continuity with the posterior capsule. At 1 year, the posterior capsule was in contact with bone. At 1 year, the group with capsulotomy and closure had no defect in the anterior capsule. The capsulectomy group had a 27% rate of persistent anterior capsular defect. The authors concluded that with DAA THA release of a portion of the posterior capsule and the conjoined tendon led to continuity of these structures to bone at short-term follow-up.

Better positioning of the implants, preserving soft tissue attachments, and minimizing soft tissue damage would inherently seem to improve gait mechanics following THA. However, several studies have failed to show a dramatic difference between DAA and PA THA.

Queen in 2013 reported on 30 subjects who underwent a THA with either PA, direct lateral, or anterolateral approach and completed a self-selected speed level walking gait assessment preoperatively, at 6 weeks, and 1 year postoperatively [36]. All patients showed improvement in walking speed, stride length, and peak hip extension during stance phase at both 6 weeks and 1 year. There were no significant differences between posterior, direct lateral, and anterolateral approaches to the hip for THA.

Rodriquez in 2014 compared 60 patients with a DAA THA with 60 patients who had a PA THA in a prospective, nonrandomized assessment of functional recovery using a variety of functional parameters [37]. Functional recovery was faster at 2 weeks in patients with the DAA THA on the basis of timed up and go test and the motor component of the Functional Independence Measure™. There were no differences in other metrics used at 2 weeks. No differences were noted between groups at 6 weeks or 1 year.

Nelms in 2020 compared 20 control subjects with 35 DAA THA patients and 34 PA THA patients in a prospective nonrandomized study using smartphone gait assessments of gait speed, step length, cadence, and center of mass displacements [38]. The DAA and PA groups were similar preoperatively. At 1 month, the DAA group had significantly faster gait speed at self-selected and fastest possible gait compared to PA. At 4 months, there were no significant differences between the 2 groups.

Results Comparing DAA to PA and Direct Lateral

As interest in less invasive surgical approaches (anterior and posterior based) grew in the early 2000s, investigators sought to determine if there was a quantifiable difference in muscle and tissue damage. Meneghini in 2006 reported on a series of 6 human cadavers that had an MIS anterior approach on one side and a MIS posterior approach on the opposite side [39]. The same implant system was used on both sides, and a surgeon experienced with the particular approach performed the cases. They found that the damage to the gluteus medius muscle was minimal with both approaches, and the tendinous portion was spared completely. The MIS anterior approach resulted in less damage to the gluteus minimus muscle versus the MIS posterior approach. The short external rotators and piriformis muscles are routinely transected with a posterior approach. The anterior approach required in 3 of 6 specimens either the piriformis or the conjoined tendon to be released as part of the femoral exposure. Some degree of damage occurred to the tensor fascia lata and rectus femoris muscle in all the anterior cases and none of the posterior cases. This study demonstrated less muscle damage to the abductor muscles with a MIS anterior approach when compared to a MIS posterior approach, but this difference may be offset by damage to the TFL and rectus femoris with the anterior approach.

Berend in 2009 reported on a series of patients who underwent THA in the 2006–2008 timeframe [40]. A less invasive direct lateral approach was used in 372 hips and a DAA THA using a standard operating room table was used in 258 hips. The same pre- and postoperative protocols, same implants, and pain management were used in all cases. The authors found the DAA THAs had a significantly improved early recovery in the form of higher Harris Hip scores and lower extremity activity scale score at 6 weeks post-op. Also, in 2009 Nakata reported a retrospective review of 195 consecutive MIS THAs [41]. There were 99 in the DAA group and 96 in the PA group. Surgeries were performed between 2003 and 2006. The same pre- and postoperative protocols were used in both groups. The DAA group was performed on a standard operating room table. The operative time was similar in both groups, and blood loss was higher in the DAA group. The DAA group had a significantly more rapid functional recovery as demonstrated by time to walk with single cane, 50 meter timed walking test, walking velocity at 3 weeks, and time to walking without assistive devices. Significantly more hips had their cups placed in Lewinnek's "safe zone" in the DAA group. The authors concluded the MIS DAA was a more useful approach for rapid functional recovery when compared to the MIS PA.

Alecci in 2011 reported a retrospective review of 419 consecutive THAs, 198 hips performed through a direct lateral (DL) approach and compared them to 221 performed using DAA [42]. They evaluated several perioperative parameters including length of surgery, blood loss, post-op pain, length of stay, and discharge destination. The surgical time was 8 min longer, which was significant for the DAA group. The DAA group had 2 minimally displaced greater trochanteric fractures. The DL group had more intra- and postoperative blood loss, which was statistically significant. The DAA group had a shorter length of stay, and higher percentage were discharged home compared to the DL group. The authors concluded the DAA was a safe and efficacious approach that accelerated functional recovery. Also in 2011, two studies were published examining the potential tissue damage done by different approaches. Bergin compared inflammatory and muscle damage markers in DAA and PA THAs [43]. They prospectively evaluated 29 patients with a DAA THA and compared them to 28 patients with a PA THA measuring serum creatinine kinase, interleukin-6, interleukin1L-beta, and tumor necrosis factor, preoperatively, in the recovery room and postoperative days 1 and 2. They found that the serum creatinine kinase a marker for muscle damage was 5.5 times higher in the PA group vs the DAA group. There was an overall trend toward lower levels of inflammatory markers in the DAA group. The authors speculated that the inflammatory cascade associated with THA may not be greatly influenced by surgical approach but is defined by bone removal and implant placement. Therefore, the inflammatory markers were not statistically different. Based on the levels of serum creatinine kinase, the authors concluded that the DAA resulted in less muscle damage when compared to the PA. In the second study, Bremer retrospectively performed MRIs at 1 year postoperatively on a group of 50 patients, 25 with a DAA THA, and 25 with a PA THA [44]. A radiologist graded changes in the abductor musculature. Detachment of the abductor insertion, partial tears and tendonitis of the gluteus medius and minimus, and fatty atrophy were significantly less pronounced and less frequent in the DAA group. There were no significant differences in damage to the tensor fascia lata between the 2 groups. They concluded that the DAA resulted in less muscle damage when compared to the PA.

Barrett in 2013 reported a single-surgeon prospective randomized study comparing DAA THA in 43 patients to PA THA in 44 patients [45]. They noted patients with the DAA had a longer incision, more blood loss, and longer operative time all of which were significant. They attributed that to the additional steps associated with use of a fracture table and C-arm. The DAA group had a statistically higher percentage of cups in Lewinnek's safe zone for both inclination and anteversion (73%) when compared to the PA group (57%). The length of hospital stay was significantly shorter for the DAA group 2.3 days vs 3 days for the PA group. Early postoperative data, including VAS pain score and walking distance, were significantly better for the DAA group. These benefits in addition to better HSS and HOOS scores persisted for up to 3 months. At 6 months and 1 year, there were no significant differences in outcomes between the groups. The authors published a 5-year follow-up study in 2019 of this same group. Two patients had been lost to follow-up in each group. The authors noted no difference in complications, survivorship, and patient function as measured by PROM scores between the 2 groups at an average 5-year follow-up. They concluded the DAA offers early (up to 3 months) benefits without compromise of survivorship at 7 years.

Zawadsky in 2014 reported on a single-surgeon retrospective series of 150 consecutive THAs [46]. The first 50 cases utilized a mini-PA, the next 50 were done through a DAA considered the surgeons learning curve, and the final 50 were the "routine" DAA using a standard operating room table and no intraoperative fluoroscopy. The pre- and postoperative protocols were the same for all groups. The hospital-based data favored the DAA groups with significantly shorter length of stay, and higher percentage discharged home. The operative time was significantly longer in the DAA learning curve group but not different for the "routine" DAA group when compared to PA group. At 2 weeks, both DAA groups had significantly better pain scores and used less narcotics versus the PA group. At 6 weeks, 84% of the DAA group were walking free of assistive devices versus 32% of the PA group. There were more complications in the DAA group all of which occurred in the first 29 cases during the learning curve. The authors concluded that the DAA allows for more rapid recovery with less pain when compared with the PA. However, they noted a significant learning curve with a higher complication rate during the first 50 cases.

Poehling-Monaghan in 2014 published "Direct anterior versus Mini-posterior THA with the Same Advanced Perioperative Protocols: Surprising Early Clinical Results" [47]. They compared 125 DAA THA cases done by one surgeon with 96 mini PA THAs done by another surgeon over a one-year period of time. The groups did not differ demographically. They found no differences in length of hospital stay, in-hospital complications, distance walked in the hospital, or discharge destination. The DAA cases took statistically longer to perform. At 2 weeks, more DAA patients required gait aids (92%) versus the PA group (68%). At 8 weeks, the DAA group had a higher Harris Hip Score (95 versus 89) with no difference between the groups with use of gait aids, narcotic use, and activities of daily living. More wound problems occurred in the mini PA group. They concluded there was no systematic advantage of one approach over the other. In a follow-up study from the same institution, Taunton in 2018 reported on a randomized clinical trial of 52 patients performed by one high-volume DAA surgeon and 49 mini PA patients performed by 3 high-volume PA surgeons [48]. All patients received the same implants and rapid recovery rehab protocols. Functional results evaluated included time to discontinue gait aids, discontinue all narcotics, independence with various activities of daily living, and PROMs up to 1 year. Early functional recovery such as walking without a walker or any aid, navigating stairs with aid, and stopping narcotics was all statistically better in the DAA group. The DAA group used less post-op pain medicine and walked farther in therapy prior to discharge. Activity monitoring at 2 weeks and 8 weeks after surgery revealed the DAA group was more active versus the PA group. PROMs at 2 months and 1 year revealed no significant difference between the groups. There were no differences in complications between the 2 groups. The authors concluded both approaches provide early functional recovery with low risk of complications.

Higgins in 2015 performed a systematic review and meta-analysis of anterior versus posterior approach for THA [49]. They included 17 studies with 2302 patients. They concluded that available evidence did not support one approach to be superior to another. They did note the anterior approach may provide potential benefits in early patient-reported pain and functional outcomes, postoperative length of stay, dislocations, and postoperative narcotic use. Additionally, the pooled results favored the anterior approach in terms of patients discharged home and percentage of acetabular components in Lewinnek's "safe zone".

Another meta-analysis in 2018 by Miller reviewed prospective studies comparing postoperative outcomes through 90 days [50]. They evaluated 13 prospective studies with 524 DAA THAs and 520 PA THAs. They found patients with DAA THA had less pain, consumed fewer narcotics, and reported better hip function according to Harris Hip Scores up to 90 days postoperatively. They noted no differences in complications (dislocations, fractures, infections, hematoma, and reoperations) between the 2 groups.

Seah in 2019 compared opioid consumption after THA in three surgical approaches: DAA, PA, and DL [51]. In a single-center retrospective observational study, they compared 179 DAA, 203 PA, and 178 DL THAs. They found that the DAA was associated with lower daily opioid use and better pain scores at 12, 24, and 72 h post-op. The DAA was associated with a 21% reduction in daily opioid use when compared to DL and 18.7% reduction compared to PA.

After reviewing the literature comparing DAA to other approaches over the last 15 years, I have concluded that the DAA offers advantages in terms of less pain, better function, and earlier return to activity when compared the either the PA or DL. These advantages are noted up to 3 months after surgery, and by 6 and 12 months, there seems to be no significant advantage in terms of the factors noted above. However, due to more accurate implant placement with use of C-arm and software programs the rate of dislocation and restoration of proper biomechanics are better than the other approaches.

Hype

With the emergence of "less invasive" surgical approaches in the early 2000s, questions arose regarding the influence of the approach, incision length, soft tissue injury, and the role of rapid rehab, advanced multimodal pain management, patient education, and management of expectations on outcomes. In 2007, Pour reported on a prospective randomized study comparing 4 patient groups: group A standard length incision with standard pre- and postoperative care; group B a small incision with standard pre- and postoperative care; group C standard length incision with preoperative counseling, accelerated rehabilitation, and multimodal pain management; and group D small incision with preoperative counseling, accelerated rehabilitation, and multimodal pain management. The same surgical approach, implants, and anesthesia were used in all cases. The 2 groups (C and D) with preoperative counseling, accelerated rehabilitation, and multimodal pain management had better functional outcomes regardless of incision length when compared to the 2 groups without the enhanced program. The authors concluded that multiple factors including patient and family education, multimodal pain management, and rapid rehabilitation protocols influenced outcome more than the length of the incision [52].

In 2015, Mohan reported on a study assessing the authorship, content, and quality of information presented on websites related to DAA THA [53]. They used 3 of the most commonly used search engines at the time using the search term "direct anterior hip replacement". At the time, they found that the online information was often incomplete and misleading. The authorship of the top 50 websites was primarily by private physicians/clinics. They found that sites readily allow the reader to see the benefits of the procedure and set up online appointments with a provider but often did not discuss potential risks, indications, or reference to peer-reviewed literature.

In 2018, Shofoluwe published a study examining the level of promotion of DAA THA on the Internet by members of the American Association of Hip and Knee Surgeons (AAHKS) [54]. At the time of the study, there were 1673 active members of AAHKS. They identified 1855 websites associated with the AAHKS members. They found that DAA THA was mentioned in 22.8% of the websites. Claims of the benefits of DAA including less invasive, muscle sparing, quicker recovery, and less pain were made on more than 40% of the websites. Potential risks such as lateral femoral cutaneous nerve trauma, fracture, or wound complications were mentioned on less than 4.7% of sites. The authors concluded that potential benefits of the procedure were highlighted 9 times more frequently than potential risks.

Summary

The DAA for THA uses a true intermuscular/internervous interval to approach the hip. It stands to reason that this approach if properly done should result in less soft tissue/muscle damage. The early results using this approach reported by Kennon, Siguier, and Matta gave reassurance it could be safely performed with a reasonable rate of complications in the hands of experienced surgeons. With interest in less invasive/minimally invasive approaches to the hip increasing approximately 15 years ago, surgeons began to explore/adopt the DAA. Studies reported after the early results included surgeon's learning curve experience. It became clear that surgeon experience, preparation, and mentoring impacted outcomes with DAA. The drawbacks of limited preparation and low surgical volume prior to adopting the DAA were revealed in the study by Woolson. The value of diligent preparation, learning, and planning was demonstrated in the study by Pirruccio. Results from more recent studies reveal some trends. DAA THA is associated with less pain, earlier functional recovery, and more accurate implant placement, which translates into a lower dislocation rate. Most of these advantages occur in the first 3 months postoperatively. The theoretical advantages of this approach have been documented by MRI and inflammatory markers. Has marketing and hype contributed to the popularity of this approach? One could argue it has played a role. However, as use has become more widespread and residents and fellows are learning the DAA as part of their training its growth is more organic versus resulting from external forces. There is a saying in orthopedic circles that orthopedic surgeons use data much like a drunk uses a lamp post more for support than illumination. In this chapter, I have tried to give a fair assessment of the available data without cherry picking only those articles that support my bias. Lastly, what do I tell my patients as to why I use the DAA for all my cases? "It is associated with less pain, a faster recovery and return to activity which in my experience lasts for approximately 3 months. Due to use of intraoperative fluoroscopy and a software program I am more accurate with my implant placement and this allows me to better address limb length and hip biomechanics (Fig. 15.3) this results in a short and long term reduction in the risk of dislocation."

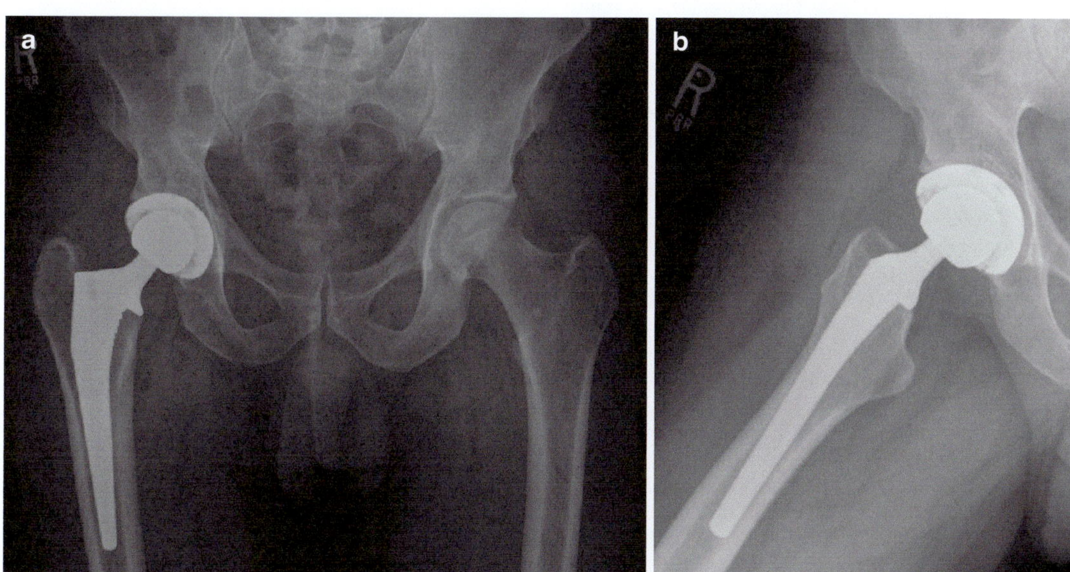

Fig. 15.3 (**a**) Post-operative AP pelvis X-ray demonstrating restoration of appropriate length and offset of hip replacement with good acetabular position. (**b**) Post-operative lateral X-ray demonstrating good cup and femoral implant position

References

1. Learmonth ID, Young C, Rorabeck C. The operation of the century: total hip replacement. Lancet. 2007;370:1508–19.
2. Markets and markets. Hip replacements market worth 5.9 billion USD by 2020. Accessed 1 Jul 2019. http://marketsandmarkets.com/Press-Releases/hip-reconstruction-devices.asp
3. Malchaur H, Bragdon CR, Muratoglu OK. The stepwise introduction of innovation into orthopedic surgery. J Arthroplast. 2011;26:825–31.
4. Kuhn TS. The structure of scientific revolutions. The University of Chicago Press; 1962.
5. Patel NM, Shah JA, Erens GA. Current trends for the direct anterior approach total hip arthroplasty. J Arthroplast. 2019;34:1987–93.
6. Judet R, Judet J. Technique and results with the acrylic femoral. J Bone Joint Surg. 1952;34B:173–80.
7. Kennon RE, Keggi JM, Wetmore R, Zatorski LE, Huo ME, Keggi KJ. Total hip arthroplasty through a minimally invasive anterior surgical approach. J Bone Joint Surg. 2003;85-A:39–48.
8. Siguier T, Siguier M, Brumpt B. Mini-incision anterior approach does not increase dislocation rate. Clin Orthop Relat Res. 2004;426:164–73.
9. Matta JM, Shahrdar C, Ferguson T. Single-incision anterior approach for total hip arthroplasty on an orthopaedic table. Clin Orthop Relat Res. 2005;44:115–24.
10. Gladwell M. Outliers: the story of success. New York: Little, Brown and Company; 2008.
11. The Anterior Total Hip Arthroplasty Collaborative Investigators. Outcomes following the singe-incision anterior approach to total hip arthroplasty: a multicenter observational study. Orthop Clin North Am. 2009;40:329–42.
12. Woolson ST, Pouliot MA, Huddleston JI. Primary total hip arthroplasty using an anterior approach and a fracture table. J Arthroplast. 2009;24:999–1005.
13. Jewett BA, Collis DK. High complication rate with anterior total hip arthroplasties on a fracture table. Clin Orthop Relat Res. 2011;469:503–7.
14. de Steiger RN, Lorimer M, Solomon M. What is the learning curve for the anterior approach for total hip arthroplasty. Clin Orthop Relat Res. 2015;473:3860–6.
15. Schwartz BE, Sisko ZW, Mayekar EM, Wang OJ, Gordon AC. Transitioning to the direct anterior approach in total hip arthroplasty: is it safe in the current health care climate. J Arthroplast. 2016;31:2818–24.
16. Stone AH, Sibia US, Atkinson R, Turner TR, King PJ. Evaluation of the learning curve when transitioning from posterolateral to direct anterior hip arthroplasty: a consecutive series of 1000 cases. J Arthroplast. 2018;33:2530–4.
17. Pirruccio K, Evangelista PJ, Haw J, Goldberg T, Sheth NP. Safely implementing the direct anterior total hip arthroplasty: a methodological approach to minimizing the learning curve. J Am Acad Orthop Surg. 2020;0:1–7.
18. Gofton WT, Ibrahim MM, Kreviazuk CJ, Kim PR, Feibel RJ, Beaule PE. Ten-year experience with the anterior approach to total hip arthroplasty at a tertiary care center. J Arthroplast. 2020;35:1281–9.
19. Christensen CP, Karthikeyan T, Jacobs CA, Cale A. Greater prevalence of wound complications requiring reoperation with direct anterior approach total hip arthroplasty. J Arthroplast. 2014;29:1839–941.
20. Watts CD, Houdek MT, Wagner ER, Sculoc PK, Calmers BP, Taunton MJ. High risk of wound complications following direct anterior total hip arthroplasty in obese patients. J Arthroplast. 2015;30:2296–8.
21. Russo MW, Macdonnell JR, Paulus MC, Kellar JM, Zawadsky MW. Increased complications in obese patients undergoing direct anterior total hip arthroplasty. J Arthroplast. 2015;30:1384–7.
22. Jahng KH, Bas MA, Rodriguez J. Risk factors for wound complications after direct anterior approach hip arthroplasty. J Arthroplast. 2016;31:2583–7.
23. Sheth D, Cafri G, Inacio MCS, Paxton EW, Namba RS. Anterior and anterolateral approaches for THA are associated with lower dislocation risk without higher revision risk. Clin Orthop Relat Res. 2015;473(11):3401–8.
24. Fleischman AN, Tarabichi M, Magner Z, Parvizi J, Rothman RH. Mechanical complications following total hip arthroplasty based on surgical approach. A large, single-institution cohort study. J Arthroplast. 2019;34:1255–60.
25. Charney M, Paxton EW, Stradiotto R, Leen JJ, Hinman AD, Sheth DS, Prentice HA. A comparison of risk of dislocation and cause-specific revision between direct anterior and posterior approach following elective cementless total hip arthroplasty. J Arthroplast. 2020;35:1651–7.
26. Lee GC, Marconi D. Complications following direct anterior hip procedures: costs to both patients and surgeons. J Arthroplast. 2015;30:98–101.
27. Barnett SL, Peters DJ, Hamilton WG, Ziran NM, Gorab R, Matta JM. Is the anterior approach safe? Early complication rate associated with 5090 consecutive primary total hip arthroplasty procedures performed using the anterior approach. J Arthroplast. 2016;31:2291–4.
28. Hart A, Wyles CC, Abdel MP, Perry KI, Pagnano MW, Taunton MJ. Thirty-day major and minot complications following total hip arthroplasty- a comparison of the direct anterior, lateral, and posterior approaches. J Arthroplast. 2019;34:2681–5.
29. Rudin D, Manestar M, Ullrich O, Johannes E, Grob K. The anatomical course of the lateral femoral cutaneous nerve with special attention to the anterior approach to the hip joint. J Bone Joint Surg. 2016;98:561–7.
30. Grob K, Manestar M, Ackland T, Filguerira L, Kuster SK. Potential risk to the superior gluteal nerve during the anterior approach to the hip joint. J Bone Joint Surg. 2015;97:1426–31.

31. McAuther BA, Schueler BA, Howe BM, Trousdale RT, Taunton MJ. Radiation exposure during fluoroscopic guided direct anterior approach for total hip arthroplasty. J Arthroplast. 2015;30:1565–8.
32. Curtin BM, Armstrong LC, Bucker BT, Odum SM, Jiranek WA. Patient radiation exposure during fluro-assisted direct anterior approach total hip arthroplasty. J Arthroplast. 2016;31:1218–21.
33. Abdel MP, Roth PV, Jennings MT, Hanssen AD, Pagnano MW. What safe zone? The vast majority of dislocated THAs are within the Lewinnek safe zone for acetabular component position. Clin Orthop Relat Res. 2016;474:386–91.
34. Hamilton WG, Parks NL, Huynh C. Comparison of cup alignment, jump distance, and complications in consecutive series of anterior approach total hip arthroplasty. J Arthroplast. 2015;30:1959–62.
35. McLawhorn AS, Christ AB, Morgenstern R, Burge AJ, Alexiades MM, Su EP. Prospective evaluation of the posterior tissue envelope and anterior capsule after anterior total hip arthroplasty. J Arthroplast. 2020;35:767–73.
36. Queen RM, Schaeffer JF, Butler RJ, Berasi CC, Kelley SS, Attarian DE, Bolognesi MP. Does surgical approach during total hip arthroplasty alter gait recovery during the first year following surgery? J Arthroplast. 2015;28:1639–43.
37. Rodruguez JA, Deshmukh AJ, Rathod PA, Greiz ML, Deshmane PP, Hepinstall MS, Ranawat AS. Does the direct anterior approach in THA offer faster rehabilitation and comparable safety to the posterior approach. Clin Orthop Relat Res. 2014;472:455–63.
38. Nelms NJ, Birch CE, Halsey DH, Blankstein M, Mcginnis RS, Beynnon BD. Assessment of early gait recovery after anterior approach compared go posterior approach total hip arthroplasty: a smartphone accelerometer-based study. J Arthroplast. 2020;35:465–70.
39. Meneghini RM, Pagnano MW, Trousdale RT, Hozack WJ. Muscle damage during MIS total hip A. Clin Orthop Relat Res. 2006;453:292–8.
40. Berend KR, Lombardi AV, Seng BE, Adams JB. Enhanced early outcomes with the anterior supine intermuscular approach in primary total hip arthroplasty. J Bone Joint Surg. 2016;91(Supplement 6):107–20.
41. Nakata K, Nishikaw M, Yamamoto K, Hirot S, Yoshikawwa H. A clinical comparative study of the direct anterior with mini-posterior approach. J Arthroplast. 2009;24:698–704.
42. Alecci V, Valente M, Crucil M, Pelligrino CM, Sabbadini DD. Comparison of primary total hip replacements performed with a direct anterior approach versus the standard lateral approach: perioperative findings. J Orthop Traumatol. 2011;12:123–9.
43. Bergin PF, Doppelt JD, Kephart CJ, Benke MT, Graeter JH, Holmes AS, Smithe HH, Tuan RS, Unger AS. Comparison of minimally invasive direct anterior versus posterior total hip arthroplasty based on inflammation and muscle damage markers. J Bone Joint Surg Am. 2011;93:1392–8.
44. Breme AK, Kalbere F, Pfirrmann CW, Dora C. Soft-tissue changes in hip abductor muscles and tendons after total hip replacement. J Bone Joint Surg. 2011;93B:886–9.
45. Barrett WP, Turner SE, Leopold JP. Prospective randomized study of direct anterior vs postero-lateral approach for total hip arthroplasty. J Arthroplast. 2013;28:1634–8.
46. Zawadsky MW, Paulus MC, Murray PJ, Johansen MA. Early outcome comparison between the direct anterior approach and the mini-incision posterior approach for primary total hip arthroplasty: 150 consecutive cases. J Arthroplast. 2014;29:1256–66.
47. Poehling-Monaghan KL, Kamath AF, Taunton MJ, Pagano MW. Direct anterior versus miniposterior THA with the same advanced perioperative protocols: surprising early clinical results. Clin Orthop Relat Res. 2015;473:623–31.
48. Taunton MJ, Trousdale RT, Sierra RJ, Kaufman K, Pagnano MW. John Charnley award: randomized clinical trial of direct anterior and miniposterior approach THA: which provides better functional recovery? Clin Orthop Relat Res. 2018;476:216–29.
49. Higgins BT, Barlow DR, Heagerty NE, Lin TJ. Anterior vs. posterior approach for total hip arthroplasty, a systematic review and meta-analysis. J Arthroplast. 2015;30:419–34.
50. Miller LE, Gondsuky JS, Bhattacharyya S, Kamath AF, Boettner F, Wright J. Does surgical approach affect outcomes in total hip arthroplasty through 90 days of follow-up? A systematic review with meta-analysis. J Arthroplast. 2018;33:1296–302.
51. Seah S, Quinn M, Tirosh O, Tran P. Postoperative opioid consumption after total hip arthroplasty: a comparison of three surgical approaches. J Arthroplast. 2019;34:2676–80.
52. Pour AE, Parizi J, Sharkey PF, Hozack WJ, Rothman RH. Minimally invasive hip arthroplasty: what role does patient preconditioning play? J Bone Joint Surg. 2007;89:1920–7.
53. Mohan R, Yi PH, Hansen EN. Evaluating online information regarding the direct anterior approach for total hip arthroplasty. J Arthroplast. 2015;30:803–7.
54. Shofoluwe AI, Naveen NB, Inabathula A, Ziemba-Davis M, Meneghini RM, Callaghan JJ, Warth LC. Internet promotion of the direct anterior approach total hip arthroplasty by members of the American association of hip and knee surgeons. J Arthroplast. 2018;33:167–70.

Difficult Cases in Primary Anterior Total Hip Arthroplasty

16

Atul F. Kamath and Linsen T. Samuel

Introduction

The anterior approach (AA) to total hip arthroplasty (THA) is a versatile surgical approach. This approach has demonstrated benefit over other approaches during the in-hospital [1], early postoperative [2–4], and later postoperative [5] periods. Further economic benefit has been demonstrated in certain populations [6]. Preoperative planning, meticulous surgical technique, soft tissue handling to respect the intramuscular/nervous intervals, and an understanding of the appropriate femoral releases [7] all prove important when performing THA from the AA.

While gaining experience and exposure to the surgical technique [8], it is important for the surgeon to understand the types of cases that may present special challenges in the primary and/or conversion arthroplasty setting. Moreover, cataloging preoperative and intraoperative tips and techniques should help to maximize perioperative outcomes. Careful templating, preparing specialized equipment, employing specialized implants if needed, and executing particular maneuvers are all vital to surgical success, regardless of surgical approach (e.g., anterior vs. other approaches [9], or variants of the anterior approach technique [10]). This chapter presents a selection of primary arthroplasty cases to highlight particular teaching points. While these cases may be performed from a variety of surgical approaches, the reader should understand the particular soft tissue, biomechanical, and functional benefits of applying the AA to these cases.

Case

This is a 37-year-old woman who presented with symptomatic bilateral hip pain. Her right hip pain was worse than her left hip pain. She was status post multiple bilateral childhood pelvic and proximal femoral surgeries. She was also status post most recently a right hip arthroscopy with labral debridement done by another surgeon. Her right hip pain worsened significantly after this most recent hip arthroscopy.

She was of short stature: Her height was 4′2″, with a body mass index (BMI) of 33. There were severe restrictions in range of motion. She has multiple prior incisions, primarily over the anterior and lateral aspects of the hip. Considerations for this proximal right hip deformity include the

A. F. Kamath (✉)
CCLCM, CWRU SOM, Hip & Knee Reconstruction, Department of Orthopaedic Surgery, Cleveland Clinic Foundation, Cleveland, OH, USA

Center for Hip Preservation, Orthopaedic and Rheumatologic Institute, Cleveland Clinic, Cleveland, OH, USA
e-mail: kamatha@ccf.org

L. T. Samuel
Department of Orthopaedic Surgery, Cleveland Clinic Foundation, Cleveland, OH, USA

J. M. Matta, A. P. Sah (eds.), *Anterior Hip Replacement*,
https://doi.org/10.1007/978-3-030-91896-5_16

varus bowing of the femur, question of versional deformity, and short/varus neck–shaft angle. She also has a highly deficient right acetabulum and hemipelvis deformity.

Consideration for surgery on the acetabular side includes low volume socket with potential need for autograft augmentation versus metallic augmentation. Version assessment was critical given the relative retroversion of the acetabulum and small volume socket. Considerations on the femoral side include small canal and issues of potential fixation problem with traditional short uncemented stem. Preparation must be made for potential proximal femoral correctional osteotomy, which can be performed either through a continuous curvilinear incision extending distally from the standard proximal AA hip incision, or through a separate lateral distal incision in a subvastus manner. The anterior approach, with the use of fluoroscopy in the supine position, allows excellent visualization of any corrective osteotomy to address proximal femoral deformity. Fluoroscopy also aids with accurate cup sizing and placement.

Intraoperative fluoroscopy views of the right hip confirm safe femoral broaching, as well as accurate implantation of the acetabular component along with augmentation autografting, fixed with cannulated screws (Fig. 16.1). Final plain radiography demonstrates satisfactory position of the components without need for a corrected osteotomy of the proximal femur (Fig. 16.1).

Case

This is a 55-year-old man, with history of multiple prior bilateral lower extremity hip and knee procedures. He has a history of remote slipped capital femoral epiphysis of the right hip, status post multiple intra- and extracapsular right hip procedures. Due to the significant right hip pain and disability, he had been wheelchair-bound for 2 months prior to presentation. He has a BMI of 36.

Considerations for right hip arthroplasty include significant capsular scarring and multiple prior incisions about the right hip and pelvis. He also has Dorr C canal and retroversional issues of the proximal head–neck segment. Planning must be made for these versional issues of the femur, as well as potential need for cemented arthroplasty given the poor bone quality. Patient has significant leg length discrepancy, with the right leg several centimeters shorter than the left. Both superficial and deep significant scarring of the soft tissues and tendons about the right proximal femur, and aggressive soft tissue mobilization, are required to reestablish normal hip biomechanics and to recreate leg length and offset.

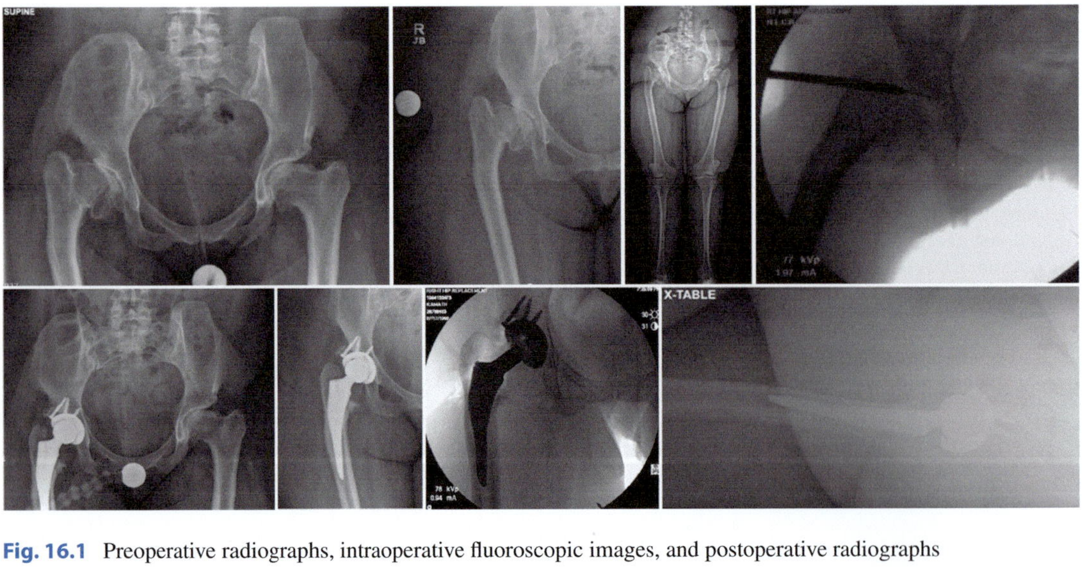

Fig. 16.1 Preoperative radiographs, intraoperative fluoroscopic images, and postoperative radiographs

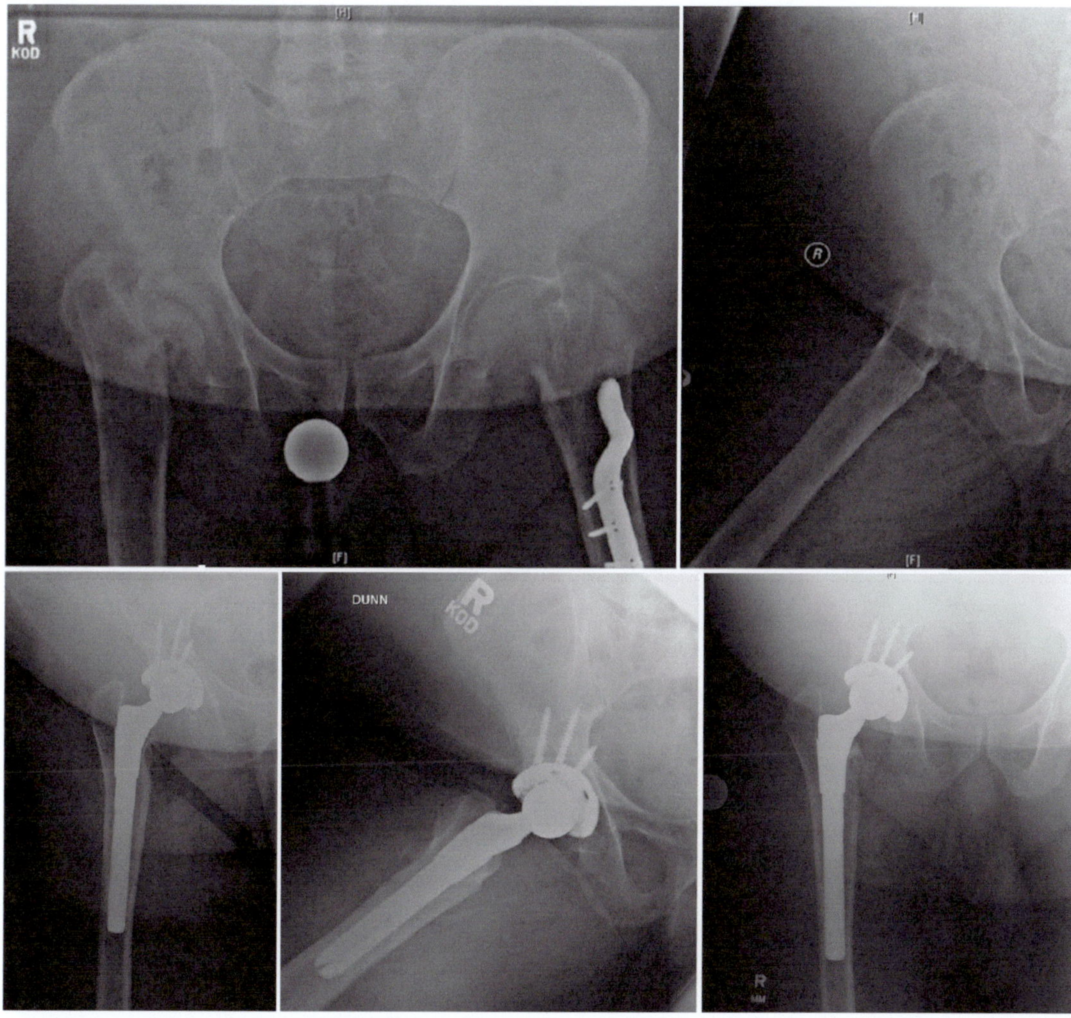

Fig. 16.2 Preoperative and postoperative radiographs

Postoperative views of the pelvis and right hip demonstrate uncemented fixation with an S-ROM prosthesis (DePuy, Warsaw, IN) to control significant retroversion deformity of the proximal femur (Fig. 16.2). Screw augmentation been placed on the acetabular side, giving obesity and to accommodate for the poor acetabular bone stock.

Other considerations in the obese patient are demonstrated in Fig. 16.3. These include appropriate taping of the abdominal pannus and closure with supplemental interrupted Nylon suture in horizontal mattress configuration. Though not routinely used by the author, an incisional negative pressure vacuum dressing may be utilized in the early postoperative period for obese patients.

Case

This is a 69-year-old woman with history of Parkinson's disease and morbid obesity, who initially presented with a severely comminuted distal femur fracture. She underwent primary distal femoral placement for a nonreconstructable distal femur fracture and severe underlying arthritis. She was subsequently lost to follow-up and had sustained an ipsilateral intertrochanteric fracture, for which a dynamic hip screw was

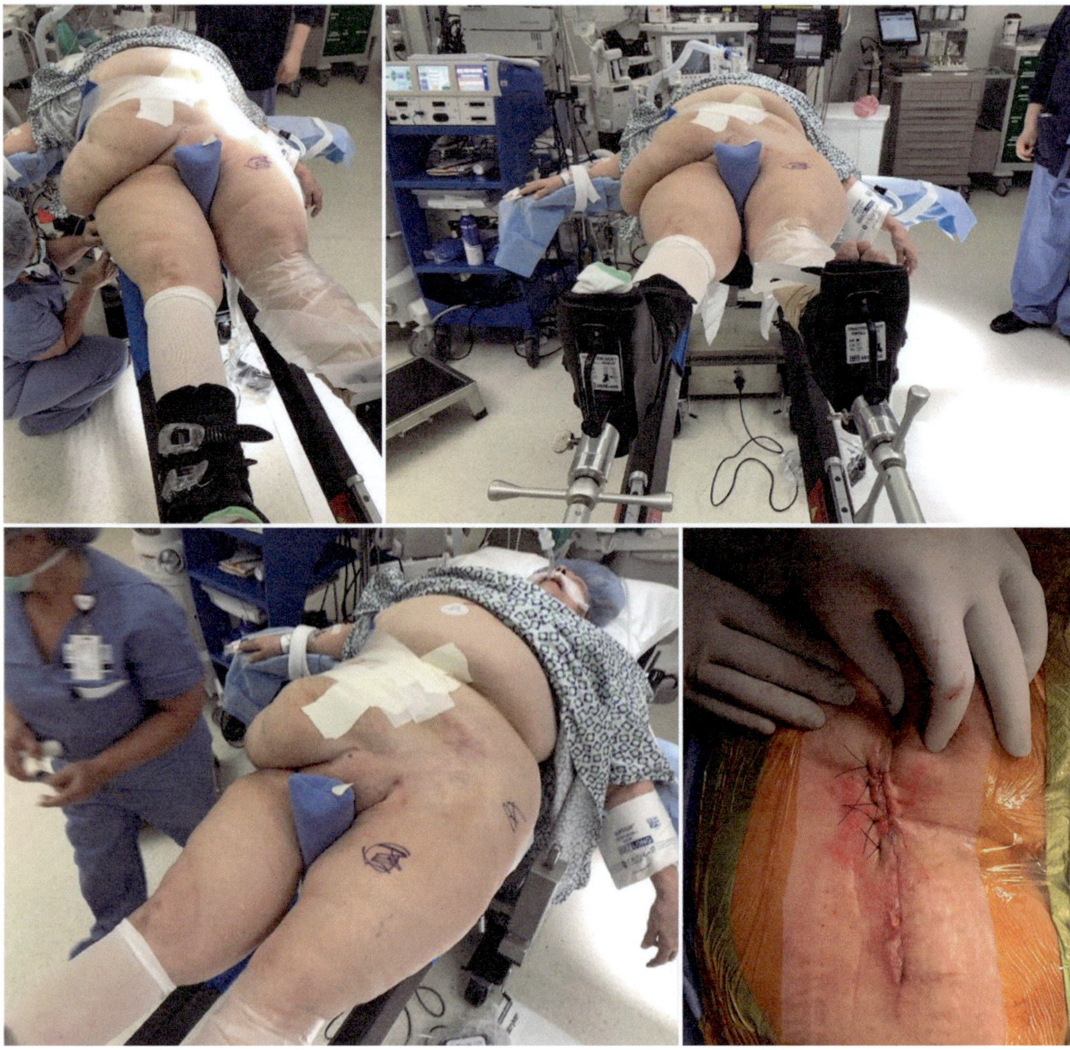

Fig. 16.3 Preoperative and intraoperative maneuvering/considerations for morbidly obese patient

placed for internal fixation at an outside institution. The hip screw subsequently cut out of the femoral head, causing severe symptomatic left hip pain and disability (Fig. 16.4). There was exuberant callous formation after healing of the intertrochanteric fracture. Workup for infection, including inflammatory markers and hip aspiration, was negative.

At the time of surgery with a posterior approach, the hip should usually be first dislocated and then relocated prior to hardware removal. However, with an anterior approach and a planned in situ neck cut, the femoral head does not necessarily need to dislocated first. There was excision of significant heterotopic bone about the intertrochanteric and lesser trochanteric regions. The plate was then cut after excision of further significant amount of heterotopic bone encasing the entire length of the plate. The dynamic hip screw was removed, and the femoral neck osteotomy can then be made in situ. A high-speed burr was used for safe access to the femoral canal. A cemented stem was placed in the setting of poor-quality bone. Sufficient bony bridging and the remnant plate segment were deemed acceptable for protection of the stress riser between the tip of the femoral stem and the proximal tip of the distal femoral replacement (Fig. 16.5). Consideration

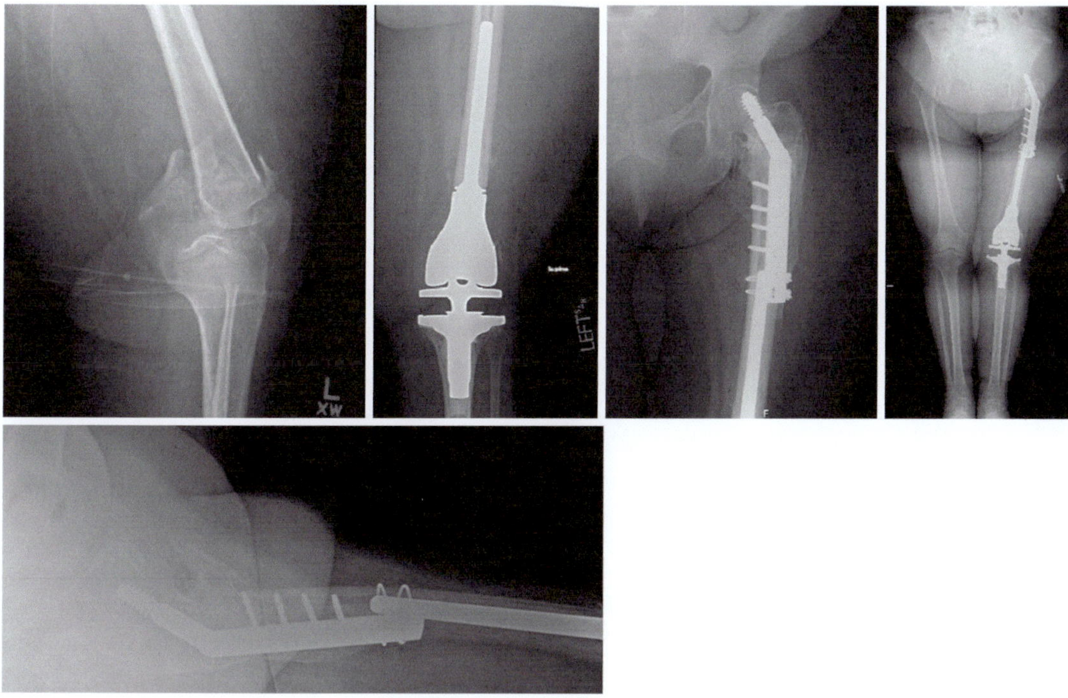

Fig. 16.4 Preoperative radiographs

can be made for supplemental strut allograft protection. Cultures taken from the time of surgery were negative for infection.

Case

This is a 61-year-old highly active man, who does recreational cycling and hiking activities. He had sustained an intertrochanteric fracture, for which a short intramedullary nail was placed for fixation at the referring institution (Fig. 16.6). He had progressive right groin symptoms, as well as abductor fatigue. He had undergone two cortisone intra-articular hip pain injections with several months of temporary relief at a time. Discussion was had regarding conversion hip arthroplasty. He understood the issues related to trochanteric fixation and abductor mechanism dysfunction, including potential for residual abductor issues. He had been worked up for occult infection, which was negative.

Preoperative computed tomography scan, including three-dimensional reconstructions obtained by the referring orthopedic surgeon, demonstrated a malunited fragment of the proximal femur (Fig. 16.6). The decision to perform conversion arthroplasty from the anterior approach in this scenario must take into account the posterior location of the malunited greater trochanteric segment, as well as any difficulties that may be encountered with mobilization and subsequent fixation of this greater trochanter, which may be challenging from an anterior-based approach. Any posteriorly based greater trochanteric malunion deformities, as well as need for potential greater trochanteric transfer, may prove difficult from an anterior Smith–Petersen approach and should be considered carefully.

At the time of surgery, the greater trochanteric segment was mobilized safely, maintaining a posterior hinge sleeve of soft tissue. The distal screw was removed through a percutaneous incision, and then, the head screw was engaged and removed through the main incision. Finally, the nail was extracted through a separate percutaneous incision. The femoral

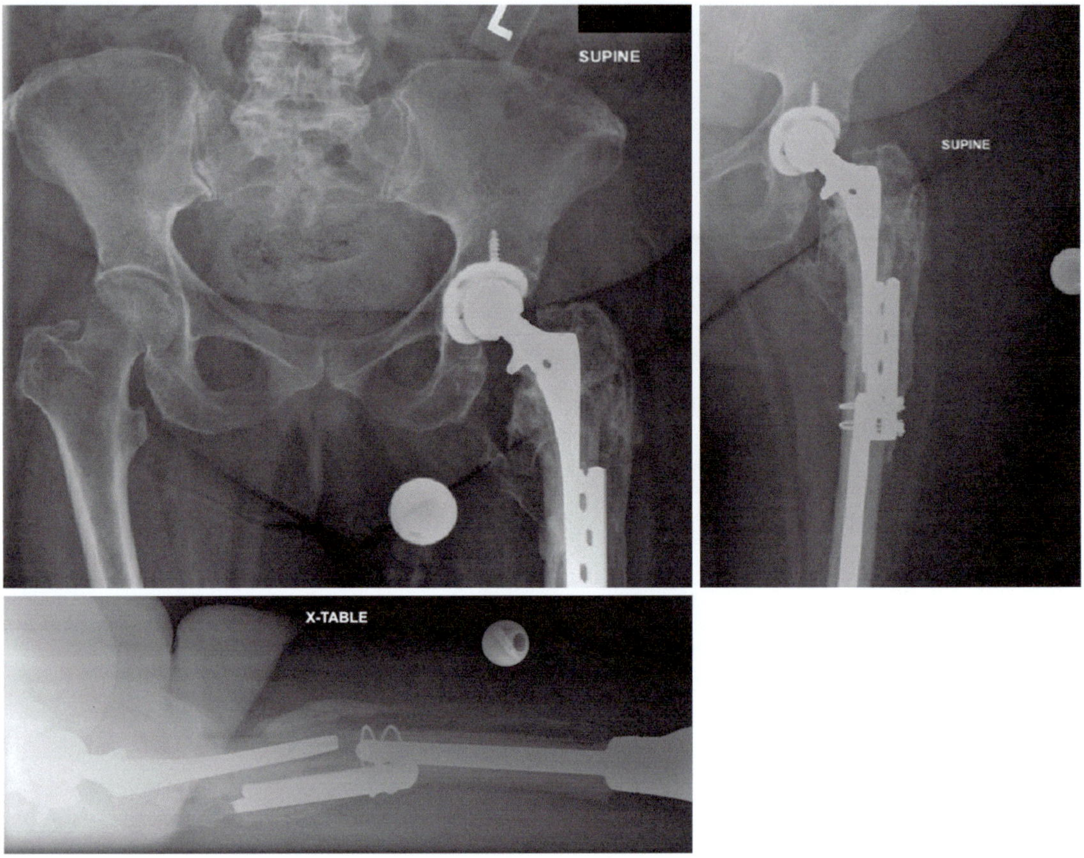

Fig. 16.5 Postoperative radiographs

neck osteotomy in situ was performed. A fully porous-coated stem was chosen to provide adequate fixation (Fig. 16.7). The author does not feel that bypassing the distal screw hole is necessary by an appreciable distance in good quality bone, as this is generally not a significant stress riser. In poor bone quality, this may be considered for longer length of fixation. The greater trochanteric piece was refixated with a double-ended Luque wire. The wire was passed through the substance of the greater trochanteric bone laterally and wrapped around the external medial proximal intertrochanteric bone. The author prefers to use cerclage wiring above the level of the lesser trochanter to avoid potential fretting and corrosion with braided cables. Alternate fixation includes an all-suture material suture as FiberTape Cerclage (Arthrex, Naples, FL).

Case

This is a 47-year-old medical assistant who sustained a left intertrochanteric fracture, managed nonoperatively for 6 months after her initial injury. She experienced progressive varus remodeling deformity of the proximal femur, with continued pain and ambulatory dysfunction. She had a 2-cm leg length discrepancy.

Anteroposterior and cross-table lateral views of the proximal femur demonstrated anterior displacement of the proximal head–neck segment compared to the long axis of the distal femoral

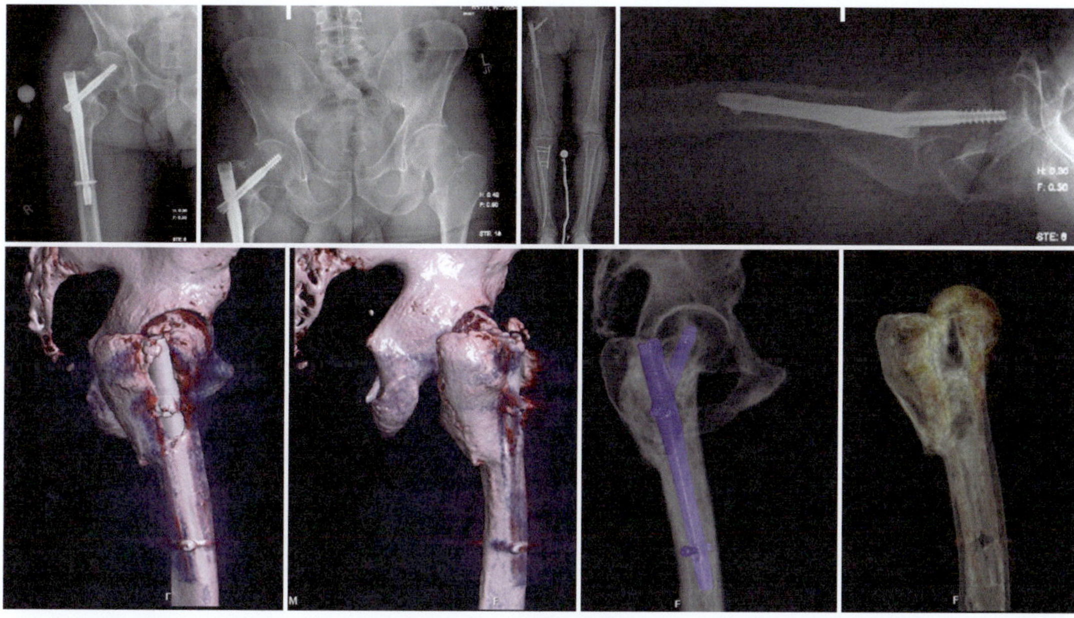

Fig. 16.6 Preoperative radiographs and computed tomography images

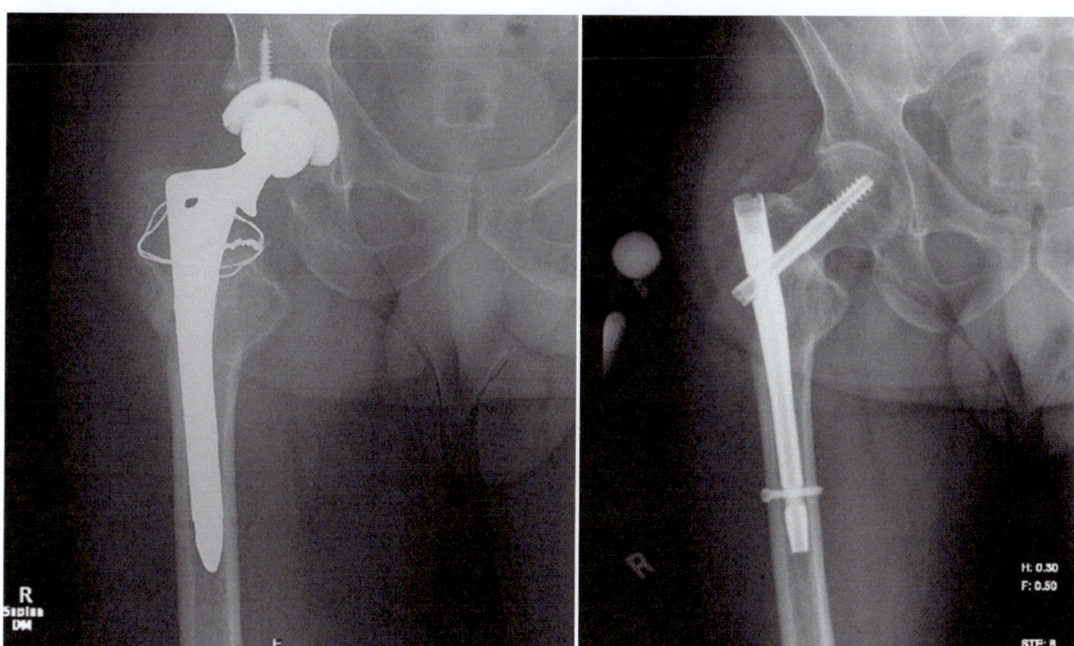

Fig. 16.7 Postoperative radiographs

intramedullary canal (Fig. 16.8). At the time of surgery, significant capsular releases were needed for mobilization the femur, as well as excision of heterotopic bone. There was also a semi-mobile nonunion of the intertrochanteric region with fibrous interposition material (Fig. 16.9). A provisional neck osteotomy was performed under fluoroscopic guidance. Standard acetabular com-

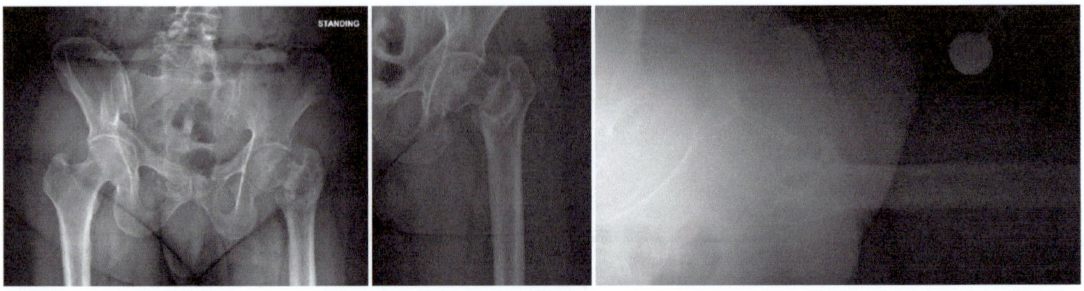

Fig. 16.8 Preoperative radiographs

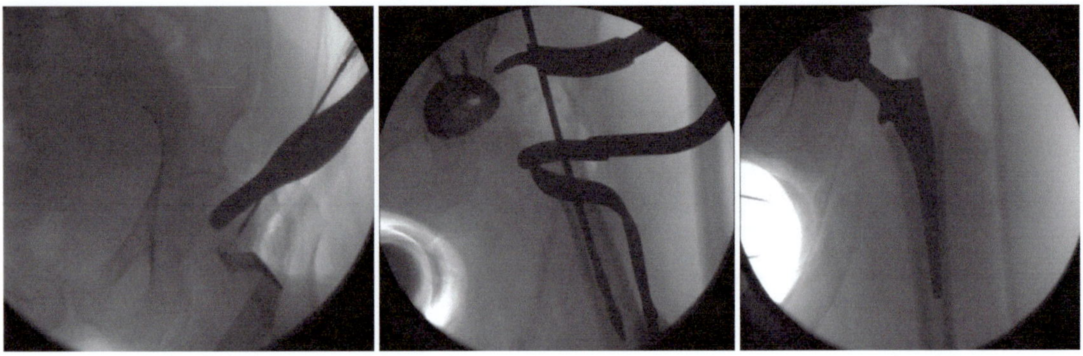

Fig. 16.9 Intraoperative fluoroscopic images

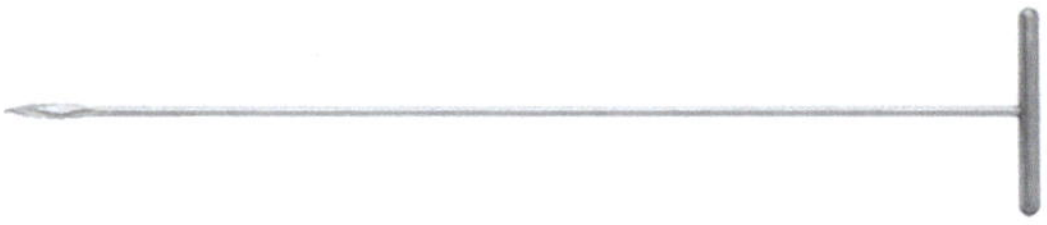

Fig. 16.10 AO T-handle reamer [11]

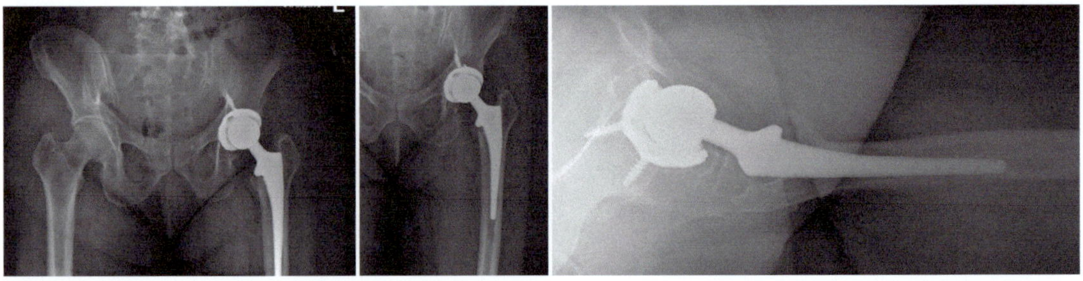

Fig. 16.11 Postoperative radiographs

ponents were placed. For access to the femoral canal, an AO T-handle reamer (DePuy Synthes, Warsaw, IN) (Figs. 16.9 and 16.10) was used to safely penetrate the chronic nonunion bony formation and to safely establish the planned intramedullary trajectory. Final radiographs demonstrate reconstruction of leg length, offset, and normal femoral inclination (Fig. 16.11).

Similar techniques can be used in the setting of a tight proximal femoral (Dorr A) canal (Fig. 16.12). The author's preferred technique is to introduce an AO T-handle reamer (Figs. 16.10

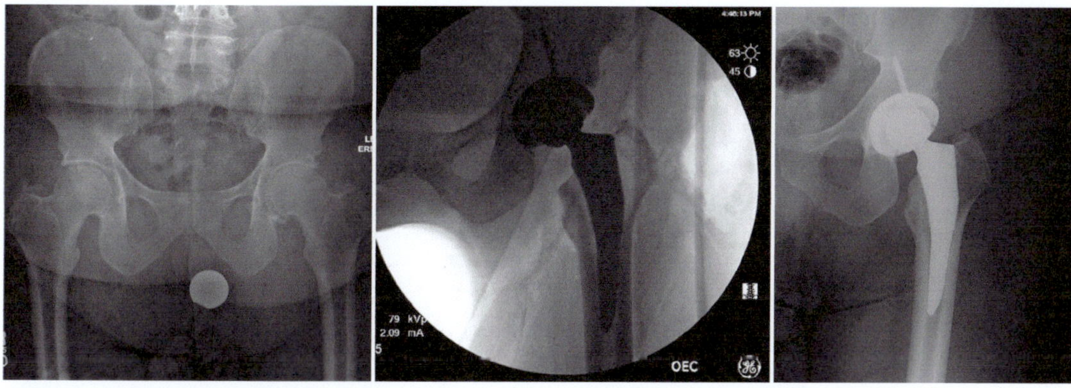

Fig. 16.12 Preoperative and postoperative radiographs

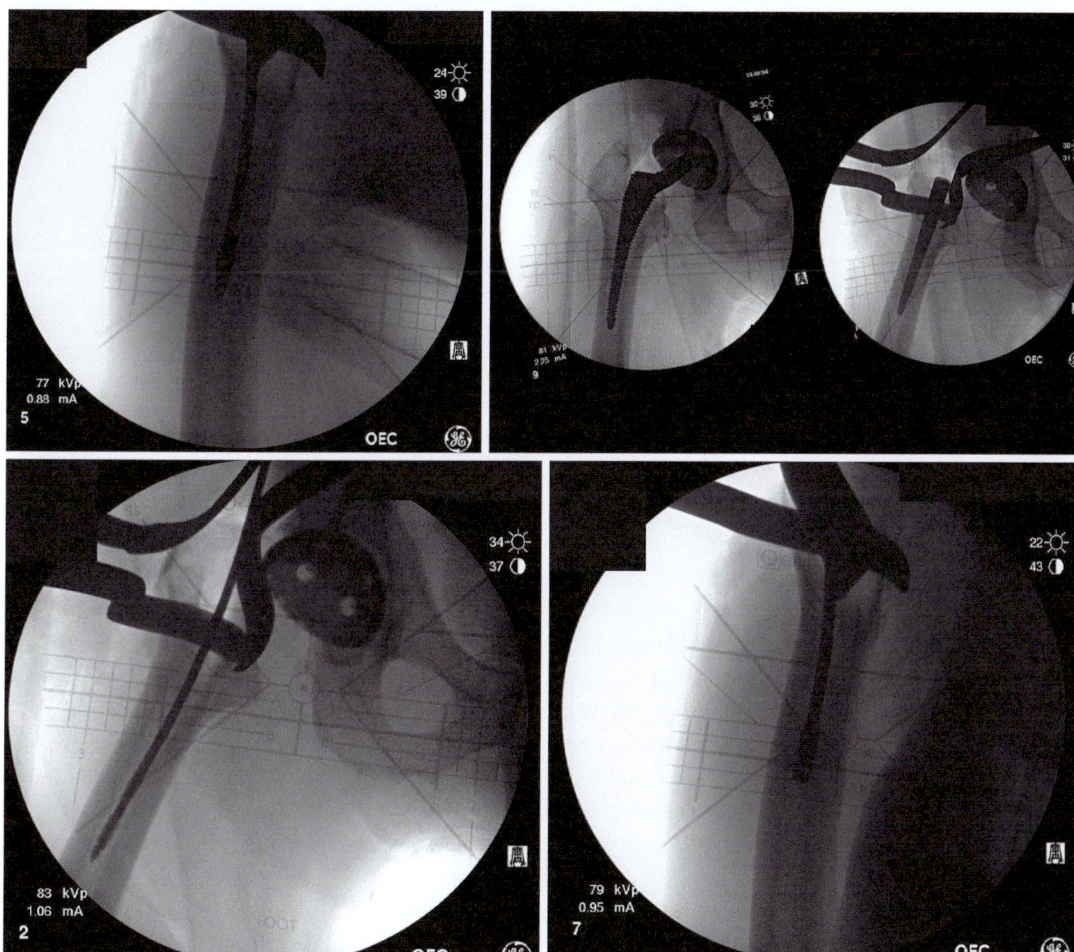

Fig. 16.13 Intraoperative fluoroscopic images

and 16.13) of the smallest diameter and manually hand ream up to an appropriate size. Depending on the planned femoral component size, monob- lock semi-flexible DePuy AML (DePuy, Warsaw, IN) thin-shaft reamers (Figs. 16.13 and 16.14) can be used to open up the canal, beginning at

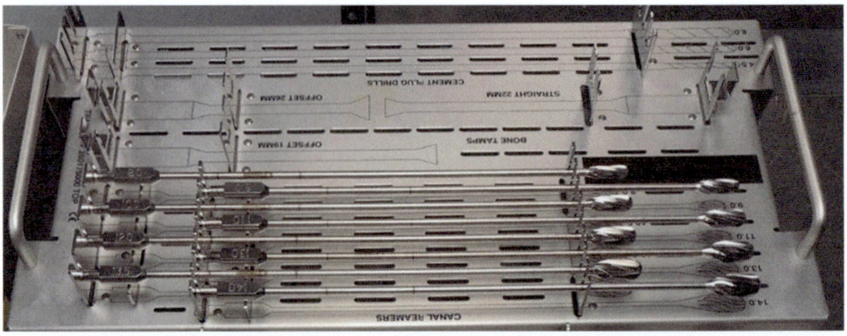

Fig. 16.14 DePuy AML thin-shaft reamers

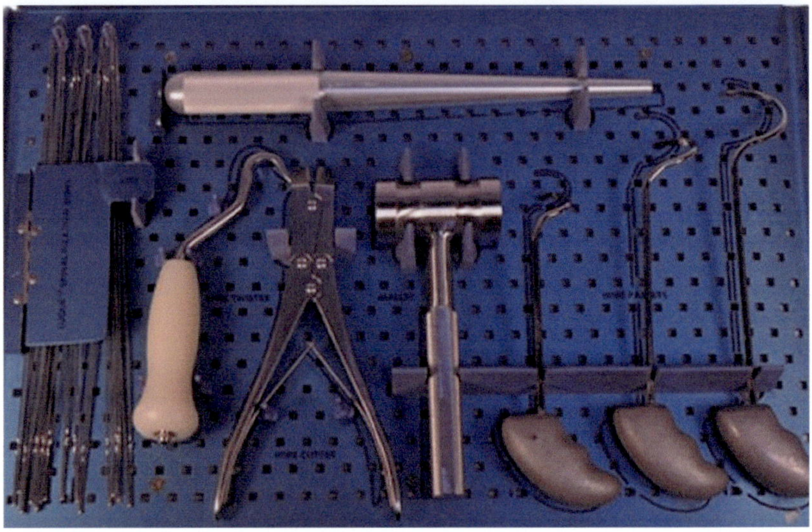

Fig. 16.15 Zimmer Cerclage wiring set [12]

size 8 mm in diameter and progressing up to the distal diameter of the planned stem.

The authors preferred technique for prophylactic fixation in a tight canal, or in osteoporotic bone, includes the Zimmer Cable Ready Set (double-ended Luque wires with manual twister) (Zimmer Biomet, Warsaw, IN) (Fig. 16.15). Reaming and subsequent broaching can be performed with intermittent fluoroscopic checks in two planes to insure safe canal trajectory without perforation or malposition.

Case

This is a 32-year-old woman with symptomatic bilateral hip pain and acetabular dysplasia (Fig. 16.16). She presented with progressive arthritis of the right hip. She had a labral tear in the left hip with preserved cartilage. Important issues with reconstruction of the right total hip replacement include establishing the normal hip center. A femoral stem with neck geometry that grows proportionally with stem size was chosen to avoid over-lengthening the limb. The acetabular cup size should remain appropriate for the native socket volume and tucked with the anterior wall, as to avoid psoas tendon impingement. Avoiding excessive anteversion of the acetabular component is important as well to reduce the risk of anterior dislocation in generally more flexible dysplastic patient population. The patient did well after the right total hip replacement (Fig. 16.17) and then was indicated for left periacetabular osteotomy to address the moderate hip dysplasia.

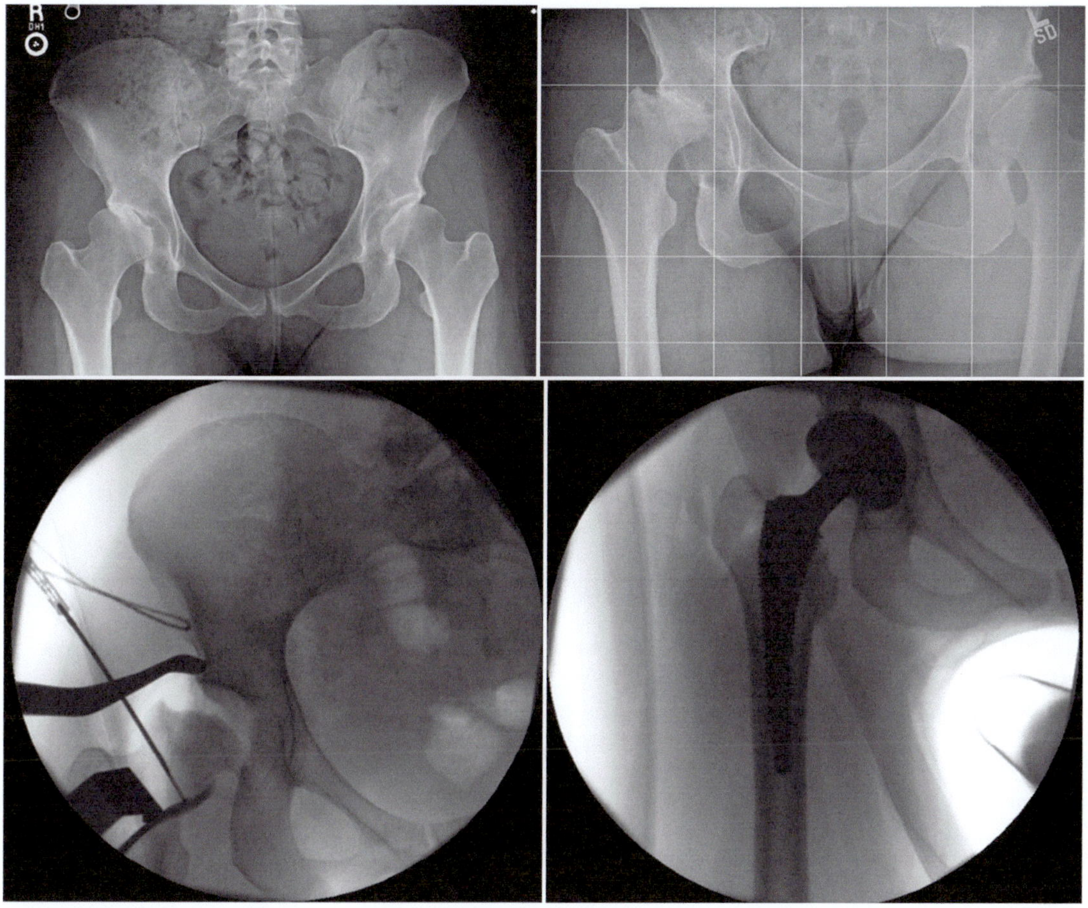

Fig. 16.16 Preoperative radiographs and intra-operative fluoroscopic images

Case

This is a 29-year-old man who presented with symptomatic right hip pain and secondary arthritis due to underlying avascular necrosis of the femoral head. He had been status post free vascularized free fibula grafting to the right proximal femur (Fig. 16.18).

At the time of surgery, it is important to understand the risk of intraoperative femoral perforation and/ or fracture if the true canal is not properly identified. A high-speed burr is often needed to penetrated the metadiaphyseal region, along with technique previously described for accessing tight canals. Any potentially obstructing hardware in the proximal femur should be navigated, or removed if it affects the final stem position (Fig. 16.18).

Another example of retained hardware requiring removal is demonstrated in Fig. 16.19. The AA approach position afforded the ability for safe removal of the retrograde femoral nail in the supine position in the same surgical procedure. A prophylactic cerclage wire was placed through the anterior hip incision (Fig. 16.20), and intraoperative fluoroscopy can aid with any hardware-related issues. An AA was also beneficial in this particular patient for stability, who was status post spinal fusion and had issues with dislocation of the contralateral THA done previously at another institution.

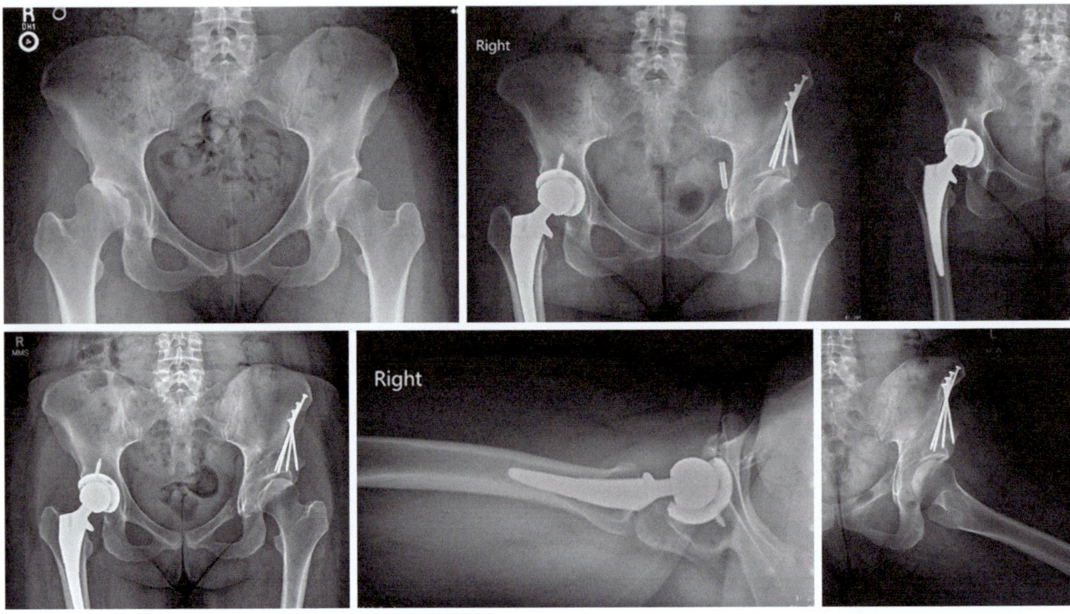

Fig. 16.17 Preoperative and postoperative radiographs

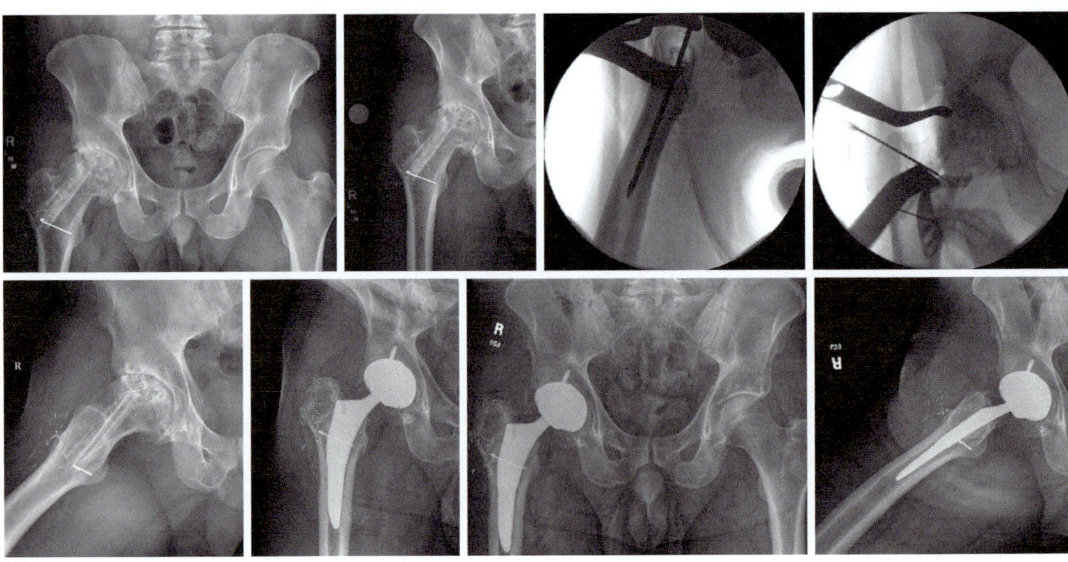

Fig. 16.18 Preoperative radiographs, intraoperative fluoroscopic imaging, and postoperative radiographs

Case

Spinopelvic deformity and its influence on THA stability and component positioning have been gaining increasing interest. This is a 74-year-old woman, status post long-segment spinal fusion, who presented with left hip pain and underlying acetabular dysplasia. Due to the stiff spine, an extreme outlet view is seen on the preoperative imaging studies (Fig. 16.21). Given the risk of instability, a dual mobility component was chosen at the time of THA through an AA (Fig. 16.22). The use of dual mobility in the author's practice is rare in the primary setting and generally reserved for patients with severe spinal disease,

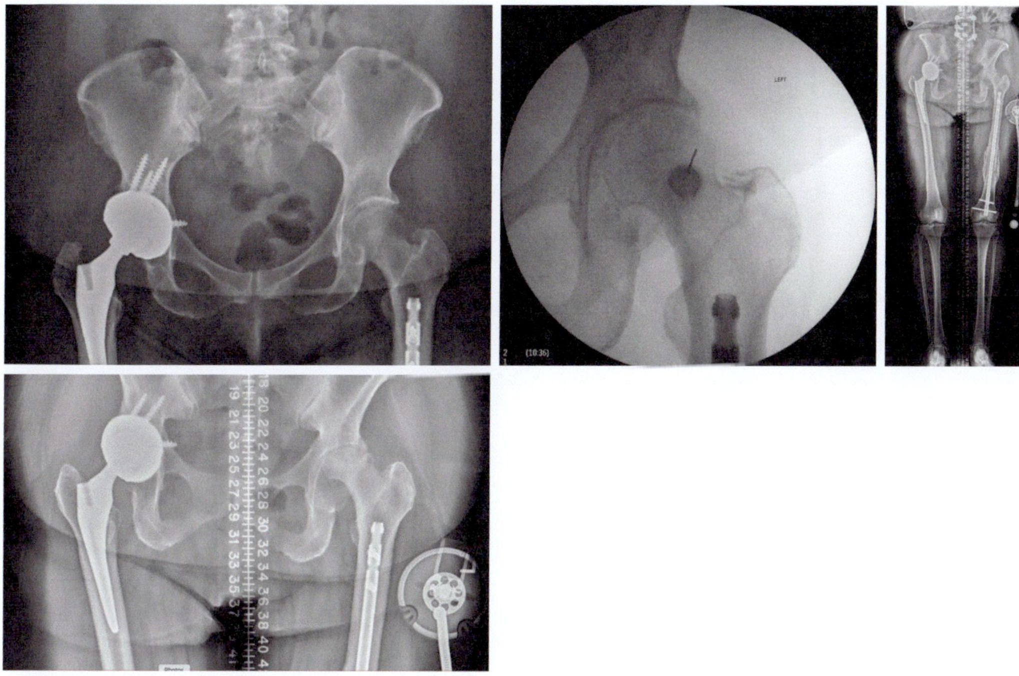

Fig. 16.19 Preoperative radiographs

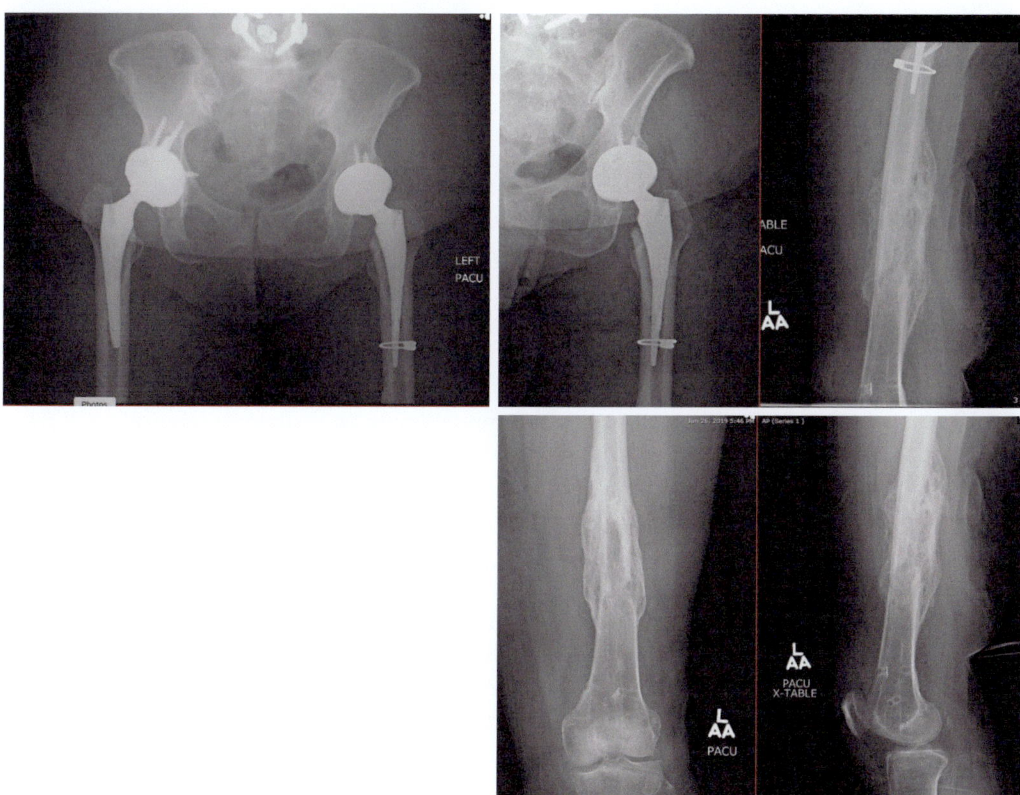

Fig. 16.20 Postoperative radiographs

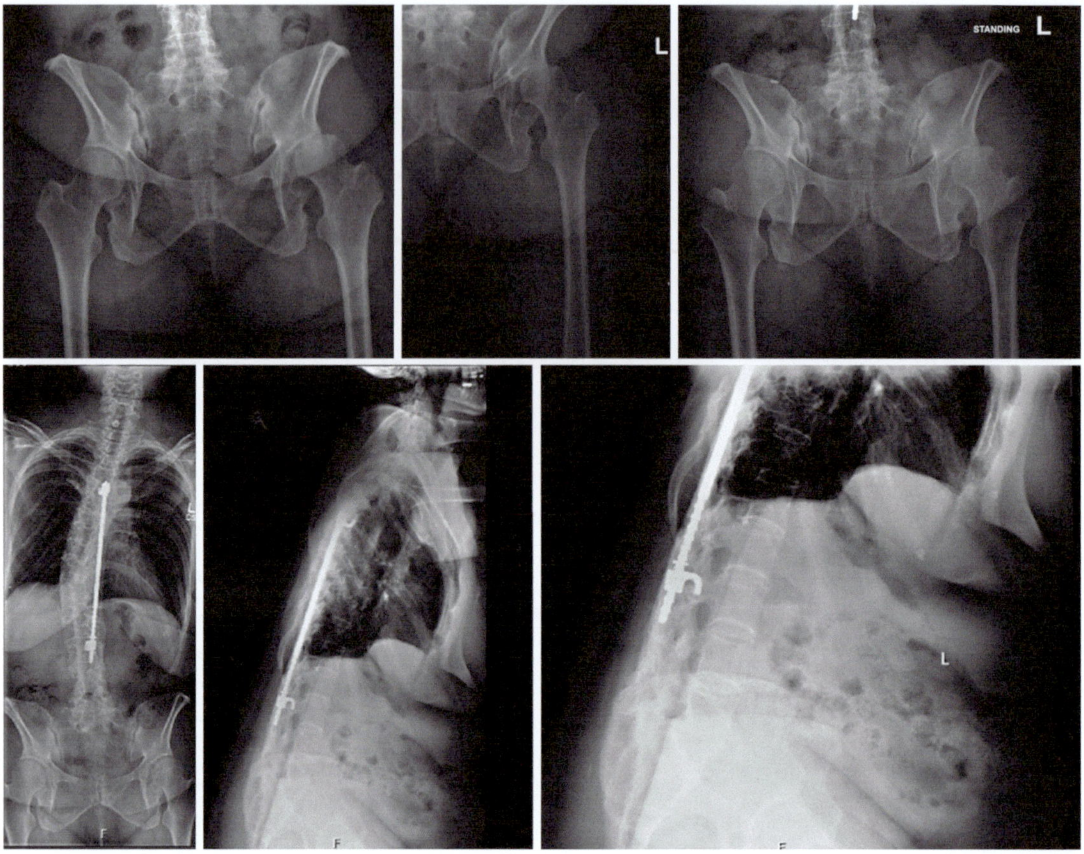

Fig. 16.21 Preoperative radiographs

significant cognitive issues, and other issues like poor abductor control.

Case

This is a 57-year-old female healthcare worker who sustained a right anterior column acetabular fracture, managed nonsurgically for 4 months at an outside institution. She was referred for THA due to significant pain and ambulatory dysfunction. Judet views of the right hemipelvis confirmed an anterior column fracture (Fig. 16.23).

At the time of surgical intervention, care must be taken when placing the anterior acetabular retractor, to avoid neuropraxia of the femoral nerve (Fig. 16.24). Intraoperative fluoroscopy is used to confirm ideal acetabular component positioning. A standard hemispherical shell can be used with supplemental screw fixation with excellent construct stability.

Similar technique is used in a more complex case of a geriatric right acetabular fracture combined with an ipsilateral femoral neck fracture (Fig. 16.25). A large hemispherical shell placed with fluoroscopic confirmation bridges the compromised anterior column/dome defect (Fig. 16.26). Autograft from the femoral head can be used to reconstitute bone stock and maintain the appropriate center of rotation. It is critical to place screws in the superior and inferior hemispheres of the socket to afford solid fixation. A cemented femoral stem was used to address the femoral neck fracture in this patient with significant osteoporosis.

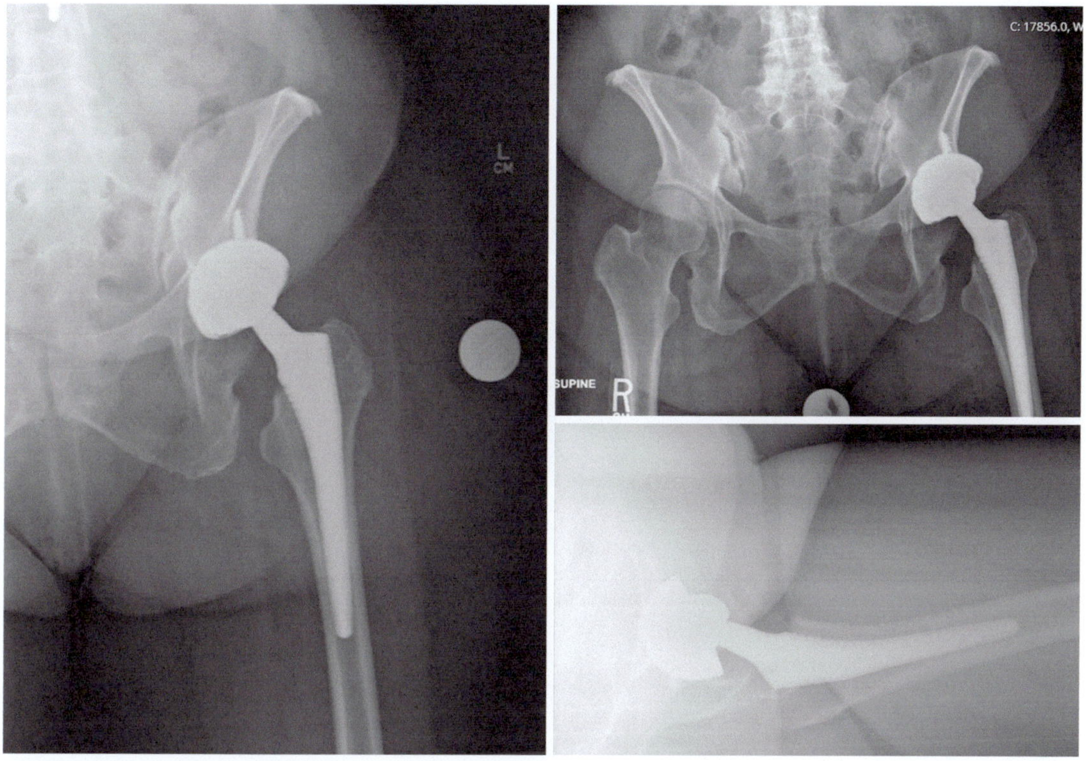

Fig. 16.22 Postoperative radiographs

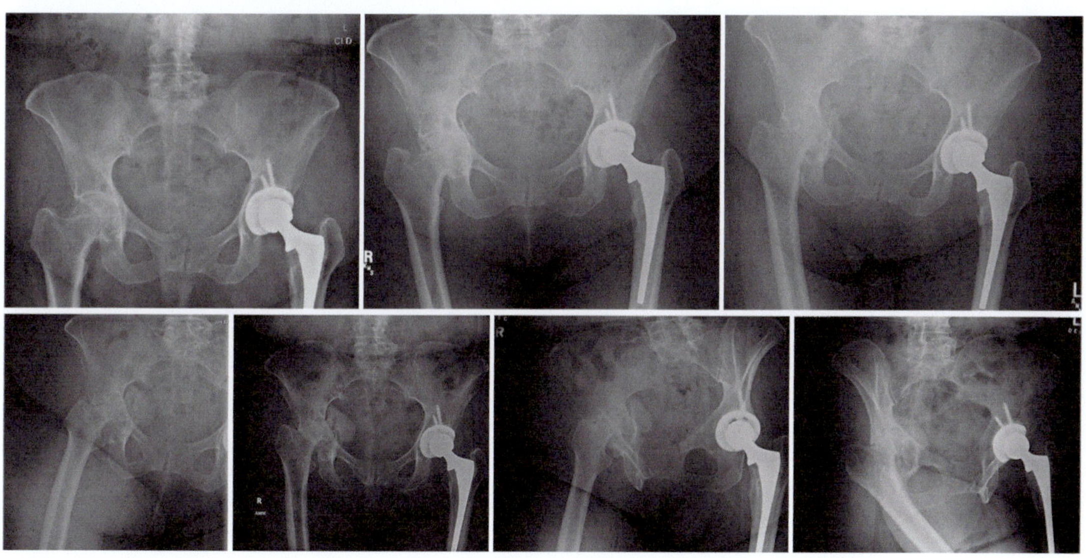

Fig. 16.23 Preoperative radiographs

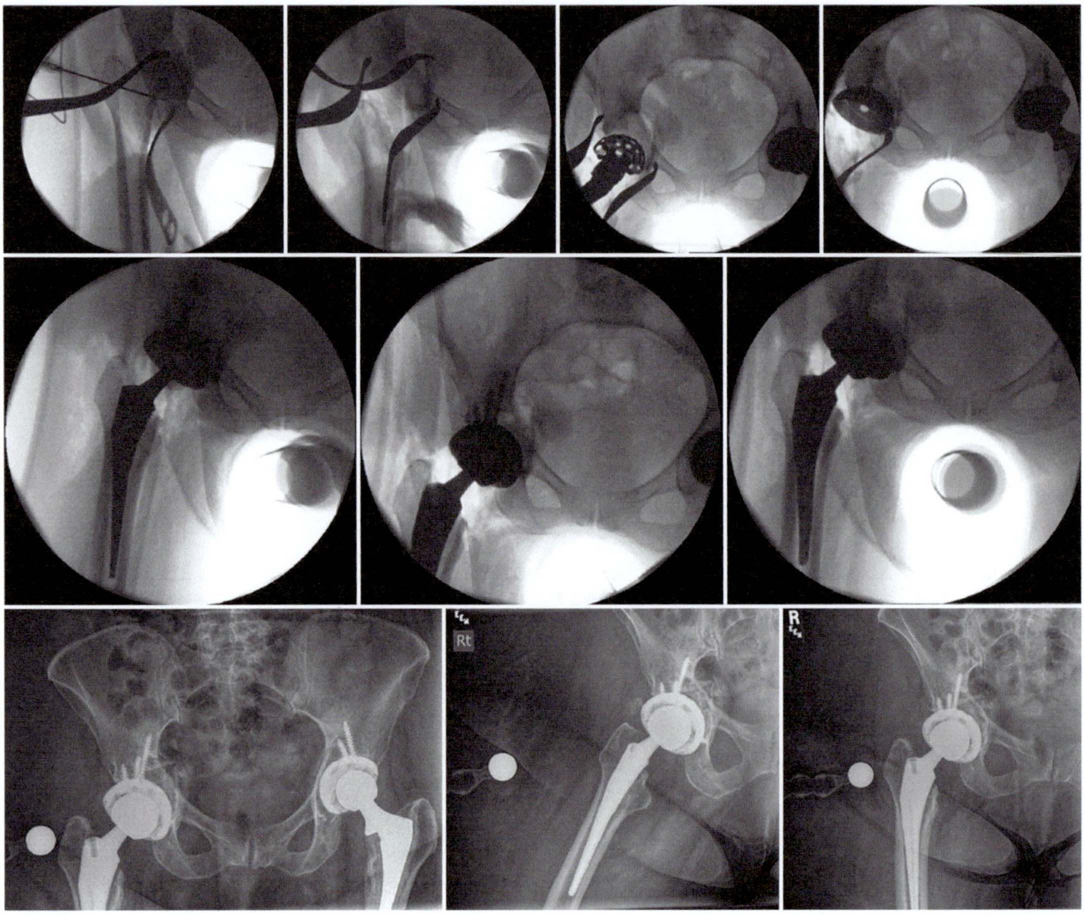

Fig. 16.24 Intraoperative fluoroscopic images and post-operative radiographs

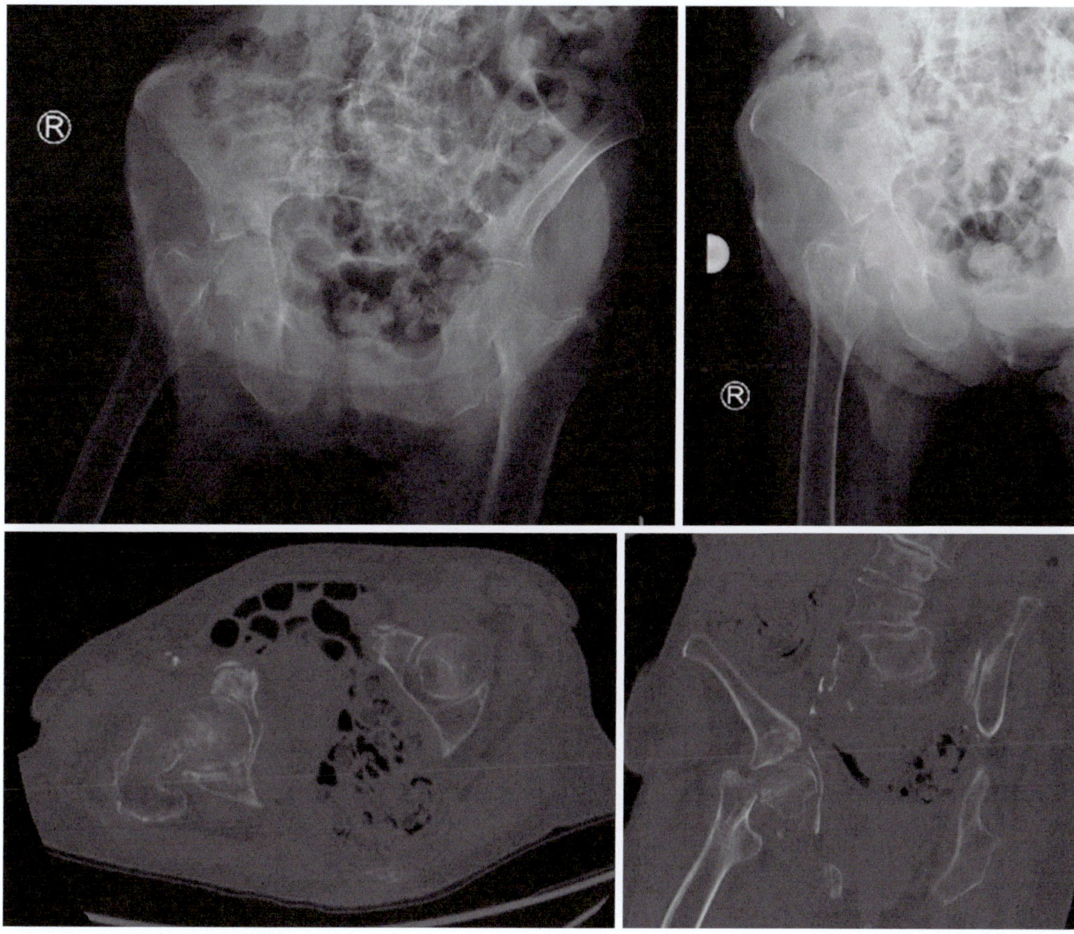

Fig. 16.25 Preoperative radiographs

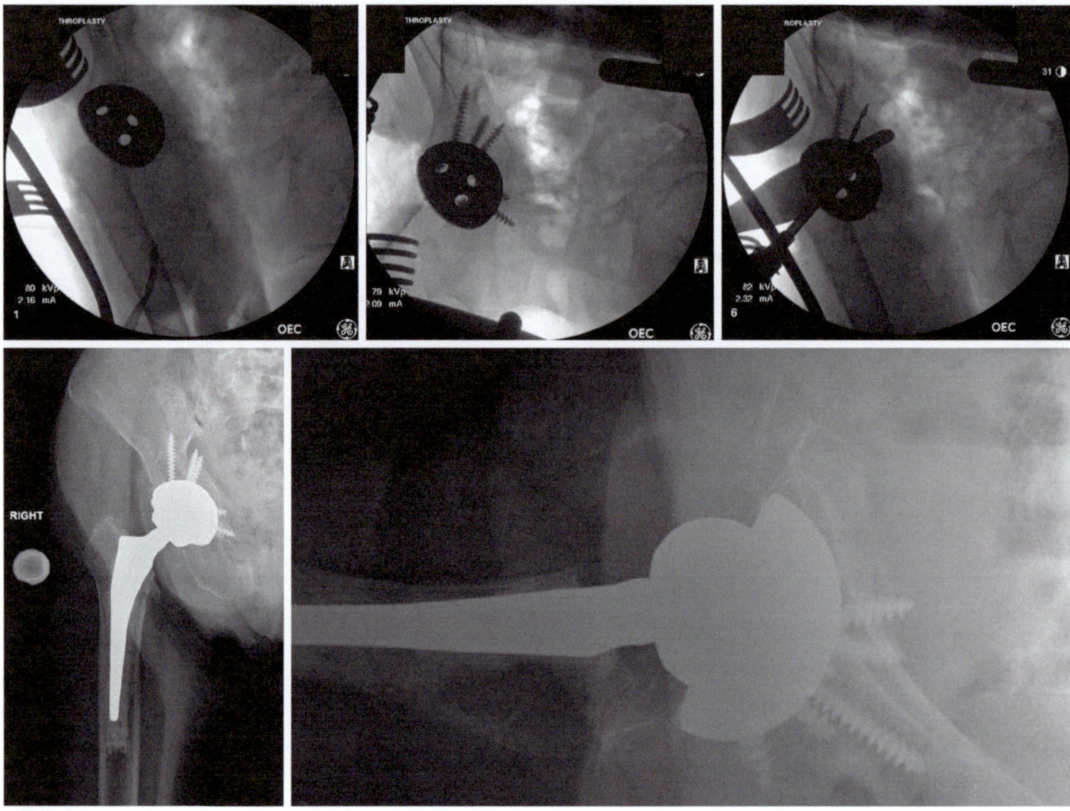

Fig. 16.26 Intraoperative fluoroscopic images and post-operative radiographs

References

1. Miller LE, Kamath AF, Boettner F, Bhattacharyya SK. In-hospital outcomes with anterior versus posterior approaches in total hip arthroplasty: meta-analysis of randomized controlled trials. J Pain Res [Internet]. 2018; Jul [cited 2019 Apr 17];11:1327–34. Available from: http://www.ncbi.nlm.nih.gov/pubmed/30214269
2. Miller LE, Gondusky JS, Bhattacharyya S, Kamath AF, Boettner F, Wright J. Does surgical approach affect outcomes in total hip arthroplasty through 90 days of follow-up? a systematic review with meta-analysis. J Arthroplasty [Internet]. 2018 Apr [cited 2019 Apr 17];33(4):1296–302. Available from: https://linkinghub.elsevier.com/retrieve/pii/S088354031730983X
3. Miller LE, Martinson MS, Gondusky JS, Kamath AF, Boettner F, Bhattacharyya SK. Ninety-day postoperative cost in primary total hip arthroplasty: an economic model comparing surgical approaches. Clin Outcomes Res. 2019;11:145–9.
4. Taunton MJ, Trousdale RT, Sierra RJ, Kaufman K, Pagnano MW. John Charnley Award: randomized clinical trial of direct anterior and Miniposterior approach THA: which provides better functional recovery? In: Clinical orthopaedics and related research. Lippincott Williams and Wilkins; 2018. p. 216–29.
5. Miller LE, Gondusky JS, Kamath AF, Boettner F, Wright J, Bhattacharyya S. Influence of surgical approach on complication risk in primary total hip arthroplasty. Acta Orthop [Internet]. 2018 May 4 [cited 2019 Apr 17];89(3):289–94. Available from: http://www.ncbi.nlm.nih.gov/pubmed/29451051
6. Kamath AF, Chitnis AS, Holy C, Lerner J, Curtin B, Lochow S, et al. Medical resource utilization and costs for total hip arthroplasty: benchmarking an anterior approach technique in the Medicare population. J Med Econ. 2018;21(2):218–24.
7. Chughtai M, Samuel LT, Acuña AJ, Kamath AF. Algorithmic soft tissue femoral release in anterior approach total hip arthroplasty. Arthroplast Today. 2019;5(4):471–6.
8. Gofton WT, Ibrahim MM, Kreviazuk CJ, Kim PR, Feibel RJ, Beaulé PE. Ten-year experience with the anterior approach to total hip arthroplasty at a Tertiary Care Center. J Arthroplast. 2020;35(5):1281–1289.e1.
9. Connolly KP, Kamath AF. Direct anterior total hip arthroplasty: comparative outcomes and contemporary results. World J Orthop Baishideng Publishing Group Co. 2016;7:94–101.

10. Connolly KP, Kamath AF. Direct anterior total hip arthroplasty: literature review of variations in surgical technique. World J Orthop. Baishideng Publishing Group Co. 2016;7:38–43.
11. Flexible Reamers for Intramedullary Nails Surgical Technique [Internet]. [cited 2020 May 9]. Available from: http://synthes.vo.llnwd.net/o16/LLNWMB8/US Mobile/Synthes North America/Product Support Materials/Technique Guides/Final Approved Technique guide Clean Copy 11-14-17.pdf.
12. Zimmer Cerclage Wiring Set [Internet]. [cited 2020 May 9]. Available from: https://a-zortho.com/item-listing-default/item/1837-zimmer-cerclage-wiring-set

Anterior Approach THA for the Treatment of Femoral Neck and Acetabular Fractures

17

Philip James Kregor

Introduction

The benefits of a direct anterior total hip arthroplasty in the patient with degenerative arthritis include accurate component positioning, avoidance of dislocation, leg length equality, and easier early rehabilitation following surgery [1–4]. In the patient with a displaced femoral neck fracture or acetabular fracture, these benefits are in fact amplified because each issue is historically more problematic. Therefore, a strong argument can be made to utilize the direct anterior total hip arthroplasty for displaced femoral neck fractures in patients approximately 55 years or older. Additionally, the technique can be useful in a small subset of acetabular fracture patients in whom traditional open reduction/internal fixation is fraught with poor outcomes.

Femoral Neck Fractures

Key questions that have emerged in the last two decades in the treatment of femoral neck fractures are as follows:

- When should internal fixation be utilized versus arthroplasty?
- If arthroplasty is utilized, is hemiarthroplasty or total hip arthroplasty preferable?
- If arthroplasty is utilized, should the femoral component be cemented or uncemented?
- If arthroplasty is utilized, is there an advantage of a given approach? (traditional posterior or anterolateral versus direct anterior approach).

Fixation Versus Arthroplasty

Bhandari et al. [5] provided a useful meta-analysis in 2003 to look at the question of internal fixation versus arthroplasty. Certainly, most surgeons would advocate internal fixation for any young individual. This meta-analysis looked at patients 65 years of age or older with a displaced femoral neck fracture who were treated with either internal fixation or arthroplasty. Compared with internal fixation, arthroplasty reduced the relative risk of revision surgery by 77%. They noted that for every six patients treated with arthroplasty rather than internal fixation, one revision surgery would be avoided. Revisions following internal fixation were often due to nonunion and avascular necrosis. Interestingly, the mean for dislocation following total hip arthroplasty was noted to be 6.9%. Additionally, the risk of infection associated with arthroplasty was slightly higher than with internal fixation, with the risk difference being 3.4%. Finally, increased

P. J. Kregor (✉)
The Hughston Clinic, HCA TriStar Skyline Medical Center, Nashville, TN, USA
e-mail: pkregor@hughston.com

J. M. Matta, A. P. Sah (eds.), *Anterior Hip Replacement*,
https://doi.org/10.1007/978-3-030-91896-5_17

blood loss and operative times were seen with arthroplasty versus internal fixation. Thus, from this meta-analysis it appears that failure of fixation can be avoided with arthroplasty, but with increased risks of dislocation, infection, blood loss, and operative times.

Hemiarthroplasty Versus Total Hip Arthroplasty

There is debate regarding the use of total hip arthroplasty versus hemiarthroplasty in patients with a displaced femoral neck fracture. In general, better hip function and quality of life are seen with total hip arthroplasty versus hemiarthroplasty. Ekhtiari et al. [6] performed a meta-analysis and saw no significant differences between these two modes of treatment in terms of revision rate at up to 5 years of follow-up and functional outcome at up to 3 years. There was superior health-related quality of life in the total hip group compared with the hemiarthroplasty group. The final conclusion was that revision rates, function, mortality, periprosthetic fracture, and dislocation at up to 5 years were no difference between the two groups. Ravi et al. [7] performed a retrospective cohort study comparing total hip versus hemiarthroplasty in the treatment of femoral neck fractures in patients 60 years of age or older. This was done in the healthcare system of Ontario, Canada. Medical and surgical complications and perioperative and postoperative healthcare costs were looked at in the first year following injury. In comparing roughly 2700 patients in each group, the risk of dislocation was 1.7% in the total hip group and 1.0% in the hemiarthroplasty group. Surgical revision rate was 1.8% in the first year following hemiarthroplasty and 0.2% in the first year following total hip arthroplasty. For this reason and possibly secondary to decreased therapy costs, total hip arthroplasty was associated with 2700 Canadian dollars *less* in expenditures in the first year following the fracture.

Lewis et al. [8] published a meta-analysis of hemiarthroplasty versus total hip arthroplasty for the treatment of femoral neck fractures. In looking at 13 randomized controlled trials in 1364 patients (660 total hips; 704 hemiarthroplasties), the evidence can be summed up as follows:

- Patents with a total hip arthroplasty have better function and quality of life in the years following their fracture;
- Fewer re-operations occur with use of a total hip arthroplasty;
- There is no difference in mortality or infection between the two modalities; and
- Dislocation rates are higher with total hip arthroplasties for the first 4 years following surgery.

Based on this, the authors recommended that total hip replacements be utilized for any patient with a life expectancy of greater than 4 years, especially if age is less than 80 years. They felt that a hemiarthroplasty *and* total hip arthroplasty were both reasonable if the patient was 80 years old or older, or their expected longevity was less than 4 years.

Recently, the HEALTH trial was published, detailing a randomized, 80 center, prospective, international trial comparing total hip arthroplasty versus hemiarthroplasty [9]. Patients 50 years or older who sustained a low energy femoral neck fracture were included. Overall, 749 patients were in the total hip group and 746 patients were in the hemiarthroplasty group. There were several key observations:

- Secondary hip procedures with 2-year follow-up were 7.9% in the total hip group and 8.3% in the hemiarthroplasty group. Overall, 33 of the 57 secondary hip procedures in the total hip group were open or closed reductions related to hip dislocation. In addition, 36 of 60 secondary hip procedures in the hemiarthroplasty group were implant revisions.
- Hip instability or dislocation was seen in 2.4% of patients treated with hemiarthroplasty and 4.7% of patients with total hip arthroplasty.
- Over a 24-month follow-up period, 13.7% of patients died, with no significant differences seen between the two groups.

- Serious adverse events occurred in 41.8% of total hip arthroplasty patients and 36.7% of hemiarthroplasty patients.
- Total hip patients had superior WOMAC total scores, indicating better hip function and less pain, but the differences were not felt to be a clinically important difference.

Cemented Versus Uncemented Arthroplasty

Historically, cemented stems have been more utilized, but recent improvements in uncemented stems have seen a significant increase in their use. In 2010, Parker et al. [10] compared cemented versus uncemented stems in 400 patients aged 61–104 years over a 5-year period. With cemented stems, they noted better mobility through 1 year postoperative and less pain up to 2 years postoperative. They noted equivalent mortality and medical complications between the two groups. Chen et al. [11] and DeRogatis et al. [12] both provided excellent recent reviews of the issue of utilizing cement for the femoral component in arthroplasty for a femoral neck fracture, noting that cemented stems are associated with improved patient-reported outcomes and decreased pain in relatively short-term follow-up (1–2 years). They are also associated with less intraoperative periprosthetic fractures. Operative times and estimated blood loss are usually increased with the use of cement. In addition, there is concern of cardiopulmonary compromise, also known as the "cement implantation syndrome," with the use of cement. Kumar et al. [13] performed a meta-analysis of six randomized controlled studies comparing the treatment of 500 patients with cemented stems and 471 uncemented stems. They noted shorter operative times and decreased blood loss with uncemented stems. With patients treated with uncemented stems, there was an increase in periprosthetic fractures, dislocation, and stem subsidence. In the end, most studies favor the use of cement for the femoral component when treating a geriatric femoral neck fracture with arthroplasty. However, the surgeon should consider the individual bone quality, functional status, and age of a given patient.

Choice of Approach: Utilization of the Anterior Approach

Direct anterior total hip arthroplasty is associated with more ease of earlier rehabilitation, [2] less muscle damage, [4] less risk of dislocation, and more accurate component positioning compared with traditional approaches (posterior and lateral) when utilized for elective arthroplasty for degenerative arthritis. While it is a natural progression to anticipate similar benefits when treating the patient with a femoral neck fracture, the actual evidence to date needs further randomized prospective trials proving its efficacy. Cichos et al. [14] investigated 90-day and 1-year outcomes of femoral neck fracture patients who underwent total hip arthroplasty via either a direct anterior approach or a posterior approach. A total of 44 direct anterior patients were compared with 99 posterior approach patients. Patients with a posterior approach had a 27% chance of being nonambulatory postoperatively, while only 11% of patients via an anterior approach were nonambulatory (p = .05). There were no differences between the two groups in terms of dislocation, joint infections, periprosthetic fractures, mechanical complications, or revision surgery. However, Carlson et al. [15] found no benefit of the direct anterior approach in terms of return to function when comparing 85 direct anterior patients with 75 patients who had a direct lateral approach for hemiarthroplasty for a femoral neck fracture.

Differences in Anterior Approach THA for Femoral Neck Fracture and Degenerative Arthritis

There are several differences which make the total hip replacement for femoral neck fractures different from that for elective hip replacement for degenerative arthritis. *Osteoporosis* is common in the setting of a geriatric femoral neck fracture. This can make excessive use of the two-prong retractor on the posterior medial aspect of the femoral neck problematic in terms of perforation or fracture propagation. It is often avoided in such cases. Instead, a common Weitlander retractor between the elevated anterior capsules in the tensor fascia lata muscle belly can be utilized. Alternatively, a plastic Yankauer suction tip can be used on the posterior aspect of the neck, as it is flexible and will not perforate the femoral neck. The osteoporosis also makes the proximal femur more susceptible to a fracture, which can occur during the relocation of the femoral head into the native acetabulum or acetabular liner. Thus, a very controlled relocation maneuver (discussed below) and appropriate release of the anterior capsule are paramount.

Dementia is common in the patient with a femoral neck fracture and often the patient cannot follow any restrictions or instructions. Of course, no "preoperative clinic" or instruction before the surgery is able to be given. Fortunately, this is not needed as the anterior approach does not require such and often in the demented patient it is simply a matter of convincing the demented patient that they simply can walk again, usually with a walker.

The patient who sustains a femoral neck fracture often is very *frail.* The benefit of the anterior approach can be advantageous in all patients but may be the most valuable in the patient with very limited physical capacity to walk. The elderly patient who sustains a femoral neck fracture is often "teetering on the edge" of being able to walk or not. Thus, after they sustain a femoral neck fracture it is helpful to have the surgery cause as little insult to their muscular envelope as possible.

Author's Step-by-Step Surgical Technique for Anterior Approach Arthroplasty for Femoral Neck Fracture (Fig. 17.1)

1. Preoperative assessment: In addition to normal preoperative laboratories, a C-reactive protein is obtained to indicate any ongoing infection. This can often be elevated in the setting of a pneumonia or urinary tract infection. If these are present, it is rare that they preclude surgical intervention, unless there are signs of systemic sepsis. Usually, appropriate antibiotics are given for a urinary tract infection and continued 5 days postoperatively.
2. Preoperative X-ray: A good quality level AP pelvis with the opposite hip internally rotated is helpful for preoperative templating. However, it is sometimes difficult to obtain in the fracture patient. Additionally, it is not uncommon for the opposite hip to have had intervention for a previous fracture. In either situation, after the patient is placed on the HANA table, a small amount of traction can be utilized on the involved hip to reduce the fracture, and the opposite hip is internally rotated. Symmetrical fluoroscopic images of both hips are then obtained and saved and can then later be used for radiographic overlay technique. In case the opposite hip has had previous surgical intervention, the overlay technique can be utilized with the "reduced hip" image or the opposite hip. It is not uncommon for the opposite hip to have, for example, a malunion with varus and shortening, and this should be recognized. The surgeon should not necessarily try to "match" the opposite hip if such is the case, but instead compare it to the "reduced hip image."
3. Patient positioning: Careful placement of the HANA boots on the patient is important. Foley catheters are not utilized unless needed for hemodynamic monitoring. Both arms are usually placed out to the side with the shoulders abducted approximately 70–80° with appropriate padding on the arm boards.
4. Incision: 10–11 cm Hueter incision is made, and the tensor fascia sheath is divided in its posterior 1/3. Small branches of the lateral femoral cutaneous nerve are looked for and avoided if possible. Finger dissection elevates the gluteus minimus off of the superolateral hip capsule and a Cobra retractor is placed in this interval, held 45° to the long axis of the torso. The fascia overlying the rectus femoris

is divided, and the lateral femoral circumflex vessels are cauterized. L-shaped capsulotomy is performed, which divides the reflected head of the rectus femoris at the upper extent of the vertical limb. The lateral capsule is released off of the saddle region of the proximal femur, and a 1.5 cm strip of lateral capsule is removed from the saddle region to the superolateral acetabulum. With a small amount of traction on the involved leg, the leg is externally rotated approximately 60–70°. The medial capsule is then released.

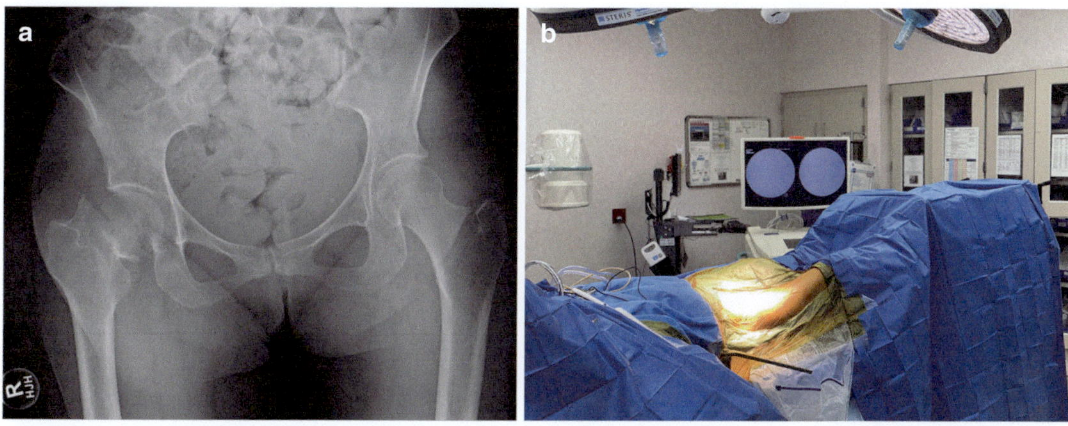

Fig. 17.1 A 37-year-old woman with a history of anorexia nervosa, depression, and diabetes mellitus presents with severe right hip pain after a stumble several days prior. Patient had significant groin pain for 4–6 weeks. Discussion regarding open reduction and internal fixation versus total hip arthroplasty was had with the patient and their mother. Putting all factors together, it was determined that a well-done arthroplasty would give her the most definitive outcome and the ability to walk on the leg immediately, which was important to her. (**a**) Initial AP pelvis radiograph; no previous films had been obtained. It was felt that her history and X-rays were most consistent with a stress fracture of the femoral neck which then displaced. (**b**) Operating room setup on the anterior hip traction table with the hips slightly flexed, and the fluoroscopy unit in the appropriate position. (**c**) Preoperative "pseudo-AP pelvis," which allows the surgeon to predict neck cut and offset choice, even if a good quality preoperative AP pelvis radiograph has not been obtained. (**d**) The anterior superior iliac spine is drawn out and the incision starts approximately 2 cm distal and 2 cm lateral to it. Depending on body habitus, the incision is usually 10–12 cm. Here, a 10 cm incision was utilized. (**e**) The tensor fascia is divided, and a finger sweep on the medial aspect of the tensor fascia muscle belly is followed by placement of the surgeon's index finger on the superolateral aspect of the hip capsule. This is then replaced by a Cobra retractor. (**f**) An L-shaped capsulotomy is then performed. The upper limb is along the superior aspect of the femoral neck and the lower limb is along the anterior intertrochanteric line of the proximal femur. A tag stitch is utilized on the corner aspect of this capsular flap to elevate the capsule during acetabular reaming and femoral head reduction. This capsulotomy is repaired at the end of the case. (**g**) The femoral neck fracture is visualized. If it is questionable if the surgeon potentially wants to perform open reduction internal fixation, it is seen that this gives appropriate visualization to do so. In this case fracture fragmentation confirmed the choice to perform an anterior total hip arthroplasty. (**h**) The femoral neck cut may be made after or before femoral head removal. Preoperative templating allows for the surgeon to plan the height of the cut above the lesser trochanter. (**i**) Slight reaming medially is first performed. If desired, this can be under fluoroscopic control. (**j**) Final reaming is performed. Usually, this is 1 mm under the outer diameter of the acetabular cup. (**k**) Initial cup insertion. (**l**) Final cup insertion. (**m**) Final acetabular cup position. This was read as 39° from the horizontal and 19° of anteversion. (**n**) Proximal femur visualization after the leg is placed into the femoral preparation position with a combination of extension, external rotation, and adduction. Here, exposure is aided by a two-prong retractor on the posteromedial aspect of the femur. If the patient has significant osteoporosis, this retractor may cause more fragmentation of the femoral neck in the setting of a femoral neck fracture. Thus, an alternative is to use a plastic suction tip on the posterior aspect of the femoral neck, also as seen here. (**o**) Final position of the trial broach. Note appropriate "fit and fill" of the proximal femur. (**p**) AP radiograph of the right hemipelvis with the trial broach in position. This can be compared by the opposite via the X-ray overlay technique or software integration with fluoroscopy data to ensure that offset and leg length have been adequately restored. (**q**) Opposite hip AP radiograph for comparison. (**r**) Final implant position. (**s**) Fluoroscopic view of the distal femoral stem to ensure appropriate position of the stem without femoral crack. (**t**) Postoperative AP radiograph of the pelvis

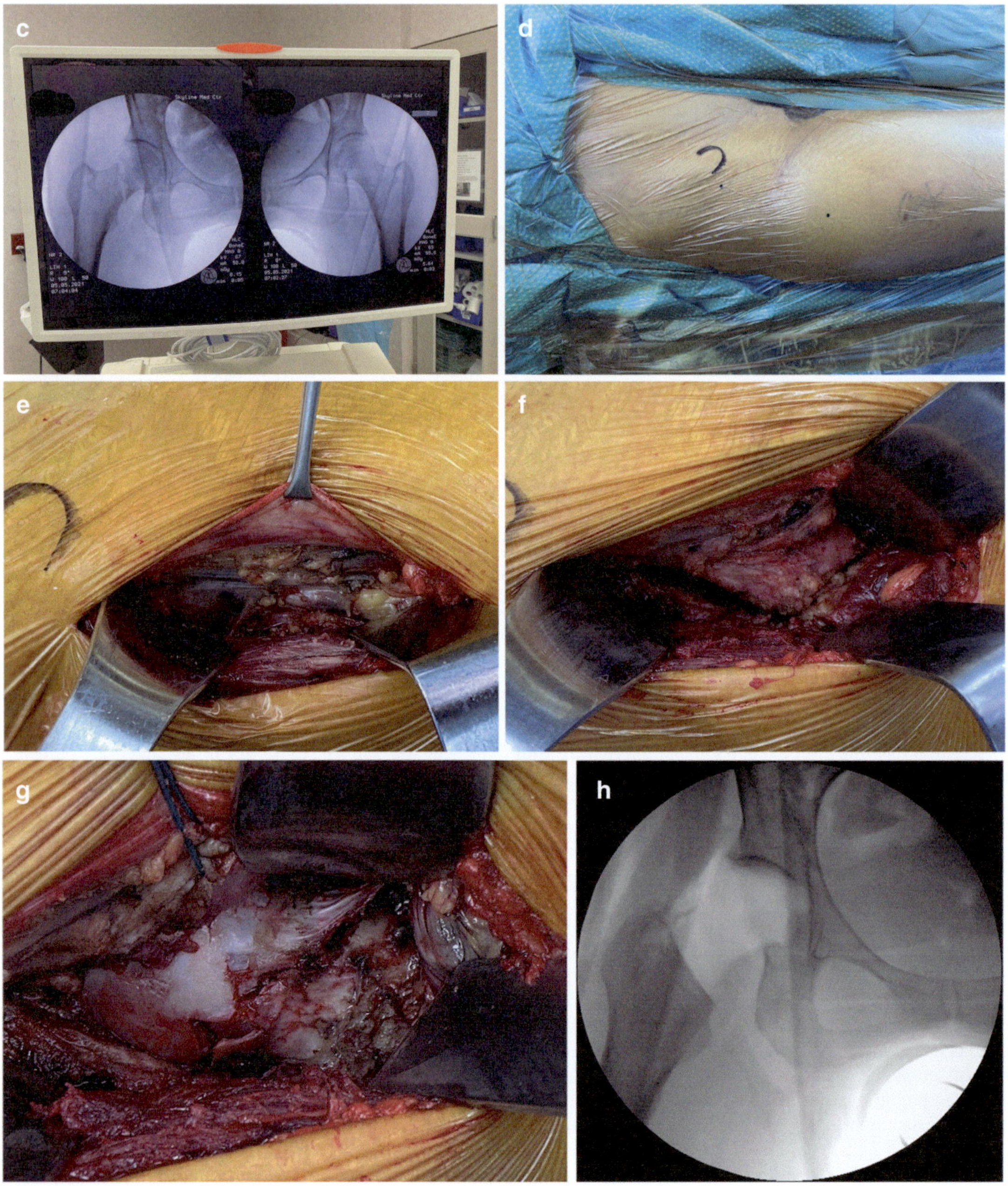

Fig. 17.1 (continued)

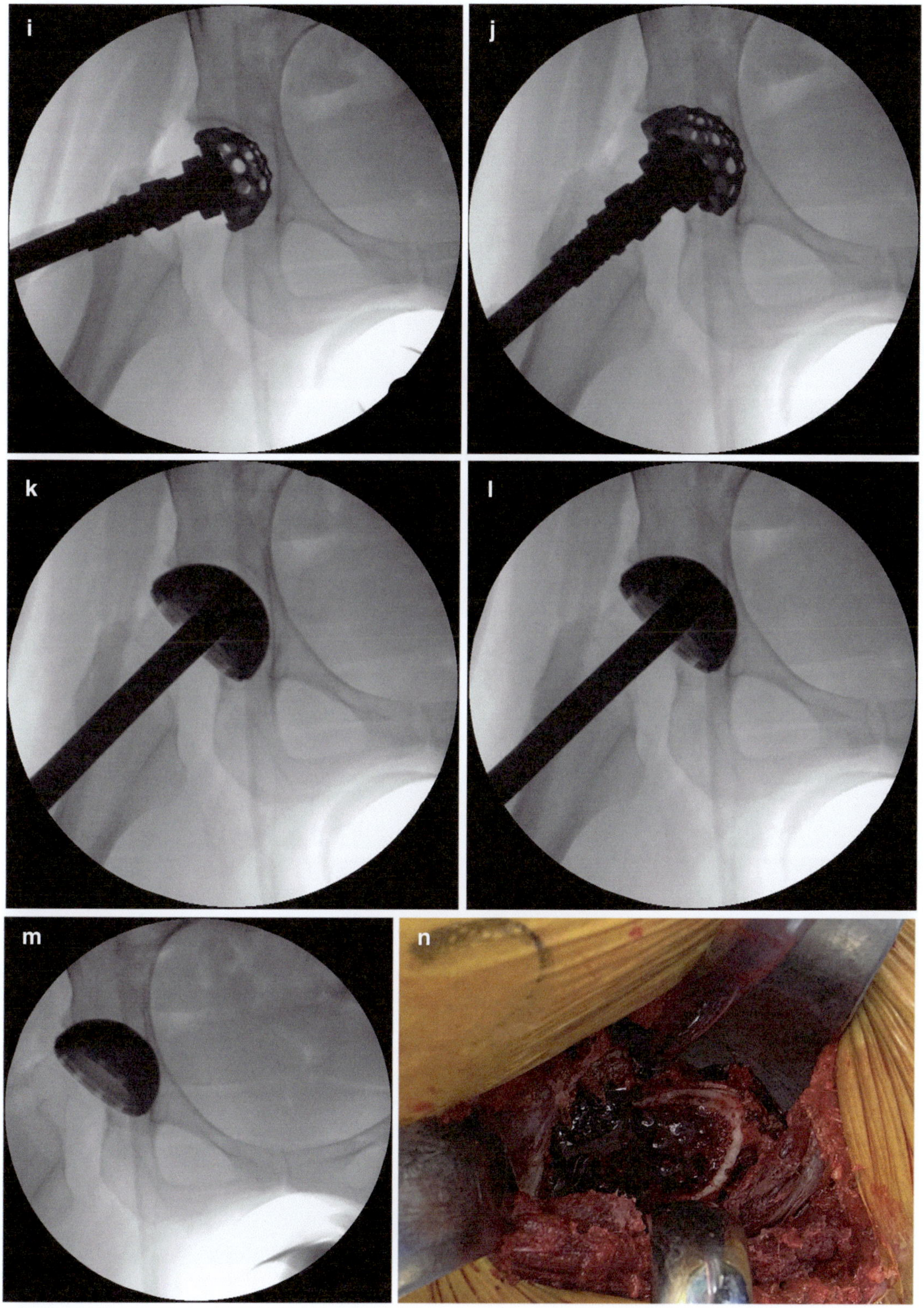

Fig. 17.1 (continued)

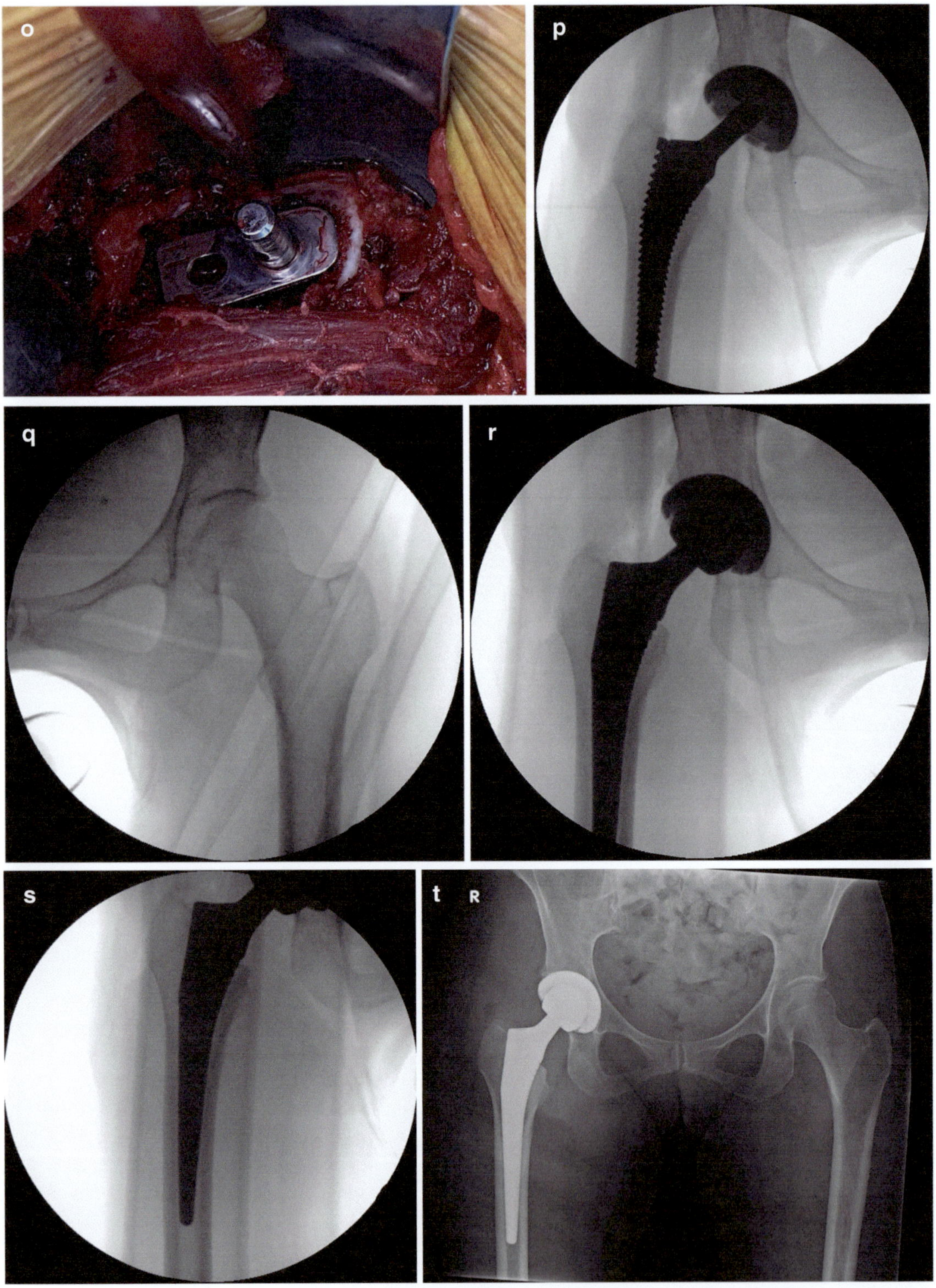

Fig. 17.1 (continued)

5. Femoral head removal: A fresh femoral neck cut is then made from the saddle region laterally to point a given distance above the lesser trochanter, as determined by the preoperative (or intraoperative) plan. The greater trochanter posteriorly wraps medially, and therefore, the saw blade should be oriented approximately 20° lateral to medial when the leg/patella is straight up toward the ceiling. This avoids a small saw cut in the greater trochanter, which can then propagate into a complete greater trochanter fracture. The intercalary fragment of the femoral neck is then removed, and the femoral head is removed with the corkscrew either entering the femoral head itself, or in the fractured surface of the femoral neck/head.
6. Acetabular reaming and cup impaction: The labrum is removed as is the ligamentum teres before reaming. The Aquamantys device is helpful to control bleeding in the fovea, along the posterior capsule and in the supra-acetabular region. Because of osteoporosis in geriatric patients, it can be easy to eccentrically ream the anterior wall. It is therefore helpful to visualize the reamer going into the center of the acetabulum and then to visualize with fluoroscopy subsequent reaming. The inferior aspect of the reamer should hug the teardrop or remain 1–4 mm lateral to it. Reaming should match the patient's normal anatomy, but in general is approximately 40° from the horizontal and in approximately 15–20° of anteversion. Usually, only one or two reamers are needed, with the first one being 0–1 mm larger than the size of the measured femoral head. Under-reaming is usually by 1 mm.
7. Acetabular cup impaction: The cup is then impacted into the reamed acetabulum. The orientation can be checked initially under fluoroscopy. It should be ensured that the surgeon is viewing a good AP of the hip. Occasionally, the acetabular cup impaction is not accompanied by a solid impaction feeling. In that case, slight additional medial reaming by 1–3 mm or lightly reaming to the size of the acetabular cup (as opposed to 1 mm under) is helpful to then allow a solid impaction. If desired, a hole eliminator is placed and the acetabular liner is impacted into position. Care is taken to visualize the cup completely circumferentially to ensure that the liner is completely down.
8. Femoral broaching: As is detailed in other chapters of this book, the femur is placed in a femoral preparation position, characterized by external rotation, adduction, and extension of the femur. Typical soft tissue releases are the lateral capsule from the saddle region and the medial capsule down to the level of the lesser trochanter on the proximal femur. In about 20–30% of cases, the piriformis and obturator internus is released from the proximal femur to allow for lateralization of the femur. The surgeon can control the rotation of the femur and should ensure that the medial aspect of the femoral neck is pointing toward the ceiling or straight up. The Hana table hook underneath the proximal femur can be used as a light handle to lateralize the femur as it is being lowered to the floor. The starter broach, a 3/8 inch curved curette, a rongeur, and a curved rasp are all instruments which help to ensure that broaching is approrpiately lateral on the proximal femur. Broaching commences up to a point where there is good canal fill, good proximal fill, and excellent rotational control of the femur via the broach handle. If there is tight canal fill distally but not good fill proximally, flexible reaming is helpful. A trial of components can then be carried out to check leg length, offset, and stability.
9. Reduction in the femoral head: It is recognized that the surgical team performing arthroplasty for a femoral neck fracture may not be a team which is performing arthroplasty every day. The author has found it helpful to have a stepwise system to reduce the femoral head (or hemiarthroplasty), which can be easily communicated, taught, and remembered. It has been reduced to four steps:
   - Step 1: Internally rotate the leg 60°. This ensures the femoral head or bipolar head

is underneath the hip capsule, which has been tagged and which is being held directly toward the ceiling.

- Step 2: Abduct the extremity while still on the floor.
- Step 3: Raise the leg to neutral height. At this point, the surgeon checks again the relationship of the femoral head to the capsule and ensures that there is a reasonable distance to relocate the femoral head viz a viz the acetabulum.
- Step 4: Traction and internal rotation by the leg spar operator. This is accompanied by the surgeon utilizing a head ball pusher if necessary.

10. Radiographic analysis of trial components: Fluoroscopy can be utilized to create a virtual AP pelvis for the surgeon to compare the operative to the nonoperative side. The overlay technique is also helpful to compare the operative side implants to the nonoperative side. The surgeon can also ensure that the femoral component is going straight down the femoral canal.
11. Dislocation: The dislocation maneuver is traction, external rotation, extension, and adduction of the leg, followed by slow release of traction. The surgeon can use their index finger around the femoral neck to lateralize the proximal femur or can alternatively use a dislocation hook to provide the same effect. The trial head and neck are then removed, and the femur is placed in the femoral preparation position.
12. Component insertion: The broach can then be removed, the canal irrigated, and the real implants impacted into place. If the surgeon is confident regarding leg length, the real head ball may be impacted onto the stem. If desired, an additional trial with the femoral head trials on the real femoral component can be carried out.
13. Stability testing: Stability testing of the hip prosthesis is generally not needed. If desired, the boot can be taken out of the leg spar and testing for posterior instability may be conducted by the surgeon. Anterior instability can be tested by lowering the leg spar approximately 1 foot, adducting approximately 20°, and externally rotating while the surgeon palpates the femoral head and its propensity to anteriorly dislocate. This is rare with this test, but if present, the surgeon should question: (1) excessive acetabular cup anteversion, (2) excessive femoral anteversion, or (3) lack of appropriate length and offset.
14. Closure: The capsule is closed with three absorbable 1–0 sutures, and the tensor fascia sheath is closed with a running 1–0 absorbable suture. The subcutaneous tissues are closed with 1–0 and 3–0 absorbable suture, and the skin is closed with a subcuticular 4–0 Monocryl, with Dermabond applied.
15. Postoperative rehabilitation: Patients are allowed full weight-bearing without restrictions. Emphasis is placed on quadriceps strengthening, ankle pumps, and ambulation training.

Author's Perspective: Implant Selection for Hip Arthroplasty for Femoral Neck Fracture

Since 2002, the author has nearly exclusively used the DePuy CORAIL femoral component in the setting of femoral neck fractures (Figs. 17.1 and 17.2). This stem is a compaction broaching, titanium alloy, hydroxyapatite-coated stem. For femoral neck fracture patients, its use may have several advantages:

- The compaction broaching and design of the stem rely on full-length "fit and fill" of the stem. Thus, if there is femoral neck comminution or fragmentation, the stem is still stable because of distal stem stability.
- The survivability of the stem in published series and personal experience has been high [16].
- The broach only technique is simple and quick, which may be important in geriatric patients.

Certainly, it is recognized and completely acknowledged that multiple other stem designs

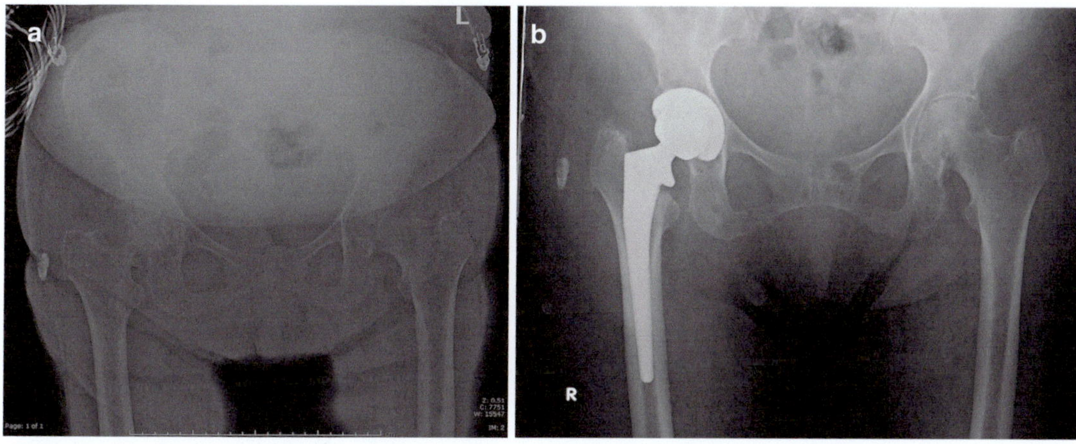

Fig. 17.2 99-year-old woman sustained a dislplaced femoral neck fracture in a fall. She had some underlying right hip/groin pain. She was fully ambulatory in her own home with an occasional use of a walker. A right anterior total hip arthroplasty was performed. (**a**) AP injury pelvic radiograph. (**b**) AP pelvis after right anterior total hip replacement

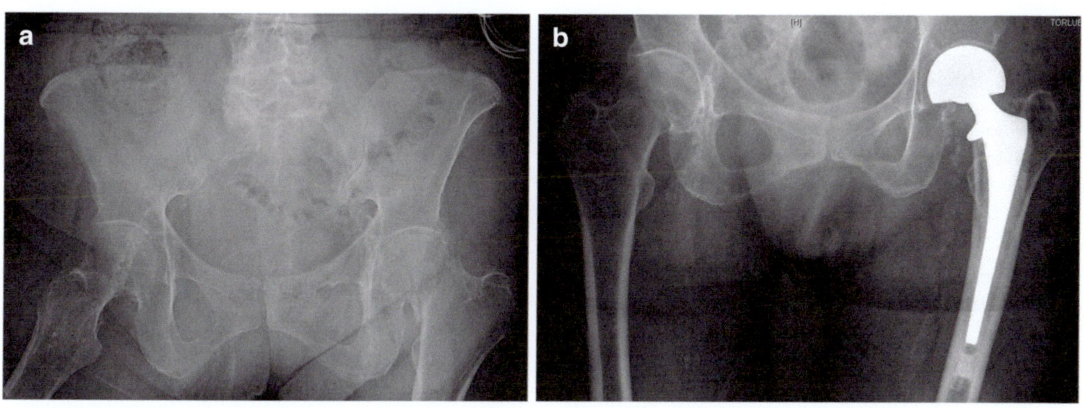

Fig. 17.3 88-year-old woman with scoliosis fell and sustained a displaced left femoral neck fracture. (**a**) Injury AP pelvis radiograph. (**b**) AP pelvis following cemented hemiarthroplasty (Case courtesy of Tania Ferguson, MD)

can be effectively utilized in the patient with a femoral neck fracture. Even in the setting Dorr type C femora, the CORAIL stem has been utilized without significant subsidence or intraoperative fracture.

In the setting of Dorr type A femora, distal intramedullary reaming may be helpful. The author has found that it turns out that intramedullary reaming to the same millimeter (or 0.5 mm greater than the stem size) as the CORAIL stem size (coincidentally) is efficacious in creating a good "fit and fill" of the canal for the full length of the stem. As in any hip arthroplasty, the surgeon wants to remove bone laterally in the proximal femur, so that the stem is not in varus and so that the stem hugs the medial aspect of the greater trochanter.

As noted above, significant evidence exists that use of a cemented stem is associated with a lower rate of intraoperative fracture during stem insertion and less pain in the years following surgery. Certainly, the anterior approach can be utilized for cemented stem insertion (Fig. 17.3).

Also as discussed above, there is increasing literature support for use of a total hip arthroplasty compared with a hemiarthroplasty. However, based on the patient's age and function level, if a hemiarthroplasty is desired to be done, it can be easily accomplished via the direct anterior approach (Fig. 17.4).

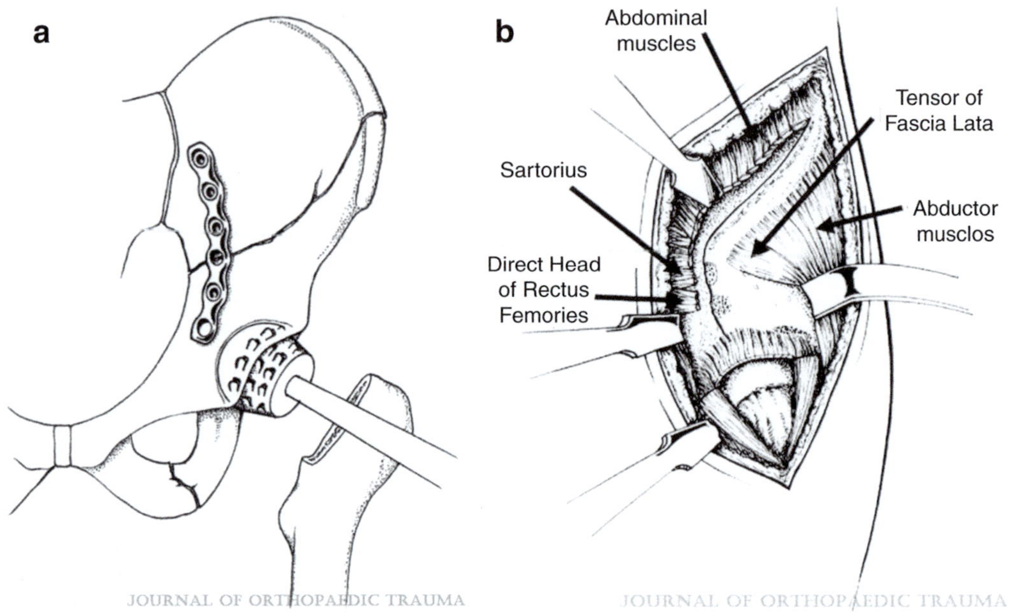

Fig. 17.4 Beaulé et al. described the technique described by Joel Matta for fixation of the anterior column family fracture followed by direct anterior hip arthroplasty, all through the Levine modified iliofemoral approach. (**a**) The anterior column, anterior wall, or anterior column posterior hemitransverse fracture is first stabilized with an undercontoured plate in the internal iliac fossa. Care is taken to ensure that the screws are outside future acetabular cup position. (**b**) A direct anterior hip arthroplasty is then performed. (Reproduced with permission from Journal of Othopaedic Trauma 18(9):623-629, October 2004, Wolters Kluwer Health, Inc)

Acetabular Fractures

The outcomes of operatively treated acetabular fractures have considerably improved since the 1960s. Emile Letournel is largely responsible for this improvement, who published his findings in *Fractures of the Acetabulum* along with Robert Judet [17]. Letournel defined the radiographic analysis of acetabular fractures and established a classification for them that still exists today. Furthermore, he elucidated the surgical approaches, reduction strategies, and fixation options for their treatment. Finally, he carefully investigated the outcome of patients treated with internal fixation.

Letournel and Judet [17] documented the outcome of 569 acetabular fractures treated within 3 weeks of injury. They initially classified their quality of reduction into perfect (all radiographic landmarks restored) or imperfect (all radiographic landmarks not restored). Secondary surgical congruence (usually occurring in the both column fractures) occurred when the articular surface around the femoral head was internally fixed as perfectly as possible, but there was malreduction between the innominate bone and the joint. They achieved a perfect reduction in 73.7% of cases, with 4.8% having secondary congruence. In 1996, Matta [18] initially reported on a series of 262 acetabular fractures. A new scale was established for the quality of reduction: anatomic (1 mm or less of displacement), imperfect (2–3 mm of displacement), and poor (greater than 3 mm of displacement). In his series, the postoperative reduction was perfect in 71% of cases, imperfect in 20% of cases, and poor in 7% of cases. Overall, 96% of the simple fracture types were reduced with an anatomic reduction, while only 64% of the associated fracture type had an anatomic reduction. The age of the patient also certainly matters in terms of how good of reduction the surgeon can obtain: 78% of patients younger than 40 years had an anatomic reduction; 57% of patients older than 40 years had an anatomic reduction. As a result, Matta established that the quality of the reduction was associated with the clinical result in the patient. Specifically, in those patients with an anatomic reduction, a good or excellent clinical outcome was achieved in 83% of cases. If an imperfect reduction was achieved, a good or excellent clinical result was achieved in only 68% of cases. Several factors predicted a worse clinical result: an imperfect reduction, traumatic injury to the cartilage or bone of the femoral head, and a patient age of 40 years or older. Tannast et al. [19] looked at the 20-year survivorship of 816 hips treated with open reduction internal fixation by Matta. Negative predictors for the need for a secondary salvage operation were as follows:

- Nonanatomic fracture reduction (greater than 1 mm displacement);
- Age of 40 years or older;
- Anterior hip dislocation;
- Postoperative incongruence of the femoral head with the acetabular roof;
- Involvement of the posterior wall;
- Acetabular impaction;
- Femoral head cartilage injury;
- Initial displacement of the fracture greater than 20 mm; and
- Utilization of the extended iliofemoral approach.

In the past, results of total hip arthroplasty after fractures of the acetabulum were compromised by high rated of loosening of the acetabular component [20]. However, with more modern acetabular cup designs coupled with stabilization of the pelvis prior to cup insertion, results have been more encouraging. The challenge for the surgeon/patient team is to determine when total hip arthroplasty (with or without additional fixation of the innominate bone) should be chosen over open reduction internal fixation.

Thus, the surgeon treating acetabular fractures does want to predict which particular patients have a high chance of poor clinical outcome with open reduction internal fixation alone. There are particular patterns which should be considered for an anterior total hip arthroplasty, with or without internal fixation. These include the following:

- Anterior column, anterior wall, and anterior column/posterior hemitransverse fractures with significant articular impaction (Fig. 17.5).
- Pipkin IV acetabular fracture dislocations (usually consisting of a combined posterior wall acetabular fracture and a femoral head fracture).
- Rarely, elderly patients with posterior wall fractures and significant articular involvement (Fig. 17.6).

The challenge in utilizing a total hip replacement in these circumstances is of course having a stable foundation for the acetabular cup. In the setting of the posterior wall acetabular fractures, the author has treated a few select cases with medializing the reaming. The cup is then impacted into position and screws are routinely used. The surgeon could perform such a total hip replacement from a posterior approach with fixation of the posterior wall followed by reaming and cup insertion. However, such an approach is associated with increased risk of dislocation, sciatic nerve injury, and inappropriate cup position. In contrast, the anterior approach total hip arthroplasty is associated with more accurate component positioning, significantly lower risk of dislocation, and a quicker early rehabilitation and recovery. Certainly, published series in peer-reviewed journals will be necessary to bring credibility to this approach.

Beaulé [21] and Matta advocated the Levine modified approach for fixation of anterior column acetabular fractures (or their variants), followed by direct anterior total hip arthroplasty (Figs. 17.3 and 17.4).

Chen [22] also described its use. This can be extremely helpful not only with fractures that have significant displacement of the anterior column, but also significant articular impaction (Fig. 17.5).

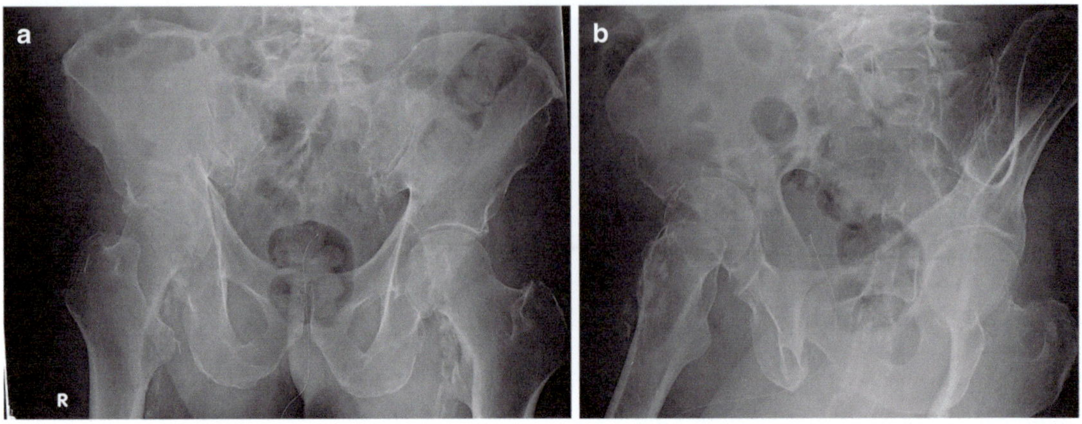

Fig. 17.5 An 88-year-old man presented to the hospital for chest pain. After further evaluation, he was noted to have an anterior column acetabular fracture with significant articular impaction. Additionally, he had an aortic aneurysm, which warranted endovascular intervention. His biggest complaint was that of right hip pain. After extensive workup and discussion with cardiology, cardiovascular surgery, and vascular surgery, it was deemed that surgical intervention on his right hip should proceed if warranted. Patient was independently living with some assistance from his family. He utilized a cane preinjury. (**a**) AP pelvis radiograph demonstrating significant articular impaction. Note the cephalad migration of the femoral head when compared to the teardrop. (**b**) Iliac oblique view of the pelvis demonstrating separate articular impaction on the top of the femoral head (arrow). (**c**) Obturator oblique view of pelvis. (**d**) CT scan. (**e**) Intraoperative view of right hip joint with traction applied to the right hip. Although in some cases this separate impaction can be reduced and supported above with bone graft and hardware, it was not felt that this was predictable in this patient, and with his medical problems. Therefore, fixation of the anterior column and subsequent total hip replacement was planned. (**f**) AP radiograph of the hip following fixation of the displaced anterior column. Note that although the anterior column is reduced, there is still articular impaction. This represents that the articular surface impaction is dissociated from the anterior column. Significant osteoporosis was noted in placement of screws. A Schanz pin was placed in the proximal femur to aid in distal/lateral traction of the femoral head. (**g**) Obturator oblique view of the right hip following internal fixation of the anterior column fracture. Two undercontoured plates were utilized to afford reduction of the anterior column. (**h**) The cartilage of the superior aspect of the acetabulum was gently reamed, and a femoral head bone graft was placed in the superior aspect of the acetabulum. (**i**) Initial stages of reaming. (**j**) Final stage of reaming. Despite the bone graft, by necessity the hip center was raised. (**k**) Impaction of the acetabular cup. A revision cup was utilized, which allowed for screws in the periphery of the acetabular cup. Multiple screws were placed. (**l**) Intraoperative iliac oblique view demonstrating screws for fixation of an anterior superior iliac spine osteotomy, the anterior column plates and screws, and screws in the acetabular cup. (**m**) Intraoperative radiograph with trial head ball. A surgical error was made here as there was traction on the leg, giving the author a false sense of equal leg length with the given head ball. As noted below, this resulted in shortening of the leg or approximately 9 mm. (**n**) Immediate postoperative AP radiograph of the pelvis. The patient was made partial weight-bearing for 6 weeks. He went on to have a coronary artery bypass grafting surgery and an endovascular aortic aneurysm repair in the next 3 weeks. (**o**) AP radiograph at 4 months. The patient was fully ambulating with a cane. His pain was minimal, and he was offered a shoe lift of approximately ¼ inch. (**p**) Iliac oblique view at 4 months postoperative. (**q**) Obturator oblique view at 4 months postoperative

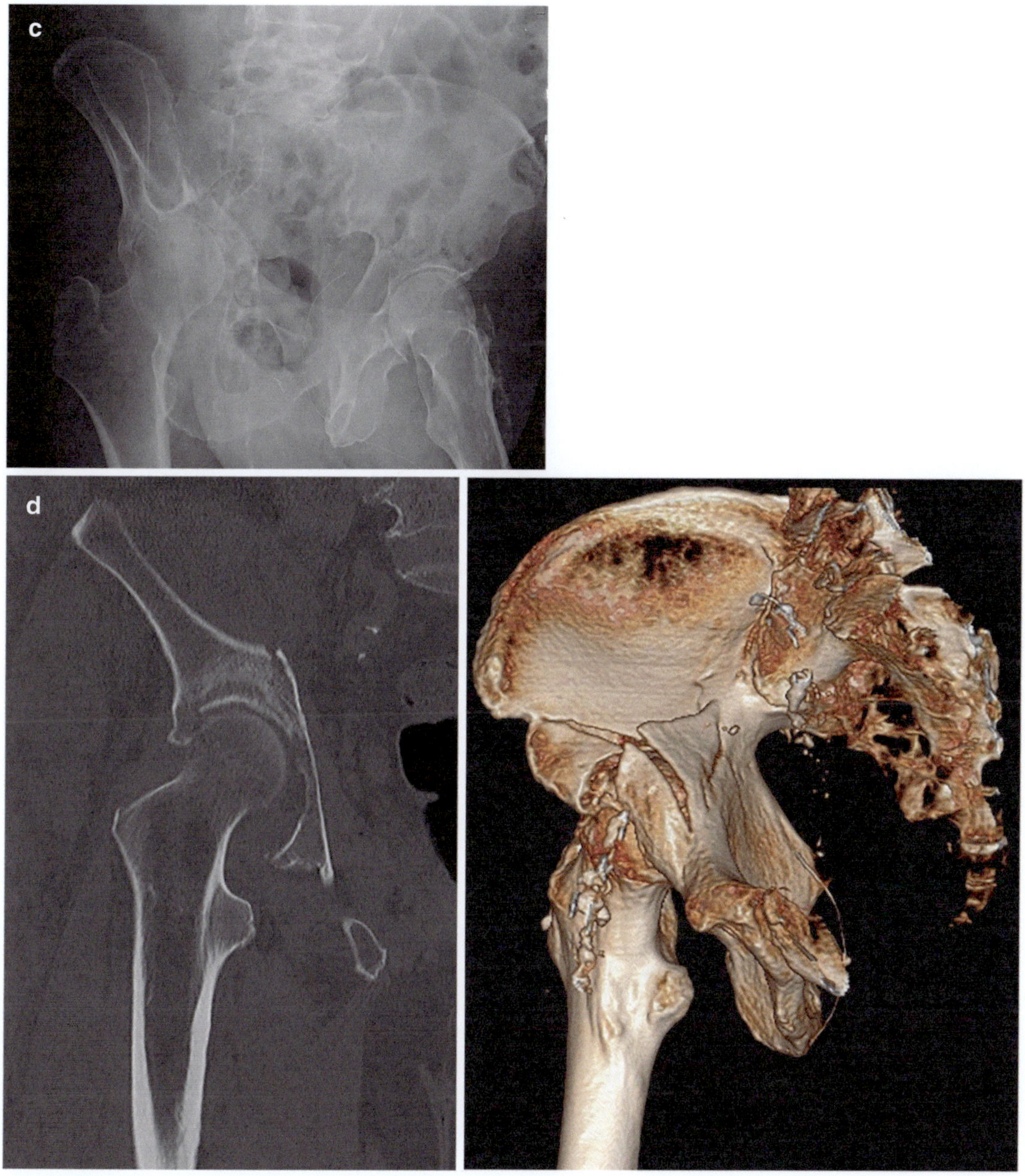

Fig. 17.5 (continued)

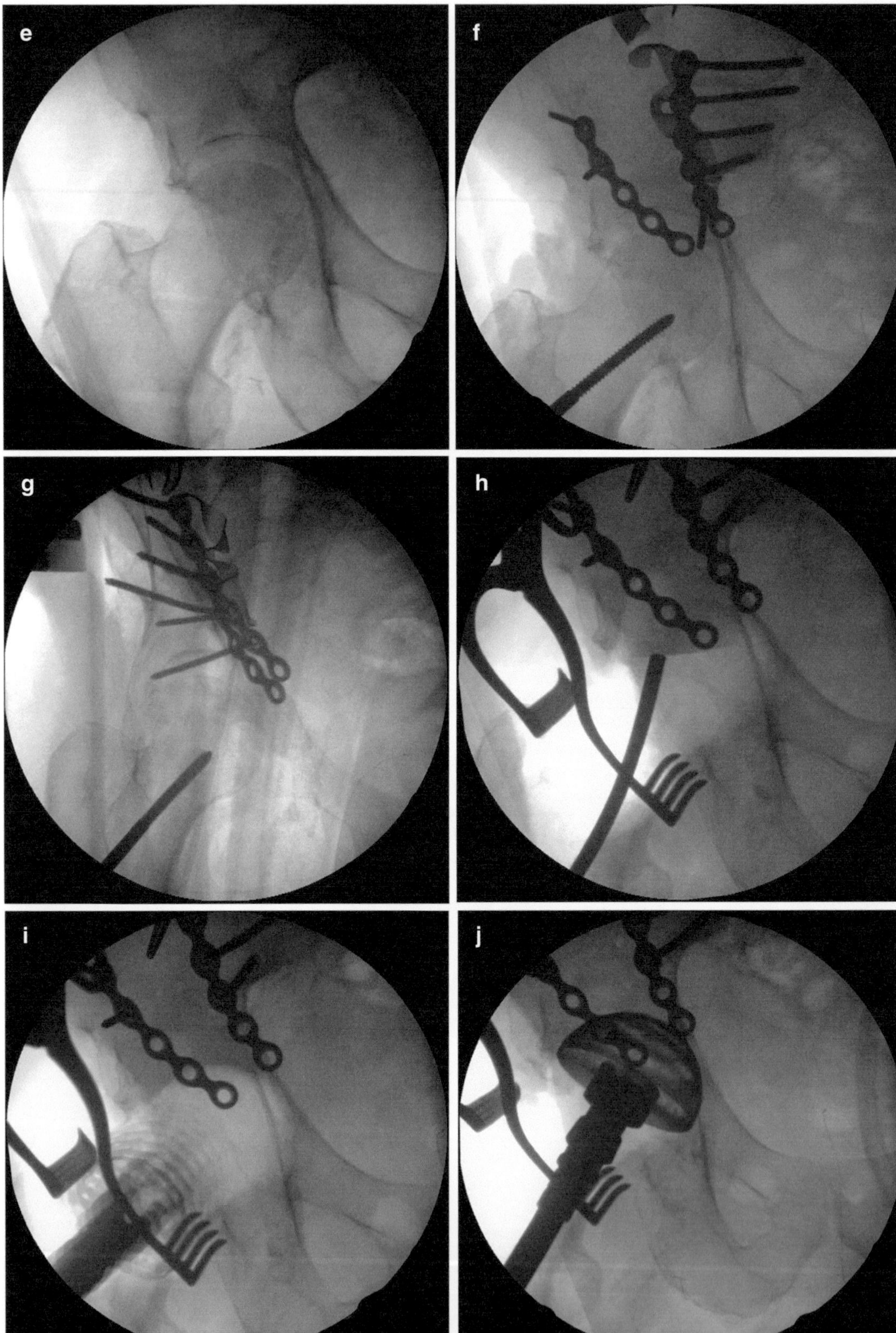

Fig. 17.5 (continued)

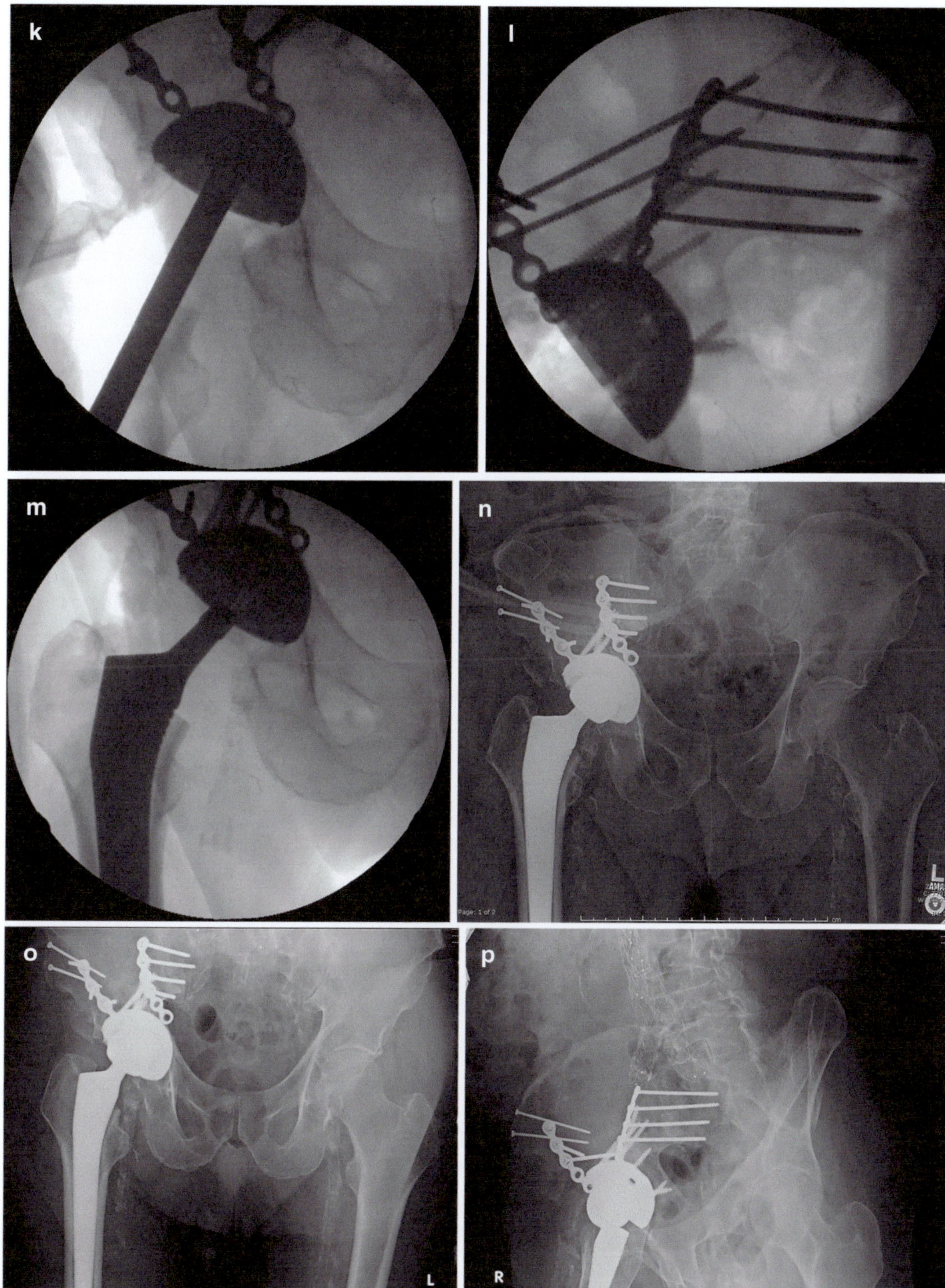

Fig. 17.5 (continued)

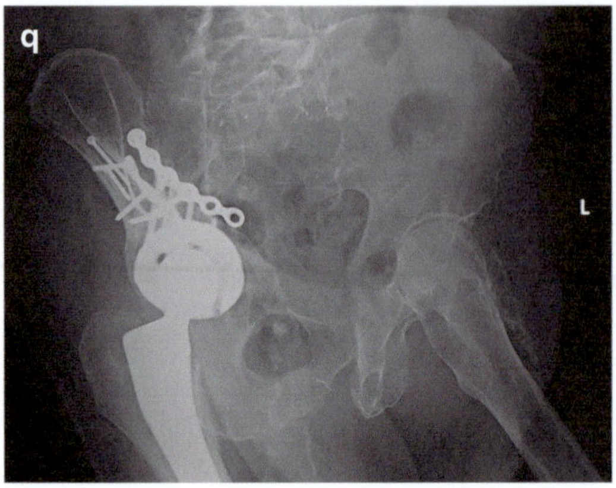

Fig. 17.5 (continued)

Femoral Head Fractures (Figs. 17.7 and 17.8)

Swiontkowski et al. [23] detailed the clinical outcome of 24 patients with at least 2 years of follow-up and noted only 2/3 had a good or excellent approach. Recently, Koerner et al. [24] reported on twenty-eight patients with greater than 10 years of follow-up and reported a 75% chance of a major complication during that time period. Thirty percent of patients required a total hip arthroplasty at an average of 6.4 years after injury. Thus, if the patient is faced with a femoral head fracture patient, a very viable option is an anterior total hip replacement.

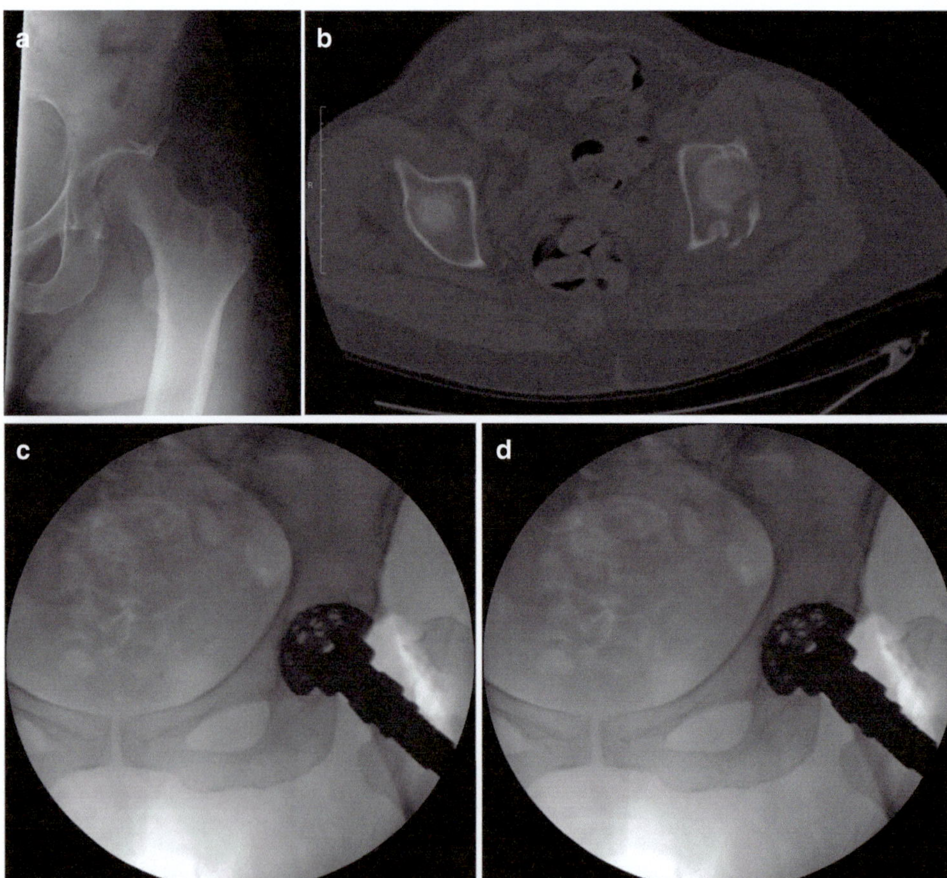

Fig. 17.6 A 77-year-old woman had a misstep while descending stairs and sustained a left posterior wall fracture dislocation. There was residual subluxation of the femoral head despite attempts at reduction in the emergency room. (**a**) AP radiograph of the left hip. (**b**) CT scan of the left hip demonstrating the posterior wall acetabular fracture and marginal impaction. (**c**) An anterior total hip arthroplasty was performed. No attempt was made to reduce or fix the posterior wall fracture. Instead, the intent was to ream slightly more medial than normal. (**d**) Final acetabular cup position. (**e**) Intraoperative iliac oblique view demonstrating good impaction of the acetabular cup into the posterior column and safe screw placement. (**f**) Postoperative AP pelvis radiograph. The patient has had a painless total hip at 4-year follow-up

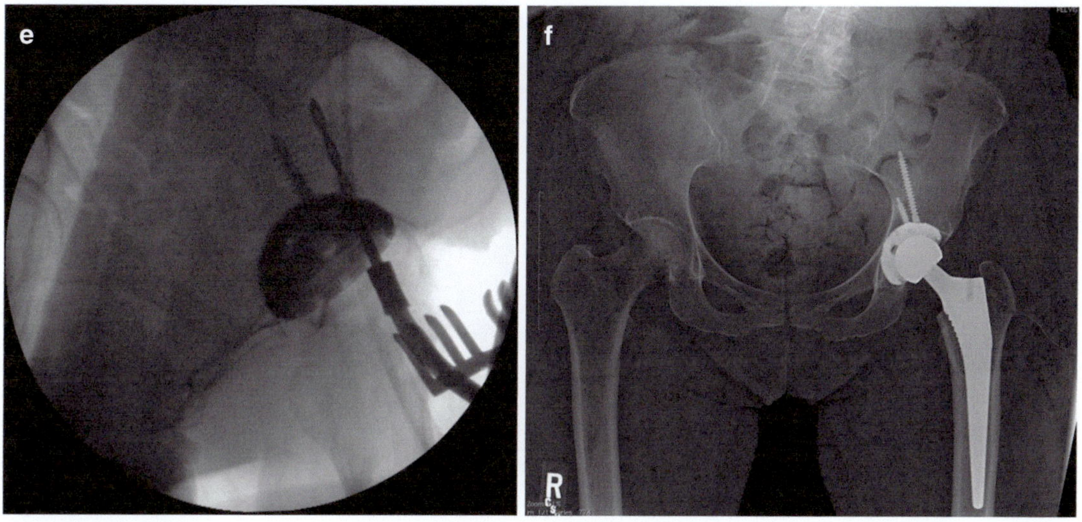

Fig. 17.6 (continued)

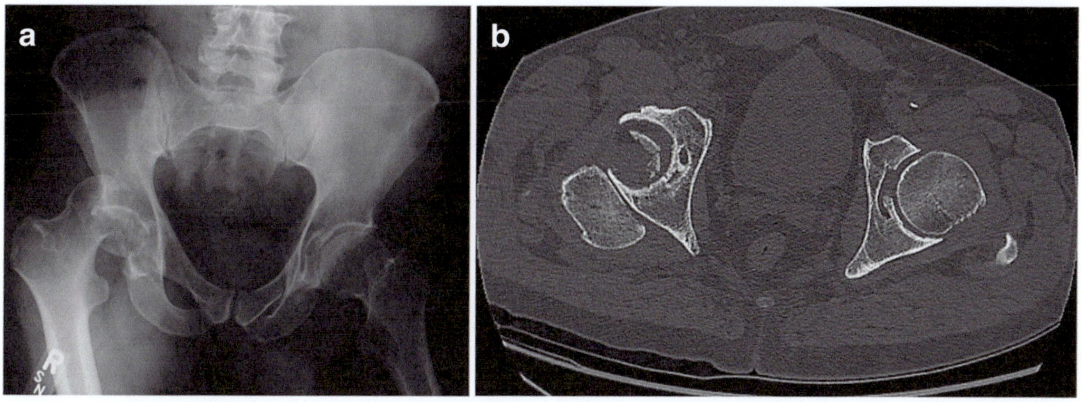

Fig. 17.7 Irreducible right femoral head fracture dislocation of the right hip in a 55-year-old carpet professional. Patient had definite radiographic signs of femoral–acetabular impingement. He noted decreased range of motion of his hip prior to the trauma but did not have pain. He owned his own floor covering business, and it was very important to get back to work as soon as possible. Putting together his desires, the natural history of a femoral head fracture with an irreducible dislocation, and his femoral–acetabular impingement, the decision was made to perform a direct anterior total hip arthroplasty. (**a**) AP radiograph demonstrating the fracture dislocation of the right hip. An attempt at closed reduction in the emergency room and at the beginning of the operative procedure was not successful. (**b**) CT scan through the hip joint demonstrating the fragmentation of the femoral head remnant in the hip joint and the posterior dislocation of the femoral head. (**c**) Intraoperative view of right hip. (**d**) A femoral neck cut was made with the femoral head still dislocated. Then, acetabular reaming and cup impaction proceeded as usual. (**e**) Final AP pelvis radiograph

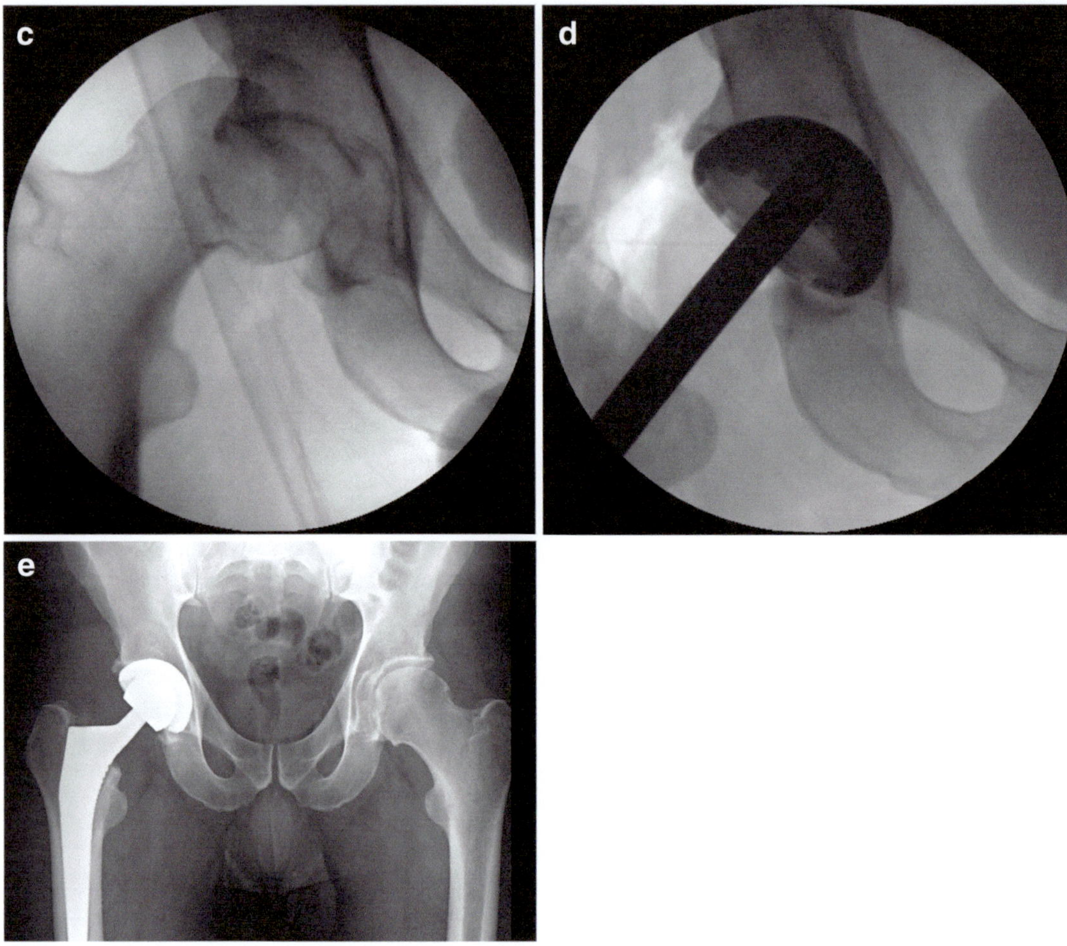

Fig. 17.7 (continued)

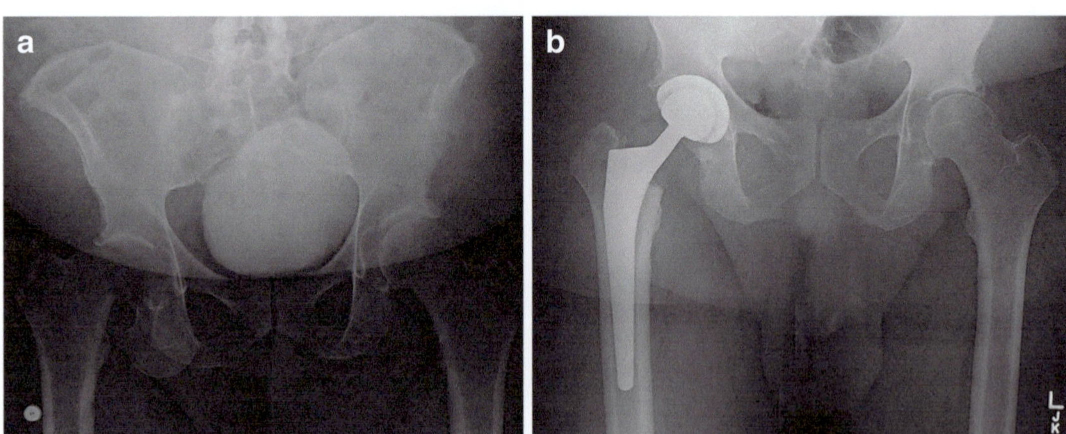

Fig. 17.8 38 year old male sustained a motorcycle accident and a right femoral neck fracture dislocation of the proximal femur. CT scan demonstrated a femoral head fracture as well. (**a**) AP pelvis film demonstrating right hip fracture dislocation. (**b**) AP radiograph demonstrating right anterior total hip replacement following removal of the femoral head/neck fragment and seperate femoral head fragments in the hip joint

References

1. Crist BD, Ivie CB, Bal BS. Total hip replacement with use of a direct anterior approach: a critical analysis review. JBJS Rev. 2014;2(6):e4. https://doi.org/10.2106/jbjs.Rvw.M.00086.
2. Barrett WP, Turner SE, Leopold JP. Prospective randomized study of direct anterior vs postero-lateral approach for total hip arthroplasty. J Arthroplast. 2013;28(9):1634–8. https://doi.org/10.1016/j.arth.2013.01.034.
3. Barrett WP, Turner SE, Murphy JA, Flener JL, Alton TB. Prospective, randomized study of direct anterior approach vs posterolateral approach total hip arthroplasty: a concise 5-year follow-up evaluation. J Arthroplast. 2019;34(6):1139–42. https://doi.org/10.1016/j.arth.2019.01.060.
4. Bergin PF, Doppelt JD, Kephart CJ, Benke MT, Graeter JH, Holmes AS, et al. Comparison of minimally invasive direct anterior versus posterior total hip arthroplasty based on inflammation and muscle damage markers. J Bone Joint Surg Am. 2011;93(15):1392–8. https://doi.org/10.2106/JBJS.J.00557.
5. Bhandari M, Devereaux PJ, Swiontkowski MF, Tornetta P 3rd, Obremskey W, Koval KJ, et al. Internal fixation compared with arthroplasty for displaced fractures of the femoral neck. A meta-analysis. J Bone Joint Surg Am. 2003;85(9):1673–81. https://doi.org/10.2106/00004623-200309000-00004.
6. Ekhtiari S, Gormley J, Axelrod DE, Devji T, Bhandari M, Guyatt GH. Total hip arthroplasty versus hemiarthroplasty for displaced femoral neck fracture: a systematic review and meta-analysis of randomized controlled trials. J Bone Joint Surg Am. 2020;102(18):1638–45. https://doi.org/10.2106/jbjs.20.00226.
7. Ravi B, Pincus D, Khan H, Wasserstein D, Jenkinson R, Kreder HJ. Comparing complications and costs of total hip arthroplasty and hemiarthroplasty for femoral neck fractures: a propensity score-matched, population-based study. J Bone Joint Surg Am. 2019;101(7):572–9. https://doi.org/10.2106/JBJS.18.00539.
8. Lewis DP, Wæver D, Thorninger R, Donnelly WJ. Hemiarthroplasty vs total hip arthroplasty for the management of displaced neck of femur fractures: a systematic review and meta-analysis. J Arthroplasty. 2019;34(8):1837–43.e2. https://doi.org/10.1016/j.arth.2019.03.070.
9. Health Investigators, Bhandari M, Einhorn TA, Guyatt G, Schemitsch EH, Zura RD, et al. Total hip arthroplasty or hemiarthroplasty for hip fracture. N Engl J Med. 2019;381(23):2199–208. https://doi.org/10.1056/NEJMoa1906190.
10. Parker MI, Pryor G, Gurusamy K. Cemented versus uncemented hemiarthroplasty for intracapsular hip fractures: a randomised controlled trial in 400 patients. J Bone Joint Surg Br. 2010;92(1):116–22. https://doi.org/10.1302/0301-620x.92b1.22753.
11. Chen KK, Nayyar S, Davidovitch RI, Vigdorchik JM, Iorio R, Macaulay W. Cemented compared with uncemented femoral fixation in the arthroplasty treatment of displaced femoral neck fractures: a critical analysis review. JBJS Rev. 2018;6(4):e6. https://doi.org/10.2106/jbjs.Rvw.17.00119.
12. DeRogatis MJ, Piatek AZ, Jacob R, Kelly SC, Issack PS. Hemiarthroplasty for femoral neck fractures in the elderly: a comparison of cemented and uncemented femoral stems. JBJS Rev. 2020;8(7):e1900192. https://doi.org/10.2106/jbjs.Rvw.19.00192.
13. Kumar P, Rajnish RK, Neradi D, Kumar V, Agarwal S, Aggarwal S. Hemiarthroplasty for neck of femur fractures: to cement or not? A systematic review of literature and meta-analysis. Eur J Orthop Surg Traumatol. 2019;29(4):731–46. https://doi.org/10.1007/s00590-019-02364-z.
14. Cichos KH, Mabry SE, Spitler CA, McGwin G Jr, Quade JH, Ghanem ES. Comparison between the direct anterior and posterior approaches for total hip arthroplasty performed for femoral neck fracture. J Orthop Trauma. 2021;35(1):41–8. https://doi.org/10.1097/bot.0000000000001883.
15. Carlson VR, Ong AC, Orozco FR, Lutz RW, Duque AF, Post ZD. The direct anterior approach does not increase return to function following hemiarthroplasty for femoral neck fracture. Orthopedics. 2017;40(6):e1055–61. https://doi.org/10.3928/01477447-20170925-08.
16. Hallan G, Lie SA, Furnes O, Engesaeter LB, Vollset SE, Havelin LI. Medium- and long-term performance of 11,516 uncemented primary femoral stems from the Norwegian arthroplasty register. J Bone Joint Surg Br. 2007;89(12):1574–80. https://doi.org/10.1302/0301-620X.89B12.18969.
17. Letournel E, Judet R. Fractures of the acetabulum. 2nd ed. Berlin: Springer; 1993.
18. Matta JM. Fractures of the acetabulum: accuracy of reduction and clinical results in patients managed operatively within three weeks after the injury. J Bone Joint Surg Am. 1996;78(11):1632–45.
19. Tannast M, Najibi S, Matta JM. Two to twenty-year survivorship of the hip in 810 patients with operatively treated acetabular fractures. J Bone Joint Surg Am. 2012;94(17):1559–67. https://doi.org/10.2106/jbjs.k.00444.
20. Mears DC, Velyvis JH. Acute total hip arthroplasty for selected displaced acetabular fractures: two to twelve-year results. J Bone Joint Surg Am. 2002;84-A(1):1–9. https://doi.org/10.2106/00004623-200201000-00001.
21. Beaulé PE, Griffin DB, Matta JM. The Levine anterior approach for total hip replacement as the treatment for an acute acetabular fracture. J Orthop Trauma. 2004;18(9):623–9. https://doi.org/10.1097/00005131-200410000-00008.
22. Chen MJ, Wadhwa H, Bellino MJ. Sequential ilioinguinal or anterior intrapelvic approach with anterior approach to the hip during combined internal fixation and total hip arthroplasty for acetabular fractures. Eur

J Orthop Surg Traumatol. 2021;31(4):635–41. https://doi.org/10.1007/s00590-020-02810-3.
23. Swiontkowski MF, Thorpe M, Seiler JG, Hansen ST. Operative management of displaced femoral head fractures: case-matched comparison of anterior versus posterior approaches for Pipkin I and Pipkin II fractures. J Orthop Trauma. 1992;6(4):437–42.
24. Koerner M, Westberg J, Martin J, Templeman D. Patient-reported outcomes of femoral head fractures with a minimum 10-year follow-up. J Orthop Trauma. 2020;34(12):621–5. https://doi.org/10.1097/BOT.0000000000001880.

Anterior Approach Total Hip Arthroplasty Following Previous Femoral and Acetabular Fractures

18

Michael J. Chen and Michael J. Bellino

Indications

Conversion total hip arthroplasty (THA) may be indicated following operative or nonoperative management of proximal femoral and acetabular fractures. While posterior approach THA is commonly performed in these scenarios, anterior approach (AA) THA is a viable alternative and is our preferred method during conversion when feasible. When used during conversion THA, the AA may have additional benefits as those observed during acute AA THA for femoral neck fracture [1–3]. We prefer using a posterior approach during conversion THA in the following scenarios: (1) if there is clinically significant heterotopic ossification (HO) in the abductors and/or external rotators that requires excision, (2) if there is erosion of the posterior wall with intra-articular translocation of a posterior plate that requires removal, (3) if there are multiple intra-articular screws placed from the retro-acetabular surface that require removal, and (4) if there is a posterior acetabular defect that requires augmentation that can otherwise not be done through the AA.

In a recent clinical trial, fractures of the femoral neck treated with internal fixation progressed to nonunion in 6% of cases, osteonecrosis of the femoral head in 7% of cases, and implant failure in 8% of cases [4]. While head-preserving strategies to manage nonunion include revision with a valgus intertrochanteric osteotomy [5], some patients may be better served with conversion THA. Such patients include those at risk for failure of nonunion repair, the elderly, and patients that cannot tolerate weight-bearing restrictions [6]. Conversion THA under these circumstances eliminates the need for fracture healing and facilitates immediate return to full weight-bearing. Other indications for conversion THA include implant-related chondrolysis from femoral head perforation of the screws or helical blade [7] and preexisting or development of hip arthritis from post-traumatic or idiopathic etiologies.

While intertrochanteric (IT) femur fractures treated with internal fixation have higher rates of union [8], malunion and implant perforation of the femoral head may result in abnormal hip biomechanics and painful arthritis of the hip, respectively [7, 9]. Malunion with limb shortening in the absence of intra-articular hip pathology may be treated with a proximal femoral osteotomy [10]. However, the presence of symptomatic hip arthritis may be an indication for conversion THA. Care should be taken to differentiate intra-articular hip pain from lateral trochanteric pain secondary to the implant backout that occurs from fracture collapse, which can be treated with implant removal once the fracture has healed [8].

M. J. Chen · M. J. Bellino (✉)
Department of Orthopaedic Surgery, Stanford University Medical Center, Stanford, CA, USA
e-mail: mbellino@stanford.edu

J. M. Matta, A. P. Sah (eds.), *Anterior Hip Replacement*,
https://doi.org/10.1007/978-3-030-91896-5_18

Other indications for conversion THA include nonunion and preexisting or development of hip arthritis from post-traumatic or idiopathic etiologies.

Acetabular fractures treated with or without internal fixation may progress to post-traumatic hip arthritis in the presence of persisting articular incongruency, intra-articular loose osteochondral debris, or from irreversible chondral damage that occurred at the time of injury [11]. Tannast et al. [11] demonstrated a cumulative 20-year survivorship of 79% in 810 acetabular fractures. Many surgically treated acetabular fractures are thus anticipated to eventually require conversion THA. Nonunion in acetabular fractures is a rare occurrence and should be managed with revision internal fixation if symptomatic [12]. Femoral head fractures that occur with acetabular fractures or hip dislocations are also at risk of osteonecrosis and post-traumatic osteoarthritis [13]. Patients with symptomatic hip arthritis that fail nonoperative management are indicated for conversion THA.

Patient History and Physical Findings

A thorough history should be elicited from the patient to identify the location of pain, activity limitations, and associated symptoms. Details regarding their postoperative course should be known especially if there was a wound issue or surgical site infection.

Pain should be localized to the hip joint and not to the greater trochanteric region, for example, which can occur from the backout of implants going into the femoral head, causing iliotibial band irritation. If there is any question as to the origin of pain, an intra-articular lidocaine injection should be administered to aid in the diagnosis. The sciatic, femoral, obturator, and lateral femoral cutaneous nerves should be tested. Distal pulses should be assessed. The incisions used for internal fixation should be inspected and their proximity to an AA hip incision noted. Hip range of motion and abductor function should be tested.

Imaging and Other Diagnostic Studies

An anteroposterior (AP) pelvis radiograph with a calibrated marker ball and a cross-table lateral radiograph of the proximal femur are obtained. Judet pelvic radiographs are obtained for patients with prior fracture the acetabulum. Full-length femur radiographs may be needed when an implant is present that extends down the diaphysis of the femur.

A computed tomography (CT) scan is obtained if there is concern for incomplete fracture union or nonunion, and to better identify acetabular bone defects that might require bony or metallic augmentation. Computed tomography can also aid in identifying intra-articular perforation of implants. This is especially helpful in posterior wall fractures of the acetabulum that were treated with a peripheral buttress plate, which can become intra-articular if the posterior wall erodes.

Magnetic resonance imaging (MRI) has little role in our experience. While it can be useful to detect early signs of femoral head osteonecrosis, metal artifacts from the internal fixation make MRI difficult to interpret without removing the implants first.

Laboratory studies including C-reactive protein and erythrocyte sedimentation rate should be drawn without hesitation if infection is suspected. Hip aspiration of the intra-articular fluid to examine the cell count and to culture is indicated in the presence of elevated inflammatory markers or high clinical suspicion for infection.

A diagnostic intra-articular hip injection with lidocaine should be performed if there is any question regarding the origin of pain. Corticosteroids should not be injected if the patient is being considered for THA to minimize the risk of infection [14].

Differential Diagnosis

The differential diagnosis includes lateral soft-tissue irritation from femoral implant back-out, nonunion, malunion of the proximal femur without osteoarthritis of the hip, lumbar back pain and spine pathology, osteomyelitis of the proximal femur or acetabulum, septic arthritis of the hip, and peripheral nerve entrapment.

Nonoperative Management

Nonoperative treatment is the same as for primary osteoarthritis of the hip and includes weight loss, oral analgesics, assistive walking devices, activity modification, and physical therapy [15].

Surgical Management

Preoperative Planning

Prior incisions and the location of internal fixation implants are taken into consideration. For example, acetabular fractures with posterior wall and/or posterior column plates and screws may be left in situ provided that the implants are not intra-articular and will not interfere with acetabular reaming and component impaction. If the aforementioned scenarios are present, a posterior approach THA should be considered to facilitate removal of the obstructing internal fixation. Alternatively, AA THA may still be performed if the intra-articular metal is able to be removed with a metal-cutting burr. The type of internal fixation implants should be determined from prior operative reports or implant recognition on the radiographs to allow for the proper implant removal equipment to be present at the time of conversion THA.

Radiographs are scrutinized to confirm union of the fracture, and CT is obtained if there is any doubt. This is more of a concern when treating osteoarthritis of the hip in the setting of a prior acetabular fracture, which requires stable anterior and posterior columns for acetabular component impaction. The AP pelvis radiograph with a calibrated marker ball and internal rotation of the lower limbs is used to assess the caput-collum-diaphyseal angle, limb length difference, and femoral offset. Templating software is used to estimate the optimal femoral and acetabular component type, size, and placement that will best restore native hip biomechanics. Acetabular bone defects may be better assessed with CT if augmentation with bone grafting or trabecular metal is thought to be needed. Contained or uncontained acetabular defects are assessed for in these scenarios. Contained cavitary acetabular defects may be treated with impaction bone grafting while uncontained rim defects may require trabecular metal augmentation [16]. Posterior acetabular defects that cannot be accessed via the AA for augmentation may be better managed through a posterior approach.

Heterotopic ossification is common after acetabular fracture surgery, especially when a posterior approach is used [17], but mostly involves the hip abductor musculature and does not interfere with AA THA. Heterotopic ossification anterior to the hip should be looked for, however, on the iliac oblique pelvis radiograph, and better evaluated with CT if excision is needed to access the anterior hip. If clinically significant HO is present in the abductors and/or external rotators, a posterior approach should be considered to allow for simultaneous excision.

Anterior approach THA may be safely performed in the setting of a prior Kocher-Langenbeck, Gibson, or ilioinguinal incisions.

Positioning

We prefer to position the patient supine on a Hana Orthopaedic Table (Mizuho OSI, Union City, CA).

Approach

The AA to the hip is performed as described by Matta et al. [18] In the presence of a prior ilioinguinal approach, the incision is started just caudal to scar leaving a 1–2 cm skin bridge. The same caudal extent of a prior iliofemoral incision can be used if present. If enhanced exposure is needed, the proximal skin incision is extended and a portion of the tensor fascia lata is released off of the anterior ilium [19].

Technical Considerations

Prior Femoral Neck Fracture

Femoral neck fractures fixed with a sliding hip screw or multiple cannulated screws present similar challenges during preparation of the femur. Internal fixation should be removed prior to AA to the hip through the same lateral incisions that they were placed through. A threaded guide pin can be used to localize and aid in the removal of cannulated screws. After the implants are removed and a capsulotomy has been performed, the femoral neck osteotomy is performed in situ or freshened in the setting of nonunion. The femoral head is then retrieved from the acetabulum. Preparation and impaction of the acetabular component then proceed in typical fashion.

The femoral hook is placed around the lateral aspect of the femur below the vastus ridge. The extremity is externally rotated, extended, and adducted. The femoral hook is attached to the femoral lift on the orthopedic table (Mizuho OSI, Union City, CA), and the proximal femur is elevated out of the wound. Adequate release of the lateral capsule is performed. Challenges may present during broaching of the femoral canal if sclerotic bone has formed around screws traversing the femoral neck. We prefer to enter the canal in these situations using a high-speed burr to remove the sclerotic bone. Once enough sclerotic bone has been removed, the femoral canal can be serially broached with a metaphyseal press fit obtained using a standard femoral stem. Care should be taken to restore offset and limb length in the setting of femoral neck collapse with medialization of the femoral shaft (Fig. 18.1). After the femoral trial component has been placed and the hip is reduced, we obtain a posteroanterior fluoroscopic image of the entire pelvis to measure the limb length and offset of both hips to ensure that correction has been achieved. Prophylactic cabling below prior screw holes is not needed as the femoral stem will typically bypass these areas.

Prior Intertrochanteric Femur Fracture

Intertrochanteric femur fractures frequently collapse during the healing process and result in loss of offset and limb shortening. These factors need to be corrected to restore the biomechanics of the hip and obtain stability.

Our approach is to first remove the internal fixation device using the prior incisions. Bony overgrowth of the implant may require the use of curettes, osteotomes, or a high-speed burr to facilitate removal. The AA to the hip is performed and the femoral neck is osteotomized in situ. After the acetabular component has been impacted, the proximal femur is gently lifted out of the wound with the femoral hook, and soft-

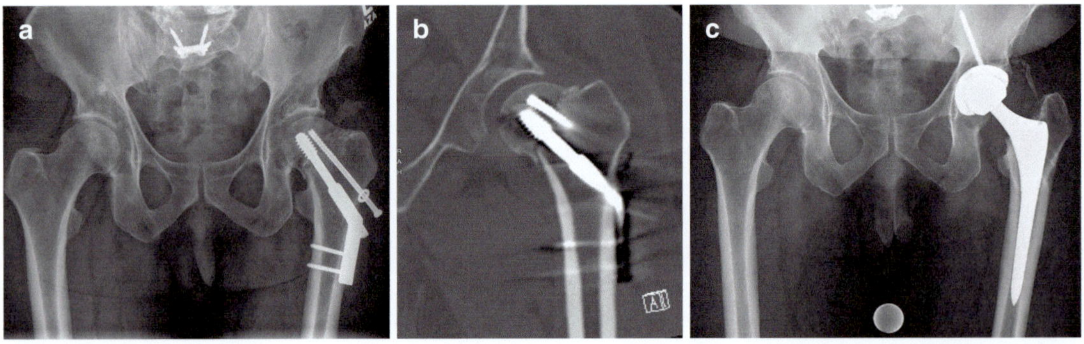

Fig. 18.1 (**a**) Radiograph of a 53-year-old man who presented with persisting left hip pain and dysfunction 10 months following internal fixation of a femoral neck fracture. The fracture had collapsed significantly with loss of femoral offset and limb shortening. (**b**) Computed tomography better demonstrating nonunion of the fracture. The patient was treated with press-fit conversion total hip arthroplasty performed through an anterior approach. (**c**) Radiograph at 1 year post-conversion showing restoration of limb length, femoral offset, and stable positioning of the acetabular and femoral components

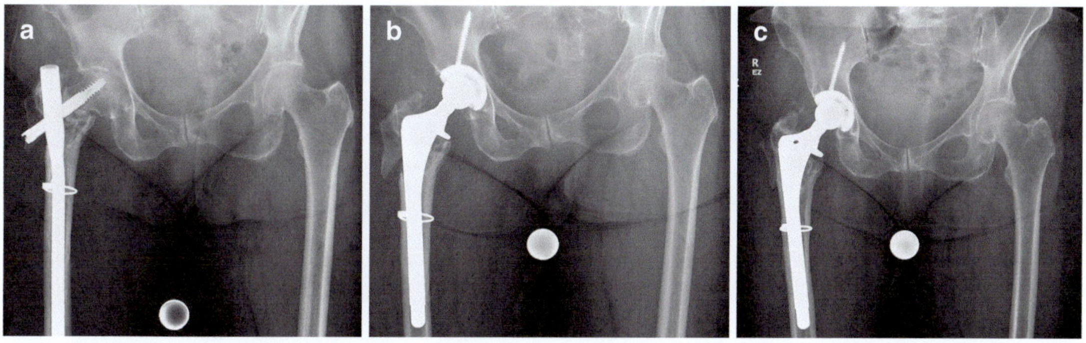

Fig. 18.2 (**a**) Radiograph of an 84-year-old woman with nonunion of a right pertrochanteric femur fracture. This patient had preexisting symptomatic osteoarthritis affecting the same hip. Conversion total hip arthroplasty was performed though the anterior approach. The femoral canal was prepared distally with flexible reamers, and a fully porous-coated revision stem was used to obtain distal fit. The greater trochanter was relatively stable due to the counter pull of the hip abductor insertion and vastus lateralis origin, and not addressed with internal fixation. (**b**) Immediate postoperative radiograph showing the reconstruction with residual displacement of the greater trochanter. (**c**) Radiograph at 2 years post-conversion showing stable position of the acetabular and femoral components. Interestingly, the greater trochanteric fracture went onto union. This patient regained excellent function of her hip with minimal pain

tissue releases are made off of the greater trochanter in typical fashion to achieve the desired access. The use of excessive force should be avoiding during this step to prevent fracture of a deficient greater trochanter.

Fractures that were treated with a cephalomedullary nail (CMN) will frequently have sclerosis of the proximal femoral canal and can be difficult to broach. We remove any remaining lateral femoral neck with a box osteotome and rongeur, and then carefully remove the sclerotic bone around the canal with a high-speed burr to dilate the proximal femur in a rectangular fashion. Care is taken not to perforate the femoral cortex. Broaching of the femur can then proceed. If the distal femoral metaphyseal canal is sclerotic and impedes insertion of the broach, the sclerotic bone should be reamed by hand until a broach can be inserted safely to the desired depth. Alternatively, cannulated flexible reaming of the femoral canal can be performed over a ball-tipped guidewire. Occasionally, the femoral canal at the distal tip of the CMN will be obliterated. We prefer to open the distal canal using a large diameter drill bit under the guidance of biplanar fluoroscopy to ensure that the trajectory of the drill is correct and will not result in cortical perforation. Our preference is to use a metaphyseal press-fit femoral stem if proximal fixation can be obtained.

If metaphyseal fit of the femoral stem cannot be obtained, consideration should be given toward using a cemented stem, a long fully porous-coated press-fit stem, or a diaphyseal engaging press-fit revision stem. This is especially needed when treating an IT nonunion with conversion THA (Fig. 18.2). If a cemented stem is selected, difficulties may be encountered during cement pressurization if the holes from removed internal fixation are not occluded.

Prior Acetabular Fracture

The type and location (i.e., posterior column, posterior wall, supra-pectineal, infra-pectineal) of internal fixation should be assessed for potential interference during preparation of the acetabulum. Internal fixation of the acetabular columns should otherwise be retained. The proximity of posterior column and/or wall internal fixation to the acetabular subchondral bone should be carefully evaluated on radiographs or CT to ensure that the acetabulum can be reamed without interference from existing plates and screws (Figs. 18.3 and 18.4). If a screw is encountered during reaming of the acetabulum, the offending portion may be removed with a metal cutting burr.

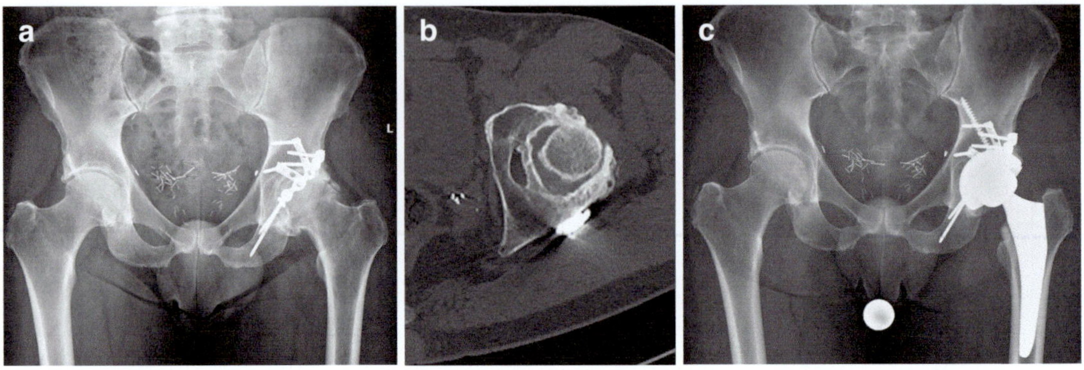

Fig. 18.3 (**a**) Radiograph of a 64-year-old man with post-traumatic osteoarthritis of the left hip in the setting of a previous posterior wall acetabular fracture dislocation that was treated with open reduction and internal fixation 15 years prior. (**b**) Computed tomography was obtained preoperatively to ensure that the posterior plates and screws would not interfere with acetabular preparation and component impaction. The patient was treated with conversion total hip arthroplasty through an anterior approach with retention of the non-obstructing posterior internal fixation. (**c**) Radiograph at 6 months post-conversion showing stable positioning of the acetabular and femoral components

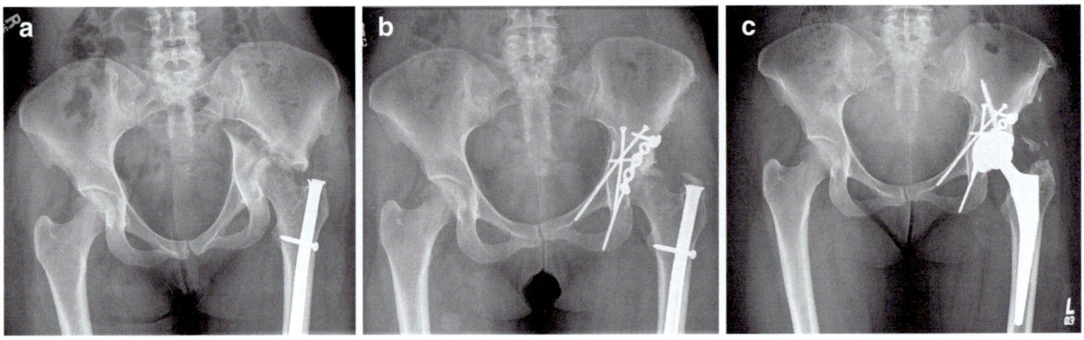

Fig. 18.4 (**a**) Radiograph of a 34-year-old woman who presented with a trans-tectal transverse acetabular fracture malunion that was initially treated nonoperatively. Successful open reduction and internal fixation were performed through an extended iliofemoral approach. However, the patient developed post-traumatic osteoarthritis of the hip, as shown in the (**b**) radiograph, and was converted to a press-fit total hip arthroplasty using the anterior approach. The prior acetabular internal fixation did not obstruct acetabular preparation or component impaction and was left in place. (**c**) Radiograph at 2 years post-conversion showing stable positioning of the acetabular and femoral components

However, if a plate has become intra-articular from bony erosion, a posterior approach to facilitate removal of the plate is our preferred strategy. Supra-pectineal and infra-pectineal plates seldom obstruct preparation of the acetabulum and should be left in place, provided that the screws were not errantly placed within the joint.

Cavitary defects on the acetabular side from articular impaction can be treated with impaction bone grafting from the resected femoral head and acetabular component implantation using standard press-fit techniques. Rim defects, on the other hand, from necrosis or erosion of the posterior wall, may require further medialization of the acetabulum to increase posterior and superior coverage of the acetabular component. Consideration should be given to using a high-offset femoral stem in these scenarios to optimize soft-tissue tensioning and restore stability. Alternatively, trabecular metal augments may be used to provide peripheral support of the implant.

The acetabular component is sized for optimal fit while preserving existing bone stock. Fluoroscopic imaging facilitates placement of the component with the correct version and inclination. We use standard liners and do not use dual mobility components routinely. Our preference is to use a ceramic head with a polyethylene liner.

A single intraosseous 6.5 mm × 50 mm cancellous screw is typically inserted through the acetabular component and directed into the sciatic buttress to obtain immediate stability while bony ingrowth occurs.

Closure

We repair the anterior capsule with a heavy running suture to obtain as much stability as possible, especially since the hip may be lax in comparison with patients with primary osteoarthritis. This is especially true when treating patients with femoral neck nonunion and less so when treating post-traumatic arthritis in the setting of prior acetabular fracture. The tensor fascia is repaired followed by routine closure of the dermis and skin.

Postoperative Care

The patient is made weight-bearing as tolerated with anterior hip precautions, and physical therapy is started the day of surgery. All other aspects of postoperative care, including venous thromboembolism prophylaxis, are routine. Heterotopic ossification prophylaxis is not used.

Complications

Complication rates are generally higher after conversion THA in comparison with primary THA. This has been shown by several authors with regard to infection, dislocation, HO, intraoperative fracture, subsidence, and aseptic loosening [20–25]. However, these complications have not been specifically studied after using the AA for conversion THA.

Outcomes

Conversion THA after acetabular fracture has a historically lower 10-year survivorship compared with primary THA at 70% versus 90%, respectively [25]. Similarly, the survivorship for conversion THA after failed femoral neck internal fixation is less than that of primary THA for treatment of femoral neck fractures [26]. These demanding procedures better resemble the complexities seen with revision THA compared with primary THA [27].

References

1. Cichos KH, Mabry SE, Spitler CA, McGwin G, Quade JH, Ghanem ES. A comparison between the direct anterior and posterior approaches for total hip arthroplasty performed for femoral neck fracture. J Orthop Trauma. 2021;35(1):41–8.
2. Dimitriou D, Helmy N, Hasler J, Flury A, Finsterwald M, Antoniadis A. The role of total hip arthroplasty through the direct anterior approach in femoral neck fracture and factors affecting the outcome. J Arthroplast. 2019;34(1):82–7.
3. Haller J, Working Z, Gililland J, Rothberg D, Kubiak E. Fewer complications performing total hip arthroplasty through a direct anterior approach for femoral neck fracture. Orthopaedic Trauma Association Annual Meeting; 2015. p. 379–80.
4. FAITH Investigators. Fracture fixation in the operative management of hip fractures (FAITH): an international, multicentre, randomised controlled trial. Lancet. 2017;389(10078):1519–27.
5. Medda S, Jinnah AH, Marquez-Lara A, Araiza ET, Hasty EK, Halvorson JJ, et al. Valgus intertrochanteric osteotomy for femoral neck nonunion. J Orthop Trauma. 2019;33(Suppl 1):S26–S7.
6. Mabry TM, Prpa B, Haidukewych GJ, Harmsen WS, Berry DJ. Long-term results of total hip arthroplasty for femoral neck fracture nonunion. J Bone Joint Surg Am. 2004;86(10):2263–7.
7. Frei HC, Hotz T, Cadosch D, Rudin M, Käch K. Central head perforation, or "cut through," caused by the helical blade of the proximal femoral nail antirotation. J Orthop Trauma. 2012;26(8):e102–7.
8. Hou Z, Bowen TR, Irgit KS, Matzko ME, Andreychik CM, Horwitz DS, et al. Treatment of pertrochanteric fractures (OTA 31-A1 and A2): long versus short cephalomedullary nailing. J Orthop Trauma. 2013;27(6):318–24.
9. Fang C, Gudushauri P, Wong TM, Lau TW, Pun T, Leung F. Increased fracture collapse after intertro-

chanteric fractures treated by the dynamic hip screw adversely affects walking ability but not survival. Biomed Res Int. 2016;2016:4175092.
10. Bartonícek J, Skála-Rosenbaum J, Dousa P. Valgus intertrochanteric osteotomy for malunion and nonunion of trochanteric fractures. J Orthop Trauma. 2003;17(9):606–12.
11. Tannast M, Najibi S, Matta JM. Two to twenty-year survivorship of the hip in 810 patients with operatively treated acetabular fractures. J Bone Joint Surg Am. 2012;94(17):1559–67.
12. Letournel E, Judet R. Fractures of the acetabulum. 2nd ed. Berlin: Springer; 1993.
13. Koerner M, Westberg J, Martin J, Templeman D. Patient reported outcomes of femoral head fractures with minimum 10-year follow-up. J Orthop Trauma. 2020;34(12):621–5.
14. Chambers AW, Lacy KW, Liow MHL, Manalo JPM, Freiberg AA, Kwon YM. Multiple hip intra-articular steroid injections increase risk of periprosthetic joint infection compared with single injections. J Arthroplast. 2017;32(6):1980–3.
15. Quinn RH, Murray J, Pezold R, Hall Q. Management of osteoarthritis of the hip. J Am Acad Orthop Surg. 2018;26(20):e434–e6.
16. Sheth NP, Nelson CL, Springer BD, Fehring TK, Paprosky WG. Acetabular bone loss in revision total hip arthroplasty: evaluation and management. J Am Acad Orthop Surg. 2013;21(3):128–39.
17. Giannoudis PV, Grotz MR, Papakostidis C, Dinopoulos H. Operative treatment of displaced fractures of the acetabulum. A meta-analysis. J Bone Joint Surg Br. 2005;87(1):2–9.
18. Matta JM, Shahrdar C, Ferguson T. Single-incision anterior approach for total hip arthroplasty on an orthopaedic table. Clin Orthop Relat Res. 2005;441:115–24.
19. Mast NH, Laude F. Revision total hip arthroplasty performed through the Hueter interval. J Bone Joint Surg Am. 2011;93(Suppl 2):143–8.
20. DeHaan AM, Groat T, Priddy M, Ellis TJ, Duwelius PJ, Friess DM, et al. Salvage hip arthroplasty after failed fixation of proximal femur fractures. J Arthroplast. 2013;28(5):855–9.
21. Zhang B, Chiu KY, Wang M. Hip arthroplasty for failed internal fixation of intertrochanteric fractures. J Arthroplast. 2004;19(3):329–33.
22. Ranawat A, Zelken J, Helfet D, Buly R. Total hip arthroplasty for posttraumatic arthritis after acetabular fracture. J Arthroplast. 2009;24(5):759–67.
23. Chen YT, Chen WM, Lee KS, Huang CK, Chiang CC, Chen TH. Diaphyseal locking hip arthroplasty for treatment of failed fixation of intertrochanteric hip fractures. J Arthroplast. 2008;23(2):241–6.
24. Winemaker M, Gamble P, Petruccelli D, Kaspar S, de Beer J. Short-term outcomes of total hip arthroplasty after complications of open reduction internal fixation for hip fracture. J Arthroplast. 2006;21(5):682–8.
25. Morison Z, Moojen DJ, Nauth A, Hall J, McKee MD, Waddell JP, et al. Total hip arthroplasty after acetabular fracture is associated with lower survivorship and more complications. Clin Orthop Relat Res. 2016;474(2):392–8.
26. McKinley JC, Robinson CM. Treatment of displaced intracapsular hip fractures with total hip arthroplasty: comparison of primary arthroplasty with early salvage arthroplasty after failed internal fixation. J Bone Joint Surg Am. 2002;84(11):2010–5.
27. Baghoolizadeh M, Schwarzkopf R. The Lawrence D. Dorr Surgical Techniques & Technologies Award: conversion total hip arthroplasty: is it a primary or revision hip arthroplasty. J Arthroplast. 2016;31(9 Suppl):16–21.

Part III

Introduction to Part III

If today we had the opportunity to design and implant the first prosthetic hip joint, would it be logical to make it a goal to duplicate normal hip biomechanics? The obvious answer is yes. From the beginning of modern THA, however, the standard methodology has often purposely changed hip biomechanics. Charnley sought to medialize the center of rotation in order to decrease joint reactive forces and wear. With posterior approach, the instruction has often been to increase the femoral offset in order to possibly add resistance to dislocation through tensioning the soft tissues as well as reducing the chance of extra-articular impingement.

Anterior approach along with improved prosthetic design is allowing us to go back to the most logical goal: restoration of normal, pre arthritic hip biomechanics specific to the individual patient. Other new technologies are also facilitating this goal.

19 Normal Hip Biomechanics

Anna Jungwirth-Weinberger
and Friedrich Boettner

Bony Anatomy

The hip is a ball in socket joint with three axes of movement constrained by the presence of the femoral neck and the contour of the acetabular socket. The hip joint is often described as a multi-axial ball-and-socket joint [1].

The acetabulum is formed by the innominate bone from the ilium, which makes up about 40%, the ischium (40%), and the pubis (20%) [2]. They are formed mainly of spongy trabecular bone [3]. Inherent stability is achieved by the hip's osseous anatomy due to the depth of the acetabular socket [4]. Additional stability is provided by the labrum and the joint capsule with its main parts such as the iliofemoral, ischiofemoral, and pubofemoral ligaments.

The surfaces of the femoral head and the acetabulum are covered by layers of hyaline cartilage, which handle the forces acting on the joint [5]. There is a central hole, which is not covered by cartilage at the femoral head, the fovea centralis.

The head of the femur is attached to the femoral shaft by the femoral neck. The length of the femoral neck depends on the size of the body but is around 5 cm long in the adult hip [6]. In the normal adult anatomy, the neck–shaft angle (CCD angle) is 125 ± 5° [7]. Normal anteversion of the acetabulum accommodates flexion of the hip and reduces impingement with high flexion [8]. Normal values of acetabular anteversion range between 15° and 20° [9]. Another important factor impacting on impingement besides acetabular anteversion is the degree of coverage of the femoral head. This can be measured on X-rays as the central edge angle of Wiberg. This angle is formed by a vertical line from the center of the femoral head and a line from the center of the femoral head to the lateral rim of the acetabulum. The normal center edge angle is 25–35° [10]. An increased center edge angle increases the risk of PINCER impingement in a native hip.

The physiologic femoral anteversion, which is defined as the angle by which the femoral neck deviates forwards from the axis of the femoral condyles, is approximately 15° [11]. Reduced or excessively increased anteversion has both contributed to impingement (Fig. 19.1).

A. Jungwirth-Weinberger
Hospital for Special Surgery, New York, NY, USA

Kantonsspital Baden AG, Baden, Switzerland
e-mail: jungwirthweinbergera@hss.edu

F. Boettner (✉)
Hospital for Special Surgery, New York, NY, USA
e-mail: boettnerf@hss.edu

J. M. Matta, A. P. Sah (eds.), *Anterior Hip Replacement*,
https://doi.org/10.1007/978-3-030-91896-5_19

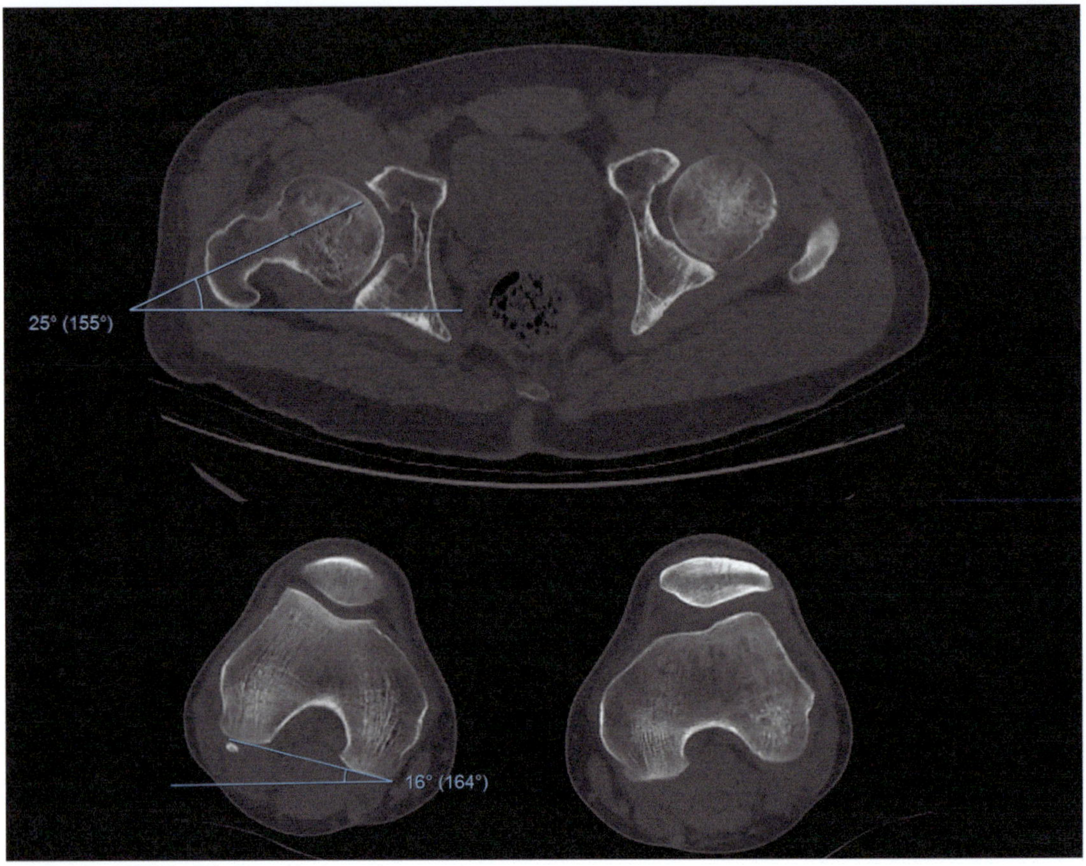

Fig. 19.1 Femoral anteversion of 41° (25° + 16°) as measured on an anteversion CT scan

Ligament and Capsule

The hip joint is surrounded by a strong ligamentous capsule. It is attached outside the labrum along the periphery of the acetabulum. A study by Tsutsumi et al. reports a distinct impression inferior to the anterior inferior iliac spine which provides an attachment site for the hip joint capsule [12]. Distally, it inserts along the intertrochanteric line and inside the greater trochanter; posteriorly, it incompletely covers the femoral neck [13, 14].

The capsule is a main contributor to stability of the hip and restrains the movement of the femoral head in the acetabulum in addition to preventing dislocation [7, 12, 15].

The hip joint is surrounded by complex ligamentous structures, which consist of ischiofemoral, iliofemoral (also known as the Y-ligament of Bigelow), and pubofemoral ligaments. They are passive structures and act by restricting movement [15].

Extension of the hip is restricted by the iliofemoral ligament. The ischiofemoral ligament has its origin at the ischial rim of the acetabulum and inserts on the posterior aspect of the femoral neck. Because of its posterior insertion, it primarily restricts internal rotation, but also restricts adduction of the flexed hip [16]. The femoral arcuate ligament is located posteriorly in the deep capsular layer. It originates at the greater trochanter, runs under the ischiofemoral ligament around the posterior femoral neck, and inserts at the lesser trochanter. It tightens the capsule at extreme positions of flexion and extension [17] (Fig. 19.2).

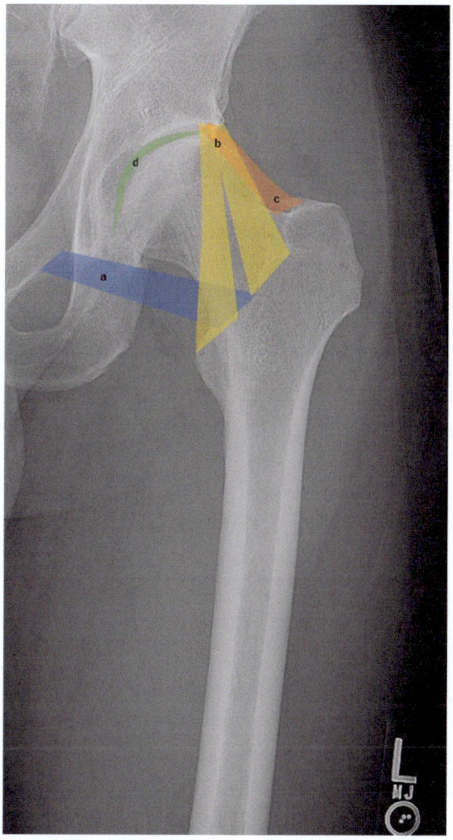

Fig. 19.2 Capsular ligaments contributing to joint stability (a = Lig. pubofemorale, b = Lig. iliofemoral, c = Lig. ischiofemorale, d = Labrum). Also contributing but not seen here: Lig. Teres)

The ligamentum teres, which lies in the fovea centralis, contains blood supply for the femoral head. It is assumed that the ligamentum teres plays an important role in the neonatal hip as a stabilizing structure and for blood supply of the femoral head [18]. According to Byrne et al., it does not contribute to the stability of the adult hip [7]. Newer studies, however, discuss a contribution to hip stability by the ligamentum teres, as it supports the femoral head inferiorly during combined flexion and abduction of the hip [19].

Acetabular Labrum

The labrum is a circular fibrocartilaginous structure that is connected by the anterior and posterior aspects of the transverse acetabular ligament and is attached to the rim of the acetabulum. At the periphery of the acetabular cartilage, it blends into the hyaline cartilage [7, 20]. The labrum plays an important role in distributing contact forces during activity [1].

The labrum increases the acetabular surface and depth of the acetabular socket [21].

It contributes to stability of the hip by increasing the containment of the joint and by the so-called suction effect. The labrum obstructs fluid flow in and out of the joint by creating a suction seal and resisting distraction of the femoral head from the acetabular socket [22] through creating a negative pressure within the joint [23].

A study by Safran et al. used a cadaveric model to analyze the relative movement of the femoral head in relation to the acetabulum, when all the soft tissue constraints are intact. Loss of the acetabular labrum results in increased translation of the femoral head and possibly can lead to instability and osteoarthritis [24].

Except for the anterosuperior region, where the collagen of the labrum runs parallel, the collagen at the junction between the articular cartilage and the labrum is oriented perpendicular. The anterosuperior region of the junction between cartilage and labrum with its parallel orientation of collagen represents a weak link due to a decrease in strength of the labral attachment [25].

Periarticular Muscles

The geometry of the hip requires muscles to augment stability and facilitate movement. 22 muscles act on the hip and provide stability and movement [7]. The muscles of the hip and the thigh lie within a continuous fibrous layer, the fascia lata. The fascia lata is attached proximally to the iliac crest, the posterior sacrum, the inguinal ligament, the iliac crest, the ischial tuberosity, and the pubis. It improves the efficiency of the muscular contractions through its inelasticity [26].

The most important hip flexor muscle is the iliopsoas. The iliopsoas muscle consists of three parts, the psoas major, psoas minor, and iliacus. Additional hip flexors are the sartorius, tensor fascia latae, and the rectus femoris. The psoas has its origin from the T12-L5 vertebral bodies and inserts onto the lesser trochanter. The sartorius origins from the anterior superior iliac spine and inserts at the pes anserinus at the medial aspect of the knee. It aids in abduction and external rotation. The straight head of the rectus femoris arises from the anterior superior iliac spine, the reflected head from the acetabulum. Together with the vastus lateralis, vastus intermedius, and vastus medialis, the rectus femoris forms the quadriceps femoris and the quadriceps tendon and insert through the patellar tendon onto the tibial tuberosity.

The most powerful extensor of the hip joint is the gluteus maximus. It runs from the surface of the sacrum, the posterior ilium, and the thoracolumbar fascia to the iliotibial tract. The deep fibers insert at the gluteal tuberosity of the femur. The gluteus maximus also helps with external rotation of the hip joint and stabilizes the femur by attaching it to the tensor fascia latae.

Abductors of the hip joint are the gluteus medius and the gluteus minimus. Both lie beneath the fascia lata. The gluteus medius has its origin at the gluteal surface of the ilium and inserts on the lateral aspect of the greater trochanter. The gluteus minimus origins under the gluteus medius on the ilium and inserts deep to the gluteus medius at the anterolateral greater trochanter.

The tensor fasciae latae arises from the anterior superior iliac spine and the iliac crest. It merges with the gluteus maximus and the fascia lata and forms the iliotibial tract. The tensor fasciae latae flexes and internally rotates the hip.

The piriformis runs from the sacrum to the greater trochanter and is an external rotator of the hip. Other external rotators are the superior gemelli, obturator externus, inferior gemelli, and quadratus femoris. They run horizontally from the ischiopubic ramus, obturator membrane, and ischial tuberosity, respectively, to the medial aspect of the greater trochanter.

Adductors of the hip include the obturator externus, pectineus, adductor longus, adductor brevis, adductor magnus, adductor minimus, and gracilis. The obturator externus has its origin on the obturator membrane and obturator foramen; it inserts into the trochanteric fossa of the femur. It also facilitates with external rotation of the hip.

The pectineus arises from the pectineal line of the pubis and runs to the pectineal line of the femur. Besides adduction, it contributes to external rotation and flexion of the hip. The adductor longus runs from the pubis and ischial tuberosity to the middle third of the linea aspera and the adductor tubercle of the femur. The adductor longus additionally helps with flexion of the hip. The adductor brevis arises from the inferior pubic ramus and inserts on the linea aspera proximal to the adductor longus and the lesser trochanter. The adductor magnus originates from the inferior pubic rami and the ischial tuberosity and runs to the linea aspera and adductor tubercle of the femur. It contributes also to external rotation and extension of the hip. The adductor minimus originates from the inferior ramus of the pubis and also inserts at the linea aspera. It helps with external rotation besides adduction of the hip.

The gracilis arises inferior from the ischiopubic ramus and inserts distal to the knee in the pes anserinus.

The muscles of the hip contribute to range of motion depending on the position of the hip, which is caused by a change of the hip's axis of rotation and the muscle's line of action [7] (Table 19.1).

Additionally, the muscles of the hip provide stability and help reduce bending stresses on the femur. When load is applied vertically to the femur, tensile and compression forces act on the medial and lateral side of the bone. The tensor fasciae latae, for example, then reacts as lateral tensioning band and reduces stress on the bone [7] (Fig. 19.3).

Movement

Because of its ball-and-socket nature, the hip provides excellent range of motion and stability. All motion between femoral head and acetabulum is rotational because of the congruency of

Table 19.1 Different muscle groups of the hip joint

Muscle group	Primary function	Secondary function
Flexors	M. iliopsoas M. sartorius M. tensor fasciae latae M. rectus femoris M. adductor longus M. pectineus	M. adductor brevis M. gracilis M. gluteus minimus (anterior fibers)
Extensors	M. gluteus maximus M. adductor magnus (posterior head) M. biceps femoris (long head) M. semitendinosus M. semimembranosus	M. gluteus medius (middle and posterior fibers) M. adductor magnus (anterior head)
External rotators	M. gluteus maximus M. piriformis M. obturator internus M. gemellus superior M. gemellus inferior M. quadratus femoris	M. gluteus medius (posterior fibers) M. gluteus minimus (posterior fibers) M. obturator externus M. sartorius M. biceps femoris (long head)
Internal rotators	N/A	M. gluteus minimus (anterior fibers) M. gluteus medius (anterior fibers) M. tensor fasciae latae M. adductor longus M. adductor brevis M. pectineus M. adductor magnus (posterior head)
Adductors	M. pectineus M. adductor longus M. gracilis M. adductor brevis M. adductor magnus (anterior and posterior heads)	M. biceps femoris (long head) M. gluteus maximus (posterior fibers) M. quadratus femoris M. obturator externus
Abductors	M. gluteus medius (all fibers) M. gluteus minimus (all fibers) M. tensor fasciae latae	M. piriformis M. Sartorius M. rectus femoris

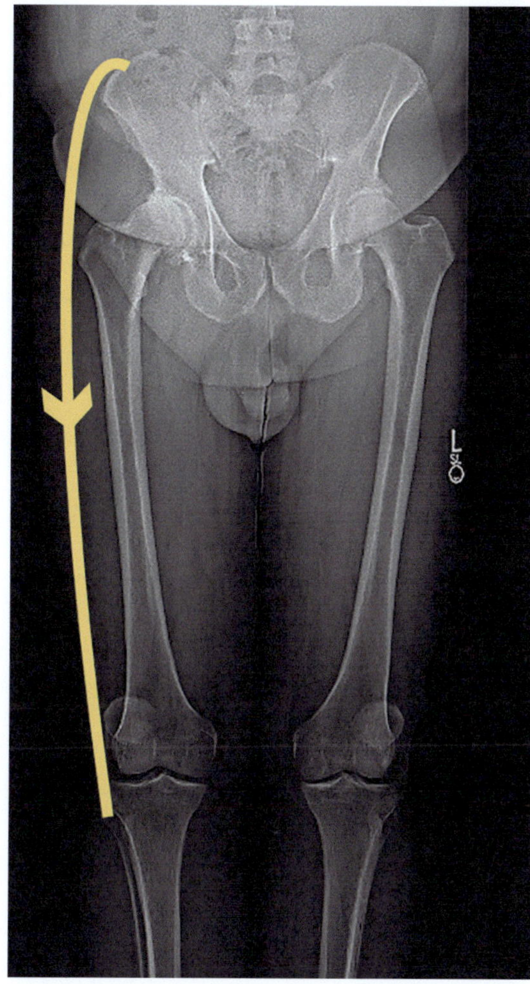

Fig. 19.3 The compression band effect of the Iliotibial band

the two articulating surfaces [4]. The depth of the acetabulum limits the range of motion due to bony impingement of the femoral neck onto the rim of the acetabulum [1].

Overall limitations of the range of motion not only result from bony impingement, but also from the capsuloligamentous and musculotendinous structures [27].

In the sagittal plane, a normal hip can reach a flexion of approximately 125 degrees (°) and an extension of 15°. In the frontal plane, it accommodates abduction of 50° and adduction of 30°. Internal and external rotations of the flexed hip range from 0° to 70° and from 0° to 90,° respectively [14] (Fig. 19.4).

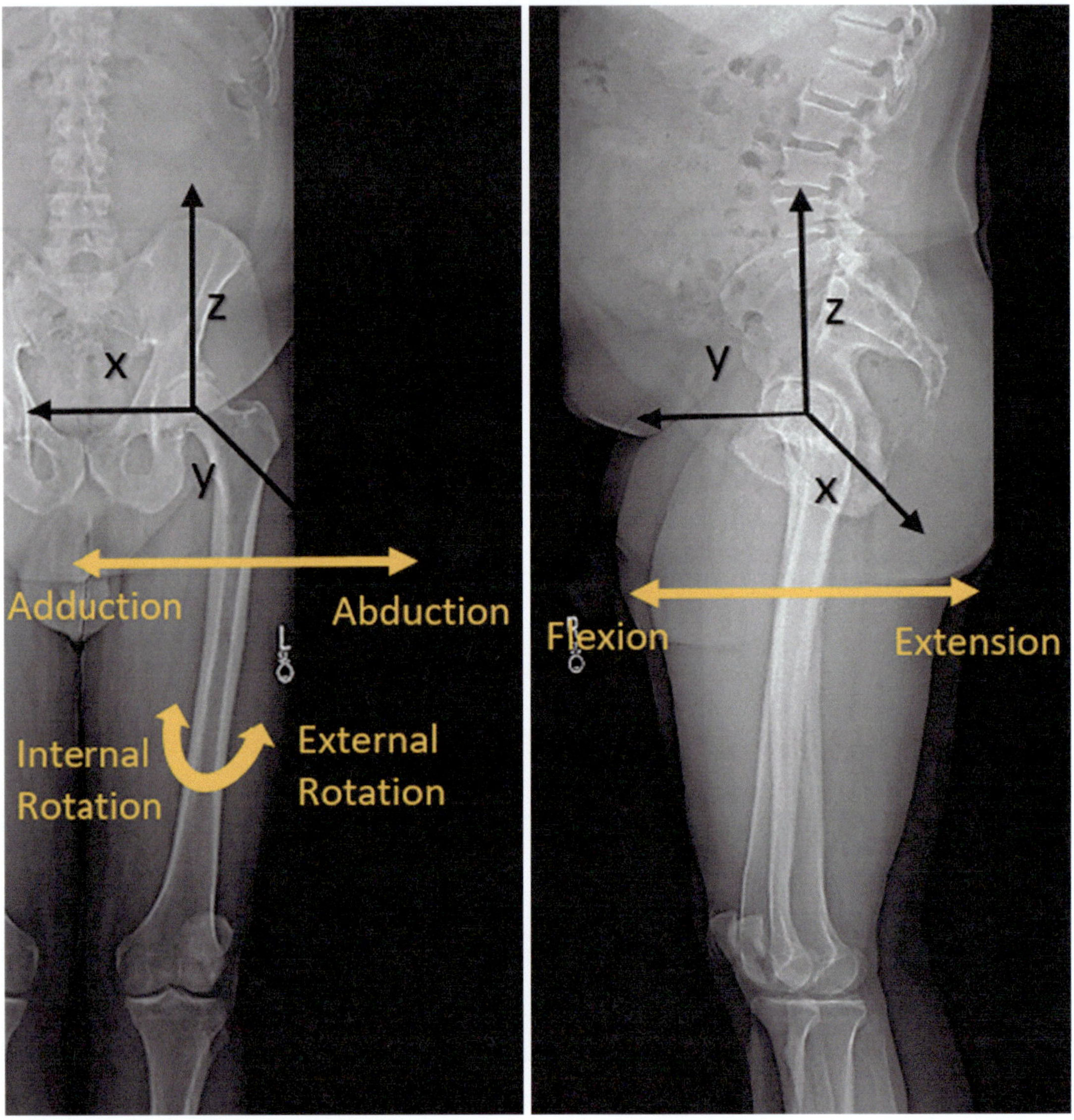

Fig. 19.4 Range of motion in the hip joint in three planes

Biomechanics

The geometry of the hip joint has an influence on the forces acting on the hip joint [28].

A residual compressive force always acts across the joint at all times, with an average magnitude approximately equal to the person's body weight [1].

Static loading of the hip joint has often been described by a two-dimensional analysis in the frontal plane [7, 15]. This model was first invented by Koch in 1917 [29] and refers to forces acting on the hip during single leg stance. The underlying principle of static analysis is that of equilibrium. A body at rest is said to be in equilibrium if the sum of all loads (i.e., forces and moments) is zero [30].

Koch assumed that the center of gravity of the body is located midline, 1 cm anterior to the first sacral vertebra body. From this point, the effect of gravity on the lower extremity was represented by a vertically oriented vector (W).

During weight bearing of the leg, the center of gravity moves distally and away from the supporting leg. The contralateral, non-supporting leg is added to the weight acting on the hip. This downward force results in a rotation through the center of the femoral head (fulcrum). Resisting forces include the abductors, who perform an isometric contraction and act with a lever arm on the femoral head [7, 29, 31, 32].

The moment arm length produced by gravity is approximately three times longer than that of the abductor muscles lever arm (A). This creates an advantage for the gravity force. To remain static, the hip joint creates a joint reaction force (F) that is equal and opposite to the sum of the forces of body weight and abductors. By reducing the lengths of the moment arms, hip joint forces may be decreased [33].

Three-dimensional models improved the concept of Koch. There are in reality three forces acting on the femur: one acting distally, one acting posteriorly, and the other acting laterally. The total joint reaction force is the resultant of those three forces acting on the hip [28, 34].

Gait and Standing

The hip is main connection of the lower extremity to the body during gait. The natural gait consists of the stance and the swing phase. The stance phase is defined as phase, during which the foot is on the ground, beginning with the initial contact of the heel until toe-off. The swing phase is defined as the period, during which the foot is off the ground and moving forward [14]. Perry divided the stance phase in 5 further phases: initial contact, loading response, midstance, terminal stance, and preswing [35].

The cycle begins with a heel strike and ends, when the same heel again contacts the ground. During gait cycle, a maximal extension of the hip occurs at heel-off and a maximal flexion during the late swing phase. During the stance phase of gait, the hip adducts and internally rotates, bringing the center of gravity closer to the hip joint. During the swing phase, the hip abducts and externally rotates. The presence of the double-support phase defines the activity of walking. In contrast, running is not characterized by a double-support phase but displays a float phase instead, when both feet are off the ground at the same time. As the speed of running increases, the duration of the float phase increases [15, 27].

Clinical Implications of Hip Anatomy

Loading of the proximal femur in total hip arthroplasty (THA) is influenced by the length and shape of the stem. In a study by Decking et al., the strains of three different stems were measured in vitro. A conventional straight stem, an anatomic stem, and a stemless prosthesis were compared. The straight and the anatomic stem led to a decrease in the longitudinal strains in the proximal femur; the stemless prosthesis resulted in an increase in strains lateral to the greater trochanter. The medial strains in this case were closer to physiological values than in the conventional and the anatomical stem [36].

In THA, decreasing joint reaction forces can be achieved by shifting the center of rotation medially. Moment arm for abduction and adduction of the abductor muscles (primarily middle fiber of the gluteus medius) increases by 10–85% with cup medialization. For flexion and extension, the effect is not always positive. Cup medialization has a greater impact on increasing the abductor moment arm in patients with less femoral antetorsion [37]. Femoral offset is defined as the distance from the center of rotation of the femoral head to a line dissecting the anatomic femoral axis. An increase in femoral offset occurs when the stem is placed in varus or offset is increased by using a high offset implant; a decrease occurs when the stem is placed in valgus or reduced offset stem is selected for the femoral component [38]. A loss of offset in total hip arthroplasty leads to a decrease in the abductor moment arm [39] and a loss of function, while an increase in femoral offset did not have an impact on postoperative outcome scores [38]. Increased offset, however, can result in increased tension on the IT band and can result in trochanteric bursitis, especially in female patients. Average and maximum abduction moment arms and forces of gluteus medius and gluteus minimus were significantly higher for increased femoral offset compared to anatomical femoral offset and decreased femoral offset. Hip joint forces were higher in decreased femoral offset compared to anatomical offset [40].

Hip contact forces change during different activities. The peak force when going downstairs exceeds the peak force when going upstairs. Walking results in higher loads than standing up from a chair and even higher loads compared to sitting down [41].

Leg length discrepancy is a common complication after THA and can lead to back problems, instability, limping, and pain [42]. In addition, patients with leg length discrepancy are reported to have a lower gait velocity, decreased hip range of motion, reduced stride length, reduced hip moment, and less dynamic hip force [43]. Lengthening of the operated leg is more frequent than shortening [42].

When increasing leg length, postoperative tensioning of the gluteus medius and minimus muscles can occur and an increase in aseptic component loosening has been reported [44, 45].

Shortening of the limb leads to significantly increased hip pain, limping, and patient satisfaction [46] and is associated with lax soft tissues, which may increase the risk for dislocation [47].

Brand and Yack [48] reported in their study that ground reaction forces are increased with increasing leg length. Shortening of the limp leads to a length tension disadvantage and a decrease in abductor strength [49].

The position of femoral and acetabular components in THA has an influence on mechanics of the hip joint and range of motion. Poor positioning can lead to impingement, wear, and dislocation [50, 51]. Femoral antetorsion plays a role in the load from the implant to the bone, and an increase in femoral antetorsion up to 30° leads to increased hip contact forces [52] and also has been associated with pain and decrease in hip external rotation. Not restoring physiologic anteversion can impact on activities of daily living, with patients with excessive anteversion usually not being able to go into a figure of four position or tying their shoes. If antetorsion is increased after THA, an increase in proximal femoral bending moments can occur, which might increase the risk of implant loosening [52].

References

1. Bowman KF Jr, Fox J, Sekiya JK. A clinically relevant review of hip biomechanics. Arthroscopy. 2010;26(8):1118–29.
2. Schuenke M, Shutle E, Schumacher U. General anatomy of the muscoloscletal system. Ross LM, Lamperti ED, editors. Thieme; 2006.
3. Radin EL. Biomechanics of the human hip. Clin Orthop Relat Res. 1980;152:28–34.
4. Buckwalter JE, Einhorn TA, Simon SR. Orthopaedic basic science: biology and biomechanics of the muscoloskeletal system. Rosemont: American Academy of Orthopaedic Surgeons; 2000.
5. Teshima R, Otsuka T, Takasu N, Yamagata N, Yamamoto K. Structure of the most superficial layer of articular cartilage. J Bone Joint Surg Br. 1995;77(3):460–4.
6. Robbins C. Anatomy and biomechanics. Fagerson T, editor. Boston: Butterworth-Heinemann; 1998.
7. Byrne DM, Mulhall KJ, Baker JF. Anatomy & biomechanics of the hip. Open Sports Med J. 2010;4:51–7.
8. Torry MR, Schenker ML, Martin HD, Hogoboom D, Philippon MJ. Neuromuscular hip biomechanics and pathology in the athlete. Clin Sports Med. 2006;25(2):179–97, vii.
9. Tönnis D, Heinecke A. Decreased acetabular anteversion and femur neck antetorsion cause pain and arthrosis. 2: etiology, diagnosis and therapy. Z Orthop Ihre Grenzgeb. 1999;137(2):160–7.
10. Wiberg G. Studies on dysplastic acetabula and congenital subluxation of the hip joint with special reference to the complication of osteo-arthritis. J Am Med Assoc. 1940;115(1):81.
11. Tayton E. Femoral anteversion: a necessary angle or an evolutionary vestige? J Bone Joint Surg Br. 2007;89(10):1283–8.
12. Tsutsumi M, Nimura A, Honda E, Utsunomiya H, Uchida S, Akita K. An anatomical study of the anterosuperior capsular attachment site on the acetabulum. J Bone Joint Surg Am. 2019;101(17):1554–62.
13. Martin HD, Savage A, Braly BA, Palmer IJ, Beall DP, Kelly B. The function of the hip capsular ligaments: a quantitative report. Arthroscopy. 2008;24(2):188–95.
14. Hughes PH, Hsu JC, Matava MJ. Hip anatomy and biomechanics in the athlete. J Sports Med Arthroscopy Rev. 2002;10:103–14.
15. Lunn DE, Lampropoulos A, Stewart TD. Basic biomechanics of the hip. Orthop Trauma. 2016;30(3):239–46.

16. Fuss FK, Bacher A. New aspects of the morphology and function of the human hip joint ligaments. Am J Anat. 1991;192(1):1–13.
17. Hewitt JD, Glisson RR, Guilak F, Vail TP. The mechanical properties of the human hip capsule ligaments. J Arthroplast. 2002;17(1):82–9.
18. Chandler SB, Kreuscher PH. A study of the blood supply of the ligamentum teres and its relation to the circulation of the head of the femur. JBJS. 1932;14(4):834–46.
19. Kivlan BR, Richard Clemente F, Martin RL, Martin HD. Function of the ligamentum teres during multiplanar movement of the hip joint. Knee Surg Sports Traumatol Arthrosc. 2013;21(7):1664–8.
20. Hartigan DE, Perets I, Meghpara MB, Mohr MR, Close MR, Yuen LC, et al. Biomechanics, anatomy, pathology, imaging and clinical evaluation of the acetabular labrum: current concepts. J ISAKOS Joint Disord Orthop Sports Med. 2018;3(3):148–54.
21. Freehill MT, Safran MR. The labrum of the hip: diagnosis and rationale for surgical correction. Clin Sports Med. 2011;30(2):293–315.
22. Crawford MJ, Dy CJ, Alexander JW, Thompson M, Schroder SJ, Vega CE, et al. The 2007 Frank Stinchfield Award. The biomechanics of the hip labrum and the stability of the hip. Clin Orthop Relat Res. 2007;465:16–22.
23. Takechi H, Nagashima H, Ito S. Intra-articular pressure of the hip joint outside and inside the limbus. Nihon Seikeigeka Gakkai Zasshi. 1982;56(6):529–36.
24. Safran MR, Lopomo N, Zaffagnini S, Signorelli C, Vaughn ZD, Lindsey DP, et al. In vitro analysis of peri-articular soft tissues passive constraining effect on hip kinematics and joint stability. Knee Surg Sports Traumatol Arthrosc. 2013;21(7):1655–63.
25. Türker M, Kılıçoğlu Ö, Göksan B, Bilgiç B. Vascularity and histology of fetal labrum and chondrolabral junction: its relevance to chondrolabral detachment tears. Knee Surg Sports Traumatol Arthrosc. 2012;20(2):381–6.
26. Moore K. Clinically oriented anatomy. 3rd ed. Baltimore: Williams and Wilkins; 1992.
27. Polkowski GG, Clohisy JC. Hip biomechanics. Sports Med Arthrosc Rev. 2010;18(2):56–62.
28. Monk AP, Simpson DJ, Riley ND, Murray DW, Gill HS. Biomechanics in orthopaedics: considerations of the lower limb. Surgery (Oxford). 2013;31(9):445–51.
29. Koch JC. The laws of bone architecture. Am J Anat. 1917;21(2):177–298.
30. Miles AW, Gheduzzi S. Basic biomechanics and biomaterials. Surgery (Oxford). 2012;30(2):86–91.
31. Santoni BG, Sanders RW. What you need to understand biomechanically about the hip fracture. Tech Orthop. 2015;30(1):2–8.
32. Fetto JF. A dynamic model of hip joint biomechanics: the contribution of soft tissues. Adv Orthop. 2019;2019:5804642.
33. Robertson DD, Britton CA, Latona CR, Armfield DR, Walker PS, Maloney WJ. Hip biomechanics: importance to functional imaging. Semin Musculoskelet Radiol. 2003;7(1):27–41.
34. Simpson DJ, Monk AP, Murray DW, Gill HS. Biomechanics in orthopaedics: considerations of the hip and knee. Surgery (Oxford). 2010;28(10):478–82.
35. Perry J, K ST, Davids JR. Gait analysis: normal and pathological function. J Pediatr Orthop. 1992;12(6):815.
36. Decking R, Puhl W, Simon U, Claes LE. Changes in strain distribution of loaded proximal femora caused by different types of cementless femoral stems. Clin Biomech (Bristol, Avon). 2006;21(5):495–501.
37. Terrier A, Levrero Florencio F, Rüdiger HA. Benefit of cup medialization in total hip arthroplasty is associated with femoral anatomy. Clin Orthop Relat Res. 2014;472(10):3159–65.
38. Cassidy KA, Noticewala MS, Macaulay W, Lee JH, Geller JA. Effect of femoral offset on pain and function after total hip arthroplasty. J Arthroplast. 2012;27(10):1863–9.
39. Rüdiger HA, Parvex V, Terrier A. Impact of the femoral head position on moment arms in total hip arthroplasty: a parametric finite element study. J Arthroplast. 2016;31(3):715–20.
40. Rüdiger HA, Guillemin M, Latypova A, Terrier A. Effect of changes of femoral offset on abductor and joint reaction forces in total hip arthroplasty. Arch Orthop Trauma Surg. 2017;137(11):1579–85.
41. Bergmann G, Deuretzbacher G, Heller M, Graichen F, Rohlmann A, Strauss J, et al. Hip contact forces and gait patterns from routine activities. J Biomech. 2001;34(7):859–71.
42. Ranawat CS, Rodriguez JA. Functional leg-length inequality following total hip arthroplasty. J Arthroplast. 1997;12(4):359–64.
43. Li J, McWilliams AB, Jin Z, Fisher J, Stone MH, Redmond AC, et al. Unilateral total hip replacement patients with symptomatic leg length inequality have abnormal hip biomechanics during walking. Clin Biomech (Bristol, Avon). 2015;30(5):513–9.
44. Visuri T, Lindholm TS, Antti-Poika I, Koskenvuo M. The role of overlength of the leg in aseptic loosening after total hip arthroplasty. Ital J Orthop Traumatol. 1993;19(1):107–11.
45. Flecher X, Ollivier M, Argenson JN. Lower limb length and offset in total hip arthroplasty. Orthop Traumatol Surg Res. 2016;102(1 Suppl):S9–20.
46. Röder C, Vogel R, Burri L, Dietrich D, Staub LP. Total hip arthroplasty: leg length inequality impairs functional outcomes and patient satisfaction. BMC Musculoskelet Disord. 2012;13:95.
47. Abraham WD, Dimon JH 3rd. Leg length discrepancy in total hip arthroplasty. Orthop Clin North Am. 1992;23(2):201–9.

48. Brand RA, Yack HJ. Effects of leg length discrepancies on the forces at the hip joint. Clin Orthop Relat Res. 1996;333:172–80.
49. Gore DR, Murray MP, Gardner GM, Sepic SB. Roentgenographic measurements after Müller total hip replacement. Correlations among roentgenographic measurements and hip strength and mobility. J Bone Joint Surg Am. 1977;59(7):948–53.
50. Renkawitz T, Haimerl M, Dohmen L, Gneiting S, Lechler P, Woerner M, et al. The association between femoral tilt and impingement-free range-of-motion in total hip arthroplasty. BMC Musculoskelet Disord. 2012;13:65.
51. Higa M, Tanino H, Abo M, Kakunai S, Banks SA. Effect of acetabular component anteversion on dislocation mechanisms in total hip arthroplasty. J Biomech. 2011;44(9):1810–3.
52. Heller MO, Bergmann G, Deuretzbacher G, Claes L, Haas NP, Duda GN. Influence of femoral anteversion on proximal femoral loading: measurement and simulation in four patients. Clin Biomech (Bristol, Avon). 2001;16(8):644–9.

20 Key Concepts and Methods for Acetabular Positioning

Jakub Tatka and Joel M. Matta

Accurate positioning of the acetabular component is of high importance. Enhancing accuracy facilitates restoration of hip biomechanics, functional range of motion, resistance to wear, and decreased dislocation risk.

The position of the acetabular component refers to center of rotation and rotational position defined by inclination and anteversion.

For hips that were previously nonpathologic, the center of the acetabulum/center of rotation should be placed as close as possible to the hip's original, predisease center of rotation. For dysplastic hips, the acetabulum should be placed in the anatomic acetabulum, which is often different from the preoperative rotation center and is more medial and distal. Wear of the acetabulum that can occur with prolonged arthritis can cause a superior bone defect that may only move the acetabulum a small distance proximal or a superior graft may be considered for significant superior wear and center of rotation restoration. It is also often necessary to prioritize placing the cup within the walls of the acetabulum for stability against host bone and to prevent soft tissue irritation against the cup's metal edge. Especially, the anterior bony rim should cover the cup to prevent iliopsoas tendon contact. Considerations of bony contact and preventing soft tissue irritation may inevitably medialize the center. Avoid aggressive reaming of the acetabular roof that can result in a too proximal cup and raised hip center.

It is the author's practice to place almost all primary cups without screws using a cup with no screw holes.

The second and more confusing factor in acetabular position is the rotational position. Target values for inclination and anteversion are not universally agreed upon and may be varied at times between patients [1]. Recommended values for inclination and anteversion, however, are close enough across published references to guide placement [2].

Past methodologies for achieving rotational position have produced inconsistent results even from experienced and expert surgeons [3, 4]. Methodologies to achieve desired acetabular rotational position (ARP) vary widely and include "eyeballing" the cup and/or insertion handle (most common), mechanical guides, range of motion and stability trials, alignment with the transverse acetabular ligament, computer guidance based on preoperative planning and relation to pelvic landmarks, intraoperative plain films, and intraoperative fluoroscopy. Essentially, all clinical data used to validate all methodologies are based on post-op X-ray (either post-op supine AP plain films or less commonly post-op CT scan) [5]. X-ray with the patient

J. Tatka (✉)
White Plains Hospital, White Plains, NY, USA

J. M. Matta
The Steadman Clinic, Vail, CO, USA

J. M. Matta, A. P. Sah (eds.), *Anterior Hip Replacement*,
https://doi.org/10.1007/978-3-030-91896-5_20

supine is therefore the final "gold standard" method for judging all methods for assessing ARP. The author therefore prefers supine X-ray as the intra-op and final method for accurate ARP. ARP is achieved with intraoperative fluoroscopy and aided with software analysis of the digital image.

ARP is achieved in relation to the ordinate axes (x, y, and z) of the body or the ordinate planes (transverse, sagittal, and coronal) and not in relation to the pelvis. These are the measures that intraoperative or post-op plain films, fluoroscopy, or CT defines. These are the measures that are also correct because they define the ARP in relation to the body and femur. It follows that while the cup should be adequately contained within the acetabulum, the patient's native inclination and anteversion should not influence prosthetic ARP.

Because of the various requirements for ARP including range of motion, wear, and stability, ARP is not ideal for all parameters or for any one hip position or function such as walking or standing. Whatever the hip position or patient activity, the ARP is rarely ideal but yet satisfactory and functional. The necessity, however, for ARP to be widely applicable emphasizes the need for accuracy so that function is still adequate at the extremes.

ARP should *not* vary in relation to the normal variations of femoral anteversion (as per the concept of combined anteversion, which the senior author contends is in large part erroneous) [6]. Cup position should be relatively consistent and will accommodate variations in femoral anteversion. If the patient has important problems the solution should be to "normalize" femoral anteversion with the femoral component.

Inclination and anteversion can be measured by either plain films, fluoroscopy, or CT. One method is not inherently more accurate than the other, and all methods depend on the proper orientation of the X-ray beam to the pelvis and acetabulum. For plain films and fluoroscopy, the X-ray should be perpendicular to the coronal plane. A lateral view of the acetabulum taken as a lateral pelvis can also measure inclination, and anteversion, however, does not add new information regarding ARP. A cross-table lateral does not give an accurate measurement for anteversion. For CT, the axial cut plane should be parallel to the transverse plane of the body. Both of these positions are much easier to achieve if the study is performed with the patient supine rather than lateral decubitus.

Operating Room Methodology

Accurate implantation of the acetabular component is crucial. Supine positioning and fluoroscopy have contributed greatly to achieving better cup position. Several fluoroscopic-based computer navigation programs have been developed to increase the accuracy and consistency of intraoperative cup positioning. In order to place the acetabular cup using DePuy's VELYS software effectively, there are several steps to follow:

1. Check to see that pelvis is level regarding roll-on PA fluoroscopy, centered over the pelvis.
2. In the VELYS software, enter value of the angle formed by two intersecting lines: the line connecting the pelvic brim to teardrop and the line connecting teardrop to teardrop
3. Next, center the C-arm over acetabulum and rotate the image to approximate a vertical pelvis
4. In the VELYS software, enter the desired values for inclination and anteversion, which creates a magenta target ellipse that is projected over the centered hip PA fluoroscopic image
5. Finally, impact the acetabular component. During impaction, vary the inserter angle as necessary to match the image of the rim of the acetabular component to the magenta target ellipse.

The VELYS process is simple and reproducible. Nonetheless, there are some fundamental concepts that, when understood, will increase the surgeon's ability to consistently insert the acetabular cup as intended with less error. The fully detailed process is as follows:

The preoperative supine AP pelvis plain film X-ray should be assessed for pelvic tilt and rotation. Note the size, shape, and symmetry of the obturator foramina for referencing intraoperatively. This preoperative image should be available in the operating room for visualization and comparison by the surgeon.

Proper assessment of pelvic position begins with patient positioning in the operating room. The patient is placed supine on the Hana table. The feet are placed into boots and attached to the table leg spars. These spars are gently flexed to approximately 3–5° in order to prevent and increase in pelvic tilt (Fig. 20.1).

During the procedure, prior to final cup positioning center the C-arm over the pelvis in order to assess if the pelvis is level regarding roll and also to assess if the pelvic tilt remains consistent with that seen on the pre-op AP supine pelvis. Several anatomic landmarks and relationships are used in this process, these can be seen in Fig. 20.2.

The pelvic rotation (rotation around the longitudinal axis) can be assessed using the primary relationships below:

1. The relationship of the central long axis of coccyx to the pubic symphysis.
2. The (medial–lateral) relationship of the ilioischial line with the acetabular teardrop comparing right to left.
3. The medial to lateral width of the obturator foramina comparing the right to the left.

If the pelvis is not level regarding roll, roll the HANA table appropriately to level the pelvis. With the pelvis level, the table roll orientation may not be level.

Pelvic tilt can be assessed with the following anatomic relationships:

1. The relationship of the tip of coccyx to the pubic symphysis
2. The vertical height (caudal to cephalad distance) of the obturator foramina

In a minority of cases, particularly in obese patients, pelvic tilt may increase as seen by a decrease in the caudad–cephalad dimension of the obturator foramina compared to the pre-op supine AP. Typically, this change is prevented by 3–5° flexion of the HANA spars during patient set-up. If a significant change in tilt is evident, angle the fluoroscope 5–10° in a caudad to cephalad direction to obtain a fluoroscopic picture that shows an obturator foramen shape similar to the pre-op X-ray.

If the teardrop–brim angle was not measured from the pre-op X-ray, the intra-op PA fluoroscopic view can be utilized. This angle value is entered in the VELYS program. This angle value orients the rotational position of the acetabulum on the VELYS screen and thereby the correct angular relation between the acetabular image and the magenta ellipse.

Prior to this fluoroscopic assessment and adjustment of pelvis position, it is the author's preference to start acetabular reaming. Prior to completion of reaming, the pelvis is leveled and if necessary a fluoroscopic tilt adjustment for pelvic tilt.

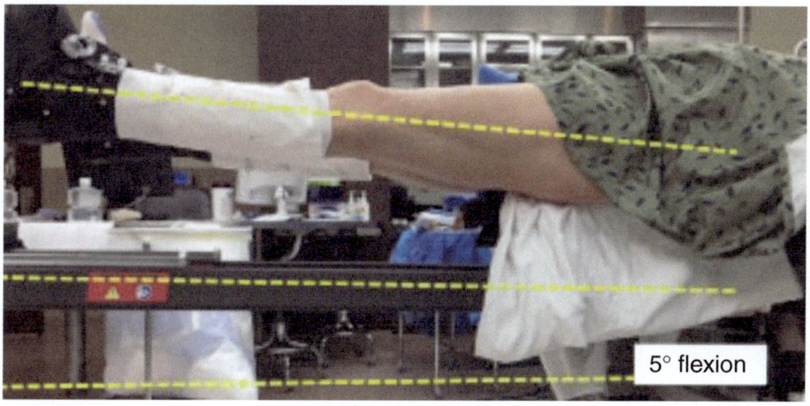

Fig. 20.1 Shows 3–5° of flexion of the table spars from the plane of the floor to prevent pelvic tilt/extension. (Photo courtesy of Joel Matta, MD)

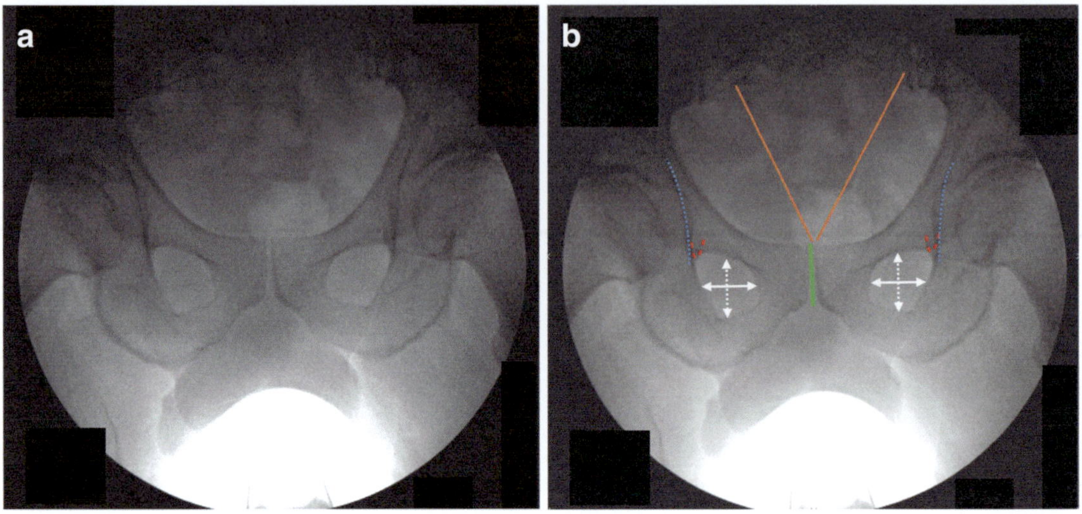

Fig. 20.2 (**a**) PA pelvis fluoroscopic image taken intraop. (Courtesy Jakub Tatka, MD). (**b**) Same PA pelvis image from (**a**) with landmarks and their relationships marked to assess pelvic rotation and tilt. They are labeled as follows: Solid orange lines outline the sacrum, blue dotted lines outline the ilioischial line, the dashed red lines outline the teardrop, the solid green line identifies the pubic symphysis, and the solid white arrows show the medial to lateral width of the obturator foramina, and the dotted white arrows show the caudal-to-cephalad distance of the obturator foramina

Next, center the fluoroscope over the acetabulum and make adjustments so that the acetabulum appears in the center of the image. If the fluoroscope has been adjusted because of an observed change in pelvic tilt, do not change this. Complete reaming as necessary and check the reamer position with fluoroscope.

Insert the cup with the Kincise impactor or by hammering, checking position during insertion, and making large or small adjustments in position as necessary. At the completion of cup insertion, the image of the rim of the cup should match the magenta ellipse created by the VELYS software. The author uses 43° inclination and 23° anteversion as the most common target values.

If the cup is not centered in the image view during impaction and assessment of ARP, parallax of the X-ray beam will give a false impression of cup position. For instance, if the fluoroscope is left centered over the center of the pelvis during cup insertion, the cup will appear to have less inclination and more anteversion than its true position (Figs. 20.3, 20.4, and 20.5).

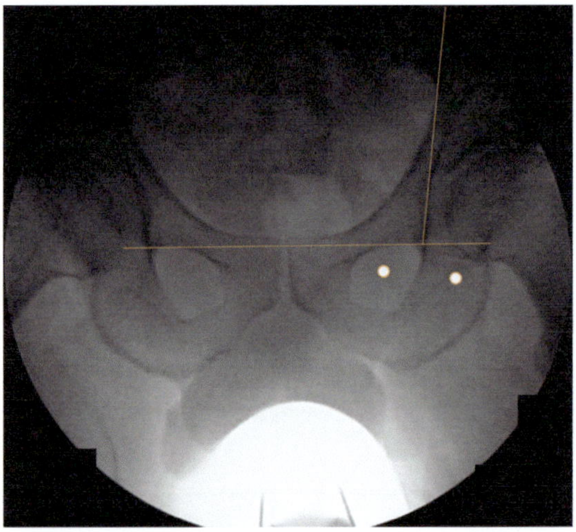

Fig. 20.3 PA pelvis from Fig. 20.2a showing VELYS pelvic angle measurement, measured as 83° in this example. The angle is formed by drawing one line from the inferior most point of each teardrop and a second lined that passes through the center of the teardrop (ipsilateral to the surgical side) and the lateral most portion of the pelvic brim. This angle is then used as the reference for inclination and anteversion of the projected ellipse

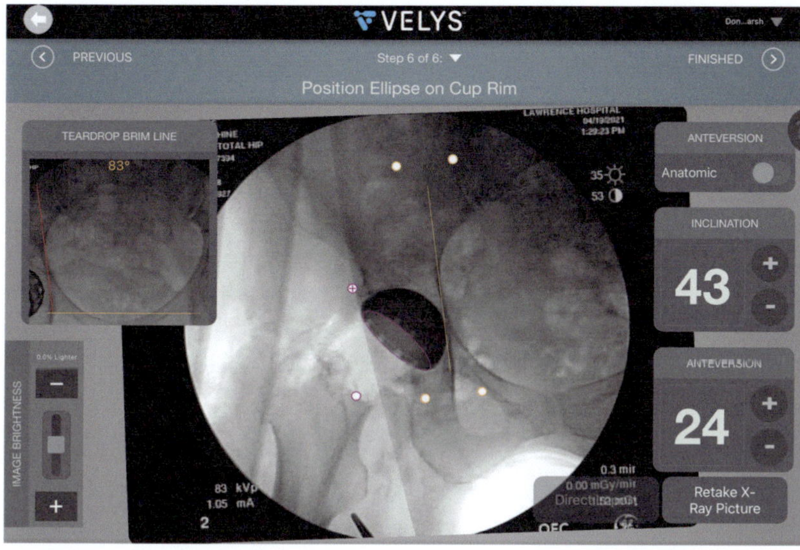

Fig. 20.4 Demonstrates VELYS (DePuy Warsaw, Indiana) software being used in conjunction with fluoroscopic images from a total hip arthroplasty case. In this mode, the software is being utilized to navigate the acetabular cup. VELYS software will project an ellipse using either Murray's anatomic or radiographic criteria that are positioned relative to a line passing through the center of the teardrop and the lateral most portion of the pelvic brim. This ellipse inclination and anteversion can be changed in one-degree increments by the surgeon or an assistant to the desired position

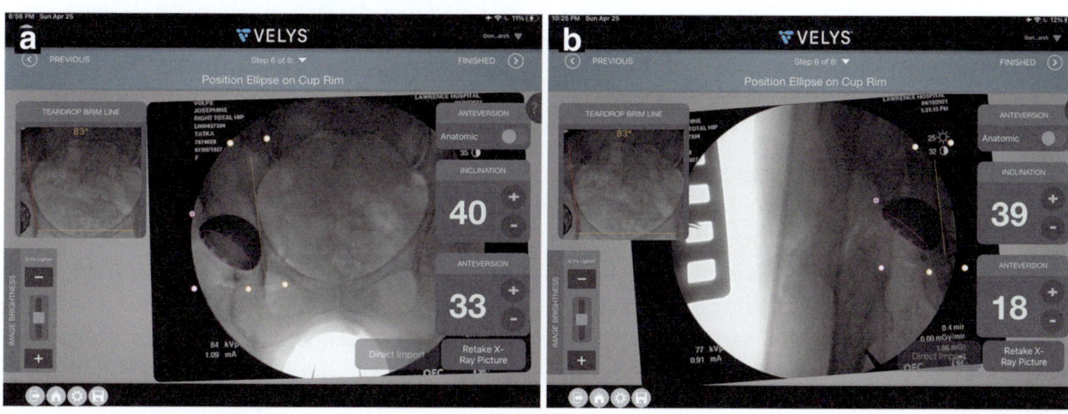

Fig. 20.5 (**a**, **b**) The parallax effect from the fluoroscope will affect the perceived acetabular cup orientation. It is important to be aware that unless the acetabular cup is centered in the fluoroscopic image, the anteversion and inclination will not be accurately represented. To illustrate this, (**a**) shows the acetabular component on the far left of the screen and 5b shows it on the far right. Both the inclination and the anteversion change as seen on the VELYS screen readout. (**a**) Positioning of the acetabular implant to the left of the screen, as seen on PA pelvis imaging. The implant appears to have increased the anteversion by 9° and decreased the inclination by 3°. (**b**) Positioning of the acetabular implant to the right of the screen, as seen on PA hip imaging. The implant appears to have decreased the anteversion by 6° and decreased the inclination by 4°

Pearls

1. It is important to be aware of the weight of the insertion handle and/or the weight of Kincise, which can roll the entire pelvis through its attachment to a well-fixed cup. Support the weight of the insertion device to prevent pelvic roll and a consequently erroneous cup image.
2. A benefit of using a specialized table with a perineal post is that it helps keep the cup centered in the fluoroscopic image because the pelvis does not translate with cup impaction.
3. During fine-tuning of cup position, it is easier to adjust before the cup is fully seated and locked in with a press fit. Cup position can then be fine-tuned as final seating is obtained. A fully seated cup in a less than ideal position can be adjusted by continued impaction with Kincise while applying angular pressure to the Kincise as appropriate.

Target Values for Inclination and Anteversion

The first widely used value range for cup inclination and anteversion was the Lewinnek "safe zone" of 40° ± 10° of inclination and 15° ± 10° as measured on a supine AP pelvis plain film [8]. Since then, there have been many challenges and disagreements to the specific target values and how they are evaluated [1, 9–12]. The table below shows a variety of suggested ARP [2].

Tables 20.1 and 20.2. These two tables are a selection of studied and suggested acetabular cup positions from various literature and textbooks. Of note, the majority of these studies primarily utilized radiographic criteria and not Anatomic criteria, with the conversion to anatomic alongside the radiographic, which illustrates the variation between the two methods. Additionally, there is the variety in the target positions or range of target positions by each publication, and there is no set consensus for what is the "best" position, either as specific target value or a target range.

The author's baseline target values are an inclination of 43° and an anteversion of 23°. These values represent acetabular rotational position (ARP). These are measured intraoperatively on an AP hip image using a fluoroscope and computer navigation software (VELYS) utilizing Murray anatomic criteria [21]. The values listed are a starting point and are adjusted as needed for specific clinical indications. Typically, the preferred values for young patients are decreased inclination and anteversion. For patients with stiff lumbar spines, the values are slightly increased inclination and anteversion.

The Argument for Murray "Anatomic" Criteria for Measuring Acetabular Rotational Position Rather than the Commonly Used "Radiographic Criteria"

Murray described 3 methods (criteria) for measuring ARP: anatomic, radiographic, and operative. This is a classic and widely quoted article that added to our understanding. On the other hand, we believe that discussion of 3 methods has introduced confusion and error into our understanding and measurement of ARP. Since all 3 methods yield different results, which one is correct? In our opinion, as there is only one definition of proximal femoral neck–shaft angle and anteversion, there should be only one definition of cup inclination and anteversion and the Murray anatomic definition should be used exclusively as femoral neck–shaft angle and anteversion uses only an anatomic definition (Figs. 20.6 and 20.7).

Table 20.1 Safety guidelines for inclination and anteversion angles from the literature

	Inclination					Anteversion				
Source	Original definitions degrees (°)	Original reference frame	Operative degrees (°)	Radiographic degrees (°)	Anatomical degrees (°C)	Original definitions degrees (°)	Original reference frame	Operative degrees (°)	Radiographic degrees (°)	Anatomical degrees (°)
Lewinnick [13]	40 ± 10° Lateral opening	Radiographic	38 ± 11	40 ± 10	42 ± 12	15 ± 10°	Radiographic	21 ± 15	15 ± 10	25 ± 18
McCollum and Gray [14]	40 ± 10° Abduction	Radiographic	36 ± 12	40 ± 10	45 ± 11	30 ± 10° Flexion	Operative	30 ± 10	25 ± 11	36 ± 19
Harris [15]	30° Abduction	Radiographic	28	30	34	20° Forward flexion	Operative	20	18	32
Pedersen [16]	<40° Tilt	Radiographic	35 ± 5	35 ± 5	36 ± 6	<10° Anteversion	Radiographic	6 ± 6	5 ± 5	10 ± 10

Table 20.2 Suggested acetabular cup inclination and anteversion angles from surgical technique in academic textbooks

	Inclination					Anteversion				
Source	Original definitions degrees (°)	Original reference frame	Operative degrees (°)	Radiographic degrees (°)	Anatomical degrees (°C)	Original definitions degrees (°)	Original reference frame	Operative degrees (°)	Radiographic degrees (°)	Anatomical degrees (°)
Jayson total hip replacement [17]	45° Open	Radiographic	45	46	45	10° Anteversion	Operative	10	10	7
Calandruccio Campbell's operative orthopaedics [18]	35°–45°	Radiographic	39 ± 6	40 ± 5	41 ± 6	10°–20° Anteversion	Operative	15 ± 5	12 ± 5	19 ± 9
Charnley [19]	45° Inclination	Anatomical	45	45	45	0° Anteversion	Anatomical	0	0	0
Muller [20]	45° Facing laterally	Radiographic	44	45	46	10° Anteversion	Operative	13 ± 3	9 ± 2	13 ± 3

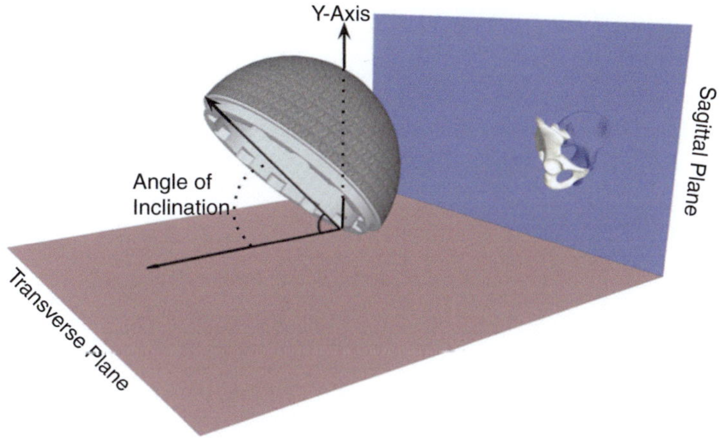

Fig. 20.6 Inclination = the angle between the plane of the cup face and a transverse plane. Anteversion is 0°, and inclination is approximately 45°

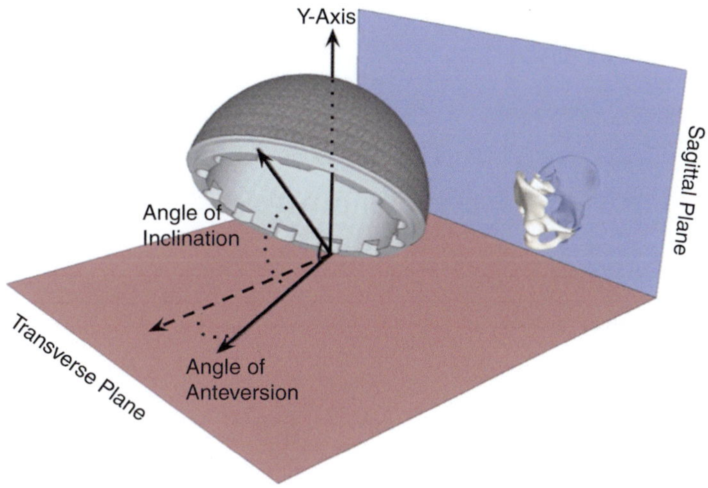

Fig. 20.7 Anteversion = the angle of rotation of the cup around a longitudinal (y)-axis. The dashed black arrow is in the coronal plane and is the reference for measuring anteversion. The solid black arrows represent the angle of inclination

If we think of femoral neck–shaft angle and anteversion, we are thinking of measurement of bony anatomy. The neck–shaft angle is a measure of the inclination of the neck and anteversion is a measure of rotation of the neck axis around the longitudinal or y-axis. To also define the position of the cup anatomically and geometrically in relation to the axes and planes of the body one must use the Murray anatomic criteria (MAC). The MAC measure inclination as the angle of the cup face to the transverse plane or y-axis and anteversion as degrees of rotation around the longitudinal y-axis (Figs. 20.6 and 20.7). MAC are therefore most intuitive and comparable to our understanding and measurement of femoral neck–shaft angle and anteversion. Paradoxically, while anatomic measurement of the femur is standard, most papers measuring ARP refer to Murray radiographic criteria (MRC) rather than the anatomically and geometrically correct MAC. Why is this? Our opinion is that there is widespread lack of understanding of how to measure MAC and lack of understanding of what the X-rays represent (Figs. 20.9, 20.10, and 20.11).

- Definitions of Anatomic

Murray radiographic inclination (MRI) defines cup inclination as the angle of the major diameter of the ellipse created by an AP view of the cup rim to a horizontal or transverse line (Fig. 20.16). The main problem with measurement of cup inclination with MRI is that for an anteverted cup, the MRI measures a value that is less than the actual

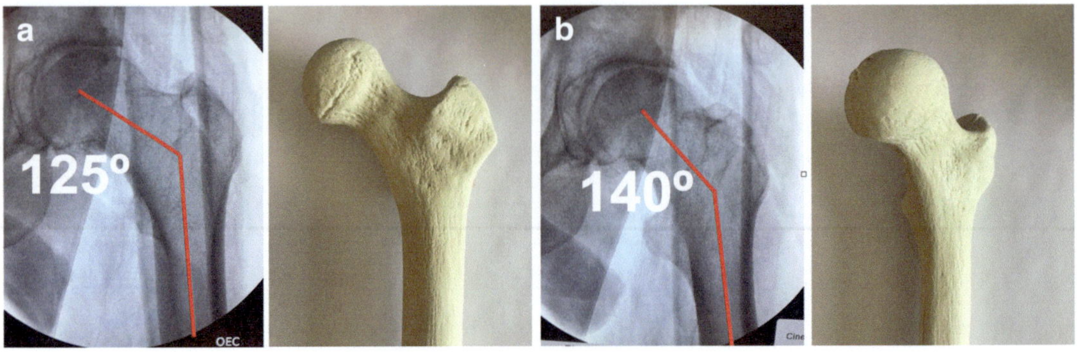

Fig. 20.8 (**a**) Accurate (maximum femoral offset) neck–shaft angle seen with x-ray perpendicular to plane of neck–shaft angle. (**b**) Inaccurate (incomplete femoral offset) neck–shaft angle (increased 15°) seen with external rotation

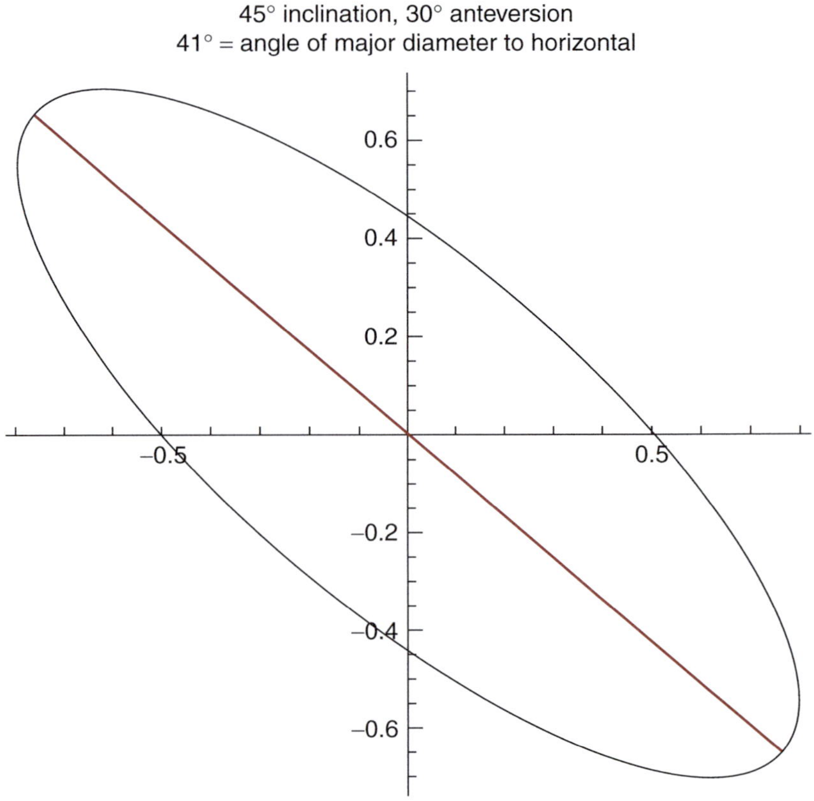

Fig. 20.9 Measuring the angle of the major diameter of the ellipse to the horizontal is the radiographic method and it always "under" measures the anatomic cup inclination. In this case on the coordinate plan, the ellipse represents an anatomic inclination, which is calculated to be 45°, but the radiographic inclination (ellipse angle) is 41°

MAC inclination. For a given degree of true inclination (the angle of the cup face to a transverse plane), increasing degrees of anteversion create a decreasing X-ray image value of the ellipse angle (MRI). The ellipse angle decreases as an exponential function from true or anatomic inclination to zero as a cup is progressively anteverted from 0° to 90°. This phenomenon is not intuitively obvious but we hope to increase understanding with the following figures. We propose that the term "radiographic inclination" be abandoned and substituted with "ellipse angle" (E).

To help the reader with understanding of how measurement of a radiographic angle does not equate to measurement of an anatomic angle, we represent the example of measurement of femoral neck–shaft angle (Fig. 20.8a, b). An X-ray view of the proximal femur will only represent the true neck–shaft angle if the X-ray beam is directed perpendicular to the plane determined by the angle between the intersection of the axes of the femoral shaft and neck. Rotation of the proximal femur and thereby this angle determined plane in relation to the X-ray beam will lead to an erroneous measurement of neck–shaft angle that is always greater than the true anatomic neck–shaft angle (Fig. 20.19a–d). Similarly, X-ray measurement of true anatomic cup inclination (measurement of the cup face angle to the transverse plane or y-axis) can only be done by measuring the cup angle for a cup with 0° of anteversion and the cup rim appears on X-ray as an oblique line. For all magnitudes of cup anteversion or retroversion other than 0, the cup rim appears as an angulated ellipse and measurement of this ellipse angle gives a lower value than true anatomic inclination (Figs. 20.9, 20.10, 20.11, and 20.19a–d).

We also argue against use of Murray radiographic anteversion (MRA) and argue for use of Murray anatomic anteversion (MAA) (Figs. 20.16 and 20.17). MRA measures the degrees of rotation around an oblique axis (the major ellipse axis). As MRA increases, therefore, the cup face becomes progressively more vertical (inclination increases). MRA is therefore not an independent variable. MAA is an independent variable that increases and decreases, while inclination remains constant (Figs. 20.6 and 20.18). MAA is also more intuitively understood because of its similarity to femoral anteversion. A further argument for use of MAA is that fluoroscopy or plain film radiographic measurement will be equal to CT measurement of cup anteversion. MRA measurements from plain films do not yield the same result as CT and lead to a falsely low value for anteversion.

The circular rim of the cup appears on X-ray as an ellipse. Both radiographic and anatomic inclination and anteversion can be calculated from the shape and position of this ellipse. The illustration of such an ellipse on a x-y-axis can be seen in Figs. 20.9 and 20.10 shows an actual acetabular component and the ellipse highlighted in dotted red, and Fig. 20.11 shows the fluoroscopic image of an acetabular component and the ellipse as projected by the rim is highlighted in dotted red.

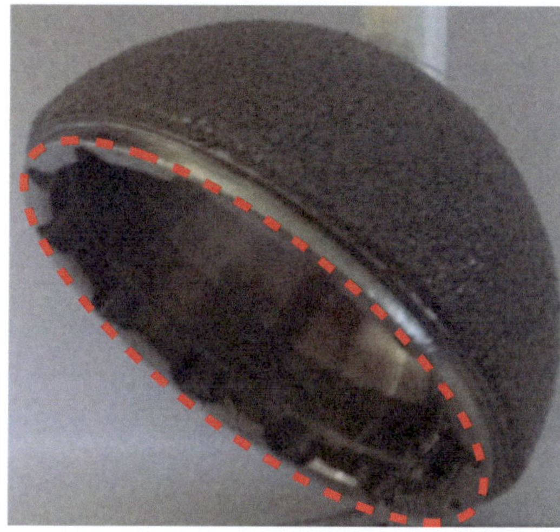

Fig. 20.10 Anatomic inclination 41° and anteversion 31°; ellipse angle = 37°

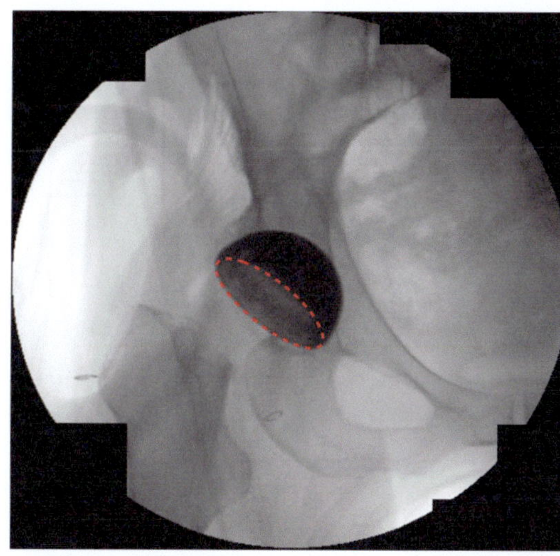

Fig. 20.11 Anatomic inclination 41° and anteversion 31°; ellipse angle = 37°

Both radiographic and anatomic inclination and anteversion can be calculated from the shape and position of the ellipse, whereas surgical criteria are evaluated by direct visualization intraoperatively. In Table 20.3 are listed the required variables and their definitions necessary to make the calculations. Figures 20.12, 20.13, 20.14, and 20.15 include the formulas that use these variables.

Table 20.3 Necessary data points that are used in the formulas in Figs. 20.12, 20.13, 20.14, 20.15, 20.16, 20.17, and 20.18 to make the calculations for acetabular cup position

Variable	Definition
A	Angle of anteversion of cup
I	Angle of inclination of cup
E	Angle of ellipse major diameter to horizontal, also described as radiographic inclination
L	Length of the major diameter of the ellipse
H	Horizontal width of the ellipse
V	Vertical height of the ellipse

$$Sin\ I = \frac{V}{L}$$

Fig. 20.12 Calculation for inclination (anatomic)

$$Sin\ A = \frac{H}{L}$$

Fig. 20.13 Calculation for anteversion (anatomic)

$$Tan\ I = \frac{Tan\ E}{Cos\ A}$$

Fig. 20.14 Calculation for anteversion (anatomic)

$$Tan\ E = (Tan\ I) \times (Cos\ A)$$

Fig. 20.15 Calculation for anteversion (anatomic)

The series of images in Fig. 20.19 depict an acetabular cup being placed in four different positions of anteversion (0°, 30°, 60°, and 90°) while maintaining the same inclination of 45°. We can see how the ellipse angle (RA) is equal to true inclination at only 0° of anteversion. As the anteversion increases, the ellipse angle decreases exponentially, from 45° to 0° as anteversion increases. This effect is akin to how the femoral rotation affects the apparent neck–shaft angle of the proximal femur on X-ray. Figure 20.19a–d.

This error of radiographic inclination measurement when compared to true (anatomic) inclination increases with increasing anteversion. Therefore, if there are 25° of anteversion in the cup position, expect 3–12° of error in the inclination radiographically from the anatomic inclination value. Figure 20.20 shows the increasing error graphically.

Problems with radiographic anteversion include the following:

- Anteversion rotation occurs around an oblique axis with the cup face becoming increasingly vertical as anteversion increases
- Does not vary independently of inclination
- Underestimates true (Anatomic) anteversion
- Does not agree with CT measurement of anteversion; however, anatomic anteversion measurement agrees with CT [23]

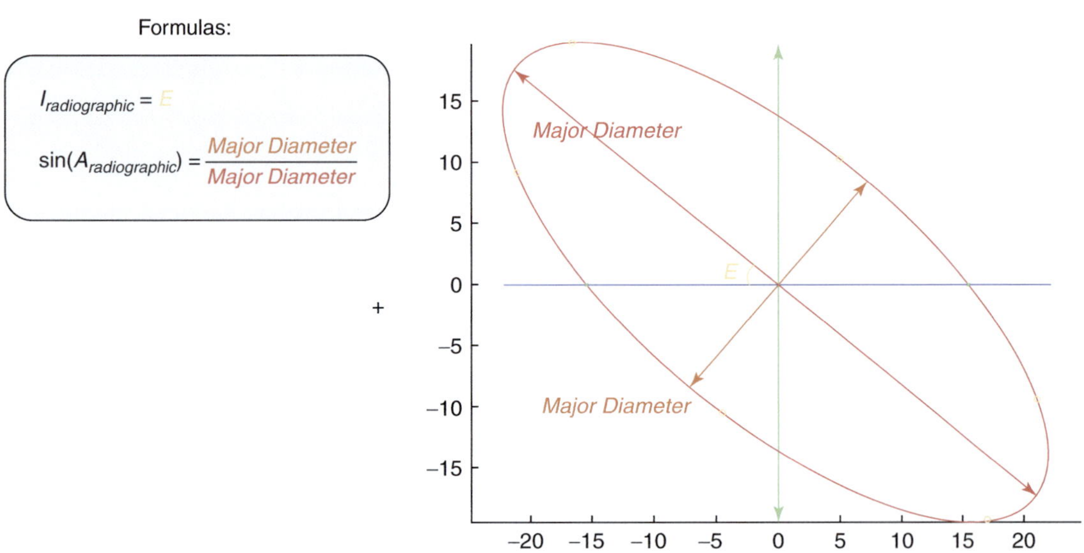

Fig. 20.16 Radiographic inclination (E) and Radiographic Anteversion

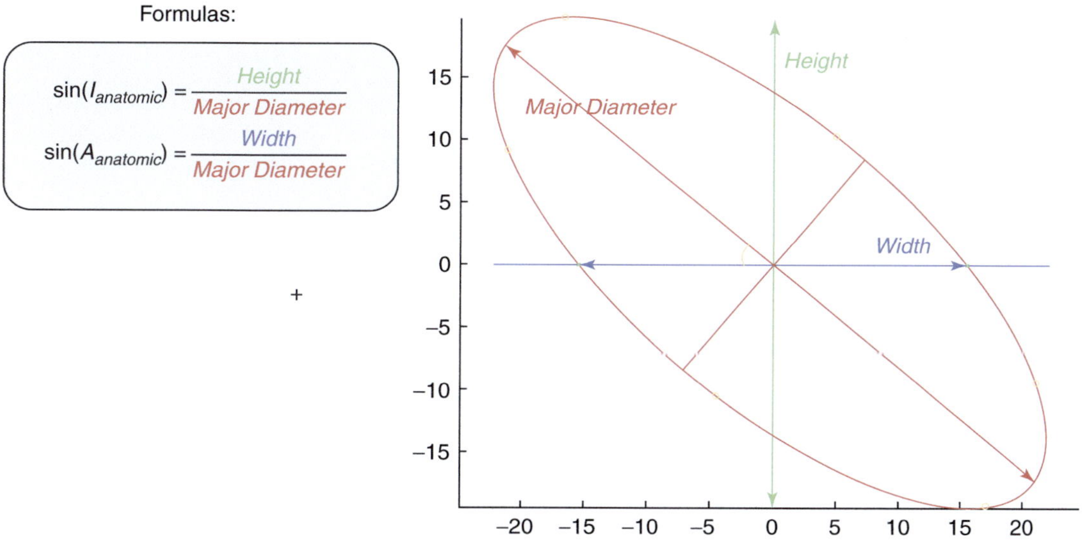

Fig. 20.17 Anatomic inclination (I) and Anteversion (A)

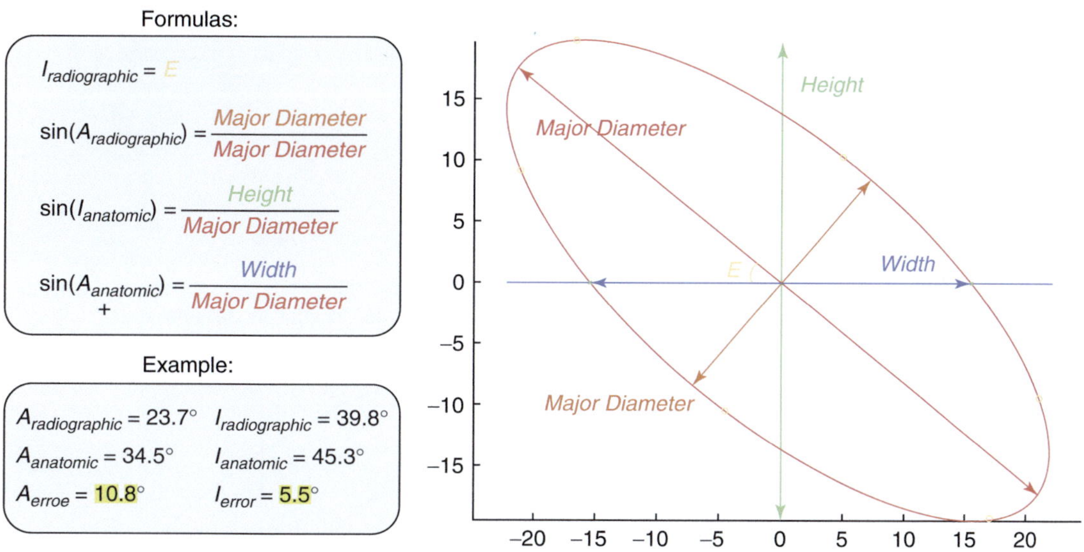

Fig. 20.18 Comparing radiographic to anatomic

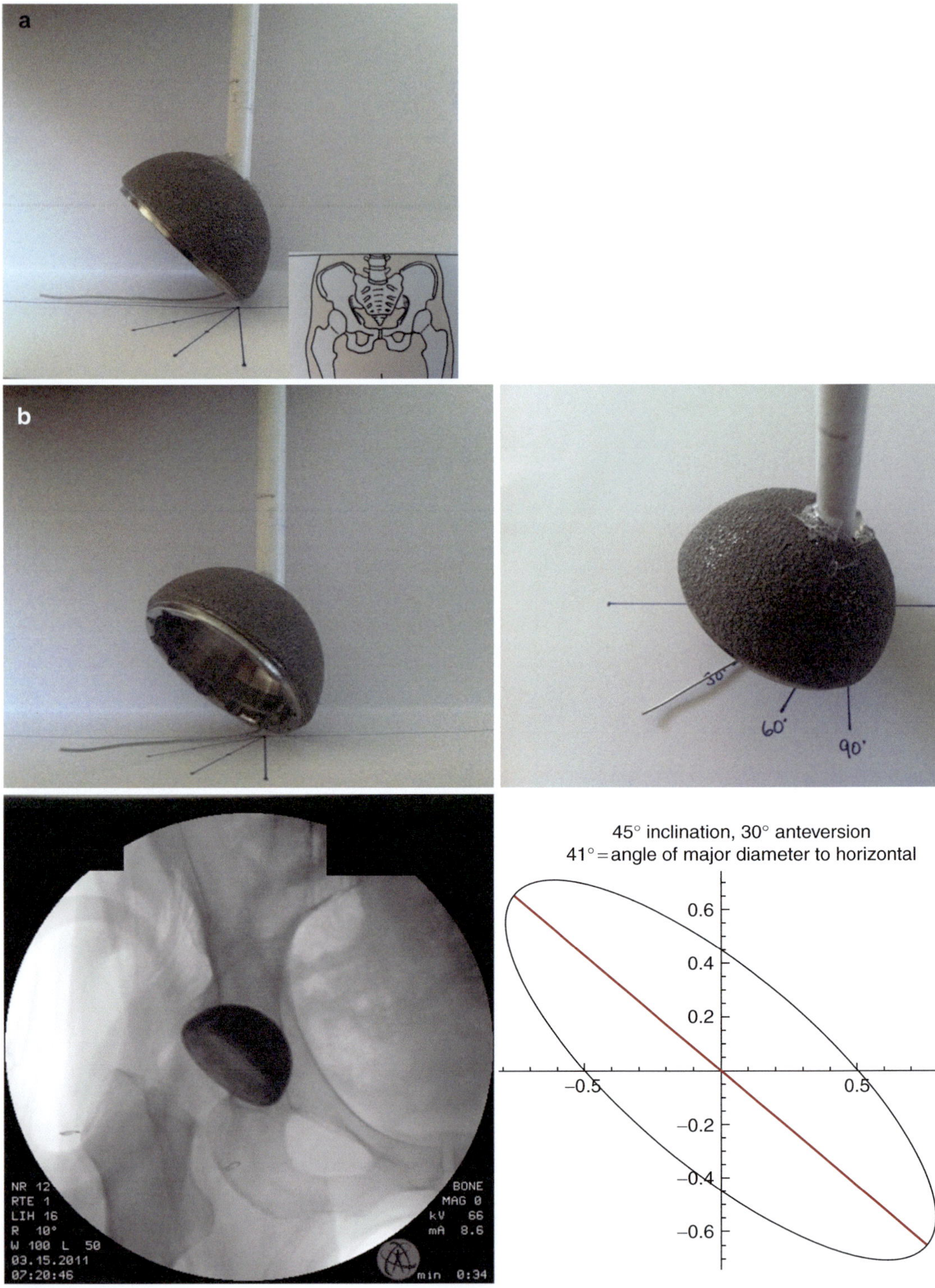

Fig. 20.19 (**a**) AP view of cup at 45° inclination and 0° anteversion. For a cup in this position, the X-ray image of the cup rim would be a line, with the anterior and posterior rims superimposed. (**b**) AP of cup that has been rotated around the white post (y-axis) 30°. View from above of the same cup. XR image of implanted cup representing the same inclination and anteversion. The projected ellipse on the x-y-axis, as would be seen on X-ray. (**c**) AP of cup that has been rotated around the white post (y-axis) 60°. View from above of the same cup. The projected ellipse of the cup rim on the x-y-axis as would be seen on X-ray. (**d**) AP of cup that has been rotated around the white (y-axis) post 90°. View from above of the same cup. The projected ellipse of the cup rim on the x-y-axis, as would be seen on X-ray

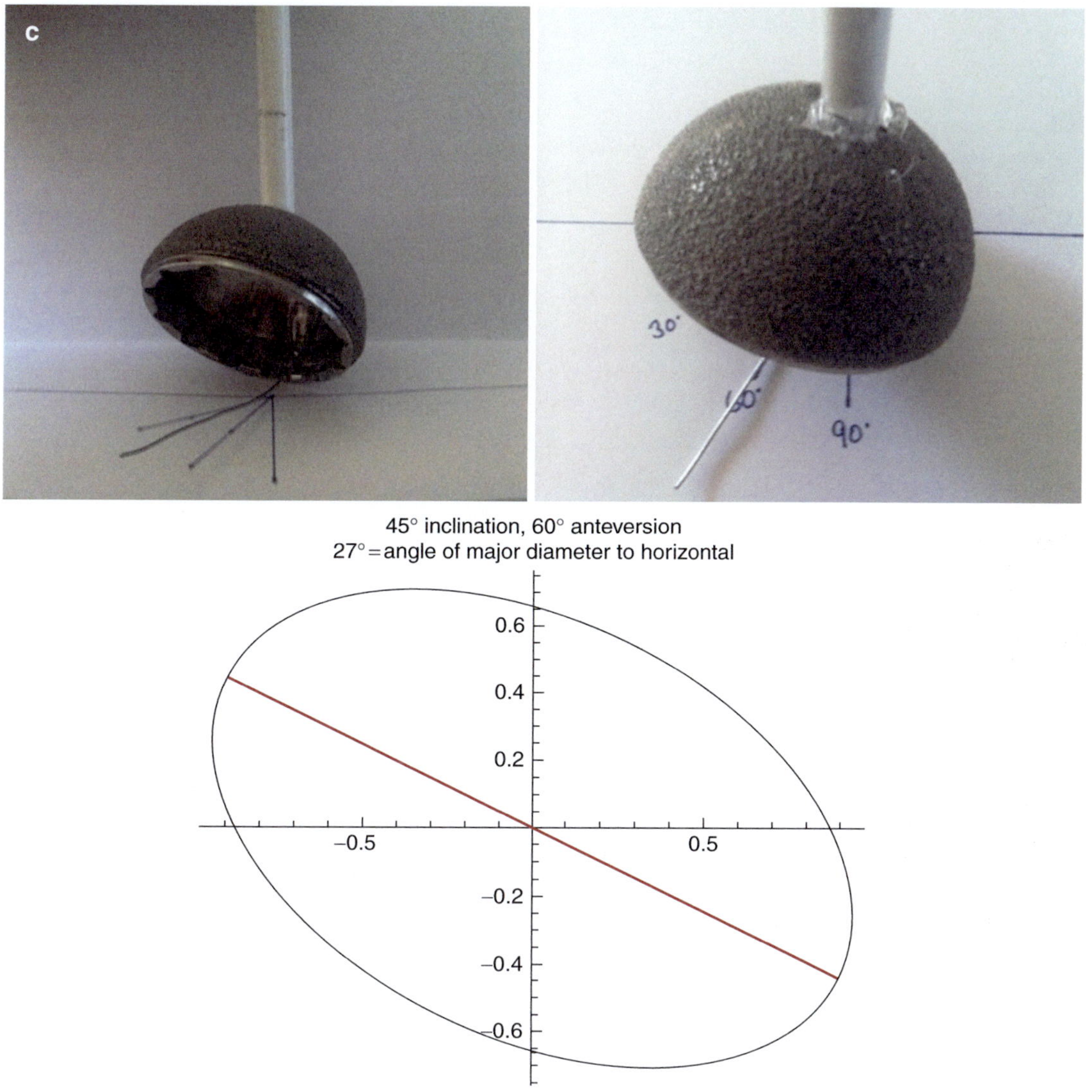

Fig. 20.19 (continued)

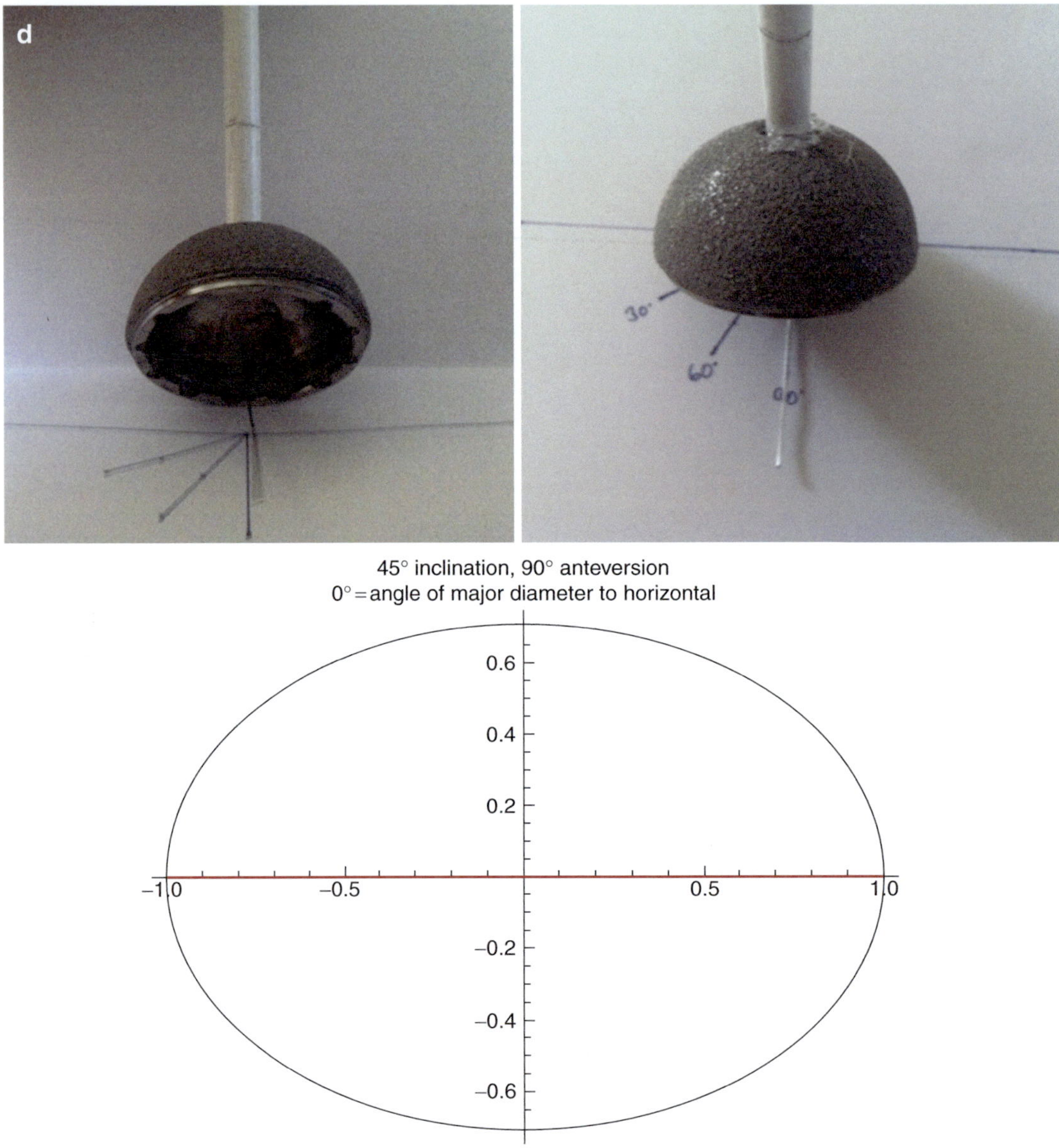

Fig. 20.19 (continued)

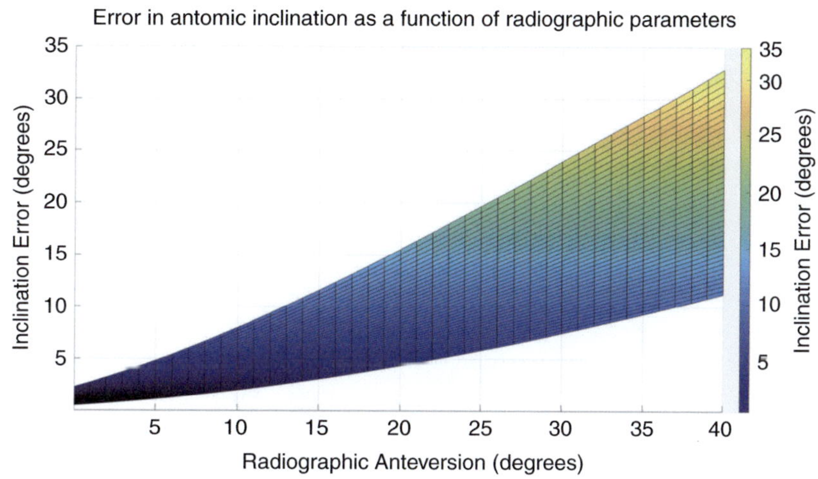

Fig. 20.20 Numerical difference between radiographic inclination and anatomic inclination as the anteversion increases

1. Controlled case study examples: Below are examples for review that show the error that is introduced when radiographic criteria are used rather than anatomic criteria. Each example shows a acetabular cup position, and both anatomic and radiographic measurements are included to show the discrepancy between each technique:

- Example 1

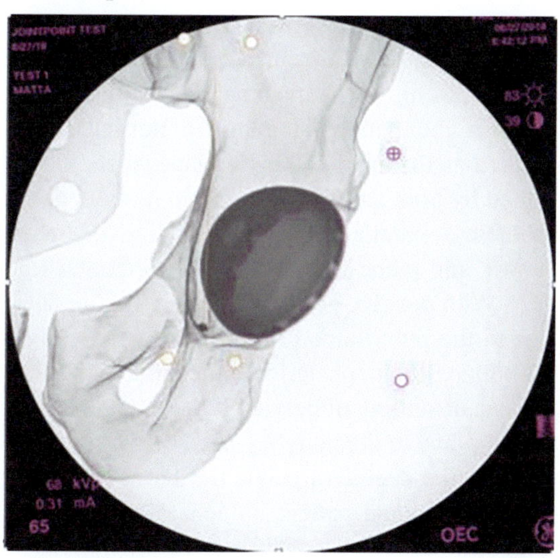

(i) Radiographic:
   1. Inclination: 51
   2. Anteversion: 33

(ii) Anatomic:
   1. Inclination: 58
   2. Anteversion: 40

(iii) Error:
   1. Inclination: 7
   2. Anteversion: 7

- Example 2

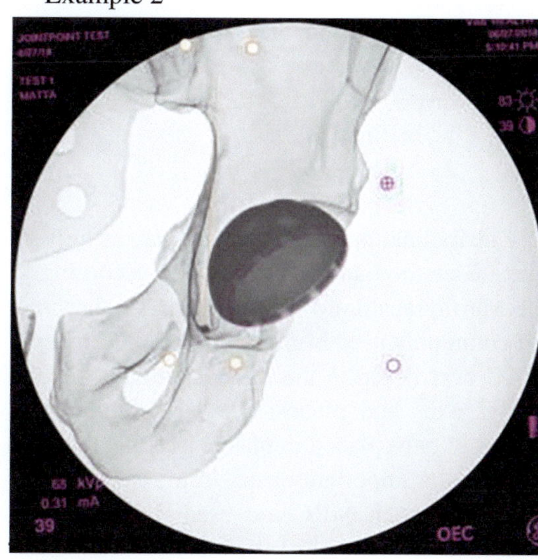

(i) Radiographic:
   1. Inclination: 34
   2. Anteversion: 26

(ii) Anatomic:
   1. Inclination: 42
   2. Anteversion: 42

(iii) Error:
   1. Inclination: 8
   2. Anteversion: 16

- Example 3

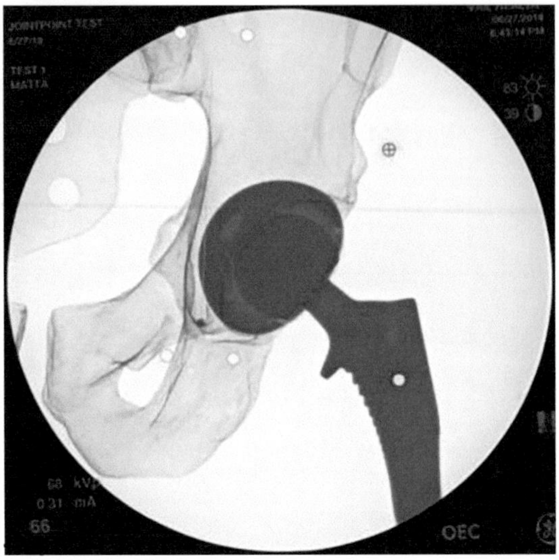

(i) Radiographic:
1. Inclination: 47
2. Anteversion: 35

(ii) Anatomic:
1. Inclination: 56
2. Anteversion: 44

(iii) Error:
1. Inclination: 9
2. Anteversion: 9

Cup inclination and anteversion are intuitively best understood and best described according to the Murray anatomic criteria (MAC) rather than the commonly used Murray radiographic criteria. MAC best describe the ARP in relation to the body's axes and planes. The preceding radiographs of cups placed in plastic hemipelvis demonstrate the important errors in measurement of true ARP when MRC are used. Even without available software, the calculation for MAC inclination and anteversion from radiographs is not significantly more difficult than for MRC. Measuring MAC inclination and anteversion requires 3 linear measurements and 2 divisions that lead to 2 sin values. Measuring MRC inclination and anteversion requires one angle measurement, 2 linear measurements, and 1 division that lead to 1 sin value. The ideal methodology, however, is widely available as software that can give accurate results during or following surgery. Real-time measurement of MAC inclination and anteversion during surgery by software is the highest standard.

Comments on Pelvic Tilt

There has been a recent emphasis on measuring pelvic tilt in patients who undergo THA. First, keep in mind that most of the research and work on this subject in relation to THA has been driven by posterior approach surgeons. Pelvic tilt is the latest "bogeyman" upon which posterior surgeons blame their dislocations [23]. With AA THA, dislocation has been almost entirely solved with the muscle preservation of AA and the accurate acetabular positioning that is possible with supine X-ray [24–26]. Despite the above, understanding pelvic tilt can help us tune things a little better and also identify a small proportion of problem cases.

Pelvic tilt refers to flexion–extension of the pelvis or rotation of the pelvis around the transverse (X) axis. Pelvic tilt can also be referred to as pelvic pitch. Positional changes in pelvic tilt (variances in tilt between, supine, standing, sitting, squatting) are an adaptive and positive function of hip and lumbar spine mobility.

With the patient standing, a normal tilt is defined as the anterior pelvic plane (plane determined by both anterior superior spines and pubic tubercles) parallel to a vertical line or when supine, the plane is parallel to a horizontal line [27]. With positive pelvic tilt, both ASIS are anterior to the pubic tubercles. With negative pelvic tilt both ASIS are posterior to the pubic tubercles. We can also think of pelvic tilt as the angle of the pelvic plane to the body's y-axis.

Does the degree of pelvic tilt that is measured for an individual patient influence the surgeon's target for acetabular rotational position (ARP)? There are exceptions, but the simple answer is no. ARP is not in relation to the pelvis (tilt or unique anatomy) but rather in relation to the body (its x-, y-, and z-axes and/or its planes: coronal, sagittal, and transverse). Pelvic tilt has been measured as average = 4.2° (range −20.5–24.5) [28]. Pelvic tilt will normally vary between individuals, however, the same methodology as described in this chapter, placing the cup according to the c-arm image and software should be utilized regardless if the individual's pelvic tilt is neutral, positive, or negative. Acetabular landmarks (anterior and posterior rim contours, transverse acetabular ligament orientation) will also vary between patients and an abnormality may be the reason for arthritis, or the original rim contour may be altered by addition of bone with osteophytes or subtraction of bone with wear. Therefore, acetabular landmarks are only a general or secondary guide to ARP and are usually ignored. The anterior bony rim should cover the anterior cup rim but achieving this is a function of depth of reaming and cup size, not changing ARP.

The degree of pelvic tilt seen on X-ray can vary between supine, standing, and sitting. The senior author often hears that the cup should be placed in the ideal position of inclination and anteversion for standing and its attendant degree of pelvic tilt because standing is the "functional" position. This argument is fallacious because the ideal position of the cup for standing would be zero degrees inclination so that weight-bearing would be perpendicular to the cup face for ideal wear and load distribution. The problem with this position is that the hip would predictably impinge and dislocate when the patient sat and flexed 90°. The fact is that the cup is not placed in an ideal position for any one hip position or activity but rather in a compromise position that accommodates a wide variety of hip positions and activities while not dislocating and minimizing wear. Since the patient is supine at surgery, using the supine pelvic position as the reference for ARP is most expeditious and logical. Also, recommendations for ARP derived from essentially all published data regarding cup position are based on supine plane films or CT so these data cannot automatically be applied to standing X-rays.

Keeping in mind the concept that pelvic tilt is the angle of the pelvic plane to the y-axis does pelvic tilt vary as an individual adopts different positions? Yes, the flexion–extension mobility of a normal lumbosacral spine leads to changes in pelvic tilt. Do these changes increase risk of hip dislocation? No, the reverse is true. Changes in pelvic tilt that are part of observed changes in hip position work to prevent dislocation. When an individual with a normal spine sits and bends the hip 90° the hip joint does not bend the full 90° but only 70–80° and the change in pelvic tilt toward negative accounts for the remainder of hip flexion.

Consider now, an individual with a long fusion of the lumbar spine to the sacrum. Despite changes in hip and body position, pelvic tilt (pelvic plane to y-axis angle) cannot change. The problem to this individual, however, is that all apparent measurements in hip flexion are due to hip motion so that sitting at 90° flexion means 90° flexion of the hip joint.

The point to keep in mind is that positional changes in pelvic tilt are normal and almost always benefit hip stability. Problems with hip stability are more common with fused or very stiff spines where pelvic tilt cannot change. These realities make one ask the question: Are preoperative films that measure changes in pelvic tilt useful? Considering that patients with positional changes in tilt are least likely to dislocate and those with fused spines have no changes but are most likely to dislocate and that when the spine is fused, no new information is acquired by different films that show no change in tilt, and I would conclude that such preoperative evaluation for all patients is not beneficial for the great majority.

For the patient in the senior author's practice that presents without significant lumbosacral spine pathology leading to important changes in spine mobility, the incidence of THA dislocation is less than .01%. How many matched cases would we need to show a statistically significant benefit to preoperative pelvic tilt evaluations?

Should cups be positioned differently for patients with fused or very stiff LS spines versus patients with flexible LS spines? It is my clinical impression that patients with reduced positional changes in pelvic tilt are more likely to experience posterior instability. Because of this clinical observation, the senior author therefore places the cups for stiff lumbar spine patients in slightly more inclination and anteversion (increase values by 2–3°). It is true, however, that the range of cup positions that produce stability is smaller with a limited motion LS spine and increasing inclination and anteversion too much could lead to anterior dislocation.

Radiographic assessment of an implanted cup shows more inclination and anteversion if the patient's pelvic tilt becomes more negative. The reverse is also true. As patients age, there is a tendency for the lumbar spine to lose lordosis and pelvic tilt to become more negative, which leads to increased inclination and anteversion. It is therefore a consideration to implant cups with slightly less inclination and anteversion in younger patients.

It is the senior author's opinion that the current terminology and measurement techniques for pelvic tilt add confusion to the subject and are not ideal. Joint motion is quantified by a measurement between body parts. Knee flexion is measured as the angle between the thigh and leg or radiographically femur and tibia. Hip flexion is measured as the angle between the torso and thigh or radiographically the change in angle between the femur and pelvic plane. It is the senior author's opinion that measuring the angle of the pelvic plane to the X-ray image is a complete departure from orthopedic measurement and also illogical because we are now measuring the rotation of the pelvic plane as it rotates in space, which is dependent on how the body rotates in space (Fig. 20.21).

The senior author proposes that, as with all other measurements of joint motion or change in position, pelvic tilt should be measured in terms of motion in relation to different anatomic parts. An existing measure that can be used is the lumbar lordosis angle (LLA). The lumbar lordosis angle is measured on the lateral radiograph as the angle between the planes of the superior endplates of L1 and S1. Since changes in pelvic tilt are a function of changes in lumbar lordosis, the measurement of positional change in LLA represents the change that occurs in pelvic tilt. LLA range between flexion and extension averages 46.2° (range 0–79.7) (Ref. [28]). Clinically measured hip flexion is the sum of hip joint flexion and lumbar spine flexion (change in pelvic tilt). A very stiff lumbar spine with a small range of LLA thereby requires the prosthetic hip joint to flex farther for a given degree of clinically observed flexion and thereby increasing the risk of dislocation. Simply put, patients with stiff spines are at higher risk of dislocation. If a stiff lumbar spine is suspected, obtain pre-op lateral flexion–extension X-rays and measure the range (observed change) of LLA. Patients with LLA ranges of 10° or less should be considered for a small increase in cup inclination and anteversion and/or a dual mobility bearing.

Fig. 20.21 Clinical hip flexion = lumbar spine flexion + hip flexion, angle of the thigh to the body. This example Illustrates clinical hip flexion of approximately 133°. The lateral X-rays show flexion of the hip joint at 94° (90° change in femur orientation +4° positive change in pelvic tilt. The lateral also shows 38° change in LLA (67–29° = 38°). Change in LLA plus hip joint flexion = 94° + 38° = 132°, which is essentially equal to observed clinical hip flexion (133°). (Reference [28])

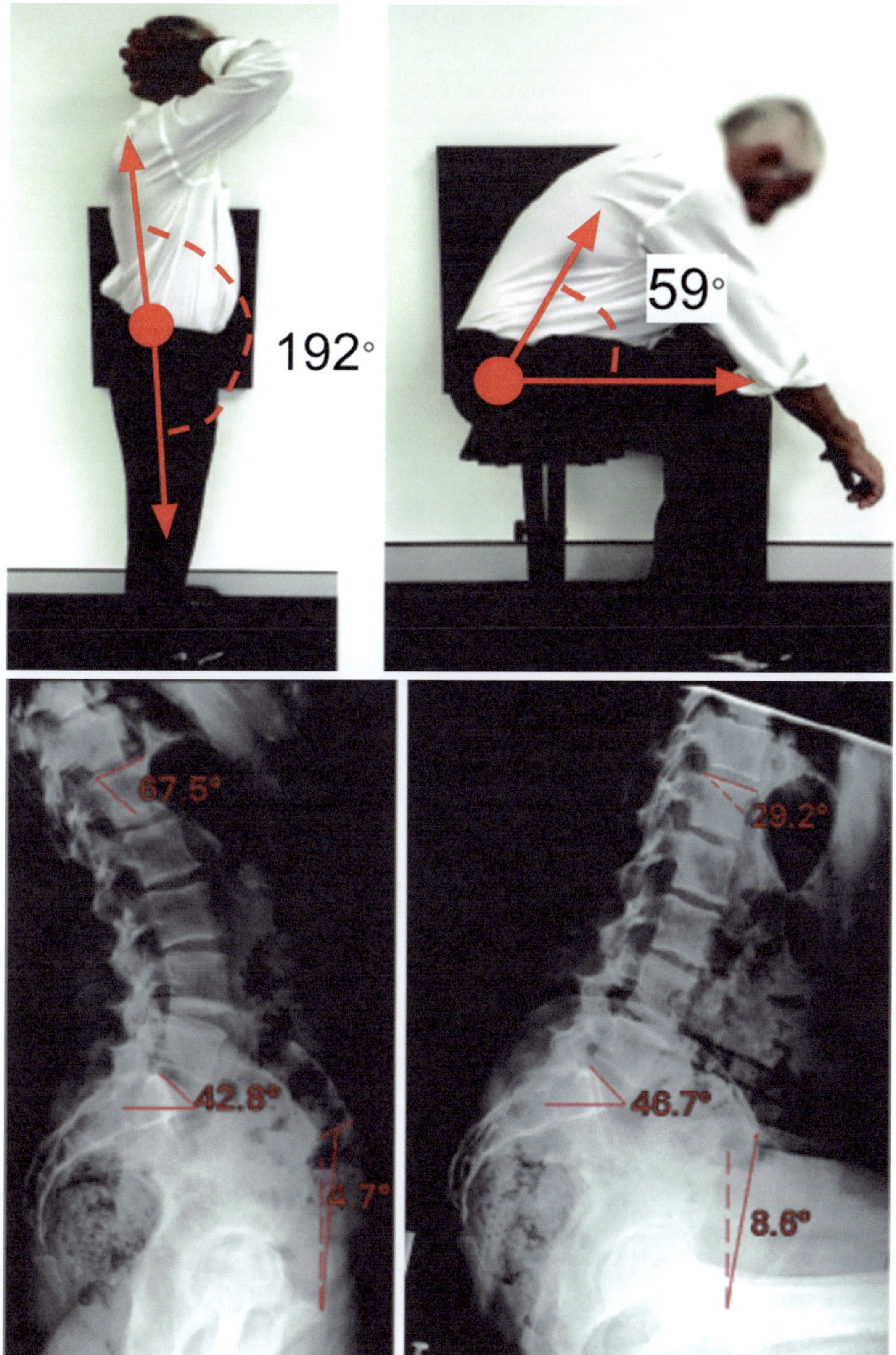
192°
59°
67.5°
42.8°
4.7°
29.2°
46.7°
8.6°

References

1. Abdel MP, von Roth P, Jennings MT, Hanssen AD, Pagnano MW. What safe zone? The vast majority of dislocated THAs are within the Lewinnek safe zone for acetabular component position. Clin Orthop. 2016;474(2):386–91. https://doi.org/10.1007/s11999-015-4432-5.
2. Harrison CL, Thomson AI, Cutts S, Rowe PJ, Riches PE. Research synthesis of recommended acetabular cup orientations for total hip arthroplasty. J Arthroplast. 2014;29(2):377–82. https://doi.org/10.1016/j.arth.2013.06.026.
3. Callanan MC, Jarrett B, Bragdon CR, et al. The John Charnley award: risk factors for cup malpositioning: quality improvement through a joint registry at a tertiary hospital. Clin Orthop Relat Res. 2011;469(2):319–29. https://doi.org/10.1007/s11999-010-1487-1.
4. Reize P, Geiger EV, Suckel A, Rudert M, Wülker N. Influence of surgical experience on accuracy of acetabular cup positioning in total hip arthroplasty. Am J Orthop Belle Mead NJ. 2008;37(7):360–3.
5. Malik A, Wan Z, Jaramaz B, Bowman G, Dorr LD. A validation model for measurement of acetabular component position. J Arthroplast. 2010;25(5):812–9. https://doi.org/10.1016/j.arth.2009.04.021.
6. Dorr LD, Malik A, Dastane M, Wan Z. Combined anteversion technique for total hip arthroplasty. Clin Orthop. 2009;467(1):119–27. https://doi.org/10.1007/s11999-008-0598-4.
7. Derbyshire B. Correction of acetabular cup orientation measurements for X-ray beam offset. Med Eng Phys. 2008;30:1119–26. https://doi.org/10.1016/j.medengphy.2008.02.001.
8. Lewinnek G, Lewis J, Tarr R, Compere C, Zimmerman J. Dislocations after total hip-replacement arthroplasties. J Bone Joint Surg. 1978;60(2):217–20.
9. DelSole EM, Vigdorchik JM, Schwarzkopf R, Errico TJ, Buckland AJ. Total hip arthroplasty in the spinal deformity population: does degree of sagittal deformity affect rates of safe zone placement, instability, or revision? J Arthroplast. 2017;32(6):1910–7. https://doi.org/10.1016/j.arth.2016.12.039.
10. Tannast M, Langlotz U, Siebenrock K-A, Wiese M, Bernsmann K, Langlotz F. Anatomic referencing of cup orientation in total hip arthroplasty. Clin Orthop Relat Res 1976–2007. 2005;436:144–50. https://doi.org/10.1097/01.blo.0000157657.22894.29.
11. Seagrave KG, Troelsen A, Malchau H, Husted H, Gromov K. Acetabular cup position and risk of dislocation in primary total hip arthroplasty. Acta Orthop. 2017;88(1):10–7. https://doi.org/10.1080/17453674.2016.1251255.
12. Bachhal V, Jindal N, Saini G, et al. A new method of measuring acetabular cup anteversion on simulated radiographs. Int Orthop. 2012;36(9):1813–8. https://doi.org/10.1007/s00264-012-1583-9.
13. Lewinnek GE, Lewis JL, Tarr R, et al. Dislocations after total hip replacement arthroplasties. J Bone Joint Surg Am 1978;60(2):217.
14. McCollum DE, Gray WJ. Dislocation after total hip arthroplasty. Causes and prevention. Clin Orthop Relat Res 1990;261:159.
15. Harris W. Advances in surgical technique for total hip replacement: without and with osteotomy of the greater trochanter. Clin Orthop Relat Res 1990;146:188.
16. Pedersen DR, Callaghan JJ, Brown TD. Activity-dependence of the "safe zone" for impingement versus dislocation avoidance. Med Eng Phys 2005;27:323.
17. Jayson MIV. Total hip replacement. Sector Publishing Ltd; 1971 0950145815.
18. Calandruccio RA. Arthroplasty of hip. In: Crenshaw AH, editor. Campbell's Operative Orthopaedics, Vol. 2. St. Louis: CV Mosby; 1987. p. 1213.
19. Canale ST, Beaty JH. Campbell's Operative Orthopaedics. 11th ed. Philadelphia, Pennsylvania: Mosby Elseiver; 2008. 978-0-323-03329-3.
20. Muller SL, Turek. Orthopaedics Priciples and Their Application 4th ed. Philadelphia: J.B. Lippincott Company, 1984. IBSN 0-397-50604-X.
21. Tatka J, Fagotti L, Matta J. Anterior approach total hip replacement (THA) with a specialized orthopedic table. Ann Joint. 2018;3:42. https://doi.org/10.21037/aoj.2018.04.07.
22. Murray D. The definition and measurement of acetabular orientation. J Bone Joint Surg Br. 1993;75-B(2):228–32. https://doi.org/10.1302/0301-620X.75B2.8444942.
23. Buckland AJ, Abotsi EJ, Vasquez-Montes D, Ayres EW, Varlotta CG, Vigdorchik JM. Lumbar spine degeneration and Flatback deformity Alter sitting-standing spinopelvic mechanics—implications for Total hip arthroplasty. J Arthroplast. 2020;35(4):1036–41. https://doi.org/10.1016/j.arth.2019.11.020.
24. Barnett SL, Peters DJ, Hamilton WG, Ziran NM, Gorab RS, Matta JM. Is the anterior approach safe? Early complication rate associated with 5090 consecutive primary Total hip arthroplasty procedures performed using the anterior approach. J Arthroplast. 2016;31(10):2291–4. https://doi.org/10.1016/j.arth.2015.07.008.
25. Matta JM, Shahrdar C, Ferguson T. Single-incision anterior approach for Total hip arthroplasty on an Orthopaedic table. Clin Orthop Relat Res. 2005;441:115–24. https://doi.org/10.1097/01.blo.0000194309.70518.cb.
26. Ji W, Stewart N. Fluoroscopy assessment during anterior minimally invasive hip replacement is more accurate than with the posterior approach. Int Orthop. 2016;40(1):21–7. https://doi.org/10.1007/s00264-015-2803-x.
27. Tannast M, Murphy SB, Langlotz F, Anderson SE, Siebenrock KA. Estimation of pelvic tilt on anteroposterior X-rays—a comparison of six parameters. Skelet Radiol. 2006;35(3):149–55. https://doi.org/10.1007/s00256-005-0050-8.
28. Pierrepont J, Hawdon G, Miles BP, et al. Variation in functional pelvic tilt in patients undergoing total hip arthroplasty. Bone Joint J. 2017;99-B(2):184–91. https://doi.org/10.1302/0301-620X.99B2.BJJ-2016-0098.R1.

Understanding Leg Length and Offset

21

Joseph M. Schwab and Kenoma Anighoro

Background

The primary goal of total hip arthroplasty (THA) is pain relief. Secondary goals include restoration of hip joint function and biomechanics. Beyond replacing degenerative joint surfaces with non-biologic materials, successful hip replacement should maximize functional range of motion, joint stability, muscular force generation, and implant longevity. Suboptimal reconstruction can lead to complications, some of which are predictable, while others may prove difficult to fully understand. Recent epidemiologic studies have shown that mechanical loosening and instability represent the most common indications for revision total hip arthroplasty, accounting for nearly 40% of all revision cases [1, 2]. Careful attention to key implant parameters will ensure mechanical optimization of the joint reconstruction and help avoid these pitfalls. In simple terms, biomechanical optimization of THA can be distilled down to optimization of two summative parameters: offset and leg length. As will be discussed throughout this chapter, however, numerous subfactors contribute to the ultimate biomechanical function of the reconstructed hip: hip center position, vertical offset, femoral offset, acetabular offset, acetabular component orientation, and femoral anteversion. Modularity of total hip components allows intraoperative decision-making and manipulation of these parameters to achieve optimal biomechanical results in the vast majority of cases. However, challenges remain. The anterior approach to the hip as described by Matta et al. [3] offers distinct advantages for optimization of these parameters.

J. M. Schwab (✉)
Department of Orthopaedic Surgery, Medical College of Wisconsin, Milwaukee, WI, USA
e-mail: jmschwab@mcw.edu

K. Anighoro
Arthroplasty & Value-Based Health Care Delivery, University of Texas at Austin—Dell Medical School, Austin, TX, USA

The Importance of Joint Reactive Force

Key predictors of long-term successful hip replacement are optimal joint reactive force, maximal joint stability through a functional range of motion, and leg length symmetry. It is important to know that these predictors are interdependent, and suboptimal management of one or more can compound problems quickly. Studies evaluating the effects of changing parameters of hip arthroplasty suggest that modifications that increase joint reactive force—such as decreased femoral offset or increased acetabular offset—result in increased polyethylene wear [4, 5].

In single-leg stance, the hip joint acts as a fulcrum for balancing the pelvis via the competing forces of abduction and body weight acting on two sides of a seesaw (Fig. 21.1). When these

J. M. Matta, A. P. Sah (eds.), *Anterior Hip Replacement*,
https://doi.org/10.1007/978-3-030-91896-5_21

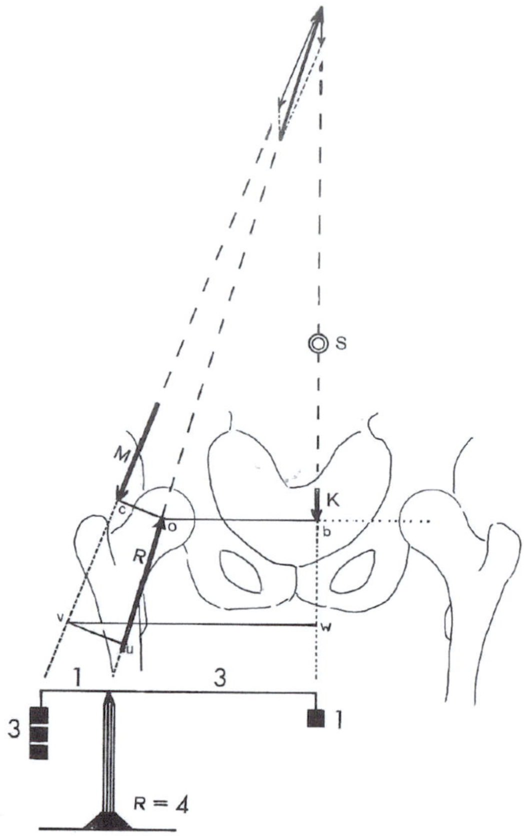

Fig. 21.1 During static load of the hip joint in single leg stance, the lever arm between the center of rotation of the hip and the body center line (o-b) leads to a downward rotational force moment (torque) toward the non-supporting leg produced by body weight. The hip abductor moment counteracts this torque with the respective lever arm (c-o) and abductor force to horizontally stabilize the pelvis—the net torque is equal to zero. The joint center experiences the magnitudes of the counteracting forces as an aggregate load, which represents the joint reactive force (R). In normal conditions, the resultant force (R) passes through the center of the femoral head and forms an angle of 16° to the vertical. The respective magnitude of the total load (R) is dependent on the body weight (K) and the length ratio of the lever arms and results in roughly four times the body weight (original figures from Pauwels) [44] (From Büchler et al. [44]—will need to request permission)

forces are in perfect balance, the hip joint has zero net rotational motion, and the pelvis is stable. The sum of these forces is still experienced by the fulcrum itself, and this combined force is the joint reactive force. Joint reactive force is reduced primarily by modifying the magnitude of

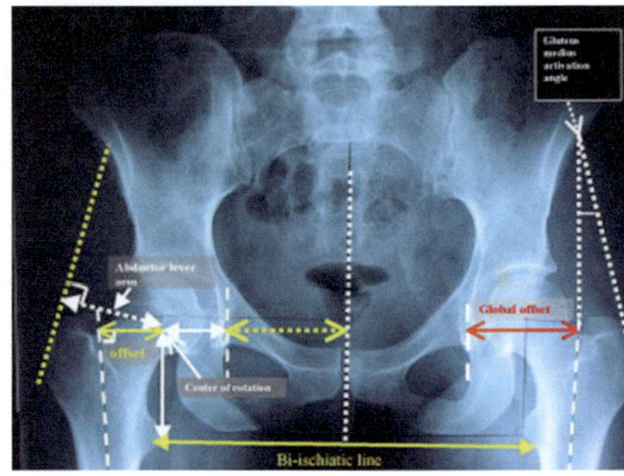

Fig. 21.2 Radiographic measures of offset (femoral and global), abductor muscle lever arm, and angle of abductor muscle activation [6]. (From Lecerf et al. [6] https://doi.org/10.1016/j.otsr.2009.03.010—will need to request permission)

abductor force. Though body weight itself does not change, the body weight moment—the product of body weight and distance of body weight from the hip center—can be modified by varying the medial–lateral position of the hip center. As the hip center is medialized, the body force moment decreases. At the same time, the competing abductor force moment required to maintain net zero torque also decreases. As a result, the joint reactive force decreases. By contrast, if femoral offset is increased while acetabular offset remains constant, lower abductor force is required to produce an appropriate abductor force moment because the lever arm for abduction is increased. This again decreases joint reactive force.

The Relationship Between Femoral Offset, Acetabular Offset, and Abductor Function

Femoral offset is defined as the distance between the center of hip rotation and a line bisecting the femoral shaft. Acetabular offset is the distance between the ipsilateral teardrop (or medial acetabular wall) and the center of hip rotation. Global offset combines these parameters and represents the total distance of the femoral shaft axis from the acetabular medial wall (Fig. 21.2) [6].

Assuming no change in the hip center of rotation, as femoral offset increases, the distance component of the abductor moment increases, conferring increased torque while minimizing change in abductor muscle force [7]. This enhances the efficiency of the abductor musculature to (1) help maintain dynamic joint stability and (2) maintain efficient muscular control of hip position throughout gait cycle. Although global offset increase also improves abductor efficiency by the same mechanism, the increase of acetabular offset by itself has a deleterious effect on abductor efficiency as it simultaneously creates a longer lever arm for body weight. In that scenario, both the abductor moment arm and body weight moment arm increase. As such, a successful reconstruction more likely results when acetabular offset is maintained, or slightly medialized, and femoral offset is optimized to reconstruct anatomic global offset. In most cases, global offset can be determined from the contralateral unaffected hip, as global offset is reasonably symmetric in non-degenerative hips. One radiographic analysis study found a normal distribution of femoral offset and that contralateral hips should fall within −4.62 to +4.62 mm with 95% confidence or two standard deviations (SD = 2.31 mm) [8]. In situations where increased offset is required and acetabular medialization is limited, offset can be modified by changing the femoral neck angle, lateralizing the femoral shaft with an extended offset option, or lengthening the femoral neck (though this also affects leg length). Implants with dual offset options are more likely to allow restoration of sufficient femoral offset because they allow independent manipulation of femoral offset without affecting leg length or acetabular offsets [9].

When abduction and body weight forces are out of balance, gait dysfunction will occur, often manifesting as a Trendelenburg gait. The Trendelenburg gait is characterized by a compensatory leaning of the body toward the side of the weak abductors during the ipsilateral stance phase of gait. This body lean decreases the effective distance of body weight from the hip center and, consequently, decreases the abductor force required to maintain single leg support. A large cohort radiographic analysis study of THA patients found that Trendelenburg-positive THA patients had significantly lower femoral offset (indexed to femoral size) compared to a Trendelenburg-negative group [10].

Cane use also helps to address Trendelenburg gait, as the ground reactive force acting on the cane reduces the net body weight affecting the hip center; this reduces the required abductor force to maintain an upright pelvis [11, 12]. In the words of Dr. Walter Blount: "Don't throw away the cane." [13].

Beyond the impact on muscle tension, a minimum amount of femoral offset is required to ensure that the bony prominences of the proximal femur do not impinge against the pelvis throughout a functional range of motion [14]. A simulation study by Hirata et al. demonstrates this phenomenon. They produced a simulation model based on CT scans of 8 patients and compared 77 hip constructs of various stem anteversion angles (0 to 70 degrees in increments of 10 degrees) and stem tilt (−5 to +5 degrees in increments of 1 degree) and measured the corresponding femoral offset, anterior offset, and max range of motion (flexion, extension, internal rotation at 90 degrees, internal rotation, and external rotation). They found that a minimum femoral offset of 32.1 mm and anterior offset of 15 mm were required to ensure sufficient range of motion without bony impingement [15]. This is consistent with other studies that have found mean native femoral offset of about 34 mm [6]. It is important to note that the simulation study did not incorporate the effects of sagittal pelvic mobility which should enable greater functional range of motion.

Hip Center Position, Vertical Offset, and Leg Length Discrepancy

Soft tissue tension is also impacted by the hip center position and height of the prosthesis. The literature is consistent with regards to which components are highlighted, but there are essentially two independent components of vertical offset: hip center position, or the vertical distance of the center of acetabulum relative to an anatomic reference point on the pelvis; and the distance between the hip center and an anatomic reference point on the ipsilateral femur (Fig. 21.2). These two factors clinically manifest as leg length.

Hip center position may be abnormal preoperatively due to pathology (e.g., developmental dysplasia) or postoperatively due to surgical technique. A hip center that is displaced superiorly will result in a decreased abductor moment arm due to shortening of the abductor length; this effect is modulated if there is also medial–lateral displacement. A biomechanical simulation study by Delp et al. showed that both superolateral and superomedial hip center positions correlate with inferior hip mechanics, but that superolateral position has markedly worse functional impact [16]. The superolateral hip center simultaneously decreases the abductor moment arm and increases the body weight moment arm, creating a substantial force imbalance.

Height of the prosthesis, as determined by the distance between the hip center and an anatomic reference point on the femur, is affected by femoral cut level, femoral stem size, neck length, and head size. Assuming as an unchanged hip center, the prosthetic height should ideally restore the length of resected bone. With near anatomic restoration of soft tissue tension, instability should be avoidable in most cases [9].

Intraoperative Assessment of Leg Length

The optimization of hip center and prosthetic height contributes to the ultimate length of the operated extremity. Leg length discrepancy is associated with worse patient satisfaction, gait abnormalities, and neurologic complications [17, 18]. Leg length discrepancy represents the second most common reason for a litigation suit in the USA, following nerve injury [19]. Leg length discrepancy is not always avoidable. Preoperative assessment may reveal pelvic obliquity due to scoliosis, distal limb length abnormalities, or even distal joint deformities that cannot be addressed.

In degenerative joint conditions, progressive wear of the cartilaginous surfaces of the femoral head and acetabulum can progress to significant bony erosion with functional shortening of the affected limb. Even when a prosthesis is appropriately placed, there can be a perception by some patients of a leg lengthening when radiographic symmetry has been achieved. Perceived leg length discrepancy is also associated with persistent negative effects on patient satisfaction [18].

There are multiple described methods to assess leg length during total hip arthroplasty. These methods range from clinical evaluations (medial malleolar positional symmetry, "shuck tests") to more complex radiographic measurements to methods requiring additional physical equipment or computer software [20–26].

The shuck test is an intraoperative clinical test to judge the gross stability of the hip and soft tissue tension. However, there are no widely accepted recommendations for appropriate shuck distance, and shuck force is expectedly variable among surgeons. Moreover, the value of a shuck maneuver in a patient under anesthetic paralysis is questionable. As such, the most reliable method continues to be radiographic assessment of leg length [22].

While no clear superior method of determining radiographic leg length has emerged in the literature, there are two methods that are worth discussing. The most commonly reported method involves using a standard pelvis radiograph (or fluoroscopic image) and evaluating the distance from a reproducible femoral landmark (e.g., lesser trochanter and greater trochanter) to a line described by two fixed points on the pelvis (e.g., inter-teardrop line, bilateral anterior superior iliac spines, obturators, or ischial tuberosities) (Fig. 21.3a, b). Reproduction of symmetric lesser trochanter distance during (or following) total hip arthroplasty suggests that vertical offset has been reconstituted. While this technique is widely used because of its simplicity and reproducibility, it is nevertheless subject to error. Any asymmetry

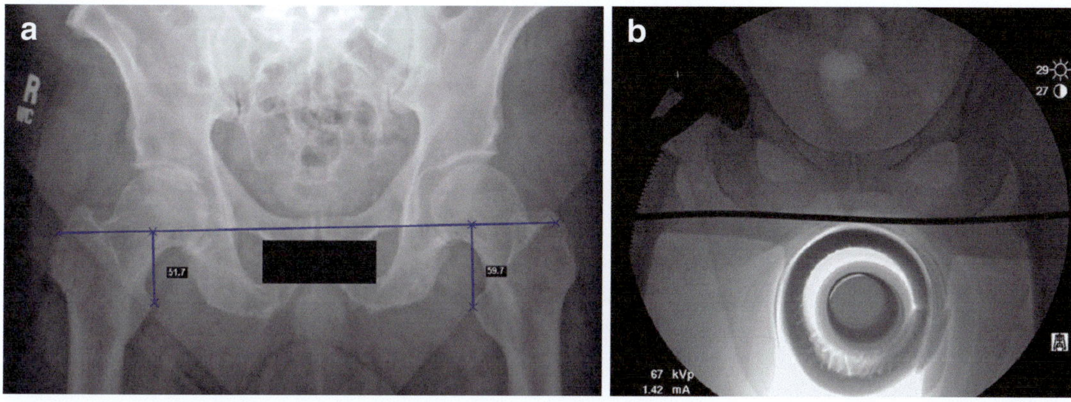

Fig. 21.3 (**a**) Radiographic measurement on standard AP Pelvis radiograph. The inter-teardrop line is marked, and the distances from that line to equivalent points on each lesser trochanter are measured. The difference between those distances is the leg length discrepancy [22]. (**b**) A similar technique to 3a is used intraoperatively by placing a radiopaque straight metal rod transversely across the inferior border of the ischial tuberosities and judging the relative intersection of the rod with the lesser trochanters [20]

inherent in the bony landmarks used in each hemipelvis can contribute to an inappropriate transverse pelvic line from which the distances are measured. Likewise, asymmetry in the femoral landmarks can also lead to unreliable measurements. Depending on the anatomic landmarks used, leg lengths measured with this technique can vary widely when performed on the same radiograph (Fig. 21.4). Finally, any asymmetry of femoral abduction or adduction will affect the reliability of this method; however, this can be corrected intraoperatively by symmetric positioning of the extremities.

Matta et al. described a novel radiographic overlay technique for fluoroscopically assisted intraoperative determination of leg length and offset (Fig. 21.5a, b) [3]. This method uses printed fluoroscopic images, obtained intraoperatively, to directly compare anatomic landmarks by overlaying the two images. This direct overlay has the advantage of being able to simultaneously evaluate changes in both leg length and offset, allowing the surgeon to easily assess and optimize both elements in order to achieve the best possible clinical outcome [27]. Depending on the clinical scenario, the surgeon has the option to overlay the operative hip onto the contralateral hip ("contralateral overlay" technique), to determine symmetry between both sides, or to overlay the operative hip onto the ipsilateral hip prior to surgery ("ipsilateral overlay" technique), to directly measure changes in offset and length from the hip's preoperative state. In cases of substantial pelvic asymmetry (prior surgery, trauma, metabolic bone disease, etc.), the options of both a contralateral and ipsilateral comparison provide greater flexibility for the surgeon to achieve the goals of surgery. While the major disadvantage to this technique is printing and physically overlaying images during surgery, computer-assisted digital implementations of this technique have been developed which both obviate the need for printing images and introduce the possibility of greater precision in leg length and offset measurement (Fig. 21.5c).

Impact of Component Orientation

To minimize risk of instability, placement of the acetabular component should rest within the traditional safe zones as proposed by Lewinnek et al.: 15 +/− 10 degrees anteversion and 40 +/− 10 degrees inclination [28]. Within this zone, it is commonly accepted that dislocation risk should be low. Subsequent studies examining arthroplasty instability have shown that the femoral component anteversion contributes to stability as well, with an ideal position within the range of 15 degrees. The version is often limited by the native

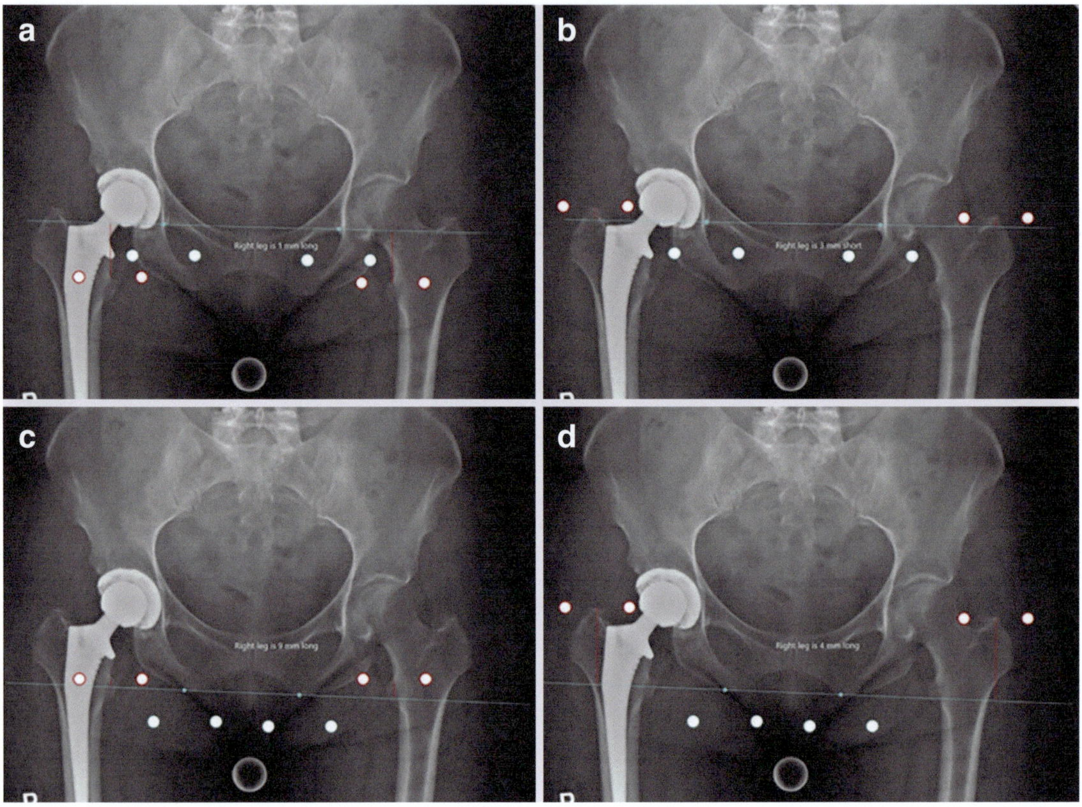

Fig. 21.4 Software evaluation of the same AP Pelvis radiograph using the transverse pelvic line method. Depending on which pelvic and femoral landmarks are used, the leg lengths measured with this technique vary from the right leg being 3 mm short to 9 mm long, a total difference of 1.2 centimeters. (Image Courtesy Dr. Andrew Cooper—used with permission)

morphology of the femoral metaphysis. The concept of combined anteversion encompasses both acetabular and femoral component positions, and numerous studies have shown lower rates of instability when constructs fall within a specific range [29, 30]. Most studies regarding combined anteversion have examined total hip arthroplasties implanted via posterolateral hip approaches, and their methods for radiographic assessment of cup anteversion were variable. For these reasons, the applicability of such recommendations in the context of the anterior hip approach may be limited.

A caveat to femoral anteversion is that the effective position of the abductor insertion is posteriorized and medialized, which functionally reduces the distance component of the abductor moment. As such, in patients with high femoral anteversion, there may be a negative impact on abductor efficiency. This can contribute to higher rates of gait dysfunction or instability postoperatively. As such, the effects of increased femoral offset on improving abductor efficiency tend to be most pronounced in patients with lower femoral anteversion.

While it is true that cup anteversion and combined anteversion are important factors for hip stability, more recent attention has been given to the sagittal clearance of the femur, as impingement can occur in this plane due to pathologic pelvic mobility. A large proportion of late hip instability may be attributable to spinopelvic factors and sagittal clearance [31]. These situations may warrant modifications of cup anteversion and/or inclination to allow for appropriate sagittal clearance of the femur.

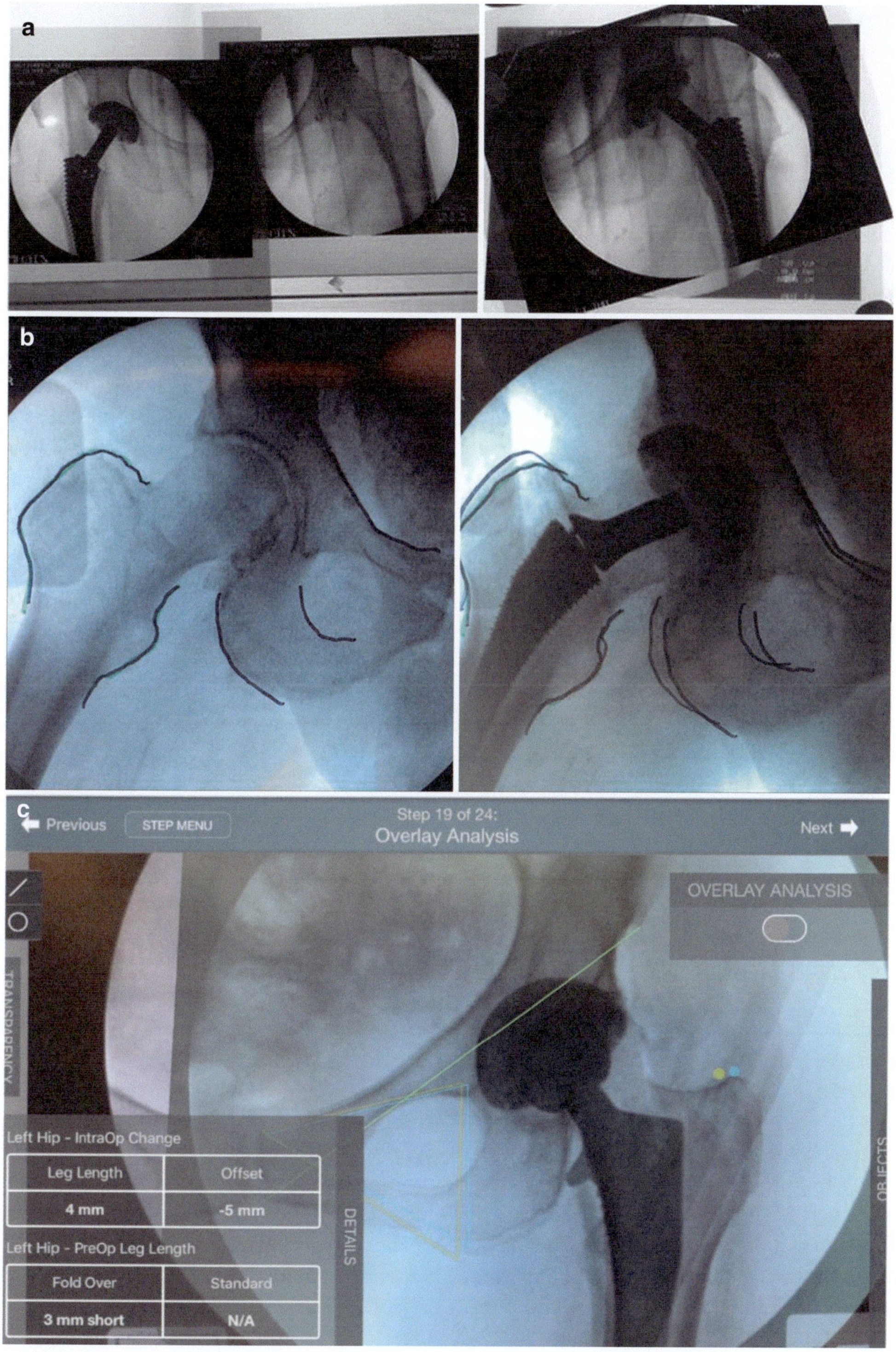

Fig. 21.5 (**a**) Direct radiographic overlay technique uses two printed intraoperative fluoroscopic images that are configured to show the same tilt and rotation of the pelvis. When the radiographs are superimposed, the pelvic anatomy can be aligned to evaluate for leg length and offset based on femoral landmarks [3]. (**b**) Similar overlay technique as illustrated in 3a, but notable pelvic and femoral anatomic landmarks have been highlighted to make comparison of leg length and offset more apparent [20]. (**c**) Digital overlay technique using computer-assisted fluoroscopic navigation. (Downloaded from https://www.jnjmedicaldevices.com/en-US/campaign/velys-digital-surgery/—Courtesy Johnson & Johnson)

Advantages of the Anterior Approach

With respect to the aforementioned considerations of mechanical force balance, limb length discrepancy, and component position, the anterior approach offers distinct advantages. The supine position allows evaluation of the joint in a neutral supine position. Supine positioning on an orthopedic table also allows easy access for intraoperative fluoroscopy. Fluoroscopy can aid with acetabular preparation to ensure appropriate cup medialization and orientation with low variability [23, 32]. Furthermore, it can aid in determination of appropriate femoral offset and leg length prior to final femoral component implantation. This enables a surgeon to use both direct visualization and radiographic evaluation to achieve the desired result.

A major benefit of anterior approach is the maintenance of soft tissue integrity, which theoretically enhances joint stability with less reliance on historical concepts such as combined anteversion employed during posterior approach arthroplasty. As mentioned earlier, inappropriately increased anteversion tends to decrease abductor tension and can cause mechanical impingement. Taken together, preserved soft tissue restraint and relatively low anteversion lends to a more mechanically efficient reconstruction. It has been shown that hip instability rates after anterior approach are low [33, 34].

Limitations of the Anterior Approach

The supine anterior approach may limit some previously routine intraoperative clinical assessments. When using an orthopedic table, for example, connection of the operative extremity to the table spar limits free intraoperative hip ranging to perform traditional stability tests. While the lower extremity boot can be disconnected from the spar to perform stability testing, this is not routinely done. In contrast, range of motion testing can be routinely performed in the lateral decubitus position during a posterior approach procedure to look for impingement or soft tissue laxity. Alternatively, by pursuing anterior approach on a standard table, with the entire extremity prepped into the surgical field, the surgeon could achieve the aforementioned soft tissue benefits while allowing access to manipulate the entire extremity. Even with these limitations, however, large multi-surgeon series show that instability rates with anterior approach are favorable compared to posterior approach [35].

There are complications that are reportedly more common in the anterior approach, such as femoral perforation, femoral fracture, and nerve dysfunction due to lateral femoral cutaneous or femoral nerve dysfunction. There is also an apparent learning curve for surgeons new to the approach, with significantly increased revision rates found patients for patient cohorts within the first set of 50 cases [36]. Early observational studies showed that complications such as periprosthetic fracture occurred more commonly with the anterior approach [37], but more recent analysis suggests that complication rates diminish with increasing surgeon experience [38].

Barriers to Implant Optimization

Optimizing the offset and length parameters of the hip reconstruction is enabled by modularity of components. The quest for biomechanical optimization has led to the development of highly modular implant designs which allow for independent variation of offset, length, and femoral anteversion. Unfortunately, many of these have been recalled due to high complication and revision [39, 40]. Recognizing these risks, there has been a shift toward streamlined implant modularity in primary total hip arthroplasty—limiting modularity to monolithic femoral stems, femoral heads, acetabular liners, and cups. Femoral neck adapters are added to allow further customization of soft tissue tension through neck length, and most modern primary hip systems have a high- and standard-offset monolithic stem option. To most accurately reproduce the biomechanical parameters described in this chapter, a higher degree of component variation incorporating a non-binary range of femoral offset options would be ideal, but obviously logistically cumbersome. Fortunately, the refined modularity of modern primary hip implants allows reasonable optimization in most cases.

Biomechanical Implications of Hip Dysplasia

In severe hip dysplasia, there may be chronic subluxation of the hip joint. Re-establishing an appropriate hip center may substantially lengthen the extremity from the preoperative state. This not only changes gait dynamics, but can also contribute to stretch neuropraxia, which may manifest as foot drop. It is advised in these cases to limit lengthening to less than 4 cm, 10% of the femur length, or to perform a concomitant femoral shortening osteotomy [41]. There also tends to be increased native acetabular and femoral anteversion. Often this can be addressed with careful attention to the orientation of both components and optimizing combined anteversion [42]. In some cases, however, very high native femoral anteversion may not be modifiable with use of standard monolithic cementless femoral stems. As mentioned earlier, anteversion tends to counteract some of the benefits of increased femoral or global offset, functionally diminishing soft tissue tension predisposing to instability. This may be compounded by increased combined anteversion from a properly placed acetabular component and natively high femoral anteversion, such that these constructs may be at greater risk for anterior dislocation in this patient population. This is particularly concerning in the anterior approach, where the anterior capsule is violated. The standard anterior approach does not explicitly recommend anterior capsular repair, and it remains unclear whether capsule management has an impact even in the case of dysplasia. To mitigate these risks, one could consider femoral derotational osteotomy, diaphyseal fixing stems with customizable anteversion, or a cemented femoral stems to allow optimization of femoral component position [6].

Central Nervous System Disorders

In a well-balanced hip where the vertical and lateral offsets of the femur are appropriate, muscular tension provides dynamic stability. In central nervous system disorders such as cerebrovascular accident, cerebral palsy, traumatic brain injury, and spinal cord injury, the muscular force balance is disrupted [43]. In such cases, even a radiographically optimal joint reconstruction can lead to suboptimal clinical outcomes. Satisfactory outcomes can be achieved by modifying the surgical plan to accommodate the pathology—select use of soft tissue releases, modular implants, dual-mobility or constrained prostheses, or cemented prostheses. Preoperative evaluation and a catered operative plan will help to diminish complications from these comorbidities. Perioperative physical therapy is of great benefit in these scenarios.

Author Experience

In the authors' collective experience, there are several key learning points about leg length, offset, and anterior approach hip replacement. First, there is inherent stability in utilizing an internervous and intermuscular approach for hip replacement as it allows minimal disturbance, release, or reflection of key hip stabilizers. The success of the anterior approach has challenged the long-standing teaching that stability comes primarily through increasing soft tissue tension via increased leg length and offset. While those tools remain in the toolbox of all hip surgeons, it is a rare event where a well-performed hip replacement from an anterior approach would benefit from increasing leg length and offset beyond normal anatomic restoration.

Second, patients undergoing anterior approach hip arthroplasty seem to be more keenly aware of even slight increases in leg length and, especially, offset. It is possible that a number of factors contribute to this perceived sensitivity including: improved preservation of periarticular proprioception, less surgical "relief" of the lateral soft tissue structures (hip deltoid and iliotibial band) compared to other approaches, lower likelihood of inappropriate lateralization of the hip center with the use of fluoroscopy, and maintenance of the medializing "pull" provided by the short external rotators. Whatever the true causes, it is important to remember that the goal of anterior approach arthroplasty is anatomic restoration.

Finally, anterior approach hip replacement enables the use of simple and effective methods to maximize anatomical and biomechanical restoration of the hip joint. The surgical technique is both effective and reproducible, and high operative consistency can be attained with the use of a dedicated orthopedic table. Additionally, the routine use of intraoperative fluoroscopy, or other more advanced navigation techniques, allows the surgeon to reliably execute an individualized plan for each patient.

Conclusion

Myriad factors influence the biomechanical stability and function of the reconstructed hip. Femoral offset and leg length optimization appear to have the most significant impact. In routine hip arthroplasty for degenerative conditions, the anterior approach to the hip offers the unique advantage of convenient intraoperative radiographic assessment of hip center, component orientation, femoral offset, and leg length. Additionally, the anterior approach allows posterior soft tissue preservation. There are important limitations, however, which should be considered before implementation, especially in arthroplasty cases complicated by neuromuscular disorders or substantial deformity.

References

1. Bozic KJ, Kurtz SM, Lau E, Ong K, Vail TP, Berry DJ. The epidemiology of revision total hip arthroplasty in the United States. J Bone Joint Surg (American). 2009;91(1):128–33.
2. Gwam CU, Mistry JB, Mohamed NS, Thomas M, Bigart KC, Mont MA, et al. Current epidemiology of revision total hip arthroplasty in the United States: National Inpatient Sample 2009 to 2013. J Arthroplast. 2017;32(7):2088–92.
3. Matta JM, Shahrdar C, Ferguson T. Single-incision anterior approach for total hip arthroplasty on an orthopaedic table. Clin Orthop Relat Res. 2005;441(&NA):115–24.
4. Sakalkale DP, Sharkey PF, Eng K, Hozack WJ, Rothman RH. Effect of femoral component offset on polyethylene wear in total hip arthroplasty. Clin Orthop Relat Res. 2001;388(388):125–34.
5. Karachalios T, Hartofilakidis G, Zacharakis N, Tsekoura M. A 12- to 18-year radiographic follow-up study of Charnley low-friction arthroplasty. The role of the center of rotation. Clin Orthop Relat Res. 1993;296:140–7.
6. Lecerf G, Fessy MH, Philippot R, Massin P, Giraud F, Flecher X, et al. Femoral offset: anatomical concept, definition, assessment, implications for preoperative templating and hip arthroplasty. Orthop Traumatol Surg Res. 2009;95(3):210–9.
7. McGrory BJ, Morrey BF, Cahalan TD, An KN, Cabanela ME. Effect of femoral offset on range of motion and abductor muscle strength after total hip arthroplasty. J Bone Joint Surg. 1995;77(6):865–9.
8. Krishnan SP, Carrington RWJ, Mohiyaddin S, Garlick N. Common misconceptions of normal hip joint relations on pelvic radiographs. J Arthroplast. 2006;21(3):409–12.
9. Bourne RB. arthroplasty CHRTJo. Soft tissue balancing: the hip. Elsevier.
10. Asayama I, Naito M, Fujisawa M, Kambe T. Relationship between radiographic measurements of reconstructed hip joint position and the Trendelenburg sign. J Arthroplast. 2002;17(6):747–51.
11. Ajemian S, Thon D, Clare P, Kaul L, Zernicke RF, Loitz-Ramage B. Cane-assisted gait biomechanics and electromyography after total hip arthroplasty. Arch Phys Med Rehabil. 2004;85(12):1966–71.
12. Krebs DE, Robbins CE, Lavine L, Mann RW. Hip biomechanics during gait. J Orthop Sports Phys Ther. 1998;28(1):51–9.
13. Blount WP. Don't throw away the cane. J Bone Joint Surg. 1956;38-A(3):695–708.
14. Jinno T, Koga D, Asou Y, Morita S, Okawa A, Muneta T. Intraoperative evaluation of the effects of femoral component offset and head size on joint stability in total hip arthroplasty. J Orthop Surg (Hong Kong). 2017;25(1):2309499016684298.
15. Hirata M, Nakashima Y, Hara D, Kanazawa M, Kohno Y, Yoshimoto K, et al. Optimal anterior femoral offset for functional range of motion in total hip arthroplasty--a computer simulation study. Int Orthop. 2015;39(4):645–51.
16. Delp SL, Wixson RL, Komattu AV, Kocmond JH. How superior placement of the joint center in hip arthroplasty affects the abductor muscles. Clin Orthop Relat Res. 1996;328(328):137–46.
17. Konyves A, Bannister GC. The importance of leg length discrepancy after total hip arthroplasty. J Bone Joint Surg. 2005;87(2):155–7.

18. Wylde V, Whitehouse SL, Taylor AH, Pattison GT, Bannister GC, Blom AW. Prevalence and functional impact of patient-perceived leg length discrepancy after hip replacement. Int Orthop. 2009;33(4):905–9.
19. Bokshan SL, Ruttiman RJ, DePasse JM, Eltorai AEM, Rubin LE, Palumbo MA, et al. Reported litigation associated with primary hip and knee arthroplasty. J Arthroplast. 2017;32(12):3573–7.e1.
20. Austin DC, Dempsey BE, Kunkel ST, Torchia MT, Jevsevar DS. A comparison of radiographic leg-length and offset discrepancies between 2 intraoperative measurement techniques in anterior total hip arthroplasty. Arthroplasty Today. 2019;5(2):181–6.
21. Bitar YFE, Stone JC, Jackson TJ, Lindner D, Stake CE, Domb BG. Leg-length discrepancy after total hip arthroplasty: comparison of robot-assisted posterior, fluoroscopy-guided anterior, and conventional posterior approaches. PMID - 26046996. Am J Orthop (Belle Mead NJ). 2015;44(6):265–9.
22. Debbi EM, Rajaee SS, Mayeda BF, Penenberg BL. Determining and achieving target limb length and offset in total hip arthroplasty using intraoperative digital radiography. J Arthroplast. 2020;35(3):779–85.
23. Gililland JM, Anderson LA, Boffeli SL, Pelt CE, Peters CL, Kubiak EN. A fluoroscopic grid in supine total hip arthroplasty: improving cup position, limb length, and hip offset. J Arthroplast. 2012;27(8 Suppl):111–6.
24. Herisson O, Felden A, Hamadouche M, Anract P, Biau DJ. Validity and reliability of intraoperative radiographs to assess leg length during total hip arthroplasty: correlation and reproducibility of anatomic distances. J Arthroplast. 2016;31(12):2784–8.
25. Keršič M, Dolinar D, Antolič V, Mavčič B. The impact of leg length discrepancy on clinical outcome of total hip arthroplasty: comparison of four measurement methods. J Arthroplast. 2013;29(1):137–41.
26. Sayed-Noor AS, Hugo A, Sjödén GO, Wretenberg P. Leg length discrepancy in total hip arthroplasty: comparison of two methods of measurement. Int Orthop. 2008;33(5):1189–93.
27. Innmann MM, Maier MW, Streit MR, Grammatopoulos G, Bruckner T, Gotterbarm T, et al. Additive influence of hip offset and leg length reconstruction on postoperative improvement in clinical outcome after total hip arthroplasty. J Arthroplast. 2018;33(1):156–61.
28. Lewinnek GE, Lewis JL, Tarr R, Compere CL, Zimmerman JR. Dislocations after total hip-replacement arthroplasties. J Bone Joint Surg. 1978;60(2):217–20.
29. Jolles BM, Zangger P, Leyvraz PF. Factors predisposing to dislocation after primary total hip arthroplasty: a multivariate analysis. J Arthroplast. 2002;17(3):282–8.
30. Nakashima Y, Hirata M, Akiyama M, Itokawa T, Yamamoto T, Motomura G, et al. Combined anteversion technique reduced the dislocation in cementless total hip arthroplasty. Int Orthop. 2014;38(1):27–32.
31. Heckmann N, McKnight B, Stefl M, Trasolini NA, Ike H, Dorr LD. Late dislocation following total hip arthroplasty: spinopelvic imbalance as a causative factor. J Bone Joint Surg (American). 2018;100(21):1845–53.
32. Lin TJ, Bendich I, Ha AS, Keeney BJ, Moschetti WE, Tomek IM. A comparison of radiographic outcomes after total hip arthroplasty between the posterior approach and direct anterior approach with intraoperative fluoroscopy. J Arthroplast. 2017;32(2):616–23.
33. Maratt JD, Gagnier JJ, Butler PD, Hallstrom BR, Urquhart AG, Roberts KC. No difference in dislocation seen in anterior vs posterior approach total hip arthroplasty. J Arthroplast. 2016;31(9 Suppl):127–30.
34. White RE, Forness TJ, Allman JK, Junick DW. Effect of posterior capsular repair on early dislocation in primary total hip replacement. Clin Orthop Relat Res. 2001;393(393):163–7.
35. Charney M, Paxton EW, Stradiotto R, Lee JJ, Hinman AD, Sheth DS, et al. A comparison of risk of dislocation and cause-specific revision between direct anterior and posterior approach following elective Cementless total hip arthroplasty. J Arthroplast. 2020;35(6):1651–7.
36. Steiger RN, Lorimer M, Solomon M. What is the learning curve for the anterior approach for total hip arthroplasty? Clin Orthop Relat Res. 2015;473(12):3860–6.
37. Lee G-C, Marconi D. Complications following direct anterior hip procedures: costs to both patients and surgeons. J Arthroplast. 2015;30(9 Suppl):98–101.
38. Investigators ATHAC, Bhandari M, Matta JM, Dodgin D, Clark C, Kregor P, et al. Outcomes following the single-incision anterior approach to total hip arthroplasty: a multicenter observational study. Orthop Clin North Am. 2009;40(3):329–42.
39. Molloy DO, Munir S, Jack CM, Cross MB, Walter WL, Walter WK. Fretting and corrosion in modular-neck total hip arthroplasty femoral stems. J Bone Joint Surg (American). 2014;96(6):488–93.
40. Nawabi DH, Do HT, Ruel A, Lurie B, Elpers ME, Wright T, et al. Comprehensive analysis of a recalled modular total hip system and recommendations for management. J Bone Joint Surg (American). 2016;98(1):40–7.
41. Nagoya S, Kaya M, Sasaki M, Tateda K, Kosukegawa I, Yamashita T. Cementless total hip replacement with subtrochanteric femoral shortening for severe developmental dysplasia of the hip. J Bone Joint Surg. 2009;91(9):1142–7.
42. Zhang J, Wang L, Mao Y, Li H, Ding H, Zhu Z. The use of combined anteversion in total hip arthroplasty for patients with developmental dysplasia of the hip. J Arthroplast. 2014;29(3):621–5.
43. Queally JM, Abdulkarim A, Mulhall KJ. Total hip replacement in patients with neurological conditions. J Bone Joint Surg. 2009;91(10):1267–73.
44. Büchler L, Tannast M, Siebenrock KA, Schwab JM. Biomechanics of the hip. In: Proximal femur fractures. 93. Springer International Publishing; 2017. p. 9–15.

Part IV

Introduction to Part IV

Anterior Approach: The Variation of Techniques and Technologies

Since the term anterior approach only refers to the incision, there is inevitably wide variation in the details of various method for AA. Part II grouped chapters on methodology together that were all similar in their use of the orthopedic table and real-time fluoroscopy for confirmation of accuracy. Anterior approach is also performed and advocated by other methods with various advocated potential advantages. A basic question that arises is: is AA best performed by changing only the incision while keeping manual extremity control and clinical assessment of accuracy or should we look at AA as a pathway to new methods and technologies including robotics, mechanical substitutes for assistants, and computer guidance?

The reader should keep in mind that when methods vary widely, each method is most likely most effective when followed in its entirety. Trying to combine pieces of different methods may have a less certain outcome.

The final future directions of AA are unknown and will probably be multiple; however, knowledge of the spectrum of variations is important. Clinical data as well as market forces will guide the future.

22 The Anterior Approach: From Robert Judet's Work to AMIS® (Anterior Minimally Invasive Surgery)

Frédéric Laude

The history of the hip anterior approach begins in Germany. Carl Hueter offers a description of it as early as in the 1870s [1]. The development of anesthesia at that time encouraged the development of most of the approaches that we know today for the various joints.

The anterior approach, which passes between the posterior muscles innervated by the gluteal nerve and the thigh muscles innervated by the crural nerve, rapidly became a classic method in hip surgery. It was Smith Petersen [2], a surgeon of Norwegian origin, who spent most of his surgical life in the USA, who popularized the approach to the point that we often speak of Smith Petersen to indicate this intermuscular, internervous approach.

This was the most commonly used approach in the first half of the twentieth century. The era of prosthetic arthroplasties had not yet begun. It is rather surprising, researching the JBJS archives, to read about Alexander Gibson [3] who was well known for his work in posterior approaches at the time, complaining about the lack of knowledge of the posterior hip approach in the USA.

In the 1930s, Henri Judet (1874–1943) developed a special table (Fig. 22.1) that allowed most orthopedic procedures. In quite a spontaneous manner, Robert Judet (1909–1980) [4, 5] and his brother Jean Judet (1905–1995) used their father's orthopedic table to perform hip surgery in 1947 [6], and, of course, through the usual approach, i.e., the anterior approach. Unfortunately, the first acrylic hip prostheses did not have the desired result whatsoever, but although the material of the prostheses has changed greatly over time, the Judet brothers have nevertheless remained faithful to Hueter's method for all their arthroplasty.

The "Hueter gaine"is one of the first modifications that Robert Judet introduced in the practice of this approach to avoid damaging the lateral nerve of the thigh. He shifted the incision toward the outer surface of the thigh by 3 or 4 centimeters by passing through the sleeve of the tensor fascia lata rather than between the sartorius and tensor muscle, thus protecting in the vast majority of cases the lateral nerve of the thigh from iatrogenic injury. The Judet brothers have developed many orthopedic devices and have tried to improve the table developed by their father, but this table, whose design is now almost 80 years old, was still being used recently by some Parisian surgeons.

In the following years, many French surgeons did not publish their work in English journals, which is highly unfortunate. The first real publication on the anterior approach was in French, in 1985 [7], and it was not even in a surgical journal. Why publish a study about a surgical procedure

F. Laude (✉)
Clinique du sport, Paris, France

J. M. Matta, A. P. Sah (eds.), *Anterior Hip Replacement*,
https://doi.org/10.1007/978-3-030-91896-5_22

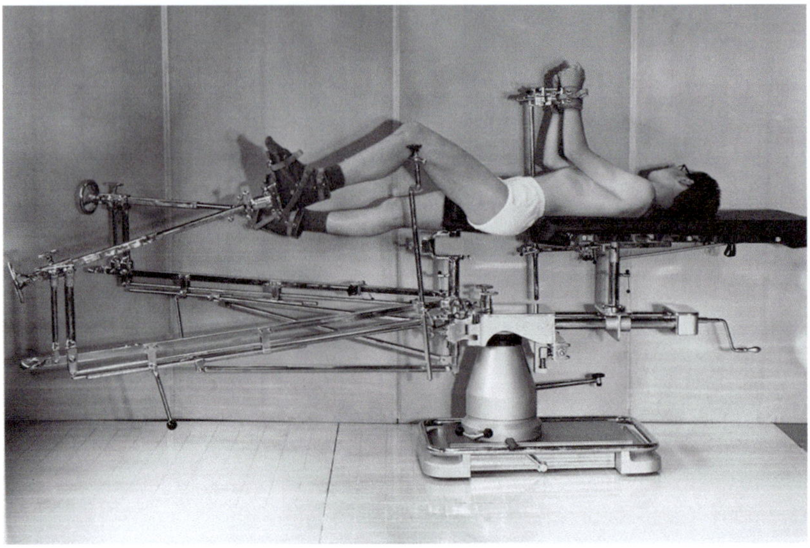

Fig. 22.1 1947: the classic Judet table (Marzet) with its deformable parallelogram design in the late 30s by Henri Judet

that had been routinely performed on a daily basis for over 30 years?

In the 1960s, the work of John Charnley [8] and the simple technique of the posterior approach became more prevalent than the anterior approach on the orthopedic table.

Robert Judet founded an actual surgical school, the Garchoise school, named after the town near Paris where the hospital was located, which became the origin of many innovations in both traumatology and orthopedics in France. The organization of a congress every year crowned the inventive spirit and the prolixity of its founder. This includes work on external fixators, especially hip prostheses. The first cementless hip [9] prosthesis and the removable femur heads on morse taper originated here [10]. Robert Judet developed many different models over the years, but unfortunately it is an understatement to say that these efforts were not always successful. The repeated failures gave quite a bad reputation to everything having to do with the implantation of a hip prosthesis in Garches, and the anterior approach certainly paid the price. The work of John Charnley [11, 12] and the competing Parisian team in Paris, the School of Cochin (Merle d'Aubigné, Kerboull), prevailed over many of the techniques developed in Garches [13]. At the time, I was an intern at Cochin Hospital, and although I did not find the inventive genius that could be found at Garches, there existed a rigor and a methodology that certainly the Judet brothers were lacking.

Robert Judet's most famous student is certainly Emile Letournel (1927–1994) [14], who revolutionized the treatment of acetabular and pelvic fractures. Emile Letournel [15], a brilliant surgeon, a hard worker, and much more rigorous than his master, also worked intensively on hip prostheses.

Disappointed by what he had seen in Garches in terms of arthroplasty and influenced by Charnley's work, he developed with his friend Jean Lagrange one of the first modern hip prostheses [16], which was a great commercial success in the 1980s in France.

Emile Letournel also developed a modern orthopedic table based on his experience (Fig. 22.2). The production of a radiolucent table, which facilitated the surgery of acetabular fractures, but which also made it possible to implant prostheses from the front, ceased in the mid-1990s, after the company that produced them went bankrupt.

It was impossible to obtain a new table for anterior prosthesis in 1995. Those who were fortunate enough to have one tried to maintain it in the best possible condition, and the others switched to the posterior approach, which had become the gold standard: the way to do

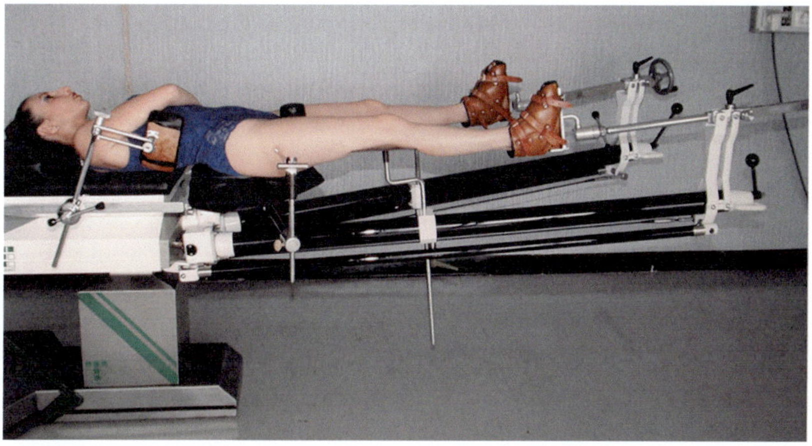

Fig. 22.2 1982: The Letournel traction table (Tasserit). Radiotransparent

everything! Letournel's table is at the origin of Joël Matta's work, who was able to improve it and to make it popular in the USA.

Although I did not meet Robert Judet, who died in 1980, I had the chance to meet Emile Letournel in 1989, 5 years before he passed away in 1994. I was immediately seduced by his very modern yet demanding vision of surgery. What seemed complicated elsewhere was simple with him.

Of course, I had seen posterior hip replacements in my training, and to say the least, this surgery did not really interest me. There is a certain "violence" in the placement of a hip prosthesis that in the end one tends to forget, but as a young intern who wanted to do hand surgery, I was not fascinated by this technique at all.

I later met surgeons who did the posterior approach elegantly, but it was too late. Most of them, by the way, switched to the anterior approach quite easily. Nothing is more elegant than a well-done anterior approach! In 1989, Emile Letournel had 40 years of experience in orthopedic table hip surgery.

He hated doing posterior approaches, and almost all the hips in his practice were operated on Judet table: prostheses, osteotomies, and acetabular fractures [17]. He had developed special tools to perform septic revisions [18], but at the time the enemies were mainly cement and polyethylene granulomas. The cementless prosthesis was in its infancy, and most revisions involved the acetabulum and the extraction of distal cement fragments.

The discovery of the anterior approach and acetabular cup surgery totally reconciled me with the hip and even made me forget about the upper limb. From hand surgery and Letournel's teaching, I have retained the fundamental respect for the soft tissue, that is, the cornerstone of any orthopedic surgery after all. In the anterior approaches, there is always an interesting and delicate dissection time. Knowledge of anatomy is important. Since I do not have an exceptionally strong build and I do not like to rely upon my assistants to do this part of the work, the table is an indispensable aid in the manipulation of the operated limb.

The 1990s is also the time when people started to talk about minimally invasive surgery. It is the beginning of laparoscopy and active arthroscopy.

Emile Letournel, who was always a step ahead of time, had bought all the equipment to do hip arthroscopy, but unfortunately he did not have time to really take an interest in it. He died rather suddenly in August 1994 when I was a young assistant in his department and, surprisingly, I was asked to replace him in the interim, while we were organizing a proper succession. Only 33 years old, I found myself at the head of one of the most prestigious departments in Paris with a large number of cases, some of which were honestly rather complex to handle.

After a few intense months, I had to do my fellowship with another student of Robert Judet, Professor Raymond Roy Camille. I became friends with his associate, Professor Jean-Pierre Benazet [19, 20], who was interested in minimally invasive spine surgery.

It was 1994, and it seemed obvious to me that we had to be able to apply these principles to the hip prosthesis. The notion of minimally invasive surgery was a totally incomprehensible concept for Emile Letournel, who did not close his patients himself. But the idea of reducing the size of the incisions (and therefore closing them more quickly), limiting bleeding, and having the patients stand more rapidly was very appealing. And the anterior approach seemed to be the ideal solution to do so. We lacked the good retractors, the good tools, but simply with what we had at our disposal, we could do a lot. All the ancillary instruments allow performing of the posterior approaches, but fortunately, as a good student of Robert Judet, Professor Roy Camille did his hip prostheses on an orthopedic table. It was not Hueter's way, but rather a kind of Watson Jones's way, which was very similar to what we will later be called the Roetinger's way [21].

Having already quite a good experience of the anterior approach, I started to perform some difficult cases like Crowe 3 and 4 dislocations [22, 23]. At the end of my fellowship, I was offered a place in an excellent institution that I could not refuse. But once I was there, I realized that it was missing the famous orthopedic table I needed to do my hip prostheses. The management of the establishment did not want to invest in it, and in any case, there was not such a table available on the market. Joel Matta's table was not yet available at this time [24] (Fig. 22.3).

I implanted a few prostheses without the table, persisting a little, but faced with the complexity of the operation and the muscular weakness of my assistant at the time, I decided that the simplest solution was to build for myself an extension that would transform any support into an orthopedic table of Judet.

I am not an engineer, but I managed to weld a few stainless steel tubes to which I attached a simple traction system. I took care to reproduce the parallelogram of a real Judet table.

A real Judet table provides a deformable parallelogram, which allows maintenance of the tension of the lower limb, independent of the position of the leg in the space.

On the Judet table, one of the centers of this deformable rectangle is the patient's femoral head and on the other side the center of the ankle. Modern tables have somewhat forgotten this ingenious principle, which is rather unfortunate. The table, or rather the table extension that I brought to the operating room in 1997, was a half-table based on this principle. The other leg is not put in traction. It is easy to transport and easy to store (Fig. 22.4).

When I brought my handiwork to the O.R., no one noticed me. At the time, the regulations, standards, and other administrative issues were much less strict than they are today. I think it would be totally impossible today!

As a young surgeon, I did not have an extraordinary group of customers, but the patients I took care of in collaboration with Professor Letournel were loyal to me, and I already had a fairly good activity.

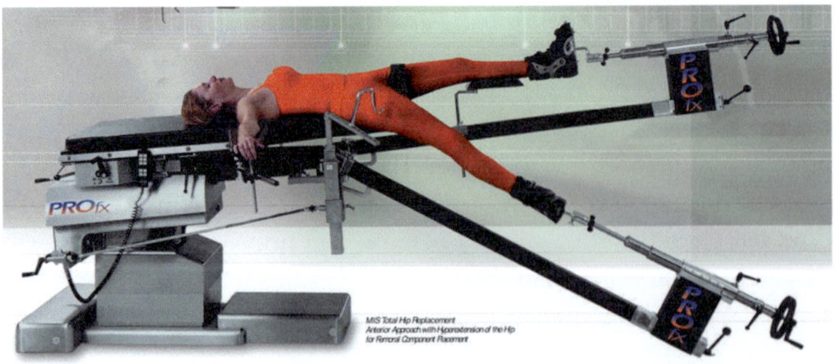

Fig. 22.3 The proFx (OSI) table design by Joel Matta: fully radiolucent for pelvic fracture and THR. The hook on the side helps to elevate the femur

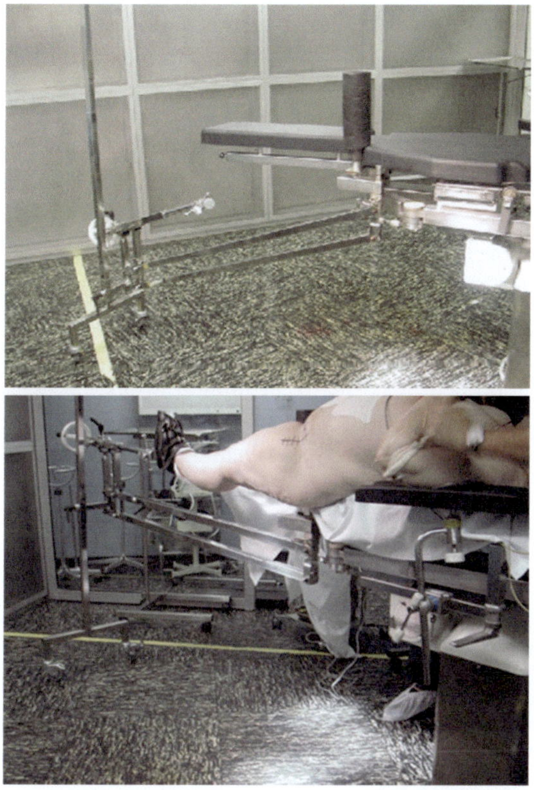

Fig. 22.4 1996: the first iteration of the AMIS table. The traction is only applied on one side. The other leg is left without traction. There is only one copy of this table

At this point, it was necessary to improve the instruments, in order to make this surgery reliable and reproductive. I found some solutions in veterinary surgery. Some retractors for our four-legged friends and especially a miniature Charnley retractor helped me greatly.

The ancillary instruments were still a problem! I had a great deal of difficulty explaining to the salesmen of the Swiss group Sulzer with whom I was working at the time that their posterior approach broach handle was a real problem for me, but finally one of them agreed, without informing his hierarchy, to modify a broach handle according to my wishes.

It is often said that minimally invasive hip surgery started with Richard Berger [25]. I am not sure if this is true, but he made many surgeons rediscover the anterior approach in 2003. We Parisian surgeons, like Marc Siguier [26] or myself, have been doing mini-invasive anterior hip surgery without really saying so for almost 10 years.

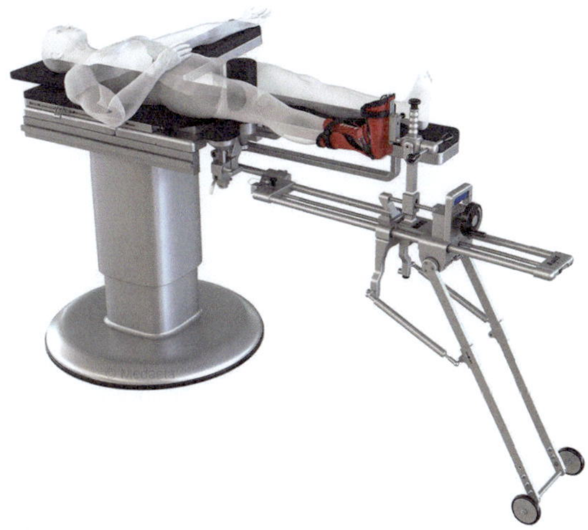

Fig. 22.5 The AMIS table (Medacta). You can plug it to a regular table. The rotation of the lower limb works with a ratchet system. The extension setting cancels the traction to avoid damaging the crural nerve

We just did not find it useful to publish our results in English in serious journals, since we were too busy managing our patients. Berger's publication, however, had an extraordinary impact on the orthopedic community, and soon, all manufacturers began to listen to the few surgeons who had experience in the field. As a young French surgeon, I did not at all have the weight of the big American majors, but I was able to develop with the young Medacta Swiss laboratory all the ancillary equipment needed to be able to do the anterior approach in an optimized, straightforward, and reproducible way. First of all, I had to explain to a prosthesis manufacturer that we needed a good extension table and that my extension table from 1997 could be copied and possibly improved.

Fortunately, they contracted out to a subcontractor who worked right next to my clinic. I was able to really get involved in this project and to develop exactly what I wanted: a light, practical table that forgives mistakes. I especially developed a table for the nurses who handle it. It is very different from Robert Judet's table with its parallelogram, but the manipulations are much more intuitive for regular operating room staff (Fig. 22.5). In 2004, the result of this collaboration led to the bird of the AMIS® (Anterior Minimally Invasive Surgery) technique and its dedicated advanced instrumentation including

- self-retaining retractors
- offset reamers and cup impactor
- 45° broach handle

contributing to facilitating the reproducibility of the anterior approach.

The past 15 years have been very rich in teaching and professional encounters. It has been necessary to train surgeons who are sometimes skeptical and not always very motivated. There is a whole world of difference between having the know-how and being able to transmit it. Many surgeons, however, have been passionate about this new way of doing things, and it is above all André Gächter whom I must thank. He was at the time chief surgeon of the hospital of St. Gallen in German-speaking Switzerland, and, with his excellent reputation, he contributed greatly alongside me to the emancipation of this technique in Switzerland and in the rest of the world. I could mention many others, but I have to admit that without the Medacta International Laboratory, which has fully believed in this approach, and in the fundamental importance of a dedicated education, we would not be here.

It was necessary to explain how to put in a primary hip replacement prosthesis, and then, gradually many colleagues understood that the anterior approach was not limited to simple cases, but that complex operations could be performed and even revisions could be done. The instrument set became more and more efficient. The technique has also evolved compared to what a Judet or a Letournel performed: introduction, more than 20 years ago, of the Bikini type incision (which I had been carrying out mainly in obese patients since 2000), drastic reduction in capsular releases (since they are totally useless in 9 cases out of 10), dedicated revision instruments [27], and addition of the computer support.

Paradoxically, the anterior approach with an orthopedic table is the oldest approach to the hip joint [1], but it does not really have a modern history. Most surgeons who perform it have not learned it during their university studies and have trained either on their own or through hasty fellowships. Many surgeons have discovered the limitations of this approach through their complication rates. Many publications have reported disappointing results, a corollary of this inadequate training. For the past 15 years, specific tables are again easily available. They are not all the same, but they do at least exist. However, the problem of the lack of expert trainers is being addressed, and thanks to the success of this approach, it is finally beginning to take hold in university centers. The anterior approach is especially appreciated by our patients, who are more and more demanding. Information circulates more and more rapidly, not to mention when it begins to be transmitted via social networks. We need to adapt to this new environment, and it is clear that the anterior approach on the orthopedic table is now in the spotlight and probably will be for a long time to come [28].

References

1. Rachbauer F, Kain MS, Leunig M. The history of the anterior approach to the hip. Orthop Clin North Am. 2009;40(3):311–20.
2. Smith-Petersen MN. Approach to and exposure of the hip joint for mold arthroplasty. J Bone Joint Surg Am. 1949;31A(1):40–6.
3. Gibson A. Posterior exposure of the hip joint. J Bone Joint Surg Br. 1950;32-B(2):183–6.
4. Robert Judet (1909-1980). Rev Chir Orthop Reparatrice Appar Mot. 1981;67(2):91–8.
5. Boutelier P. Robert Judet. Chirurgie. 1994;120(11):11–8.
6. Judet J, Judet R. The use of an artificial femoral head for arthroplasty of the hip joint. J Bone Joint Surg Br. 1950;32-B(2):166–73.
7. Judet J, Judet H. Anterior approach in total hip arthroplasty. Presse Med. 1985;14(18):1031–3.
8. d'Aubigne M, et al. Total prostheses of the hip. Rev Chir Orthop Reparatrice Appar Mot. 1967;53(8):803–8.
9. Judet R. Total hip endoprosthesis made of porometal without cement anchoring. Z Orthop Ihre Grenzgeb. 1975;113(4):828–9.
10. Judet R, et al. A noncemented total hip prosthesis. Clin Orthop Relat Res. 1978;137:76–84.
11. Charnley J. Total hip replacement by low-friction arthroplasty. Clin Orthop Relat Res. 1970;72:7–21.
12. Charnley J. Long-term results of low-friction arthroplasty. Hip. 1982:42–9.

13. Olsson E, Goldie I, Wykman A. Total hip replacement. A comparison between cemented (Charnley) and non-cemented (HP Garches) fixation by clinical assessment and objective gait analysis. Scand J Rehabil Med. 1986;18(3):107–16.
14. Johnson EE, et al. A tribute to Emile Letournel, MD (1927-1994). Clin Orthop Relat Res. 1995;310:281–2.
15. Johnson EE. The life and contributions of Emile Letournel, MD, 1927-1994. J Orthop Trauma. 2019;33 Suppl 2:Sii–Siii.
16. Lagrange J, Letournel E. The "L.L." total hip prosthesis. Int Surg. 1975;60(1):21–4.
17. Letournel E. Fractures of the acetabulum. A study of a series of 75 cases. Clin Orthop Relat Res. 1961;1994(305):5–9.
18. Letournel E. Trochantero-iliac coaptation. Treatment of suppurative total arthroplasty. Rev Chir Orthop Reparatrice Appar Mot. 1975;61 Suppl 2:115–9.
19. Lazennec JY, et al. Possibilities of anterior approach to the lumbar spine by minimal retroperitoneal access. Anatomical bases. Technical principles and initial results. Chirurgie. 1997;122(8–9):468–77.
20. Benazet JP, et al. Treatment of complete lumbar disk herniation by percutaneous discectomy. Chirurgie. 1991;117(1):59–67.
21. Rottinger H. Minimally invasive anterolateral surgical approach for total hip arthroplasty: early clinical results. Hip Int. 2006;16(Suppl 4):42–7.
22. Viamont-Guerra MR, et al. The direct anterior approach for total hip arthroplasty for severe dysplasia (Crowe III and IV) provides satisfactory medium to long-term outcomes. J Arthroplast. 2020;35:1642.
23. Viamont-Guerra MR, Saffarini M, Laude F. Surgical technique and case series of total hip arthroplasty with the Hueter anterior approach for Crowe type-IV dysplasia. J Bone Joint Surg Am. 2020;102:99.
24. Matta JM, Ferguson TA. The anterior approach for hip replacement. Orthopedics. 2005;28(9):927–8.
25. Berger RA. Total hip arthroplasty using the minimally invasive two-incision approach. Clin Orthop Relat Res. 2003;(417):232–41.
26. Siguier T, Siguier M, Brumpt B. Mini-incision anterior approach does not increase dislocation rate: a study of 1037 total hip replacements. Clin Orthop Relat Res. 2004;426:164–73.
27. Mast NH, Laude F. Revision total hip arthroplasty performed through the Hueter interval. J Bone Joint Surg Am. 2011;93(Suppl 2):143–8.
28. Anterior Total Hip Arthroplasty Collaborative, I., et al. Outcomes following the single-incision anterior approach to total hip arthroplasty: a multicenter observational study. Orthop Clin North Am. 2009;40(3):329–42.

23 The History of the Direct Anterior Approach in Innsburck

Michael Nogler

Before the DAA

The Anterolateral–Transgluteal Approach with Long Skin Incision

Professor Rudolf Bauer introduced hip arthroplasty in Innsbruck [1, 2]. From the beginning, he used an anterolateral transgluteal approach, which he published and popularized in the 1970s and 80s. This approach became very well known in the center of Europe, and it was the standard approach comparable to the posterior approach in the UK and the USA. This "Bauer" approach was of course the one and only approach at the Department of Orthopaedic Surgery in Innsbruck. It was used for both primary and revision surgeries. Using any other approach, like a posterior one, was a rare case and needed a special indication. So, everybody trained in Innsbruck was trained in the transgluteal approach performed in supine positioning of the patient. This was also true for the author who received his training in the mid-1990s. A traditional Bauer approach of that time had a 20–30 cm skin incision. Gluteus medius and vastus lateralis were split, and all short external rotators were removed to get good exposure. The credo was as one of the senior surgeons told me more the one time: **"Open wide enough to see everything. If you do not see well, open more."** As all surgeons in the area were trained in Innsbruck, all of them followed the same philosophy and saw the same outcome.

M. Nogler (✉)
Department of Orthopaedic Surgery, Medical University of Innsbruck, Innsbruck, Austria
e-mail: Michael.nogler@professor-nogler.at

Some Problems Seen

Advantages and disadvantages of approaches had been published at that time as they are still discussed in the literature. The rational for professor Bauer's preference was a reduced dislocation rate of the transgluteal anterolateral approach compared to the posterior one. Muscular defects at the gluteus medius–vastus lateralis junction, trochanteric pain, and some slight limping were accepted and ignored. All patients in our geographical area with problems after hip replacement would hear that this was not with hip arthroplasty and had to be accepted. And as all arthroplasty surgeons were trained in our institution, they would hear them same from everybody as this was a firm belief. I have seen quite a number of such patients. I have also seen dislocations in patients following primary THA, though not as many as published for the posterior approach, but closed reductions in primary THAs happened on a weekly basis and every resident was quite familiar with treating them, while this is more of an exception nowadays with the DAA.

J. M. Matta, A. P. Sah (eds.), *Anterior Hip Replacement*,
https://doi.org/10.1007/978-3-030-91896-5_23

Muscle Damage Seen in Revisions

Failed THAs following a primary THA that were performed through a Bauer approach were also revised through the same approach. All surgeons were trained to perform revisions through the anterolateral transgluteal approach with the patient in supine position. An extension of the approach was performed laterally with a further splitting of the vastus lateralis and a dissection of this muscle from its fascia at its dorsal border. Thus, the lateral aspect of the femoral diaphysis was exposed and could be opened with a small lateral window or a large anterior window according to Wagner.

For those of us who did such revisions, it was quite usual to see the anterior part of gluteus medius and vastus lateralis, e.g., the part anterior to the splitting of theses muscles that was performed in a transgluteal approach, severely damaged and fatty atrophic. Muscle degeneration following this approach is a published phenomenon [3]. Yet, despite these findings, most patients did well and showed no limping after the primary THA as enough of the gluteal function was preserved to avoid the development of a gluteal deficiency. It can be reasoned though that limping might have occurred more often after revision surgery since more muscle was destroyed in such a more extended procedure.

Supine Position and No Extension Table

As mentioned above, we always performed THAs in supine position. All patients were placed on a standard operating table, and no special devices were used for leg positioning. As Innsbruck was a traditional orthopedic department, no acute trauma cases were done, except periprosthetic fractures. Extension tables were not used very often. They were hardly available, and if one was needed and brought in from the trauma department, nobody from the OR teams really felt familiar or comfortable using it. Therefore, it never came to our mind to use any extension device for joint replacement.

A Revelation at the European Hip Society Meeting in Baveno, Italy

Equipped with this experience and with the strong belief that THAs are performed by us in the best possible way, we focused on research around the support of total joint replacement with navigation devices and robots. CAOS, computer-aided orthopaedic surgery, was the focus of our study group, and approaches were by no means of any deeper interest. At one of these CAOS meeting, we are asked what we thought about the new idea of minimally invasive THA. Well, we had never heard about that before and therefore had no answer to that question. I remember that I was a little surprised to hear that notion as everybody seemed to work on robots and navigation like we did since the mid-1990s. Therefore, although it sounded nice, we all did not give the topic of minimal invasiveness a real thought. It was just not in our minds—not yet. It might be the case of disruptive ideas that most people react to it when they hear about it the first time with little understanding. It might take a while until this reaction changes to the feeling, why nobody had thought of it earlier as it seems so natural, so obvious.

This happened to me in June 2002 at the European Hip Society's Domestic Meeting in Baveno, Italy. It struck me when I attended the lecture on the double-incision, minimally invasive approach to THA by Richard Berger. I knew this was it, the concept that we had to work on immediately, that we had to have the focus on as soon as we went back home. I talked to Martin Krismer, the professor and head of our department, and professor Franz Rachbauer the head of the tumor and joint replacement teams. We spent the rest of the meeting discussing how we could proceed (Fig. 23.1).

Different Concepts Are Discussed

The three of us, with me being the junior in the team, were in total agreement that a dual incision and using a C-arm to perform a total hip arthroplasty were not acceptable for us. It was just too far away from our current practice, we were looking for an approach that was short, and it had to be a single incision. Yet, more importantly we wanted an approach that was truly muscle sparing. Saving muscle structures and protecting as much soft tissue from any kind of damage were our definition of minimal invasiveness. The length of incision undoubtedly mattered, but it was secondary to the true soft tissue damage. Franz Rachbauer came up with the proposal to use a Smith–Petersen approach [4], an anterior approach that was well known and developed. The interval was first described by Carl Hüter [5], a German surgeon in the late 1880, and later popularized by Smith–Petersen for hip and pelvic surgery. This approach is truly intermuscular and therefore muscle sparing. It is possible to reach the hip joint in an interval between sartorius and rectus muscles medially and tensor fasciae latae laterally. One of the major advantages we felt was the fact that this approach was also truly internerval as all muscles medial to it are supplied by the femoral nerve and all lateral muscles are supplied by the gluteal nerve. With the experience of the transgluteal approach in mind, we were especially eager to avoid any damage to the gluteal abductor function as this was in our minds the most important approach-related damage with extreme negative effects for the patients (Fig. 23.2).

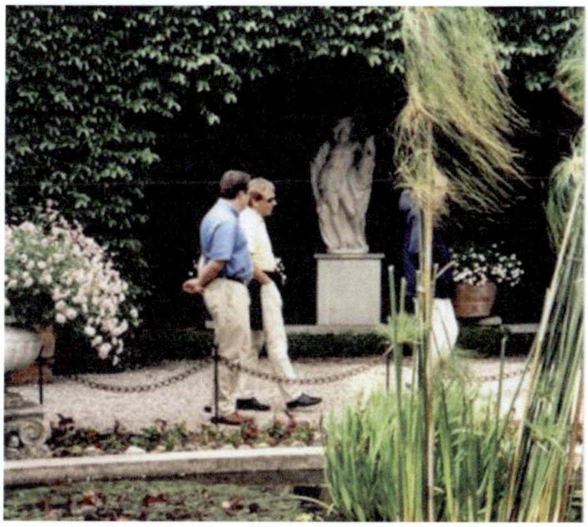

Fig. 23.1 Martin Krismer and Michael Nogler discussion minimally invasive hip concepts in Baveno, Italy 2002

Cooperation with the Anatomy Department

Traditionally, Innsbruck has a strong anatomy department. The student training in cadaver laboratories is excellent. The orthopedic department always had a very intense and productive cooperation with this department under the lead of Professor Helga Fritsch. Therefore, we approached her, and we started a series of cadaver surgeries in which we tried to explore the possibilities to utilize the anterior interval for hip arthroplasty.

What we experienced was very different from the kind of hip surgery we were used to. We kept the incision at around 9 cm, and the hole that we created was deep and dark. The standard straight retractors that we used were impeding our view into the wound, and all our instruments had no

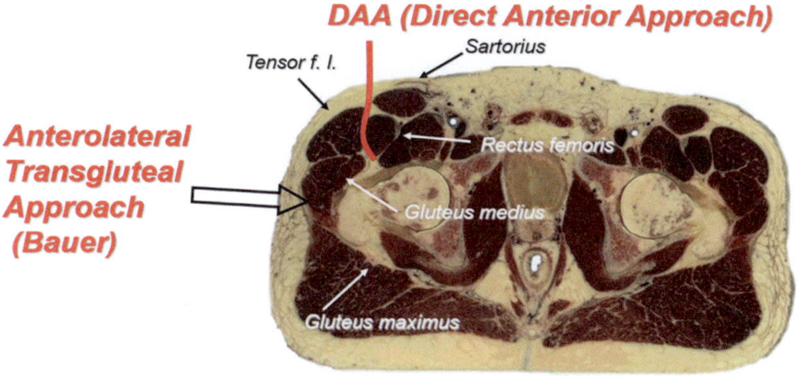

Fig. 23.2 Bauer approach vs DAA ´

angle or offset. It was clear to us from the very beginning that although the anatomy of the approach was easy to understand it was absolutely necessary to design a couple of instruments with the right offset that would allow us to get into the bone (Fig. 23.3).

We initiated a cooperation with Stryker (Mahwah, NJ, USA) a long-time partner in different fields. We set up a couple of laboratories to identify the instruments that we would need. For retraction, we developed a set of curved retractors and had them custom-made and CE marked for us by a local vendor. They are still in use in our department. We also created an offset reamer handle, which we received a US patent for. While we worked on the design of some specific instruments, we looked at the available instruments in different markets and found some that were suitable for what we wanted to do. Eventually, we put a set together that we thought would work (Figs. 23.4, 23.5, and 23.6).

First Cases

We were ready to perform the first surgery in January 2003. Under the lead of Professor Krismer and Dr. Franz Rachbauer, we implanted a relatively long straight stem (Omnifit, STRYKER). The surgery took over 2 hours, and we were exhausted. The implants were in good position, and muscle damage was moderate compared to what we were used to from the standard open approach. Yet, in the debriefing we were not sure if the effort was justified. At the late afternoon, though we were surprised how easily and with how little pain the patient got up from his bed and walked. This was impressively different from what we were used to, and we decided to keep going with the DAA. By February 2003, we had already reported 4 cases that we had successfully performed at the AFOR meeting in Pontresina. We received some very positive feed-

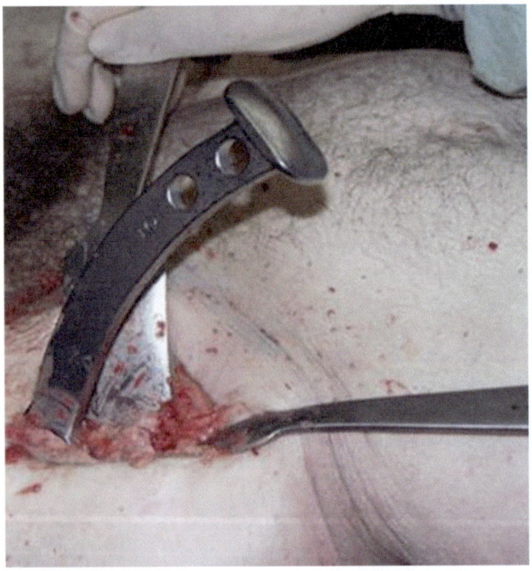

Fig. 23.3 First cadaver trials with standard instruments

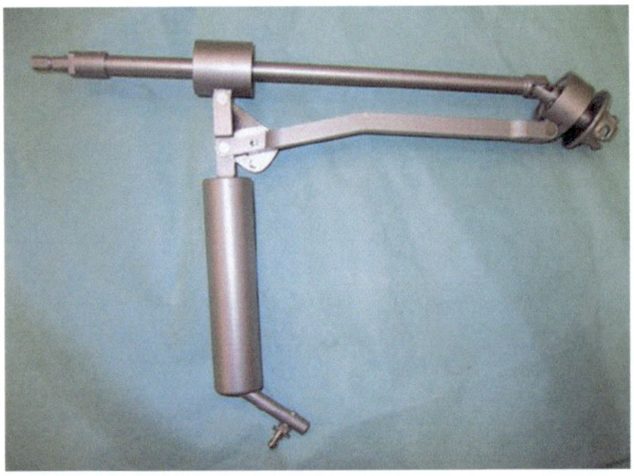

Fig. 23.4 Angular reamer handle with a navigation attachment

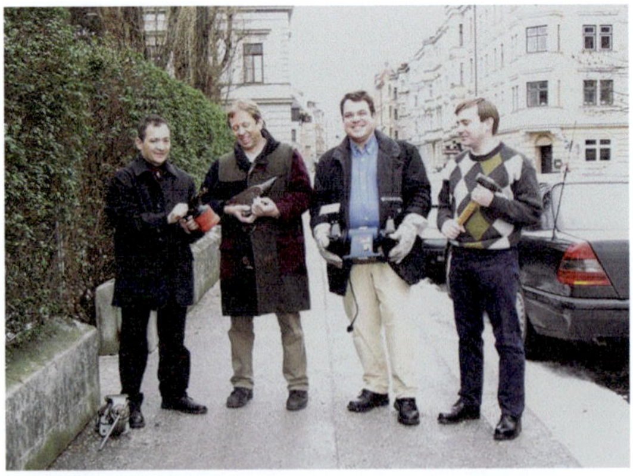

Fig. 23.5 from right: Franz Rachbauer, Michael Nogler, Martin Krismer, Jose-Luis Mocetzuma de la Barrera (STRYKER) in front of the Anatomy building at the first cadaver laboratory in Fall 2002

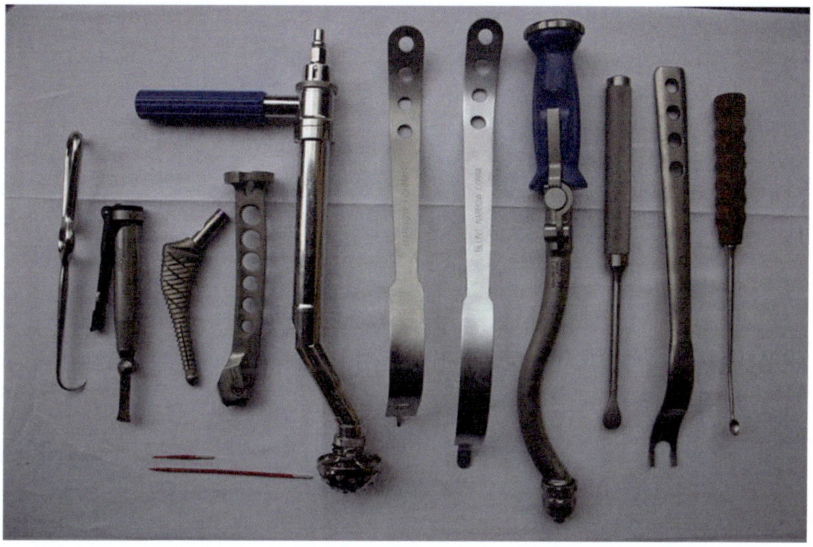

Fig. 23.6 First instrument set

back from colleagues and continued our surgical experience. We were asked to present our technique and got several requests for site visits in Innsbruck.

Better Instruments and Light

Despite the immediate success that we saw in our patients, we understood that the instrumentation and the implants were not ideal. We felt it was too early for defining a consistent technique yet. After careful consideration, we thought that a tapered stem with a cutoff shoulder would be ideal for the DAA. The Accolade I (Stryker) was the femoral component of choice. On the cup side, we had no big issues. A hemispherical press-fit cup, like the Trident (Stryker), was easy enough to use. The instruments for cup implantation were available and had curvatures and offset that were sufficient, and they could even be navigated [6]. These instruments were eventually produced by OEM companies in Switzerland and New Zealand and worked well. The tapered stem also showed immediate advantages and was much easier to ream and introduce. Nonetheless, the broach handle was never ideal. It had anterior offset, but we could show in laboratories that a double-offset broach handle would be of much help in accessing the femur with ease and little soft tissue releases. We pushed our development partner Stryker hard to create a double-offset broach handle for their broaches. Eventually, we were successful and received the instrument in early 2004 and could publish our design and clinical experience in 2006 [7].

As we realized from the very beginning, surgical cavities that we created were deep and dark. Extra light seemed to be necessary. We started out with head-mounted lights for the surgeons and had good success with them. Over time, we changed to surgical helmets with battery-powered lights that gave us both light and protection against blood and debris.

Double Offset and No Traction Table

At the beginning, I mentioned the fact that we were used to do THAs in supine position with no traction table. We kept this standard and never tried to use a traction table. Like for all other variations of DAA techniques, the preparation of the femur seems to be the technically more demanding part of the procedure. Traction table-based techniques focus on the correct lever arm and different leg positions in order to bring the proximal femur as much out of the wound as possible trying to recreate a surgical exposure that is as close to a wide-open approach as possible. In our technique, we avoid this. We place the leg in slight adduction, hyperextension, and external rotation. We avoid any major force applied to the leg. We use retractors to open the wound and support the proximal femur underneath the greater trochanter. We do not release a lot of the dorsal capsule and we do not want to release the short external rotator in the intertrochanteric fossa. With this technique, we do not aim to bring the femur up and out of the wound, and we do not necessarily look for a straight access to the femoral canal. We work inside the surgical site and angulate the instruments into the wound. Given this fast and straightforward concept, a broach handle with dual offset, e.g., anterior and lateral offset, is of huge help and allows for an easy and fast preparation of the femoral canal. The design became popular, but it was also argued that it gave a different feeling to a straight impactor—which is obviously true. We studied and published the mechanical properties of this type of design, which gives you a slightly different feeling but is nicely working anyway [8] (Fig. 23.7).

Teaching and Training

Learning and teaching usually go hand in hand, and both are the core duties of universities. Over the course of the years 2003–04, we developed our core technique. We improved on the implant choices and techniques for cemented and uncemented implants and continued to develop instruments. Eventually, we came up with a final surgical technique and made the DAA to the standard approach for THA that was performed by our entire hip surgeons, except one older colleague who wanted to stay with his standards. We also decided to only train the DAA for our residents. We repeatedly reported on our growing experience with the DAA and gained more interests and request from colleagues worldwide who wanted to learn from us. We decided to install a formal training program. As a course for the DAA had to be mostly soft tissue-related, we understood that cadaver training should be at the core of such a course. We used our cooperation with the anatomy department again and designed a course that consisted of a lecture part, a printed surgical technique, the presentation of a cadaver preparation, and a hands-on part in which the participants could exercise the technique in cadaver specimen. As these were the first DAA cadaver courses, we also felt that we had to prove that what we thought was not only possible in the cadaver laboratory but would also be performed in an OR setting. With the strong support of the university hospital, we got a video system installed in one of our ORs. We integrated the presentation of two live surgeries in the course concept (Fig. 23.8).

The first course was held in April 2004 in Innsbruck. It was attended by more than 60 surgeons from all over Europe and was well received. Since then, we have held over 300 DAA courses with over 3500 surgeons from 56 nations in Innsbruck, thus becoming one of the leading

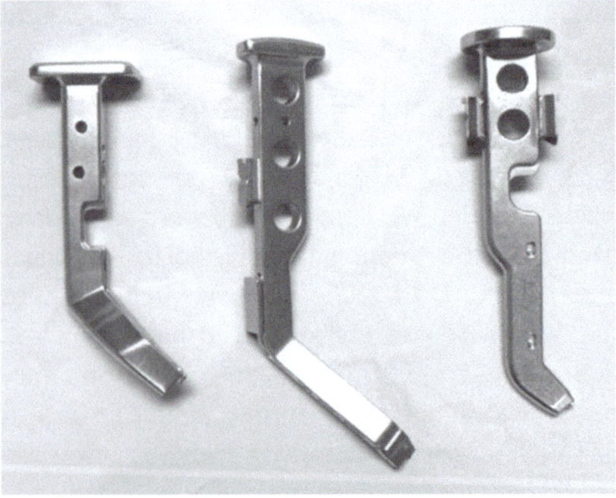

Fig. 23.7 Double offset A, double offset B, and single offset broach handle

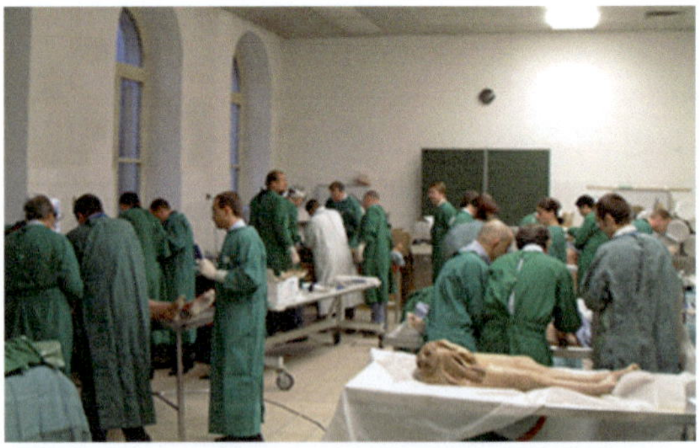

Fig. 23.8 First DAA cadaver training in April 2004

training institutions on DAA globally. Additionally, I trained over 5000 surgeons at international courses all over the world, in the USA, Asia, Australia, South America, and Europe spreading the story of the DAA (Fig. 23.9).

As learning is fundamental to teaching, teaching always is also a process of learning. With every interaction with other surgeons, we added understanding and knowledge to our practices and introduced and added it to the concept of the Innsbruck DAA technique. In one of the first surgeries that I was invited to assist, I learned from Dott. Cammarano and Dott. De Peppo, in Rome, Italy, to put an adhesive at the proximal corner of the wound. This became my standard technique for the next 2 decades (Fig. 23.10).

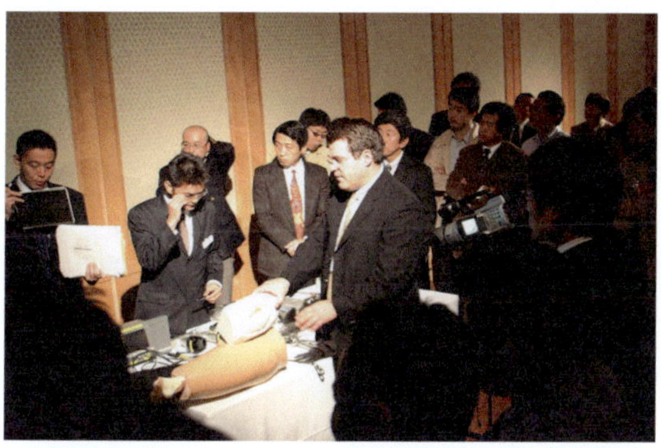

Fig. 23.9 First DAA demonstration and training in Japan in fall 2004

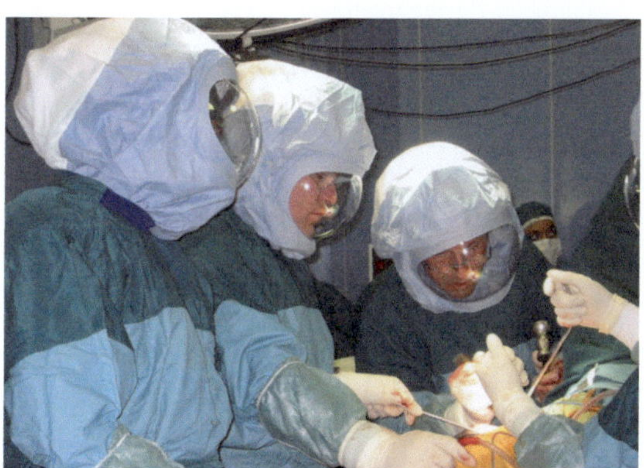

Fig. 23.10 First DAA surgery with Drs. Cammarano and de Peppo in Rome, Italy, April 2004

Since 2019, the ICJR holds an annual international DAA master course in Innsbruck in February as their second DAA center with Houston, Texas, being their center for the fall DAA course.

Revision with the DAA

For every hip surgeon who was either using a posterior approach or any form of lateral access to the hip, it was totally clear that it was possible to extend these approaches distally to perform revision surgery through them. In the first years of the history of the DAA, it, even by the most excited users of the DAA, agreed upon that the DAA was a primary THA-only approach. A direct distal extension was not possible because the nerve fibers of the femoral nerve are crossing from medial to lateral distal to the lesser trochanter. Yet, after 3 years of extensive experience we felt that doing cup revisions through the DAA was entirely possible. We started with simple liner exchanges, found no significant difficulties, and quickly started to do all our cup revisions through the DAA in 2006. The next natural step was to try to replace femoral components from proximally. This was successful in some cases, and we would only switch to the lateral approach in those cases in which the stem could not be retrieved proximally.

Nevertheless, I remember well the very first case in which I performed a revision with a laterally extended DAA in a female patient who fractured her hip in an accident 3 weeks after she had received her primary implantation. I opened the recent DAA wound and extended it laterally in a—what we later called—“lazy S” curve to reach posterior to the lateral vastus to the femoral diaphysis. It could successfully reconstruct her femur and replace her components with a long stem revision system. We could prove that it was possible to do even complex THA revision with an extended version of the DAA. We have published our comprehensive technique and its use for revisions, fractures, and infections since 2012 [9–14].

DAA a Journey

Well, the DAA is just an approach to the hip. Yet, many surgeons all over the world have dedicated two decades of their professional career developing, learning, and training DAA as a better alternative to other existing approaches. At the beginning, we faced as much interest as animosities. We constantly had to prove that it was safe and acceptable to do something new. In more recent years, this was no issue anymore and we could focus on the advantages and benefits for patients in our discussion around the approach. For myself, I am convinced that it was worth the effort. We surely have made a difference in the lives of thousands of patients all over the world, not only with the DAA itself, but also with the constant discussion on minimally invasiveness. If we compare how much tissue we have cut 20 years ago and how little we destroy and how much we focus on preserving everything we can in joint replacement I am sure we have created some impact with this journey through the past decades. I am proud to be among so many dedicated DAA surgeons.

References

1. Bauer R, Spitzer G. Operative Zugangswege in Orthopädie und Traumatologie. 2nd ed; 1990.
2. Bauer R, Kerschbaumer F, Poisel S. Operative Zugangswege in Orthopädie und Traumatologie; 1986.
3. Pfirrmann CWA, Notzli HP, Dora C, Hodler J, Zanetti M. Abductor tendons and muscles assessed at MR imaging after total hip arthroplasty in asymptomatic and symptomatic patients. Radiology. 2005;235:969–76. https://doi.org/10.1148/radiol.2353040403.
4. Smith-Petersen M. A new supra-articular subperiosteal approach to the hip joint. J Bone Joint Surg Am. 1917;15:592–5.
5. Hueter C. In: Hueter C (Hrsg) Grundriss der Chirurgie.: Fünfte Abteilung: Die Verletzung und Krankeiten des Hüftgelenkes, neunundzwanzigstes Kapitel. Leipzig: Vogel, Leipzig; 1883.
6. Nogler M. Navigated minimal invasive total hip arthroplasty. Surg Technol Int. 2004;12:259–62.
7. Nogler M, Krismer M, Hozack WJ, Merritt P, Rachbauer F, Mayr E. A double offset broach handle for preparation of the femoral cavity in minimally invasive direct anterior total hip arthroplasty. J Arthroplast. 2006;21:1206–8. https://doi.org/10.1016/j.arth.2006.08.003.
8. Putzer D, Mayr E, Haid C, Hozack W, Nogler M. Force transmission in offset broach handles used for hip replacement: comparison of three different designs. Hip Int. 2013;23:187–92. https://doi.org/10.5301/HIP.2013.10730.
9. Krismer M, Nogler M. Revisionsendoprothetik des Hüftgelenks : Der anteriore Zugang. Orthopade. 2017;46:121–5. https://doi.org/10.1007/s00132-016-3376-0.
10. Nogler M, Mayr E, Krismer M. Der direkte anteriore Zugang in der Revisionshüftendoprothetik. Oper Orthop Traumatol. 2012;24:153–64. https://doi.org/10.1007/s00064-011-0113-z.
11. Thaler M, Dammerer D, Leitner H, Lindtner RA, Nogler M. Mid-term follow-up of the direct anterior approach in acetabular revision hip arthroplasty using a reconstruction cage with impaction grafting. J Arthroplast. 2020;35:1339–43. https://doi.org/10.1016/j.arth.2020.01.004.
12. Thaler M, Lechner R, Dammerer D, Leitner H, Khosravi I, Nogler M. The direct anterior approach: treating periprosthetic joint infection of the hip using two-stage revision arthroplasty. Arch Orthop Trauma Surg. 2020;140:255–62. https://doi.org/10.1007/s00402-019-03317-1.
13. Thaler M, Dammerer D, Krismer M, Ban M, Lechner R, Nogler M. Extension of the direct anterior approach for the treatment of Periprosthetic femoral fractures. J Arthroplast. 2019;34:2449–53. https://doi.org/10.1016/j.arth.2019.05.015.
14. Nogler MM, Thaler MR. The direct anterior approach for hip revision: accessing the entire femoral diaphysis without endangering the nerve supply. J Arthroplast. 2017;32:510–4. https://doi.org/10.1016/j.arth.2016.07.044.

The Direct Anterior Approach on a Standard Table in Zurich

24

Hannes A. Rüdiger and Michael Leunig

Rational for DAA

For decades, the pioneers of modern hip surgery in Switzerland have used the direct lateral also called transgluteal approach (DL) as standard technique for total hip arthroplasty (THA). Despite low dislocation and revision rates, some major concerns remained until today, including the necessity of partial weight-bearing, persistent abductor weakness, and limping. As a result, the DL approach has lost its popularity in the late nineties and early 2000.

While some high-volume arthroplasty centers in Switzerland adopted the posterior approach, several surgeons were looking into anterior approaches including Watson–Jones type of techniques (e.g., Roettinger [1]) and the direct anterior approach (DAA, i.e., Hueter approach [2]). Major teaching hospital opted for the DAA, due to the fact that it is a truly intermuscular, intervascular, and internervous approach. In addition, dislocation rates appeared lower and component positioning in supine position easier. This together with promotion of the technique by an industry looking for innovation led to a rapid spread of the DAA in Switzerland. According to the Swiss national arthroplasty registry SIRIS, the proportion of DAA for primary total hip arthroplasty has been increasing from 42% in 2015 to 53% in 2020.

While some initial experience was gained by the use of a traction table (or leg holder) for DAA, the technique on a standard table also became popular. For many orthopedic surgeons, this positioning is closer to what they were used to. Moreover, the fact that both legs are freely movable allows for facilitated testing of anterior and posterior stability and leg length. Due to the use of various landmarks combined with functional test intraoperatively an image intensifier is not required. Rare exceptions may include large acetabular defects with complex reconstructions or repositionings of the acetabular center of rotation, or intraoperative complications, or revision surgery.

Patient Positioning and Draping

The patient is positioned on a standard OR table, which is breakable at the level of the greater trochanter. This will allow for a hyperextension in the hip for a better exposure during femoral broaching.

During THA through a DAA, the operated leg might have to assume several positions to facilitate femoral and acetabular exposure and for functional testing of trial and definitive implants. Such positioning may require alterations in table height and angulation, creating the risk of

H. A. Rüdiger · M. Leunig (✉)
Hip Surgery - Schulthess Clinic, Zürich, Switzerland

J. M. Matta, A. P. Sah (eds.), *Anterior Hip Replacement*,
https://doi.org/10.1007/978-3-030-91896-5_24

inadvertent drape contamination. Consequently, a variety of complicated draping systems have been proposed for DAA THA [3–5]. Such techniques often require prepping both legs, rolling on or rolling off multiple stockinettes, and serially applying sterile half-sheets every time the leg or table is lowered and raised again. In our high-volume DAA practice, we noted that such complicated prep-and-drape routines prolong case time, require experienced personnel, increase the risk of glove contamination,[6] and make maneuvering the operated leg and checking leg lengths more difficult over the course of the procedure.

In response to the above concerns, in 2011 we devised a novel DAA preparation, and draping protocol, which can be applied in far less time as required for draping both legs, is easy for both nurses and residents to reproduce, requires fewer personnel (3 versus 5), and facilitates leg positioning and leg length evaluation. To assess the advantage of this draping technique, we compared operative setup time, total operating time, superficial or deep periprosthetic joint infection (PJI) risk, and cost between the two draping techniques.

Our draping technique, which is similar to a horizontal draping used for hip fractures or the DAA technique using a fracture table, requires the one-time manufacturing of a U-shaped stainless steel frame (Fig. 24.1), which is then attached to the proximal half (proximal to the breaking joint) of the operating table via standard linking clamps prior to patient positioning. Due to this proximal fixation of the frame, it does not alter its position when the legs are lowered and hence does not interfere with draping, operating, or manipulating the lower limbs.

Once the patient is positioned, antithrombotic below-knee stockings are placed on both lower extremities and the patient is then brought into the operating room (OR). The surgical site, comprising of the proximal half of the thigh only, is prepped with alcohol-based povidone–iodine paint. No additional skin outside of this area is disinfected. After the povidone–iodine has dried, two 80 cm × 145 cm antimicrobial incise drapes (Ioban 2, 3M, Maplewood, MN) are applied over the area. Next, a custom 517 cm × 290 cm impermeable, disposable drape (Promedical AG, Glarus, Switzerland) is applied. This "Schulthess" drape is centered over the surgical incision, where a 35 cm × 20 cm transparent adhesive layer is located. In fact, we apply three layers of adhesive transparent foils over the incision site in order to achieve a solid protection of the skin including the wound edges, which is particularly important during femoral broaching. Once this window is adhered, the remainder of the drape is then unfolded, with redundant portions purposely tucked between the edge of the table and the U-shaped steel frame. The drape is then clamped to the steel frame using sterile clips. The distal two-thirds of the drape is transparent, permitting full visualization of both lower extremities.

The redundant folds of the drape between the table and the frame permit lowering of the distal table portion and manipulating both legs for femoral exposure and trialing without risking contamination of the operative site. The surgeon can also clearly visualize leg lengths through the transparent drape. The drape can be rapidly removed at the end of surgery.

Evaluation of Setup Time and Cost

To evaluate setup time and cost-effectiveness of our draping system, we reviewed a cohort of 756 patients undergoing THA by a single surgeon at our institution between 2008 and 2014. The cohort included 448 patients receiving the "new draping" as described above, which were compared to 308 patients who were draped conventionally using a stockinet-based method [4].

In our institution, patients are brought into the OR already positioned on the table and anesthetized. Following surgery, the patient is woken from anesthesia after leaving the OR. The operating staff records the time of patient entry into the OR, the time of the surgical incision, the duration of the surgical procedure, and the time the patient leaves the OR. These data were retrieved for all patients, and the setup and draping time was defined as the interval between the patients' entry into the OR and the time of the surgical

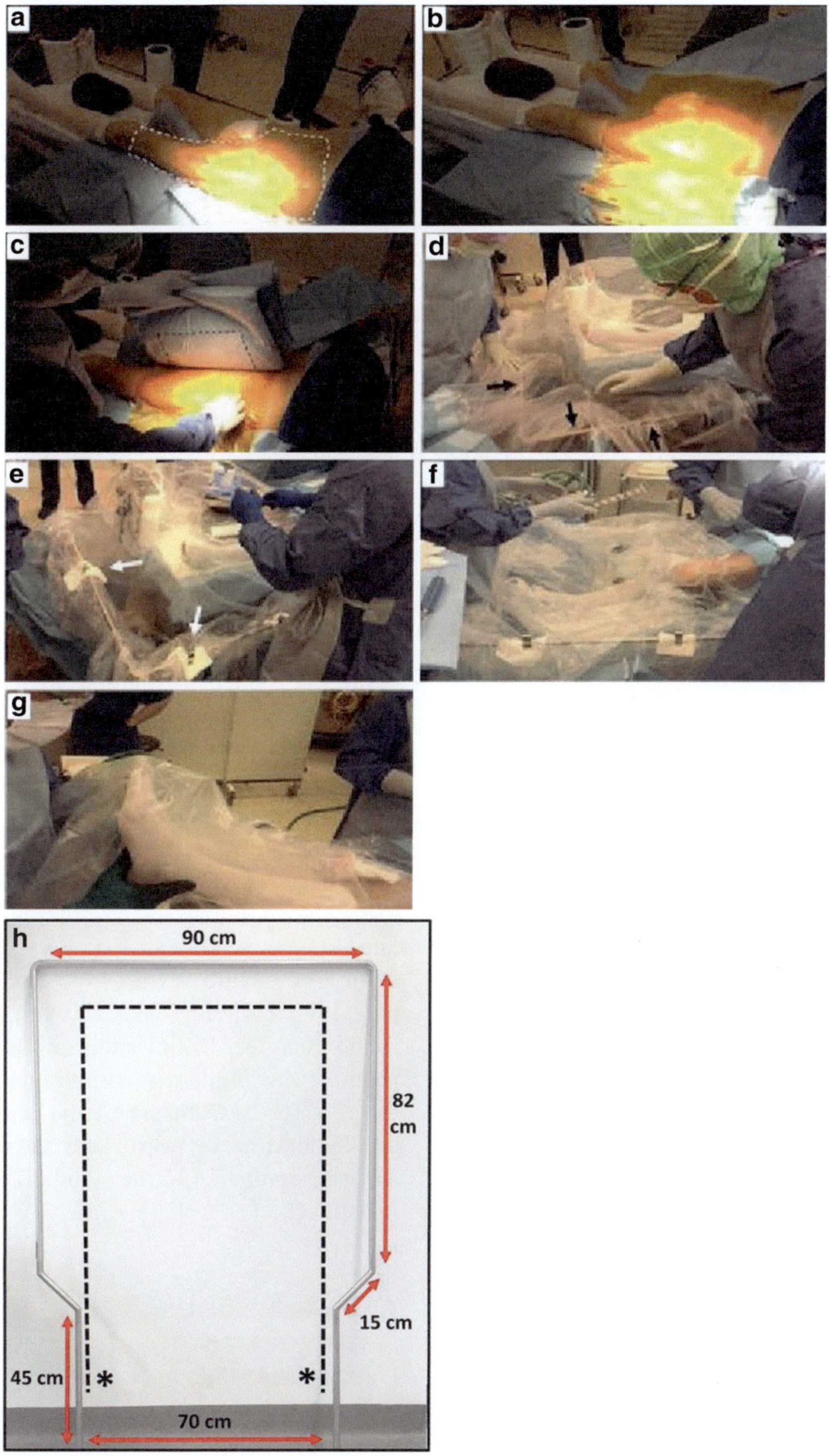

Fig. 24.1 (**a**–**h**) Our draping technique: The surgical site is disinfected and covered with a double layer of Ioban foils (**a**, **b**). The drape is the placed, with the transparent window over the surgical site (**c**). The distal transparent part of the drape is fixed with clamps to the frame (**e**). Redundant drape is placed between the drape and the table, allowing for free maneuverability of both legs. The metal frame (**h**) is fixed to the proximal part of the table. This will allow the table to break (i.e., lower the legs), while the frame remains horizontal and keeping the drape up. This draping technique allows free positioning of the legs (e.g., figure of four) (**f**) and, due to its transparency, visual assessment of leg length (**g**)

incision. To account for a decrease in surgical time over the years due to increasing expertise with the DAA, the percentage of OR time utilized for setup was calculated for both groups (setup and draping time divided by total operative time). To calculate cost savings associated with time reduction, we determined that our approximate cost per minute of OR time within each DAA THA was $51.50 USD (51 CHF). We derived North American costs using the figure of $62 per minute of OR time that has been reported in the literature [6].

With regard to intraoperative results, the use of the new drape was associated with a 30% reduction in setup time (33.5 ± 13.0 minutes) compared to conventional draping (47.67 ± 13.2 minutes; $p < 0.0001$). This reduction also decreased the overall percentage of OR time allocated for setup and draping, despite the senior author's decreasing surgical time over the study period (new draping: 22.08%, conventional draping: 26.72%, $p < 0.0001$). There were no significant differences in patient demographics or comorbidities, or the incidence PJI between the two groups (data not shown). In the conventional drape group, one early and one late deep PJI occurred requiring component revision, as well as one superficial infection treated successfully by irrigation and debridement. Two early deep infections occurred in the new drape group that was successfully treated with irrigation and debridement with liner and head exchange.

With regard to cost savings, despite the slightly higher price for the new drape ($27.24), we calculated that the new draping technique saves $693.76 per case in our institution. In North America, we have determined that this technique could save $840.76 per DAA THA.

We conclude from these data that the new draping technique significantly decreases OR setup time overall intraoperative time while improving operative leg maneuvering and leg length assessment. Furthermore, this draping technique costs less to implement, requires fewer OR personnel to set up, is easy to learn, and does not increase the risk of subsequent superficial or deep infection. This technique avoids the need for surgical stockinettes and allows the surgeon to clearly see the position and relation of both feet throughout the procedure due to the transparency of the drape.

Skin Incision

The classic skin incision of the Hueter approach is longitudinal in line with the fibers of the TFL. It starts slightly distal and lateral to the anterior superior iliac spine and aims slightly lateral toward the fibular head. A length of about 8–10 cm is usually sufficient for primary hip arthroplasties.

As this incision is perpendicular to Langer's skin tension lines and the shear forces in the groin are in line with the incision, the cosmesis of the scar is often not optimal. We have therefore introduced a transverse "Bikini" incision in 2013 along the inguinal skin fold, which can be identified by flexing the hip [7]. The incision is usually less than 8 cm in length and lateral to the ASIS to avoid proximity to the lateral cutaneous femoral nerve. At the level of the superficial TFL fascia, the approach follows the description below unrelated to type of skin incision.

In a comparative follow-up study with 964 patients undergoing THA through a DAA, we found that the Bikini incision did not compromise the implant positioning nor increase the risk for dysesthesia of the lateral cutaneous femoral nerve, while scar satisfaction was superior compared to the standard longitudinal incision [8].

Approach

For the DAA, the hip is in neutral position. To reduce flexor muscle tension, a mobile cushion may be placed underneath the knee to flex the hip slightly. The fascia of the tensor fascia lata muscle (TFL) is incised longitudinally in line with the muscle fibers. The muscle belly of the TFL is retracted laterally, and the anterior trochanteric tubercle is palpated. With a Cobb periosteal elevator, the anterior capsule proximal to it is identified and the adhesions of the gluteus minimus muscle (GMi) are separated. A blunt Hohmann retractor may be placed in this space. A second sharp Hohmann retractor is placed within the trochanteric bursa on the level of the vastus lateralis ridge. With a Cobb elevator, we follow the capsule underneath the iliocapsularis muscle around the calcar and place a blunt Hohmann retractor to retract the rectus and iliocapsularis muscle medially. Extensive dissection between the iliocapsularis muscle and capsule is to be avoided to prevent scar formation and ectopic ossifications.

Some small perforating branches of the lateral circumflex artery to the rectus muscle are coagulated. The innominate fascia is incised, and the branches of the lateral circumflex artery are exposed in the precapsular fat using a Cobb elevator. These vessels are coagulated and/or ligated. The precapsular fat is then removed, exposing the capsule within a triangle consisting of the rectus and iliocapsularis muscles medially, the vastus intermedius of the quadriceps distally, and the GMi and TFL laterally. The anterior portion of the GMi is then separated from the lateral capsule. A Hohmann retractor is then placed around the greater trochanter to retract the TFL laterally. The reflected head of the rectus is transected in stiff hips to facilitate medial retraction of the rectus muscle.

Capsulotomy

We use an inverse T-shaped capsulotomy with a large medial flap based on the anterior acetabular wall. The capsulotomy starts slightly lateral at the reflected head of the rectus and runs along the most anterior fibers of the gluteus minimus or slightly medial to the trochanteric tubercle. From the latter, the iliofemoral capsulotomy follows the anterior intertrochanteric line along the origin of the vastus intermedius to the calcar. For better exposure, the triangular medial flap may be retracted medially with a holding stitch. The lateral part of the capsule is then detached from the medial aspect of the greater trochanter, exposing the base of the femoral neck. Hohmann retractors are now replaced from extra- to intracapsular around the neck. A segmental "wedge" osteotomy of the neck removing a slice of about 1 cm thickness can be performed. Alternatively, the head can be dislocated using a corkscrew performing a single neck osteotomy to remove the head.

Release

We complete the femoral release prior to the acetabular preparation as the femur is more easily retracted posterolaterally after the capsular release, which facilitates acetabular exposure. To complete the capsular release, the leg is positioned in a lazy figure of four position (i.e., external rotation with a light hip flexion). First, the pubofemoral ligament is released from the anterior intertrochanteric line medially and posteromedially to the lesser trochanter, allowing for maximal external rotation. Second, lateral release is performed: The lateral capsular flap is further detached from the medial aspect of the greater trochanter. In external rotation, a bone hook is placed into the osteotomy site of the femoral neck, which is pulled anteriorly to tighten the posterolateral capsule. Depending on the degree of the release, the conjoint tendon (i.e., internal obturator and gemelli muscles) with the lateral capsule might be released. The piriformis tendon is rarely released, and the obturator externus tendon is almost always preserved as a release of these two structures hardly improves femoral exposure but these tendons are important for posterior joint stability.

Acetabular Exposure

A large curved Hohmann retractor ("easy rider") is placed medial to the anterior inferior iliac spine onto the anterior wall. The tip of this retractor is pushed between the labrum and the capsule on the anterior wall. Care is advised during this maneuver as the tip of the retractor is close to the femoral vessels and nerve. The medial capsular flap protects the rectus muscle. A large Hohmann retractor is placed around the inferior posterior wall, pushing the femur laterally and dorsally. The pubofemoral part of the capsule is incised from the lesser trochanter to the transverse acetabular ligament. A long narrow Hohmann is placed around the teardrop figure. Sometimes, incision of the inferior capsule down to the teardrop can improve visibility.

Acetabular Preparation

The labrum is removed for better exposure of the acetabular rim. The pulvinar is resected for visualization of the floor of the fossa and its border. An offset reamer may avoid a conflict of the reamer with lateral soft tissue (TFL) and skin in the Bikini incision and hence may help to avoid excessive anterior reaming. Now reaming can be started depending on surgeon's preference. We start reaming with a large diameter to facilitate concentricity (typically 2 to 4 mm below templated cup size). The first reaming is aimed medially in direction of the teardrop figure down to the floor of the fossa. In the presence of a coxa profunda, we avoid reaming to the floor of the fossa to avoid over-medialization of the cup and thinning of the already fragile medial acetabular floor. We then increase the reamer size millimeter-wise, pushing the reamer in direction of the expected final cup axis. Excessive anterior or posterior reaming has to be avoided to prevent thinning (and shortening) of the anterior and posterior acetabular walls. A good indicator for the anteroposterior position of the reamer is the step of the posterior facies semilunata and the teardrop compared to the step of the anterior facies semilunata to the teardrop. If these two steps are symmetric (or both completely flattened), the acetabular center of rotation is in general in a good anteroposterior position (Fig. 24.2). The cup is then impacted using an offset cup handle. Several landmarks are used to verify an optimal cup position: (1) center hole to judge depth/seating of the cup; (2) orientation of the cup handle (an angle of 38° to 45° between the handle and the line between the anterior superior iliac spine in the horizontal plane for abduction; the angle between the handle and the horizontal plane (floor) for cup anteversion); (3) the special relation of the lateral edge of the cup and the acetabulum for cup inclination; (4) the relation of the medial edge of the cup and the teardrop for cup inclination; and (5) the relation of the equator of the trial head (135° trial neck) and the liner for both inclination and anteversion. It is important to aim for bony coverage of the anterior rim of the cup to avoid painful irritation of the psoas tendon. Osteophytes are resected. In the vast majority of cases, the posteroinferior part of the facies semilunata exceeds the rim of the cup if the latter is placed in a correct position. After insertion of the polar screw and the inlay, all retractors are removed.

Femoral Preparation

The leg is placed in a real of lazy figure-of-four position. A curved Hohmann retractor is placed medially around the posterior wall of the femoral metaphysis. Using a bone hook at the calcar, the femur is mobilized anteriorly. A large double-tipped Hohmann is placed behind the greater trochanter in the bare area between the gluteus minimus and medius insertion to push the femur even more forward. Only if the mobilization of the femur is sufficient, the leg is hyper-extended by breaking the table. In case of an insufficient femoral mobilization, the capsular release has to be extended.

During hyperextension, it is pivotal to avoid that the greater trochanter is caught behind the posterior acetabular wall to avoid a fracture. For optimal exposure of the neck osteotomy, the hyperextended leg is also adducted by an

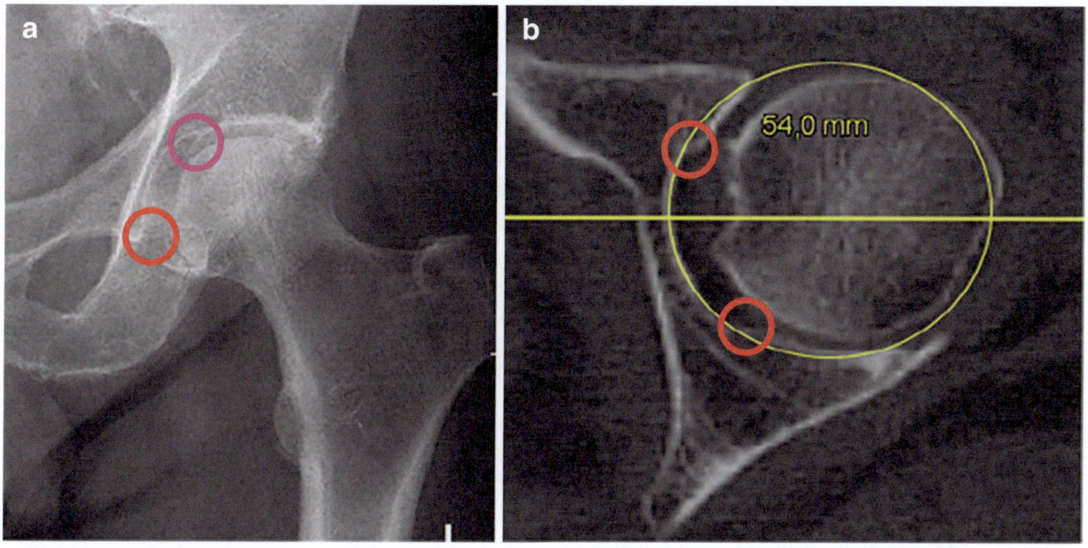

Fig. 24.2 Optimal positioning of the final reamer may be guided by the edges of the fossa. (**a**) The distance of the reamer to the teardrop (red circle) is helpful to estimate the mediolateral position. The apex of the fossa (purple circle) is helpful to estimate the superior/medial position. For example, in presence of a coxa profunda a bony step at the level of the apex of the fossa is desired, while in most other cases reaming should completely level out this area. (**b**) Axial CT scan through the center of rotation of a left hip. To estimate the anteroposterior positioning of the reamer, the bony step between the anterior fascines semilunata (anterior red circle) should be symmetric to the respective step posteriorly. After the final reamer, both steps should be completely flattened in most cases

assistant from the opposite side. In some cases (particularly in femoral revisions through DAA), the femoral exposure may be further improved by extending the approach proximally: The TFL is hereby detached from the anterior superior iliac spine and the anterior iliac crest. The femur is then broached using angled and/or offset broach handles according to the manufacturer's guidelines. With the leg in a figure-of-four position (i.e., the knee in close to 90° of flexion with the tibia parallel to the floor), the antetorsion of the broach is accurately assessable as the femur is in a standardized externally rotated position.

We do comment on evaluating the femoral prosthetic center of rotation and the technique of trialing in the "Surgeons perspective on LLD and Offset."

Closure

After implantation of the definitive stem and head, the hip is reduced and the table is brought back to a neutral position. The anterior capsulotomy is then closed with 2 to 4 absorbable sutures as is the reflected head of the rectus if transected. Next, the superficial fascia of the TFL is closed. Skin closure is performed with a barbed resorbable suture.

Postoperative Care

The patient is mobilized at the day of surgery and is allowed for immediate full weight-bearing with two crutches until a secure gait is achieved. Flexion is limited to 90° for 6 weeks to allow for optimal soft tissue healing.

DAA for Revision Surgery

DAA has proven useful in selected revision cases. This approach has several important advantages: The patient is in supine position and the pelvis hence in a more standardized position. This makes implant positioning easier and allows for better imaging using an intensifier. The approach is intermuscular, and most posterior structures including capsule and short external rotators can be preserved in most cases. In addition, while bilateral interventions are possible without repositioning or redraping, this might be considered for sterility reasons. We use this approach for most isolated cup revisions and also for selected stem revisions.

Case Example 1: Cup Revisions with Proximal Extension of DAA

Cup revision particularly with defects of the anterior wall, superior around the anterior inferior iliac spine or central cavitary defects, is usually well accessible through a DAA. Posterior column defects, large ischium defect, or pelvic discontinuities are more challenging and potentially easier accessible through a posterior or transfemoral approach.

This 59-year-old male avid runner presented with increasing groin pain 9 years after hip resurfacing (Fig. 24.3). While range of motion was normal, he showed clinical signs of an irritation of the psoas tendon. The plain X-ray showed no signs of implant loosening or osteolysis with a correct cup inclination. Serum cobalt level was 1137 nmol/L. The MRI with metal artifact reducing sequences revealed large cystic soft tissue lesions in line with an adverse reaction to metal debris. Conversion to a total hip was performed through a direct anterior approach. As the soft tissue lesion significantly extended around the anterior wall, a medial extension of the DAA was performed for better visualization: A chevron-shaped osteotomy of the anterior superior iliac spine was performed and the iliacus muscle was detached from the iliac crest and sub-periosteally elevated, allowing for retraction of the inguinal ligament and the Sartorius muscle medially. This gives an excellent view on the anterior inferior iliac spine and the direct and reflected tendon of the rectus muscle. The latter may be detached at its insertion to allow for optimized exposure of the anterior wall and the lateral aspect of the pubis. The pseudotumor was then resected, and the resurfacing was converted to a THA. The rectus tendon is reattached to the anterior inferior iliac spine with transosseous sutures, and the anterior superior iliac spine is anatomically reattached with a 3.5 mm screw.

Case Example: Bilateral DAA (R: Primary and L: Cup Revision with Autograft)

This 71-year-old woman presented 3 years after left THR elsewhere with increasing pain in her right hip and a progressive shortening of her left leg (Fig. 24.4). Plain X-ray revealed a cup migration medially with a cavitary but contained defect and an intact acetabular rim. Her right hip presented with osteoarthritis.

As symptoms were bilaterally and on the left side bone grafting of the cavitary defect was necessary, we opted for a bilateral intervention during the same anesthesia: First, standard THR is performed on the right side followed cup revision on the left during the same anesthesia. The femoral head of the right side was thereby used as a bulk autograft in the left acetabulum. A primary press-fit cup was then implanted with a solid rim fit, not necessitating additional screw fixation. As repositioning of the acetabular center of rotation is challenging, the use of an image intensifier is advised in such cases. Both procedures have been performed through a DAA without repositioning or redraping of the patient between the two interventions. This bilateral strategy allows the use of the best possible graft (nonfrozen autograft) in a fairly large quantity.

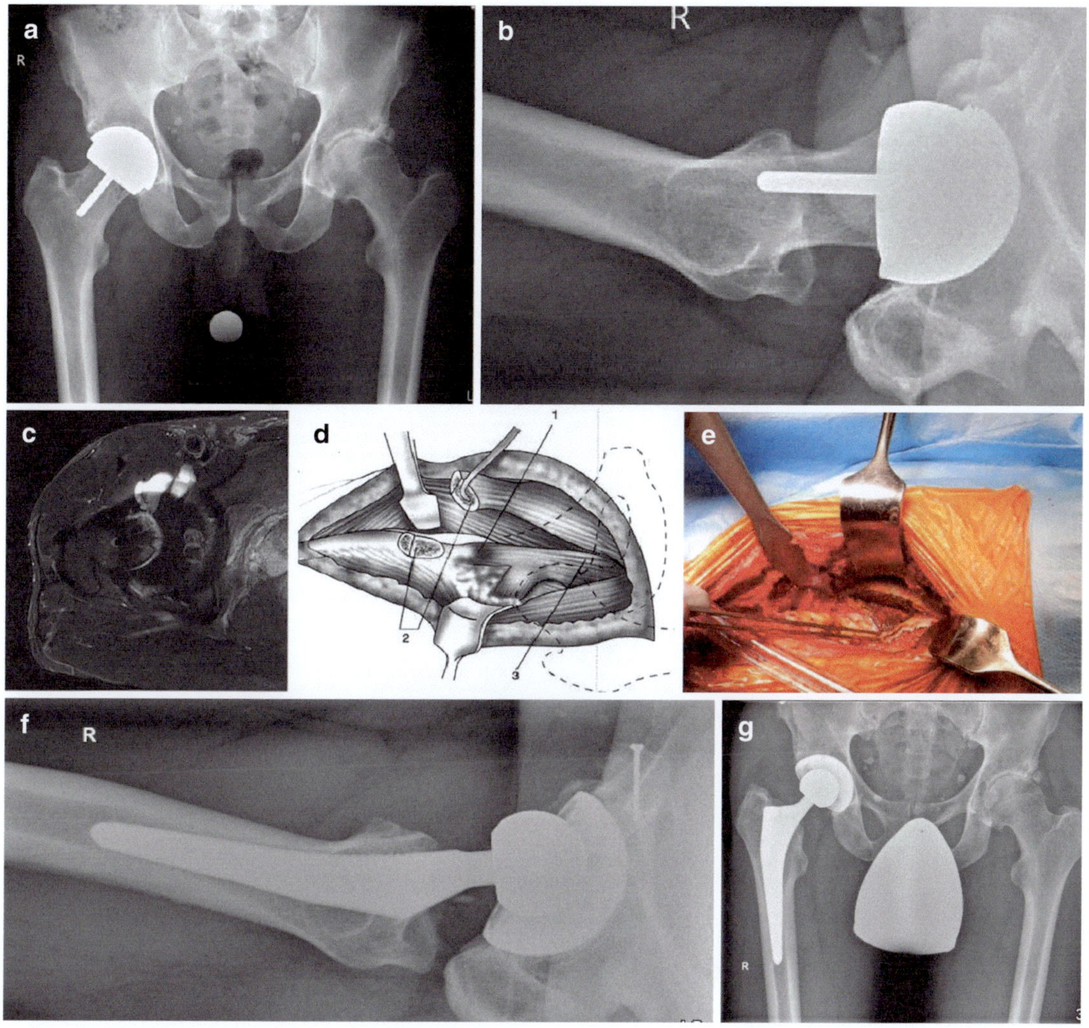

Fig. 24.3 (**a–g**) 59-year-old man with adverse reaction to metal debris (ARMD) after hip resurfacing (**a–c**). To access the cysts anterior to the anterior acetabular wall, the ASIS is osteotomized and retracted together with the origins of the inguinal ligament and the sartorius muscle medially (**d**, **e**). After implantation of the total hip prosthesis, the ASIS is reduced and fixed with a 3.5 mm steel screw

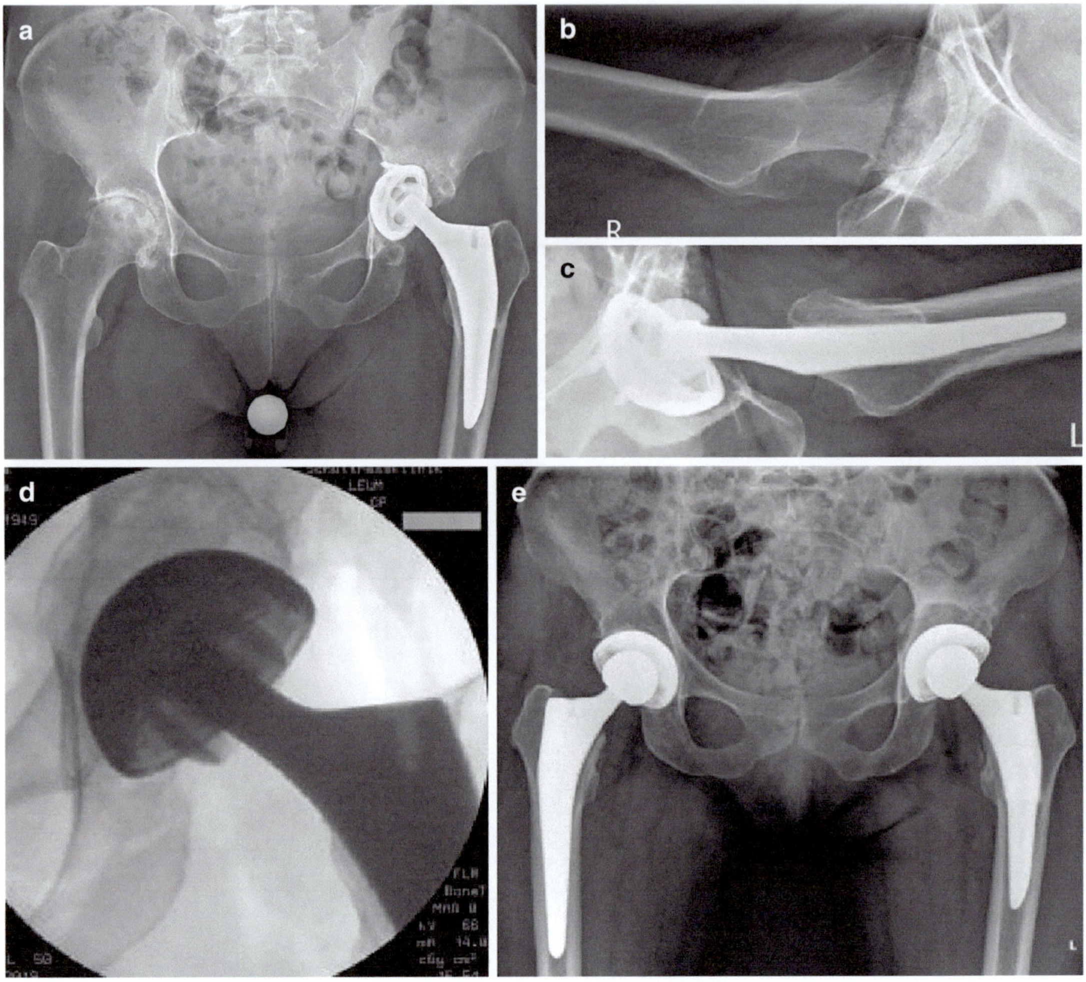

Fig. 24.4 (**a**–**e**) 71-year-old woman. Plain X-ray reveals osteoarthritis on the right hip and cup migration on the left. After THR on the right through a DAA cup revision on the left hip was performed during the same anesthesia. The femoral head of the right hip was used as an autograft on the left hip. Image intensifier was used to control cup placement (D)

References

1. Bertin KC, Rottinger H. Anterolateral mini-incision hip replacement surgery: a modified Watson-Jones approach. Clin Orthop Relat Res. 2004;(429):248–55.
2. Hueter C. Grundriss der Chirurgie. 2nd ed. Vogel, F.C.W; 1883.
3. Keggi KJ, Huo MH, Zatorski LE. Anterior approach to total hip replacement: surgical technique and clinical results of our first one thousand cases using non-cemented prostheses. Yale J Biol Med. 1993;66(3):243–56.
4. Lovell TP. Single-incision direct anterior approach for total hip arthroplasty using a standard operating table. J Arthroplast. 2008;23(7 Suppl):64–8.
5. Bender B, Nogler M, Hozack WJ. Direct anterior approach for total hip arthroplasty. Orthop Clin North Am. 2009;40(3):321–8.
6. Macario A. What does one minute of operating room time cost? J Clin Anesth. 2010;22(4):233–6.
7. Leunig M, Faas M, von Knoch F, Naal FD. Skin crease 'bikini' incision for anterior approach total hip arthroplasty: surgical technique and preliminary results. Clin Orthop Relat Res. 2013;471(7):2245–52.
8. Leunig M, Hutmacher JE, Ricciardi BF, Impellizzeri FM, Rudiger HA, Naal FD. Skin crease 'bikini' incision for the direct anterior approach in total hip arthroplasty: a two- to four-year comparative study in 964 patients. Bone Joint J. 2018;100-B(7):853–61.

25 A Hybrid Technique with a Standard Table and Mechanical Leg Holder

Joshua C. Rozell, Dimitri E. Delagrammaticas, and Raymond H. Kim

The anterior approach for hip arthroplasty has gained popularity primarily for its benefits in early recovery, minimally invasive nature, and soft tissue preservation. The approach preserves the posterior capsule, external rotators, and abductors implicit in normal hip biomechanics helping to mitigate dislocation risk. The preservation of the hip deltoid, comprised of the abductors, gluteus maximus, and tensor musculature, facilitates early functional recovery and mitigate hip abduction weakness [1, 2]. Typically, the approach is performed in the supine position where adequate positioning of the supine pelvis in three-dimensional space during surgery is critical to establish the appropriate cup position. While the target for acetabular inclination and anteversion has yet to be standardized [3], the anterior approach allows for consistent pelvic position and facilitates the use of fluoroscopy to better understand component placement.

Anterior approach for hip arthroplasty can be performed with or without the use of an orthopedic table. For the purposes of this chapter, the standard operating table will be discussed. Benefits of a standard operating room table include cost savings, no requirement for an assistant outside of the sterile field to reposition the leg throughout the case, and the ability to clinically evaluate stability and leg lengths with the legs freely draped. Both methods are amendable to fluoroscopic access during the case [4, 5]. The specialized table facilitates more hip extension but less adduction, whereas the standard table allows more adduction and less extension. Depending on the desired access, nature of the procedure (i.e., the need to access the femur versus the acetabulum, or both, for revision), anatomic variability, or implant and patient factors, one set up may be preferential to another.

The surgical technique for both primary and revision approaches using a standard table includes positioning the patient on the table such that the pubic symphysis is at the level of the break in the bed. This facilitates femoral exposure once the foot of the bed is lowered. The patient should be positioned centrally on the bed to limit overlap of the bed frame in the fluoroscopic field. Lastly, the nonoperative leg should be draped into the field to allow access to both feet and ankles for assessment of leg lengths. During femoral exposure, the nonoperative leg is positioning high on a surgical stand to allow for

J. C. Rozell
Department of Orthopaedic Surgery, NYU Langone Health, New York, NY, USA
e-mail: Joshua.rozell@nyulangone.org

D. E. Delagrammaticas
Central Coast Orthopedic Group, San Luis Obispo, CA, USA

R. H. Kim (✉)
Department of Orthopaedic Surgery, The Steadman Clinic, Vail, CO, USA
e-mail: rkim@thesteadmanclinic.comz

J. M. Matta, A. P. Sah (eds.), *Anterior Hip Replacement*,
https://doi.org/10.1007/978-3-030-91896-5_25

adduction of the operative leg. Alternatively, the leg may be abducted on a large arm board. Proximally, draping should extend above the iliac crest to allow for extension of the incision if needed. To facilitate femoral elevation during femoral preparation, a stack of surgical towels may be wrapped into a cylinder, and the size of a soda can be placed slightly laterally and proximally under the proximal femur.

Once the patient is appropriately positioned on the bed, the positioning arm is attached and clamped to the bed and placed at the level of the mid-tibia in the "pre-home" position with both logos parallel with each other. As the arm is adjusted into the home position, the arm appears in the shape of an "s" (Fig. 25.1). The home position facilitates proper sterile draping. The sterile draping kit contains the padding for the leg holder, Coban to affix the padding to the operative leg, and the sterile drape. The cover is slipped over the arm and pulled all the way down to the attachment on the table. A second drape is wrapped around the base of the arm to seal off the interface and eliminate concerns for sterility.

The padding for the leg bracket is placed over the patient's operative leg. The padding has malleable backing to assist with securing it to the metal bracket. There are also markings, and directionality prompts on the foam to place and mold the pad correctly. The pad is contoured around the leg and secured in place under a sterile metal bracket. The distal aspect of the padding is contoured to the dorsal aspect of the patient's foot. The Velcro loops are strapped around the leg and foot, securing the leg holder in place. Coban is then applied over the padding to further secure the leg holder, out of the way of the quick connect mechanism so as not to obscure this interface.

The adapter bracket for the leg holder is placed onto the positioning arm using a screw mechanism. The arm is now ready to be positioned onto the leg. By squeezing the handle, this frees the arm and allows multiple degrees of freedom. The arm is attached via a quick connect mechanism to the leg bracket, where two locations of attachment for the positioning arm are available for connections: anteriorly and medially. The arm is initially connected to the anterior adapter (Fig. 25.2) and is transferred to the medial adapter during femoral preparation so as to obtain adequate external rotation of the leg during this part of the operation.

A second positioning arm can be attached and draped on the contralateral side of the table at the level of the pelvis to facilitate assistant-free surgery if desired or may also securely hold the nonoperative leg. The arm is outfitted with a retractor coupler to allow for attachment of the two retractor holders (Fig. 25.3). While standing at the operative site, the surgeon has full control of both positioning arms to facilitate seamless operative flow (Fig. 25.4).

The first position of the leg holder for skin exposure is defined by a neutral leg position with the hip flexed slightly (Fig. 25.5). After the skin

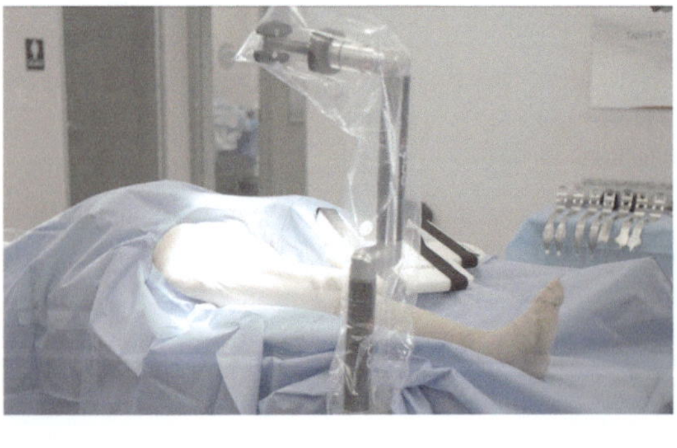

Fig. 25.1 Home position

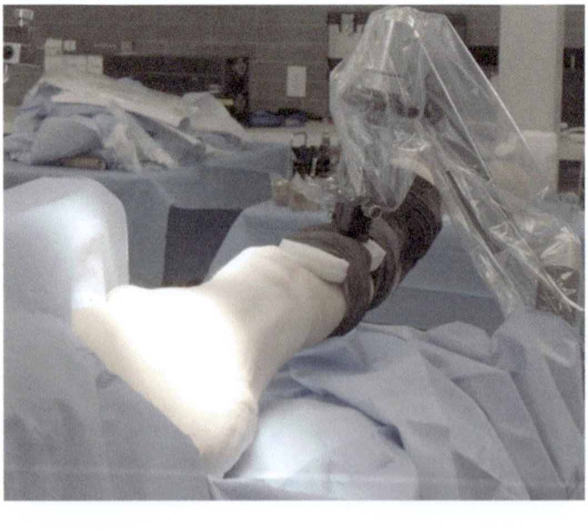

Fig. 25.2 Foot position before case

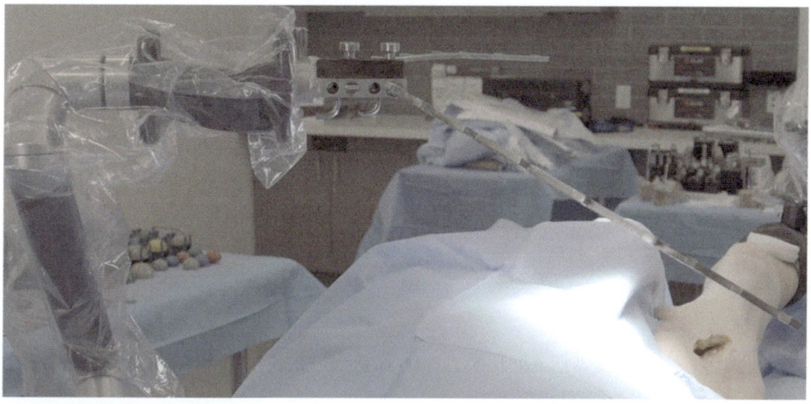

Fig. 25.3 Contralateral positioning arm

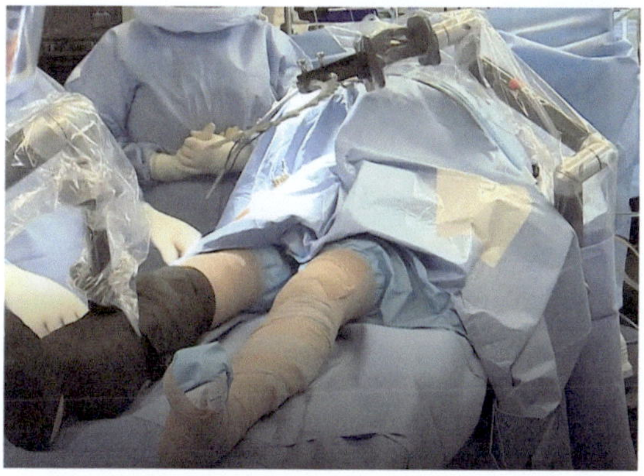

Fig. 25.4 Post draping

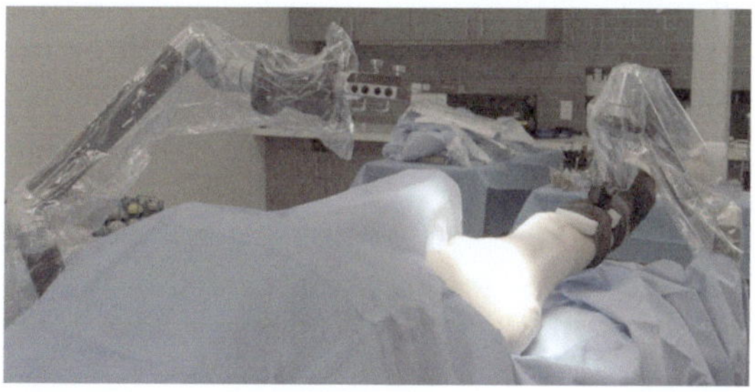

Fig. 25.5 Prior to incision

incision is made, a rake can be held in the skin by the contralateral positioning arm. Once the surgeon releases the handle on the positioner, the arm becomes locked in space with minimal toggle. The retractor wings can be attached to the coupler, one in the proximal direction and the other distally. The first retractor is placed under the tensor fascia lata along the superior aspect of the femoral neck. The second retractor is placed medially under the inferior femoral neck. Both retractors can be held by the contralateral positioning arm with appropriate tension. A third retractor is typically placed along the anterior acetabular rim beneath the rectus femoris to fully expose the hip capsule prior to capsulotomy (Fig. 25.6). Careful placement of this retractor is imperative so as to limit injury to the femoral nerve. Yoshino et al. recently performed a cadaveric study dividing the acetabulum into 360° based on a line drawn from the anterior superior iliac spine through the center of the acetabulum. They found that the femoral nerve was within 16.6–33.2 mm of the acetabular rim at points from 0° to 150° and was closest to the rim at 90° [6]. A capsulotomy or capsulectomy is then performed based on surgeon preference. Fluoroscopy may be utilized with the retractors in place to verify the position of the femoral neck osteotomy if desired (Fig. 25.7). After the osteotomy, the ipsilateral positioning arm can be moved into a position of slight traction and external rotation to facilitate removal of the femoral head (and the intercalary segment of femoral neck if a napkin ring osteotomy is performed).

Once the femoral head is removed, attention is then turned toward placement of the inferior and posterior acetabular retractors. The posterior retractor is placed between the acetabulum and the greater trochanter of the femur (Fig. 25.8). An assessment of the resection depth of the femoral neck is essential, as leaving too much remaining neck will make reamer insertion difficult. The surgeon should be able to visualize the posterior

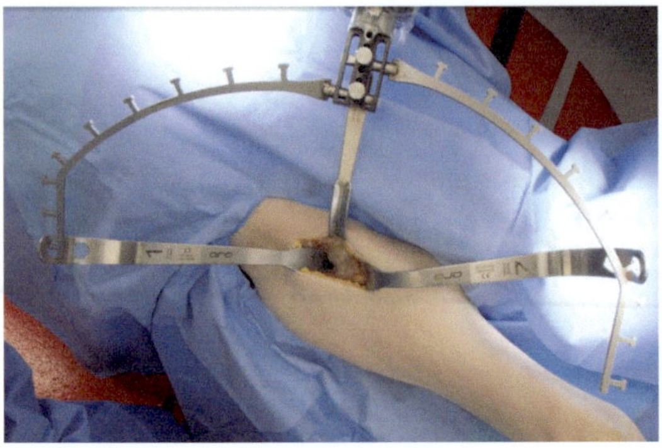

Fig. 25.6 Prior to femoral neck cut

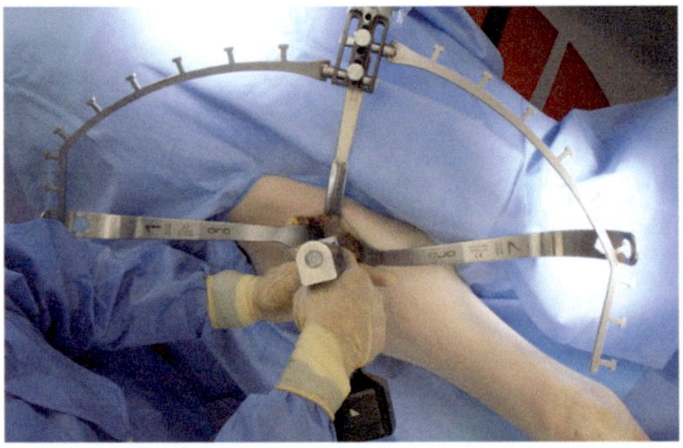

Fig. 25.7 Neck cut

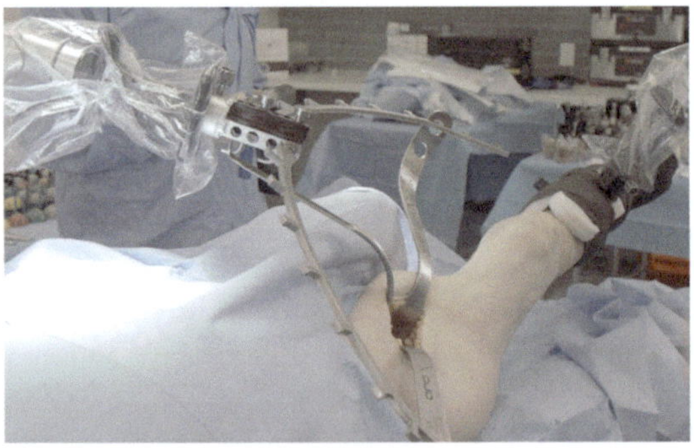

Fig. 25.8 Acetabular exposure

capsular sling, which indicates sufficient resection. Some longitudinal traction and external rotation may be applied via the ipsilateral positioning arm to aid in acetabular reamer insertion and removal. Fluoroscopy can also be used with the reamer in place to assess positioning and medialization.

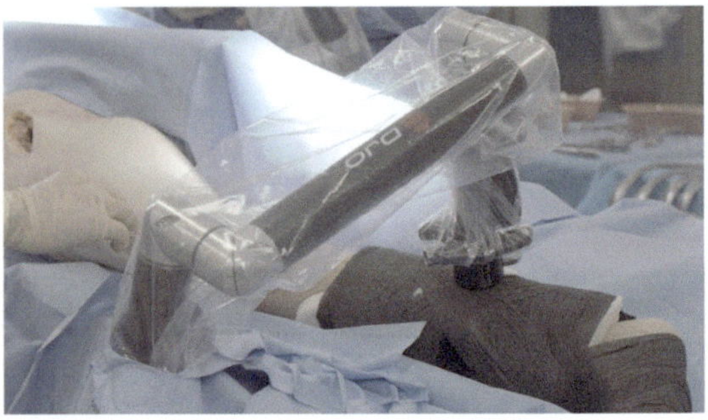

Fig. 25.9 Start of femoral exposure leg position

Once the acetabular shell and liner have been inserted, the retractors are removed, and the leg is position for femoral preparation. The bed is first placed into slight Trendelenburg, and the foot of the bed is lowered to facilitate leg extension. The traction on the leg is removed, and the positioning arm quick connect is disengaged from the operative leg. The leg can be positioned in the figure of four positions to confirm that the inferior medial femoral release of the pubofemoral ligament is complete to the level of the lesser trochanter. After this release is confirmed, the operative leg is returned to neutral and the non-operative leg may be flexed and positioned with an additional positioning arm out of the way for adduction of the operative leg. The quick connect of the operative leg is transferred to the medial attachment to guide extension external rotation and adduction (Fig. 25.9).

Retractors are then placed to facilitate femoral broaching (Fig. 25.10). A blunt retractor is placed medially around the posterior femoral neck. The contralateral positioning arm holds this in place. The bump is then placed under the proximal femur to facilitate femoral elevation out of the wound. A second wide retractor is placed between the abductors and the femur behind the greater trochanter to retract the TFL and allow superior capsular release on the femur to further allow the proximal femur to be delivered out of the wound. If required, a bone hook may be used to pull the proximal femur up out of the wound and laterally to visualize the tight superior capsule in order to titrate the release. Additionally, if the tensor is robust, the surgeon can trace the origin back to

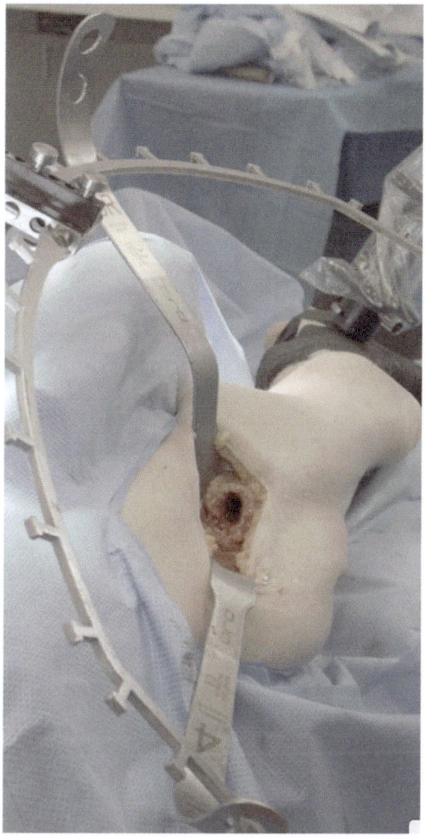

Fig. 25.10 Femoral exposure for broaching

the anterior superior iliac spine and release some of the insertion site sharply. Once the femur is adequately exposed, femoral broaching can begin in the standard fashion. It is important that exposure of the femur is sufficient such that the introduction and removal of instruments and broaches do not abrade the proximal skin of the incision as this may cause wound issues postoperatively. If the retractor holder is getting in the way of broaching, it can be repositioned or removed for this portion of the procedure and an assistant on the opposite side of the table may hold the trochanteric retractor manually.

Once an appropriately sized trial broach is in place, a trial head and neck are applied. The retractors are removed, and the leg is released from the quick connect distally. This allows for the surgeon to both reduce the hip and clinically and radiographically check leg lengths. Fluoroscopic views and clinical stability testing should confirm the appropriate restoration of leg length and offset, while also verifying component positioning and sizing. The hip is dislocated, trials removed, and the final femoral stem and head are then impacted in place.

The anterior approach has been shown to have a steep learning curve [7, 8], and complications reported with this approach compared to other approaches include higher rates of femoral fracture, periprosthetic infection, and wound break down [9, 10]. However, surgeon experience beyond the learning curve coupled with the use of an efficient and utilitarian positioning device can provide consistent and reliable leg positioning to facilitate exposure, decrease operative time, blood loss, and ultimately mitigate these risks.

References

1. Taunton MJ, Mason JB, Odum SM, Springer BD. Direct anterior total hip arthroplasty yields more rapid voluntary cessation of all walking aids: a prospective, randomized clinical trial. J Arthroplast. 2014;29(9 Suppl):169–72.
2. Kreuzer S, Matta JM. Single incision anterior approach for total hip arthroplasty: Smith-Peterson approach. In: O'Connor MI, editor. Limited incisions for total hip arthroplasty. 1st ed. Rosemont: AAOS; 2007.
3. Abdel MP, von Roth P, Jennings MT, Hanssen AD, Pagnano MW. What safe zone? The vast majority of dislocated THAs are within the Lewinnek safe zone for acetabular component position. Clin Orthop Relat Res. 2016;474(2):386–91.
4. Matta JM, Shahrdar C, Ferguson T. Single-incision anterior approach for total hip arthroplasty on an orthopaedic table. Clin Orthop Relat Res. 2005;441:115–24.
5. Lovell TP. Single-incision direct anterior approach for total hip arthroplasty using a standard operating table. J Arthroplast. 2008;23(7 Suppl):64–8.
6. Yoshino K, Nakamura J, Hagiwara S, Suzuki T, Kawasaki Y, Ohtori S. Anatomical implications regarding femoral nerve palsy during a direct anterior approach to total hip arthroplasty: a cadaveric study. J Bone Joint Surg Am. 2020;102(2):137–42.
7. de Steiger RN, Lorimer M, Solomon M. What is the learning curve for the anterior approach for total hip arthroplasty? Clin Orthop Relat Res. 2015;473(12):3860–6.

8. Meermans G, Konan S, Das R, Volpin A, Haddas FS. The direct anterior approach in total hip arthroplasty: a systematic review of the literature. Bone Joint J. 2017;99-B(6):732–40.
9. Aggarwal VK, Elbuluk A, Dundon J, Herrero C, Hernandez C, Vigdorchik JM, et al. Surgical approach significantly affects the complication rates associated with total hip arthroplasty. Bone Joint J. 2019;101-B(6):646–51.
10. Pincus D, Jenkinson R, Paterson M, Leroux T, Ravi B. Association between surgical approach and major surgical complications in patients undergoing total hip arthroplasty. JAMA. 2020;323(11):1070–6.

26 My Continuous Evolution in Using Anterior Approach

Stefan W. Kreuzer

My journey to use direct anterior approach (DAA) hip replacement started when I observed Dr. Joel Matta over 5 cases in 2003. My first exposure to the DAA was observing him utilizing the Matta table. That observation was very impactful, and I anticipated great potential for DAA to be used as the primary approach I would use in my practice. While returning home, I continued reviewing my notes from the observation, and without hesitation, I performed my first case using DAA with the OSI ProFx table. That was a turning point in my practice, and I have been using DAA since then on all my patients.

I started my practice with OSI ProFx table because it was one of the commonly used DAA tables at the time. My first case took a very long time relative to my cases that I currently perform. However, the outcome was very positive, and the patient depicted excellent postoperative clinical performance. My second case by using DAA was done within 2 days after my first case. The patient informed me that she was able to "walk" into church only 4 days after surgery without using any assistive device! I was told that her friends speculated that she did not receive her hip surgery as her gait pattern looked very normal. This story was somehow circulated in the community and ended up being broadcasted on local evening news, and this was a jump-start to my practice.

While clinical data on DAA and postoperative data were limited back in 2003, those early cases I performed and their excellent outcome had given me the confidence that DAA would be a game-changing approach in the field of hip arthroplasty. Within the next year, I increased the number of treated patients from 50 to 170 per year only 2 years after finishing my fellowship in reconstructive joint replacement. Since that time, I have performed more than 6000 DAA hip replacements and my practice has grown to perform over 1000 total joint replacement cases per year. One of the early comments I received from my colleagues, particularly those not familiar with DAA, was their concern about the high cost of marketing to promote anterior approach to patients. However, my experience was completely different; all my patients were referred to me by primary care physicians and other previous patients who had excellent experience with the DAA hip replacement. Often patients were surprised by their rapid recovery with their surgery, as many had previous interaction with other family members who underwent hip replacement with a different approach and had to spend several months on recovery.

In my evolution of DAA hip replacement, I have gone through four distinct phases. In the first phase, I have spent many hours thinking about the approach and evaluating different

S. W. Kreuzer (✉)
INOV8 Orthopedics, Houston, TX, USA
e-mail: skreuzer@inov8hc.com; stefan@inov8hc.com

J. M. Matta, A. P. Sah (eds.), *Anterior Hip Replacement*,
https://doi.org/10.1007/978-3-030-91896-5_26

aspects of the surgery including exposure, management of the capsule, reaming the acetabulum, proper placement of the acetabulum cup, management of the femur and avoiding complications, and physical therapy as well as postoperative care. I focused on proper location of the incision, soft tissue preservation, proper handling of the tensor fascia lata, and proper releases to mobilize the femur. In addition, my approach evolved to improve reaming technique by incorporating the C-arm to assist in reaming and cup position. Broaching the femur became easier as I improved the release technique and I further advanced in cementing techniques. My evolution in DAA hip replacement continued by figuring out how to increase accuracy in predicting leg length by utilizing the C-arm. I continued the improvement of leg length accuracy by adding a protocol to obtain an AP pelvis x-ray. There was a significant learning curve within the first 100 cases, and after that, the surgical time and the complication rate significantly decreased in my cases.

During the second phase, I started utilizing advanced technologies such as computer navigation and later robotics. To enter this phase, I started to replace the C-arm with computer navigation, but an AP pelvis radiograph was obtained after the implant placement. In this phase, I also started to establish a measure of offset with the navigation tool to further improve the accuracy of the anatomic reconstruction of the hip center. The result of these changes further improved our quest for optimal implant position, leg length reconstruction, and proper offset.

I entered the third phase of my evolution in DAA hip replacement by significantly increasing the number of treatments in younger patients who needed hip replacement. To achieve better results specifically in this population, I explored various implants that were better suited for these groups of patients to accommodate a more active postoperative lifestyle. Specifically, I started utilizing hip resurfacing and neck preserving implants as well as ceramic-on-ceramic bearing surfaces for my younger patients. I based my decision on evidence in the literature indicating that age- and BMI-matched cohorts showed resurfacing and neck preserving implants resulting in better performance in patients with high level of activities. In this phase, I shifted away from cementing and utilized press-fit implants only. I was able to perform more complex revision cases through the DAA including stem revision and cage reconstruction and finally migrated to anterior revision only.

The fourth phase of my evolution of DAA hip replacement started with focusing on further improving pain protocols, shortening length of stay, and the migration of inpatient model into an outpatient total joint replacement approach. Over 95% of my primary and revision hips stayed only one night in the hospital, and I have now performed more than 450 anterior hip replacements in an ambulatory surgical center with an average length of stay of only 6 hours. Due to the COVID-19 pandemic, I now utilize a protocol to discharge 70% of my inpatient cases performed at the hospital on the same day. In addition, I started to incorporate the large body of new knowledge of functional position of the acetabulum and the impact of spine on pelvic motion and on hip stability. At this time, I have performed more than 1000 cases by using the optimized position system (OPS, Corin Inc., USA) in conjunction with computer navigation to further optimize patient-specific acetabular targets of inclination and anteversion. I continued to expand the indication for complex revisions, and currently, I perform over 99% of complex primary and revision total hip replacement through the anterior approach. Despite decrease in hip cementing in phase three, I have resumed cementing hips in patients with type-c bone and I expect the percentage of hip cementing increases over the next few years.

In my journey through DAA hip replacement, I also started contributing to the field by utilizing educational live broadcasting of my surgeries by using a new platform called Proximie. I also started implementing a 3D virtual OR (Medoptic

TM—Immertec) to further expand my ability to teach the tricks of DAA to other hip surgeons and their surgical team. My goal is to improve the outcome and further expand the usage of this DAA in hip replacement cases.

My journey through DAA hip replacement has been very interesting and rewarding, and I encourage all surgeons to explore this approach for treatment of their patients. I am always grateful to Dr. Joel Matta for encouraging me to start this journey in 2003.

Part V

Introduction to Part V

Controversies Regarding the Basics (Pro vs Con)

Regarding differences in methods for performing anterior approach, certain variations have come up repeatedly as essential or at least beneficial or not beneficial. It is my observation that surgeons often get "entrenched" in their own methodology and thinking. Ideally, we should be open minded and receptive to facts and logic in order to move AA in positive directions. Pro and con arguments are presented here to invite the reader to do this.

The Orthopedic Table Versus the Standard OR Bed for the Anterior Approach

27

Nicholas H. Mast, Michael Nogler, and Michael Leunig

The Orthopedic Table

Nicholas H. Mast

A common misconception of surgeons as they approach hip surgery is related to the use of the orthopedic table. Over the past 50 years of orthopedic surgery, the typical North American exposure to hip surgery on a specialized table involved a hip pinning or femoral nailing procedure performed on a large, sometimes cumbersome table such as the "Chick Table." These tables were commonly called the "fracture table" or "traction table" as they were utilized predominantly when traction was required as the most important manipulation required to reduce a displaced fracture.

Internationally, the experience of using the "fracture table" and fluoroscopy was reserved for the traumatologist. Typically, the orthopedist was performing surgery without such tools at a different center. In many places, the lineages were not typically mixed as fracture surgery was a distinct entity of trauma or general surgery, while orthopedics was largely dedicated to reconstructive efforts. The equipment needs in each venue were vastly different, allowing for very little comingling of techniques and technologies.

A different linage of "orthopedic tables" was introduced in France in the twentieth century as pioneers in acetabular fracture management required more functionality of existing tables. From this was born the concept of a mobile spar, to allow for flexion and extension in addition to the more traditional adduction and abduction of the hip. The Judet table was one of the first orthopedic tables that allowed for this functionality (Fig. 27.1), with more recent models (Tasserit, Gron, FR) incorporating carbon fiber composites to allow for intraoperative fluoroscopy. These tables were much better suited to the techniques of hip arthroplasty, but because of difficulties obtaining tables, and commonly parts to service these devices, they achieved poor adoption worldwide.

For many years, these newer "orthopedic tables" were reserved for management of complex trauma such as pelvic ring and acetabular fractures. Outside of France, these tables were rarely used for arthroplasty. In their own right, for arthroplasty, these first tables did not offer much more than a well-placed bump behind the thigh and the ability to extend the hip. However, in the early 2000s additional modifications of the

N. H. Mast (✉)
The Hip and Pelvis Institute, San Francisco, CA, USA
e-mail: doctormast@sfhips.com

M. Nogler
Department of Orthopaedic Surgery, Medical University of Innsbruck, Innsbruck, Austria
e-mail: michael.nogler@professor-nogler.at

M. Leunig
Hip Surgery - Schulthess Clinic, Zürich, Switzerland

J. M. Matta, A. P. Sah (eds.), *Anterior Hip Replacement*,
https://doi.org/10.1007/978-3-030-91896-5_27

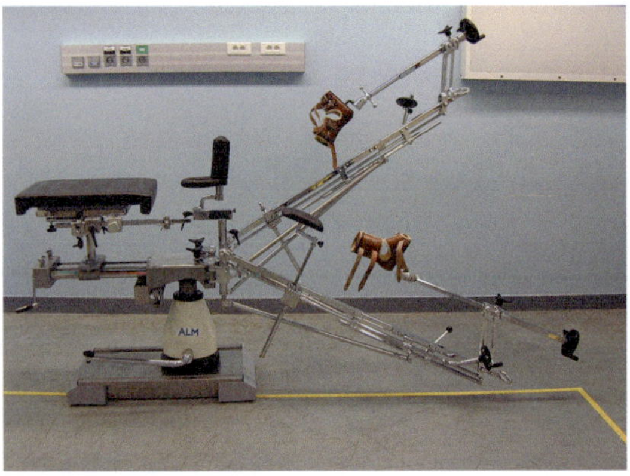

Fig. 27.1 Photograph of the original Judet table with the mobile spar, note the bump for position behind the thigh that can be used to raise or lower the femur during the procedure. (Photo courtesy Joel Matta)

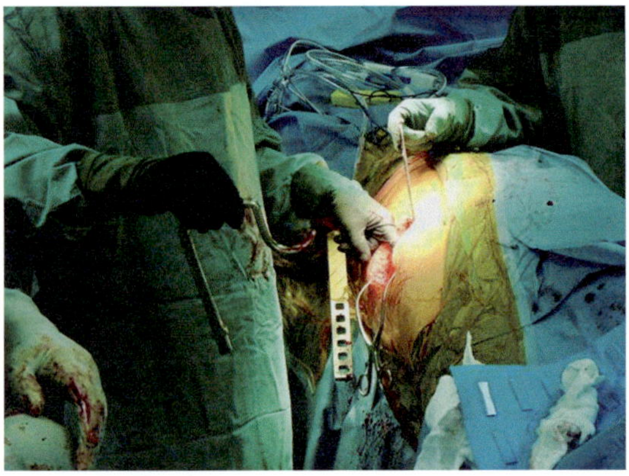

Fig. 27.2 Photograph of the original femoral hook for the orthopedic table circa 2001. (Joel Matta pictured)

table included a femoral hook that would be attached to a lift at the side of the table (Fig. 27.2). This modification allowed one to independently lift the femur for exposure without compressing the surrounding soft tissues. This facilitated the exposure and replaced a scrubbed assistant who was commonly called upon to elevate the femur with the large bone hook.

The modern "orthopedic table" is a purpose-built engineering feat. It is designed with smaller footprints, durable parts, improved radiolucency, and power controls to elevate the femur and or the extremity during surgery. The Hana table (Mizuho OSI) is the prototypical table with modern functionality for anterior approach surgery. A dizzying array of tables and table adapters are now commercially available, to facilitate anterior approach surgery using concepts pioneered by these early surgeons.

The "orthopedic table" currently employed in this regard is worlds different from the "fracture tables" or "traction tables" of prior generations. Traction is one of the functions, but arguably the least important during anterior approach hip replacement surgery. The table functions analogously in the hip to current extremity positioners used commonly in shoulder surgery.

No one would argue that a shoulder surgery performed using a McConnell arm positioner is any different than one performed using a padded mayo and a scrubbed assistant; however, these extremity positioners are commonly employed by most surgeons with more than a passing interest in complex shoulder surgery. Where it matters, these "extremity positioners" substitute for a scrubbed assistant and reduce the workload for the surgeon. While technical "work-arounds" exist to allow for techniques to be applied to the standard table, they give up some of the benefits that the orthopedic table affords.

The most common benefits of the orthopedic table in the anterior approach are standardization of pelvic and extremity position making access to the hip more reproducible, facilitation of the use of intraoperative fluoroscopy making intraoperative control of implant positioning more reliable, and reduction in the need for scrubbed assistants making overall cost of the procedure more economical.

Operating the patient in the supine position is one of the fundamental benefits that the anterior approach affords over lateral approaches to the hip. With the patient in the supine position, correct positioning of the acetabular component in the axial plane is facilitated by the table. Flexion and extension of the pelvis and axial rotation can be easily controlled for. This advantage is true for techniques that employ the standard and orthopedic tables alike. However, there is greatly improved "radiographic" standardization that can be employed using the increased radiolucency afforded by the carbon fiber cantilevered structure of the orthopedic table. The center of the sacrum and symphysis can be aligned flexion and extension of the hip controlled for radiographically, which translates to improved understanding of pelvic position during the case. This certainly can aid the surgeon when physical landmarks are not reliable (such as in the obese, the complex primary, the post-traumatic deformity, and the revision circumstances). Surgeons may argue that the setup is cumbersome when using the orthopedic table, but with proper staff and surgeon training, we find the opposite is true. For example, many surgeons that perform the technique on the standard table must sterile prepare and drape both extremities free, when using the orthopedic table, once the patient is correctly positioned on the table sterile prepping and draping of the involved surgical field is usually all that is required.

Access to the hip is improved during the surgical approach when performed on the orthopedic table. The table in this manner serves as the "silent assistant" allowing the extremity to be manipulated and held in position to facilitate exposure during the course of the procedure. The case unfolds in a very standardized fashion, with certain positions being preferred during portions of the case. The various positions used are detailed (Figs. 27.3, 27.4 and 27.5). As the exposure is facilitated by the orthopedic table and position of the extremity, surgical releases can be titrated to the need of the case, which minimizes surgical trauma and potentially minimizes the potential for prosthetic instability.

During complex primary and revision circumstances, the improved fluoroscopic control facilitated by the orthopedic table improves reliability of implant position. The ability to visualize the AP pelvis, 45° of oblique views of the pelvis, as well as the entirety of the operative and the non-operative femur, can be helpful in complex reconstruction (Fig. 27.6).

Most of the detractors of the technique argue against the operative table in that it prevents direct clinical assessment of limb length. Typically, it is argued that the best way to measure the length of the limb is by manual palpation of the medial malleoli, I would argue that one can be much more sensitive to minor alterations in implant position by the use of intraoperative radiographs or fluoroscopy. For example, alterations of global offset can affect patient perceptions of limb length. Offset is a much more difficult parameter to evaluate and reconstruct using manual palpation. However, with the improved control afforded by the orthopedic table and fluoroscopy, one can be much more precise with reconstruction of this parameter.

Another argument commonly levered at those that use the orthopedic table and table extensions is that the orthopedic table adds an unnecessary expense to a procedure. This is true if you do not take labor into account as a cost. One must not neglect that the major expense in an orthopedic practice is the skilled labor it employs. A typical surgeon employing the anterior approach on a standard table requires 2 scrubbed assistants. A physician assistant or scrubbed assistant can easily draw the cost of an orthopedic table in a year. When looked at from the total cost of the procedure and amortized over the life of the orthopedic table, there can be profound cost savings in terms of labor cost to the procedure.

Fundamentally, I do not believe the anterior approach performed on the standard operating table or on the orthopedic table are any different. However, there are some compelling advantages that the orthopedic table provides. For these reasons, I believe the marketplace will adopt the orthopedic table technique and be the preferred technique of the next generation of hip surgeons.

DAA with a Trauma Table

Michael Nogler

The previous surgeon perspective provides a wonderful overview on the history of traction tables in Orthopaedics and Trauma Surgery. I do not use a distraction table in hip arthroplasty (I sometimes use it for other procedures). The only one that I can use is a table from our trauma department, which I suppose has its focus on trauma, but it does what it is meant for—it holds the leg and distracts the hip if I wish so.

Over the past 20 years though, I have been involved in discussions on the use of specialized tables in DAA. I am quite sure that I have heard and given all the arguments on both sides of the debate regarding use of the the various specialized orthopaedic tables available. My colleague Dr.

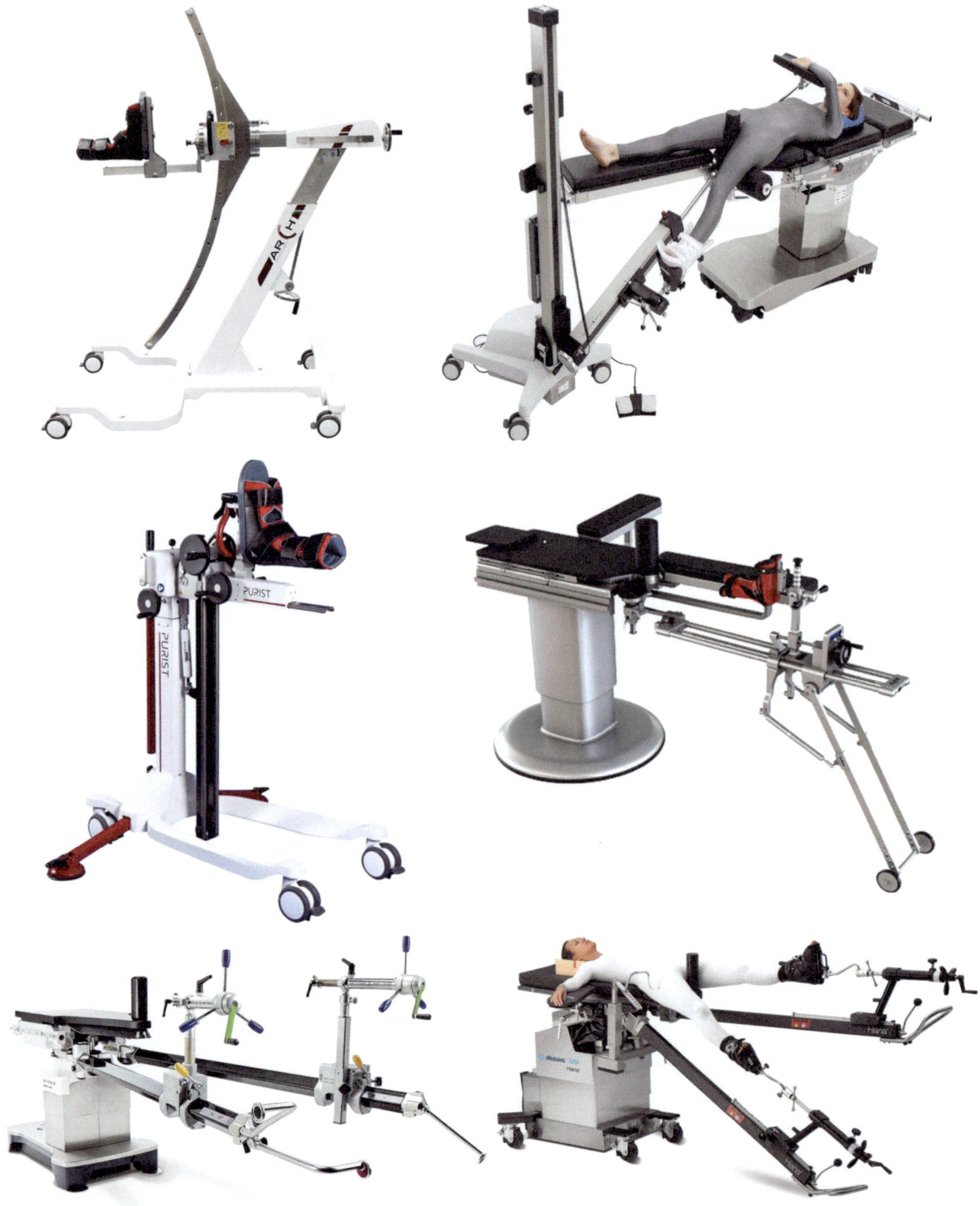

Fig. 27.3 Images of current designs of orthopedic tables and table adaptors suited to the anterior approach for hip replacement available at time of publication. From top left, The "arch table", Innovative Orthopedic Technologies, "Condor MedTec", "RotexTable®". The "Purist table extension", Innovative Orthopedic Technologies, The "Medacta table extension", Medacta International, Switzerland, The Maquet "Yuno" table, Getinge AB and the "Hana" table, MizuhoOSI, Union City, CA shown bottom right

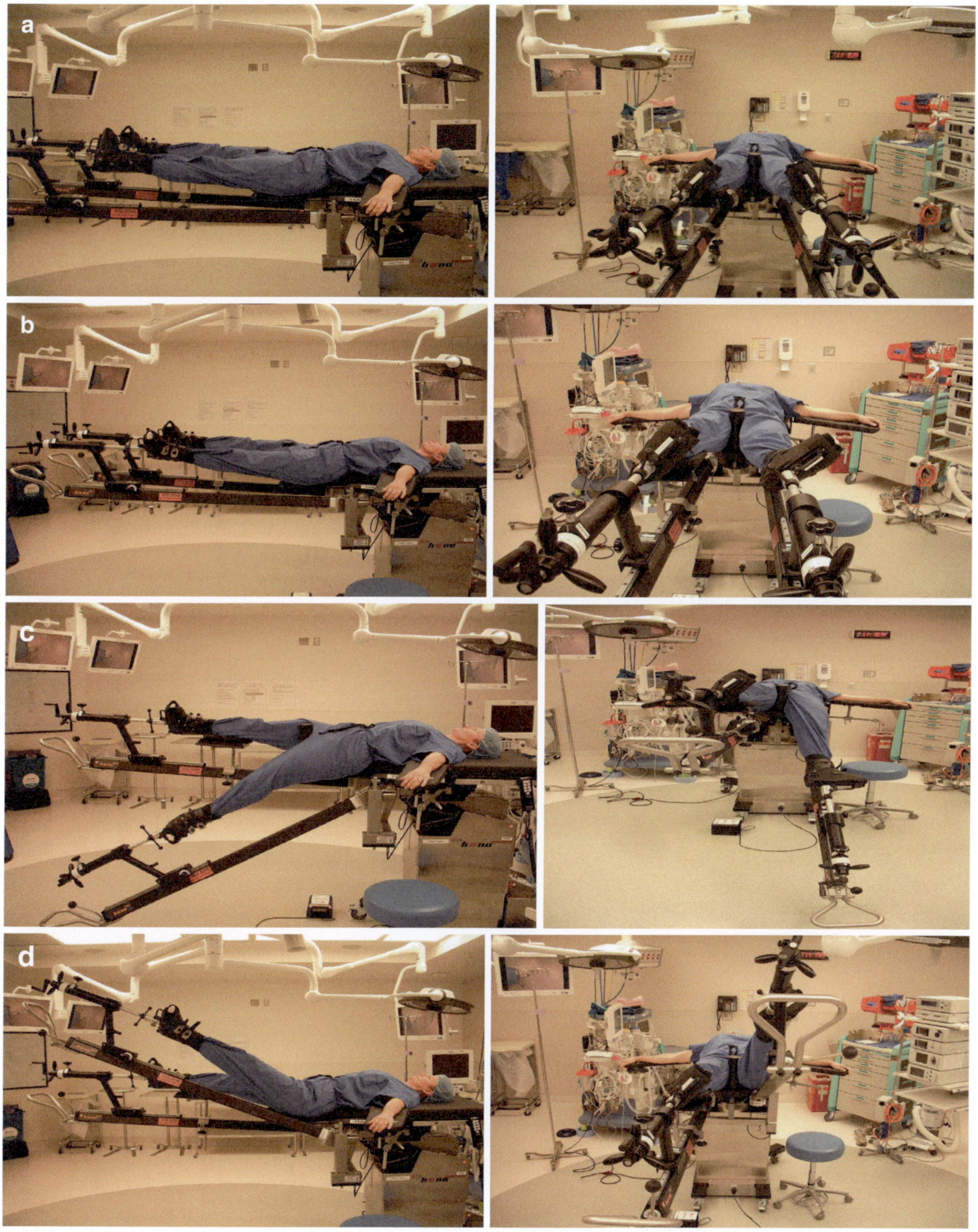

Fig. 27.4 Generally, there are 4 positions employed during the performance of the anterior approach on the orthopedic table. These are referred to in sequence as positions "A" thru "D" These are depicted in the following slides. Position "d" seen at bottom is generally reserved for revision hip surgery or cases where one must work "over the top" of the prosthetic or native femoral neck

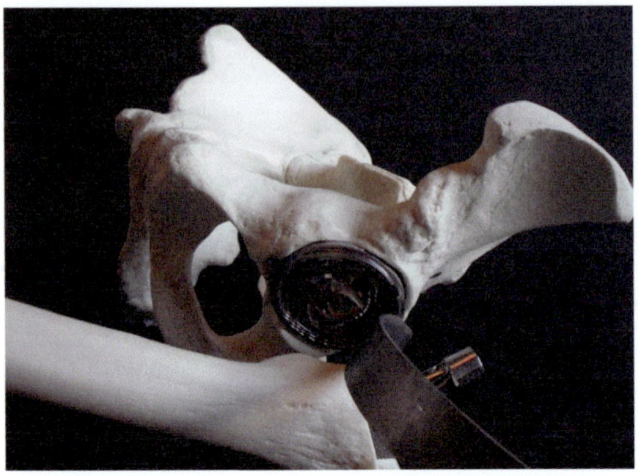

Fig. 27.5 Schematic of retractor placement in figure “d” allowing the surgeon to work “over the top” of the prosthetic femoral neck during revision surgery of the hip

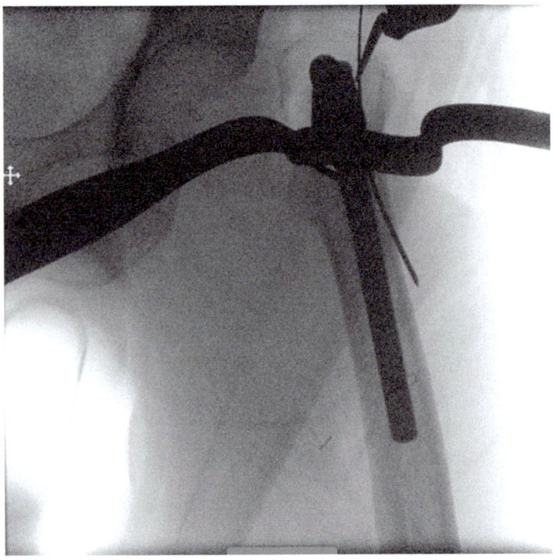

Fig. 27.6 Intraoperative visualization of a flexible osteotome exiting the cortex prematurely. This radiographic control can be helpful when performing complex or revision arthroplasty. This control is facilitated with the orthopedic table

Mast has discussed most of them, and he is right, and there are great benefits of using a traction table as there are great benefits of doing the DAA on a standard OR table. Those in favor of non-table solutions point toward lower costs, smaller footprints, and faster setups. Opponents raise the potential imitations that are specific to the device such as potential traction problems at the ankle or difficulty in testing final hip stability.

I do not want to reiterate all arguments pro and contra here. That has been done so many times and still there remains a split DAA world of surgeons who use a specialized table and those who do not. And this is typically for our surgical profession, while purists of one or the other methods try to convince all of us to only use their respective technique, we all still use different ways of performing the same surgery.

If one has the chance to travel and see colleagues doing what they do in their ORs the one thing that you learn is that there are always many ways to do it right. And this is the only thing that really matters, the question if a procedure works well for the patients. That is proven for different DAA techniques. They work, and they are beneficial to our patients compared to other approaches no matter if we use a traction device or a standard table. The wide variety of ways to do the DAA proves the fact that there are multiple ways to do the DAA successfully.

The fact that one surgeon uses a specialized table and the other does not is triggered by multiple reasons like who he trained with and what this surgeon used and what company he works with, if his background is trauma or adult reconstruction or sports. Also, if the surgeon really wanted to change to the DAA or felt pressured by his local marked and hoped that an expensive tool would make his life easier. Certainly, the number of assistants that are available in a specific environment and their costs are a substantial reason to have a table there that holds the leg instead of a human being.

The issue of “leg holding” has recently been addressed by a company that developed an “on-table leg holder” transforming a standard table into something that holds a table and tries to blend some of the benefits of both worlds (“Adaptable” DJO Surgical, Louisville, TX, USA). Maybe a compromise? Do we need one? No, we do not. Both ways work—so let us keep them and not be religious about it. It is nice to use a standard table, you get a fast setup a reliable and standardized position, no real problem with fluoroscopy, and you do not have to spend a second on how you test for stability. Your patient will do great.

As much as I agree with most of what Dr. Mast says, I completely disagree with his assumption: “… I do not believe the anterior approach performed on the standard operating table or on the orthopedic table are any different." That is not entirely true. Whenever a traction table is used, the lever arm is utilized to bring the proximal femur up to recreate an almost "normal" exposure and allow the surgeon to use straight instruments. Non-table users do not aim for this kind of a proximal exposure at all. They accept that the proximal femur remains deep inside the wound. They adjust their technique and their instruments to prepare the femur down there. I agree with Dr. Mast that both ways work well in the right hands—but this difference requires a different mindset of the surgeon and different instruments.

A summary for a beginner might be: *Both techniques work well.*

Choose one and learn the technique properly. Learn it from a master and copy the master in the beginning. Do not change the technique before you did the first case, but exercise what you learned. Do not mix different techniques. In a well-developed technique, every single step has its importance and cannot easily omit or change. That also means that you should look for a technique that you can transfer to your environment. There is no reason to learn a technique on a fancy table if you will never get this table into your OR.

And in response to Dr. Mast summary, I do not think the techniques are not any different—they are. And if he really thought so he would not conclude that the orthopedic table would be adopted by the marketplace due to some compelling advantages. I believe that our DAA world will remain split—and that is no problem at all—or maybe no problem for us non-table surgeons as we do not have tables to sell.

Enjoy the DAA and give it to your patients one way or the other—they will be grateful.

Tips and Trick for Doing the DAA Without a Special Table

The surgeon should change one's expectations with regard to what the approach looks like. While it is the same portal, doing the DAA without a special table one should expect the proximal femur to remain deep inside the wound. Any recommendations such as releases of the external rotators neglect that fact. After the surgeon has accepted that, everything else comes almost naturally. To prepare the femur in the depth of the wound without releases, you need to:

1. Open the femoral cavity proximally first, to create room to maneuver the first broach in—a curved curette is enormously helpful for that
2. Start with the smallest broach available
3. Use a double-offset broach handle
4. Push the broaches in manually until they are fully aligned with the femur
5. Have the other hand at the upper leg to use your proprioception to get the correct direction
6. Have the proximal femur well supported with a femoral elevator, but do not use it to lever the femur up
7. Have the leg in abduction, external rotation, and around 40° of hip hyperextension
8. Keep the knee straight to get the least tension of the quadriceps.

DAA on a Standard Table

Hannes A. Rüdiger and Michael Leunig

In its original description by the Judet brothers from France, the direct anterior approach (DAA) for total hip arthroplasty (THA) was performed on a fracture table. With the widespread adoption of the DAA over the past two decades, particularly in the USA but also in Switzerland, it was assumed that this approach is only possible using a special table. In Switzerland, the DAA has today become by far the most widely used approach for THA with 50% in 2019 and its share continues to increase, as reported by the Swiss national joint registry SIRIS [1]. The use of a special table (by some referred to as "leg holder") was at least in part attributable to marketing initiatives by implant manufacturers attempting to sell not only implants, but also "complete solutions" including special tables, retractors, surgical techniques, and implants.

However, the DAA for THA on a standard table is gaining increasing popularity in Switzerland compared to the traction table (or leg holder) techniques. Several centers (and the first author of this chapter) initially used a leg holder-based technique for DAA THA and later converted to a standard table-based method due to its specific advantages and simplicity. In the following, we will outline some of the specific advantages of DAA on a standard table vs an orthopaedic table.

A key difference in the technique with a standard table is that neither of the legs is fixed in a leg holder/traction device. This allows for easy and unlimited intraoperative mobilization of both hips, allowing for functional intraoperative soft tissue tension and stability assessment as well as the evaluation of leg length. While anterior joint stability may be assessed on a traction table, the assessment of posterior stability is difficult, if not impossible, on most devices. Although theoretically possible, only few surgeons remove the leg from the traction device to allow for the same assessment (except leg length) as possible with our technique. The proponents of the leg holder-based technique argue that joint stability is achieved if cup positioning, leg length, and offset are reconstructed anatomically, all factors which may be controlled using intraoperative imaging (i.e., image intensifier with increasingly sophisticated analysis software available) and that functional testing is overrated.

We strongly disagree with this line of reasoning. As long as intraoperative imaging is restricted to two dimensions (i.e., anteroposterior projection), important parameters are not assessed, and therefore, it is therefore insufficient to evaluate joint function in its entire complexity. The most important "overlooked" parameters include torsion of the femoral stem, extra-articular impingement (e.g., pelvic-trochanteric or ischiofemoral), trans-articular soft tissue tension, or anteroposterior positioning of the acetabular center of rotation. All these aspects are not captured by a simplified anteroposterior image-based evaluation of the reconstruction. However, each of these factors alone or any combination thereof may contribute to joint instability. Intraoperative functional testing as we perform it routinely in every case allows for accurate testing of prosthetic joint stability and leg length.

Femoral torsion is readily assessable in a standardized "figure-of-four" position with the knee in about 90° of flexion, a position that is difficult or impossible to achieve with most leg holder devices. Alternatively, some surgeons performing THA with leg holder devices use the posterior cortex at the level of the neck osteotomy to check the torsion of the stem. However, while this trick might allow for anatomical reconstruction of the native femoral torsion, it does not give a sufficiently accurate qualitative impression of the absolute torsion of the femoral reconstruction (i.e., in a patient with excessively high native antetorsion the torsion of the reconstruction might be underestimated).

Leg length discrepancy (LLD) *(Reference to our Chap. 29: surgical perspectives LLD by Leunig/Rüdiger)* continues to be a key factor determining patient satisfaction and the major reason for malpractices claims. In our opinion, there are two (or three) tools minimizing the risk of LLD: preoperative templating, intraoperative testing, and, if necessary, intraoperative imaging. While preoperative templating (typically performed on standard AP pelvic views) and intraoperative imaging allow assessment of length at the level of the hip with sufficient accuracy, factors affecting LLD distal to the hip joint are typically not taken into account. Such factors include asymmetries of the native anatomy (e.g., differences in tibial and/or femoral lengths), functional LLD (e.g., flexion contraction of the knee), posttraumatic LLD (e.g., shortening of long bones after healed fractures), and others. All these factors are assessable if both legs are easily accessible and not fixed in a holding device. A transparent drape allows not only the evaluation of LLD by palpation of the medial malleoli but also by visual assessment of malleoli and heels.

Of note, our technique with a standard table with the patient in supine position does not at all exclude or even impair the use of intraoperative imaging (or the use of imaging analyzing software) compared to techniques utilizing leg holders. While our standard algorithm for primary THA does typically not include the use of image intensifier in every case, we do occasionally use this tool in more complex cases (e.g., revisions, complex deformities, or intraoperative complications).

To convert from a leg holder-based technique to a standard table technique, there are no fundamental changes in the actual technique of surgical approach needed. While some argue that a more complete release of the capsule is necessary (mainly posterolateral) for a DAA on a standard table compared to leg holder-based techniques, we neither share this impression, nor are we aware of any solid quantitative data on the extent of the release in the different techniques. We do not think that the visualization of the joint is any difference between the two types of techniques.

We do currently perform THA with one surgeon, one surgical trainee, one medical student, and one scrub nurse. However, as we are a training center, we are less restricted in terms of surgical assistance compared to other (private) facilities. However, we do not think that a DAA standard table requires more surgical personnel than leg holder-based techniques. Standard table techniques have been described with one or even without surgical assistants by others using various types of self-retractors. In contrast, the technique with a standard table does not require a trained theatre technician to operate the table during surgery and therefore potentially reduces the number of staff involved during surgery.

While DAA can be performed on standard non-breakable table, we do prefer breakable tables, which have a joint at the level of the greater trochanter permitting hyperextension of the hip. This allows for a more "straight shot" to the femoral diaphysis and a less extensive release. However, excessive hyperextension may lead to increased soft tissue tension of the hip flexor muscles, impairing access to the joint. Positioning of the tibia underneath (rather than over) the contralateral leg usually improves femoral access in our hands.

In view of the ever-increasing economic pressure on healthcare systems, we do believe that the most cost-effective technique is to be preferred as long as compromises on outcomes are avoided. As standard tables are usually simpler and available in all surgical facilities, there are no initial costs when starting with a standard table-based technique. Positioning of the patient on a leg holder device is more time-consuming and therefore costly. Complications specifically associated with leg holder devices such as ankle fractures and pressure sores, which are typically not captured in national THA registries, are avoided.

In summary, after having converted from a leg holder-based technique, we do not believe that the surgical approach per se is significantly different. However, the standard table technique offers important advantages over leg holder-based techniques. These include easier and quicker patient positioning, intraoperative assessment of anterior and posterior joint stability, leg length, and range of motion. The high cost of a specific table can be avoided. The standard table technique does not impair the use of intraoperative imaging if needed. Based on all the above, it is hard to argue for the use of a fracture table when performing DAA THA.

Reference

1. Swiss National Hip & Knee Joint Registry. Report 2020. www.swiss-medtech.ch/news/siris-report-2020.

Handling the Hip Capsule with the Anterior Approach: Repair Versus Capsulectomy

28

Tania A. Ferguson and Raymond H. Kim

Capsular Maintenance in Anterior Approach Total Hip Replacement

Tania A. Ferguson

Maintaining (and at time augmenting) the hip capsule during and after the anterior hip replacement is my preferred technique for several reasons.

1. Maintenance of the hip capsule during the operation allows the surgical work and retractors to occur within the capsule, preventing any disruption or trauma to the periarticular hip musculature (particularly the anterior muscles) during the operation. It is protective and acts as a retractor itself during the case, preventing trauma to the overlying rectus femoris and iliocapsularis and iliopsoas.
2. After surgery, the capsule allows for a continued barrier between the anterior muscles and the intra-articular environment. This is important for the protection of the muscular envelope post-surgically and inhibits the development of muscular adhesions to the osseous anterior rim of the acetabulum and from muscular entrapment within the hip during certain movements. My experience has been that these phenomena, particularly in the young patient population, can lead to protracted anterior hip pain when capsular insufficiency occurs.
3. While uncommonly relevant, patients with unique anatomical or physiological features may benefit from the stability associated with the capsular containment of the hip joint.

   For example, patients with hypermobility syndromes such as Ehlers–Danlos syndrome (EDS) and some dysplastic conditions may benefit from the additional restraint to dislocation associated with the capsular maintenance, and occasionally even reinforcement via capsular plication.

In order to for these benefits to be realized, the technique of capsular handling is critical. One must be cognoscente not to injure the relationship between the muscles and the anterior hip capsule. My technique has evolved to ensure that there is no disruption of the anterior hip muscles and the anterior hip capsule, and capsular contractures and pathological thickenings are addressed, and that the capsule is repairable at the end of the operation.

Capsular Exposure and Capsulotomy

The benefits of capsular preservation are dependent upon precise capsular exposure and retractor

T. A. Ferguson (✉)
Nashville Hip and Pelvis, Nashville, TN, USA

R. H. Kim
Department of Orthopaedic Surgery, The Steadman Clinic, Vail, CO, USA
e-mail: rkim@thesteadmanclinic.comz

J. M. Matta, A. P. Sah (eds.), *Anterior Hip Replacement*,
https://doi.org/10.1007/978-3-030-91896-5_28

placement prior to the capsulotomy. While the anterior hip musculature (the sartorius, rectus femoris, and iliocapsularis or capsular origin of the iliopsoas) needs to be mobilized medially to expose the hip capsule for capsulotomy, my goal is to do so with little to no disruption of the muscular relationship with the anterior hip capsule.

A narrow Cobra retractor is placed in the interval between the superior/lateral capsule and gluteus minimus, retracting the tensor and the gluteus minimus laterally and exposing the superior hip capsule in the vicinity of the reflected head of the rectus femoris. In my early career, the next step was to place an elevator directed distally and medially to mobilize the musculature from the anterior capsule, making a path for a second narrow cobra to be placed over the inferomedial capsule (Fig. 28.1). This maneuver nicely exposed the anterior hip capsule for arthrotomy but at the cost of disrupting the capsular–muscular interface.

In order to minimize or eliminate disturbance of the relationship of these muscles and the anterior hip capsule, I now longer place a retractor over the anterior capsule. After the narrow cobra is applied posterolaterally under the posterolateral acetabular rim, a narrow Hohmann is placed under the lateral most edge of the rectus. This retractor reflects the edge of the rectus just enough

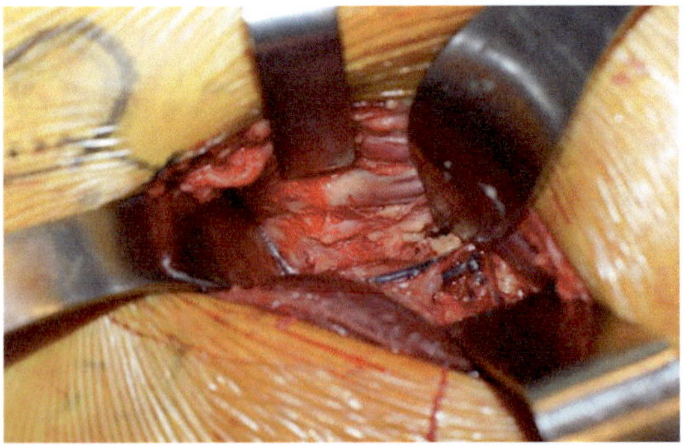

Fig. 28.1 Capsular exposure utilizing a cobra placed over the capsule, between the anterior muscular envelope and the capsule itself. This technique interferes with the relationship between the muscles and the capsule

to access the capsule. Alternatively, a Hibbs retractor can be used medially to elevate/lift the lateral rectus (Fig. 28.2a) exposing the capsule just enough for the cranial limb of the L-shaped capsulotomy (Fig. 28.2b). The anterior and the lateral capsular flaps are then tagged with a strong suture, and the retractors are placed inside the capsule (Fig. 28.2c). The patient's lower extremity is then externally rotated (via the leg spar) to allow the capsule to be elevated from lateral to medial along the intertrochanteric line, with direct observation of the cranial origin of the vastus lateralis and the pericapsular vessels (which can be coagulated without difficult). The limb is returned to a neutral position, and the anterior narrow Hohmann is replaced with a narrow cobra in preparation for the next steps of surgery.

Acetabular Exposure

The benefit of maintaining a barrier between the trauma of surgery and the retractor placement is next experienced with acetabular exposure. Regardless of retractor choices and placements, the maintenance of the hip capsule allows the surgeon to protect the periarticular musculature from surgical trauma (Fig. 28.3).

My technique involves a narrow cobra retractor placed posteriorly with the tip on the mid-posterior rim external to the labrum but within the hip capsule. A bent Hohmann retractor is carefully placed over the distal anterior rim of the acetabulum between the capsule and the acetabular labrum, taking care to keep the Hohmann tip on the bone to avoid perforation of the capsule or injury to the overlying iliopsoas and extra-articular soft tissues. Alternatively (and preferably), the contemporary Capsular retractor can be placed within the anterior and posterolateral capsular flaps. This retractor has the benefits of being self-retaining, avoiding disruption or trauma to the anterior hip musculature, and providing retraction during the reaming and acetabular component insertion.

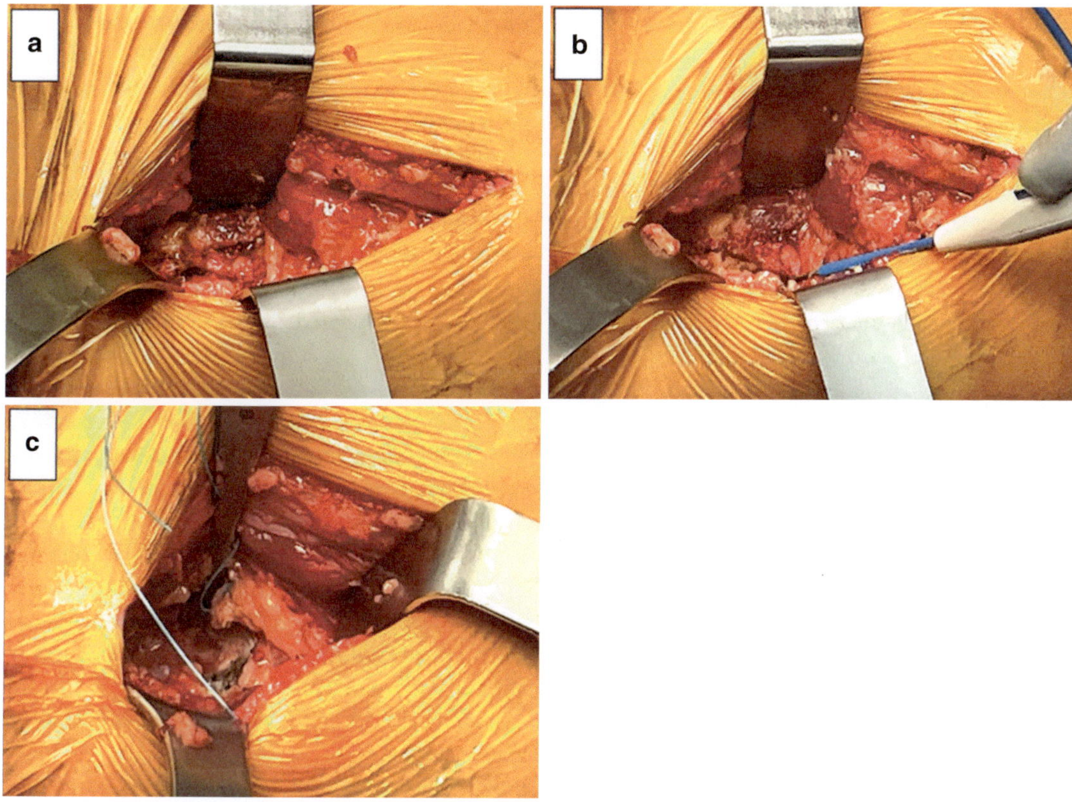

Fig. 28.2 (**a**) A Hibbs retractor elevates the lateral edge of the rectus off the capsule just enough to expose the capsule for capsulotomy. (**b**) Cranial limb of the capsulotomy is performed just lateral to the AIIS, continuing distally parallel to the neck toward the anterior tubercle of the greater trochanter at the lateral extent of the anterior intertrochanteric line. (**c**) Once the cranial limb of the capsulotomy has been performed, a retractor can be placed within the capsule around the inferior neck, and the capsule subsequently reflected from lateral to medial along the intertrochanteric line

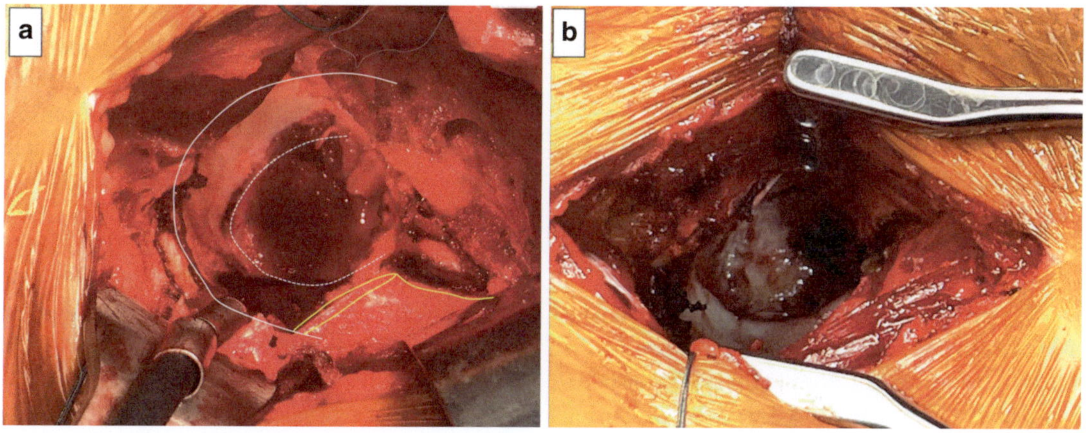

Fig. 28.3 Retractors for acetabular preparation are completely within the capsulolabral fold and do not disrupt the muscles on the external surface of the capsule. (**a**) demonstrates a narrow Hohmann placed within the capsule under the inferolateral aspect of the posterior rim, with a modified/bent narrow Hohmann placed under the anterior horn of the acetabulum. (**b**) demonstrates the newer capsular retractor, placed as a self-retainer between the anterior and posterolateral capsular flaps

Summary

In summary, I prefer to maintain the capsule for protection of the muscles around the hip during the operation. I believe having a barrier between the arthroplasty and the muscles post-surgically is advantageous as long as the capsule has been carefully handled throughout surgery. In patients with connective tissue (such as EDS or Marfan syndrome), I believe there may be some advantage in capsular plication to tighten the capsule and reorient the surrounding capsular fibers to enhance the joint stability.

Surgeon Perspective—Capsulectomy in Total Hip Arthroplasty

Joshua C. Rozell,
Dimitri E. Delagrammaticas and
Raymond H. Kim

In anterior approach, total hip arthroplasty, exposure of the hip joint, and femoral neck require an initial capsulotomy. There continues to be debate on the ideal management of the capsule and whether the anterior hip capsule should be repaired or excised during the procedure. Capsulectomy facilitates femoral and acetabular exposure, potentially decreasing operative time, but a persistent capsular defect may theoretically predispose patients to anterior instability [1]. The hip joint is reinforced by three primary fibrous capsular ligaments (iliofemoral, ischiofemoral, and pubofemoral), and each serves distinct functional roles to stabilize the native joint [2, 3]. The iliofemoral ligament reinforces the capsule during external rotation and extension, the most susceptible position of instability after anterior total hip arthroplasty. The ischiofemoral ligament inserts onto the ischium, posteroinferior to the acetabular rim, and attaches to the posterior intertrochanteric line to reinforce the capsule during internal rotation and flexion. The pubofemoral ligament inserts in the superior pubic ramus and converges with the medial iliofemoral and inferior ischiofemoral ligaments to insert into the femur [4, 5]. While these ligaments are some of the strongest in the body, their utility following direct anterior total hip arthroplasty has not been determined.

Sequential and specific release of the capsule is necessary to gain exposure and facility mobility of the femur for acetabular and femoral preparation. However, even after release, the capsule, whether thickened or as a result of the capsulotomy location, can occasionally impede visualization and/or limit mobility of the femur. Retraction of the residual capsule can be cumbersome, and anterior capsulectomy ensures that full release of the capsule has been completed and that the capsule that would otherwise need to be retracted to facilitate the exposure is no longer in the way. Additionally, true anatomic repair of the capsule is unlikely given the direct release from the proximal femur, and experience from revision anterior approach often reveals a scarred pseudocapsule that reconstitutes even week after the index surgery. In the circumstance of revision through an anterior approach, the thick pseudocapsular scar can make mobilization and visualization much more difficult than in the primary setting and defining clear normal capsular planes may be difficult. Therefore, routine capsulectomy in this circumstance can improve efficiency and enhance exposure.

By leaving the posterior capsular tissue and external rotators attached to the femur, combined with optimal neck length and offset, patients can still achieve appropriate soft tissue tension and stability without the need to retain or repair the anterior capsule. Furthermore, redundant remaining capsular tissue or inappropriate tensioning may lead to restricted range of motion or greater risk of soft tissue impingement postoperatively. An ongoing clinical trial evaluating the two approaches is currently underway [6]. With appropriately placed total hip arthroplasty components verified using anatomic landmarks, intraoperative stability testing, fluoroscopy, and/or other assistive technologies, the risk of dislocation can be mitigated. Even a well-repaired capsule will not provide an adequate checkrein for anterior dislocation if the components are not well-positioned or the soft tissues are not tensioned appropriately.

References

1. McLawhorn AS, Christ AB, Morgenstern R, Burge AJ, Alexiades MM, et al. Prospective evaluation of the posterior tissue envelope and anterior capsule after anterior total hip arthroplasty. J Arthroplast. 2020;35(3):767–73.
2. Bedi A, Galano G, Walsh C, Kelly BT. Capsular management during hip arthroscopy: from femoro-acetabular impingement to instability. Arthroscopy. 2011;27(12):1720–31.
3. Martin HD, Savage A, Braly BA, Palmer IJ, Beall DP, Kelly B. The function of the hip capsular ligaments: a quantitative report. Arthroscopy. 2008;24(2):188–95.
4. Telleria JJ, Lindsey DP, Giori NJ, Safran MR. A quantitative assessment of the insertional footprints of the hip joint capsular ligaments and their spanning fibers for reconstruction. Clin Anat. 2014;27(3):489–97.
5. Geoffrey KC, Jeffers JRT, Beaule PE. Hip joint capsular anatomy, mechanics, and surgical management. J Bone Joint Surg Am. 2019;101(23):2141–51.
6. https://clinicaltrials.gov/ct2/show/NCT02121964.

Judging Leg Length and Offset with the Anterior Approach: Clinical Evaluation Versus Fluoroscopy

29

Michael Leunig and Juan C. Suarez

LLD and Femoral Offset: A Surgeon Perspective

Michael Leunig and Hannes A. Rüdiger

Total hip replacement (THR) is the most successful procedure in orthopedics and has been even called the operation of the century (Ian Learmonth). While most patients have a high rate of satisfaction after THR, in some patients despite a significant improvement in pain and function they remain dissatisfied. Leg length discrepancies (LLDs) and trochanteric pain as a result of a lateralized trochanter are not uncommon after THR. While LLD can be quantified using clinical and imaging modalities, it is more difficult to link trochanteric pain to an increased offset. Not infrequent, however, both occur together. Nevertheless, if LLD or trochanteric pain occurs, patients often question how this could have happened and mistrust the quality of the work performed by the surgeon. Despite the fact that large differences over 10 mm, which might even lead to malpractice consequences, even smaller differences can be quite dissatisfying for patients despite the rest of the procedure went quite well and the patient is pain-free. A surgeon should always avoid to tell the patient that getting a sufficient stability was difficult to achieve, and therefore, a leg lengthening was required.

Why do the problems occur? In most cases of so-called primary hip OA, the arthritic process leads to superior joint space loss and most of the patients with OA-related hip pain particularly with an eccentric joint space narrowing have a LLD, being shorter at the hip on the OA side. Patients with medial OA such as in protrusion more rarely show a significant shortening of the hip length due to their OA. While this may be considered as the rule in most patients, some patients might, however, even be longer on the arthritic side due to muscular contractures. Moreover, many patients do have some preexisting leg length differences, which also need to be considered when performing THR.

How are the complex patients to be treated with respect to leg length and offset? In general, female patients are more prone of being dissatisfied by their leg length and offset due to their anatomical properties. This is mainly due to the fact that they are smaller, as the LLD-induced pelvic obliquity is more pronounced if distance between the two hip centers is closer together. In addition, women also have a tendency for laxity compared to male patients. Red flags for the occurrence of LLD and offset problems are short stature (less 160 cm), small socket size (<48) not allowing for 32 mm heads, varus hips with a high lesser and/or

M. Leunig
Hip Surgery - Schulthess Clinic, Zürich, Switzerland

J. C. Suarez (✉)
Miami Orthopedics and Sports Medicine Institute, Baptist Health South Florida, Miami, FL, USA

J. M. Matta, A. P. Sah (eds.), *Anterior Hip Replacement*,
https://doi.org/10.1007/978-3-030-91896-5_29

greater trochanter, and degenerative back problems such as scoliosis, spinal fusion, femoral neck fractures, or AVN patient. Particular challenges include Perthes disease with a radiologically significantly shortened hip. These hips are at an increased risk of overlengthening as pelvitrochanteric impingement has to be avoided.

Intraoperative fluoroscopy has been proposed as a low-cost and simple-to-use technique for improving component positioning including leg length and offset. Despite the potential pros of direct visualization of the hip implants, no functional information is provided by fluoroscopy and we rather functionally assess the hips during surgery. In the following, we will describe how we perform DAA THR with a high precision for correct component positioning without the routine use of a C-arm. In revisions or if there remains uncertainty on the implant positioning, we always have the option to use a C-arm.

To avoid dissatisfaction in particular due to LLD and offset problems, preoperative planning/templating is essential. The following saying by Benjamin Franklin also holds true for hip surgery: "If you fail to plan, you are planning to fail."

Step 1: In the preoperative consultation, it is important to ask the patients for their perceived leg length and whether they feel a difference. If this is in accordance with the clinical finding regarding the LLD and shorter on the OA side, it is unlikely that problems occur. Frequently, however, due to their abductor weakness and subsequent limping, patients perceive their OA leg too short, which might not be the case, but also preexisting differences in the length of the leg, sometimes due to trauma or even scoliosis leading to a pelvic obliquity needs to be appreciated.

Step 2: If patients feel it differently to that what you find clinically, a CT or EOS (ideally whole-body view for assessment of scoliosis) measurement might be ordered to address the finding.

Step 3: The informed consent needs to address LLD and trochanteric pain, but does only help if a problem occurs with respect to malpractice issues.

Step 4: Preoperative templating is key for assuming the expected implant sizes and position and change in leg length.

For templating, a correct taken ap view without rotation (coccyx and symphysis should be aligned) and if possible with internally rotated hips/legs should be used. In OA hips, internal rotation is frequently not possible, and therefore, the pelvic ap will be in external rotation. This will lead to a misleading appearance of the femoropelvic offset. Some surgeons therefore use CT for templating their hips, which we do not do routinely. The nonarthritic contralateral side can be used for assessing offset, and if both hips are arthritic, one has to assume that the offset is rather larger than estimated from the X-ray. For determining the femoral rotation, the appearance of the greater trochanter is helpful, which should appear as a small tip rather than being very wide medially. Recently, our group has looked to the trochanteric double contour sign, to help for judging on femoral rotation (Fig. 29.1). Today, mostly digital templating software programs are used, where the positioning/sizing of the acetabulum and femur can be easily performed. Based on the information from the clinical assessment, it can be planned to not change the hip length, or mildly lengthen (3–5 mm) as it is done in the majority of the patients with preoperative superior joint space loss. More rarely, more lengthening on the template is required. Shortening is more difficult, as one loses soft tissue tension potentially posing the hip more unstable. In cases of more severe shortening, one has either to convince the patient that this is not potentially destabilizing or one has to use socket providing more stability for example a double mobility system. If you have templated (planned) your hip, measure distances, which can be reproduced during surgery, such as the upper border of the lesser trochanter and the trunnion, or the lateral shoulder of the prosthetic stem and the tip of the greater trochanter or the external obturator footprint [5].

The second key issue is the surgical technique. As approach, we prefer the direct anterior approach (DAA) without a fracture table. The patient is placed supine on a regular table with the option to break the table under the hip. The supine position allows access to both anterior superior iliac spines (ASIS) and both legs (Fig. 29.2). Before even

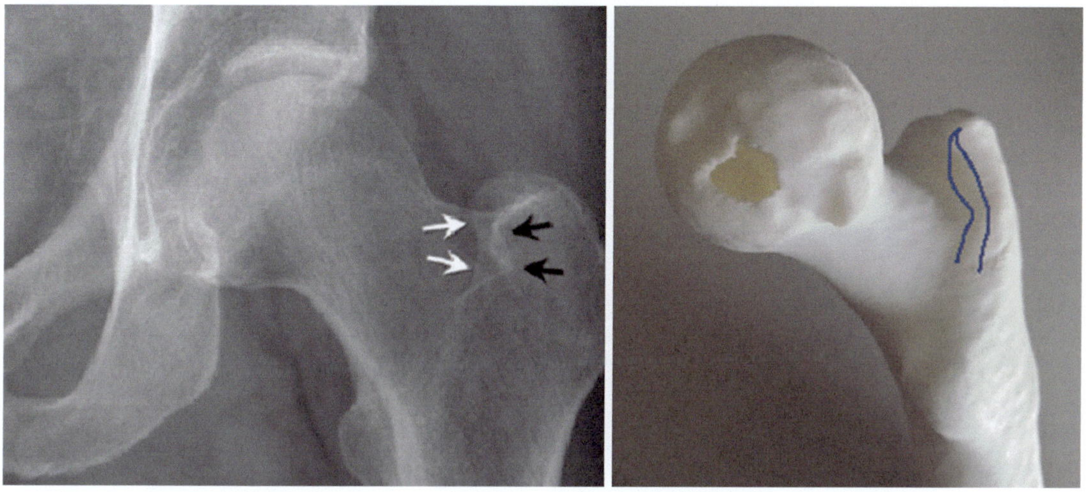

Fig. 29.1 Trochanteric double contour: The two contours visible on the posteromedial tip of the greater trochanter are indicative of the femoral projection (i.e., rotation). If these two contours are superimposed, or very close, an underestimation of the femoral offset is very unlikely (unpublished data)

draping the patient, planned incision (bikini vs. longitudinal) can palpate both ASIS and medial malleoli or heals. Now one can compare the preoperative information (patient perception and measured leg length in clinic) and the finding in anesthesia. During the surgical procedure, the quality of soft tissues can be noticed. Men are frequently stiffer and require a more pronounced capsular release, compared to women. This release is always performed in a stepwise fashion, with the capsule and short external rotators being released more frequently compared to piriformis and obturator externus, which rarely or even never released and also not helpful for exposure. Keeping the release to a minimum will increase your stability specifically in women, who sometimes tend to be hypermobile.

To obtain an optimal position of the femoral center of rotation, preoperative templating is essential. Femoral length is assessed using multiple landmarks including (1) the distance between the base of the lesser trochanter and the tip of the trunnion of the broach or stem, the relation of the stem shoulder to (2) the anterolateral base of the femoral neck and to (3) footprint of the external obturator tendon in the piriformis fossa [1]. It is helpful to check leg length with the trial implants in place. As the patient is in supine position and both legs are free underneath the transparent drape, leg length can be accurately checked by assessing the levels of the medial malleoli. Since the pelvis might have moved during surgery, palpation of both ASIS helps in judging on pelvic obliquity. This is an important advantage of this technique without the use of a traction table, where the leg is fixed in a holding/traction devise, which significantly reduces its accessibility for trialing. The choice of the neck type (i.e., offset, CCD) is based on preoperative templating and the intraoperative trans-articular tension, stability, and leg length.

Trialing

A major advantage of the DAA in supine position on a standard table in combination with our draping system is the accessibility of both legs for trialing. For anterior stability, we hyperextend the leg to about 10–15° and apply external rotation to the femur. Of note, it has been observed in CT-based collision models and some rare clinical cases of instability that a conflict of the greater trochanter with the ischium may lead to an anterior instability in slight hip flexion and external rotation (personal communication Moritz Tannast, Fribourg/Switzerland). For posterior stability, the leg is brought to various degrees of flexion and internal

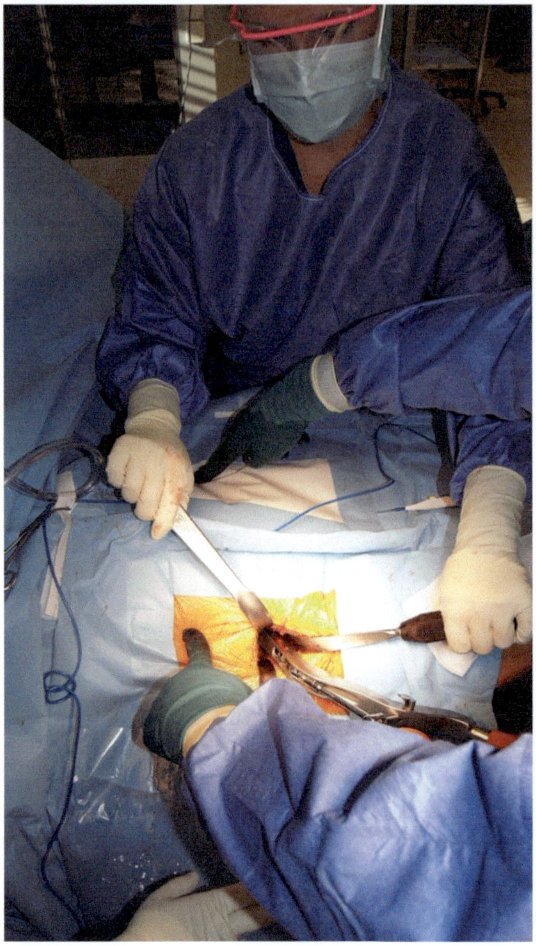

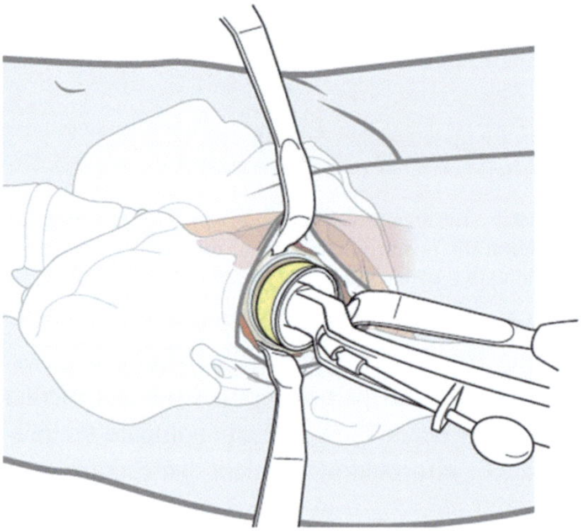

Fig. 29.2 For cup alignment and leg length testing, the surgeon has to be aware of possible pelvic rotation in the frontal plane, which might occur during the procedure (e.g., head extraction). The two anterior iliac spines are palpated (left image), and pelvic rotation is corrected if needed. Cup orientation may be estimated according to the orientation of the cup holder in relation to an imaginary line between the two ASIS (for abduction) and the table (for cup anteversion)

rotation. Leg length is assessed by comparing the level of the two knee cabs or both malleoli (Fig. 29.3), which are visible and palpable through the transparent drape. Pelvic obliquities have to be taken into account and judged using both ASIS. We routinely use the equator of the trial head on a 135° neck for a final check of the cup orientation (Fig. 29.4). The equator is brought in line with the acetabular liner. To achieve that, the femur has to be brought in slight flexion and internal rotation to correct for both the femoral antetorsion and acetabular anteversion.

With the preoperative templating and the intraoperative comparison to the anatomical landmarks, one has a good judgment on the execution of the templated lengthening. Intraoperative trialing using the Shuck test for assessing soft tissue tension, but even more the ROM maneuver and palpation of the knee caps, malleoli and/or heels will allow for verification of the correct length. The offset is more difficult to assess directly, but again soft tissue tension after using the templated implants will help for providing most optimal solution for the patient.

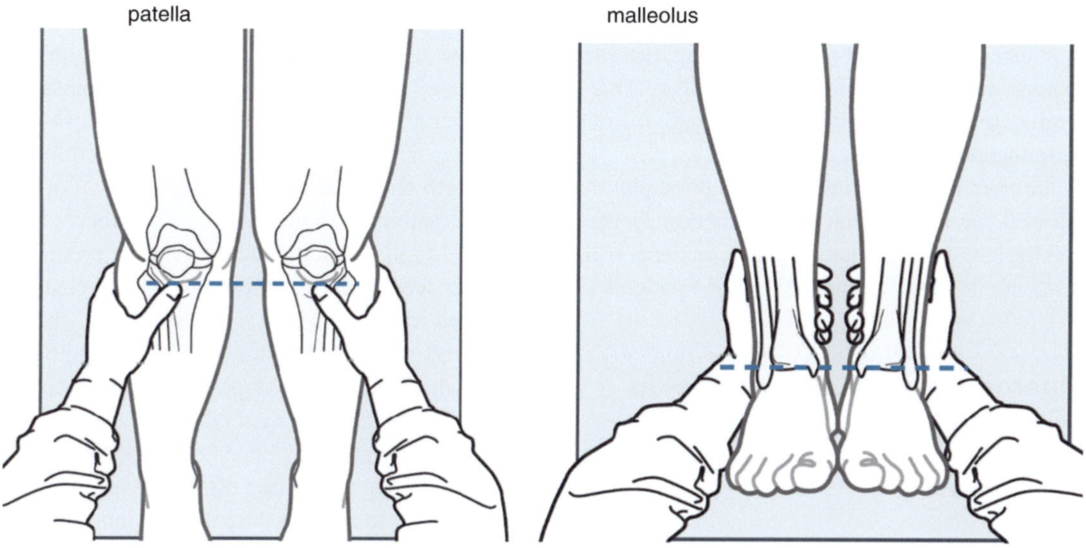

Fig. 29.3 Patellae and malleoli, are easily visible and palpable through the transparent drape and are used for judging leg length. This is always in combination with soft tissue tension and THR stability

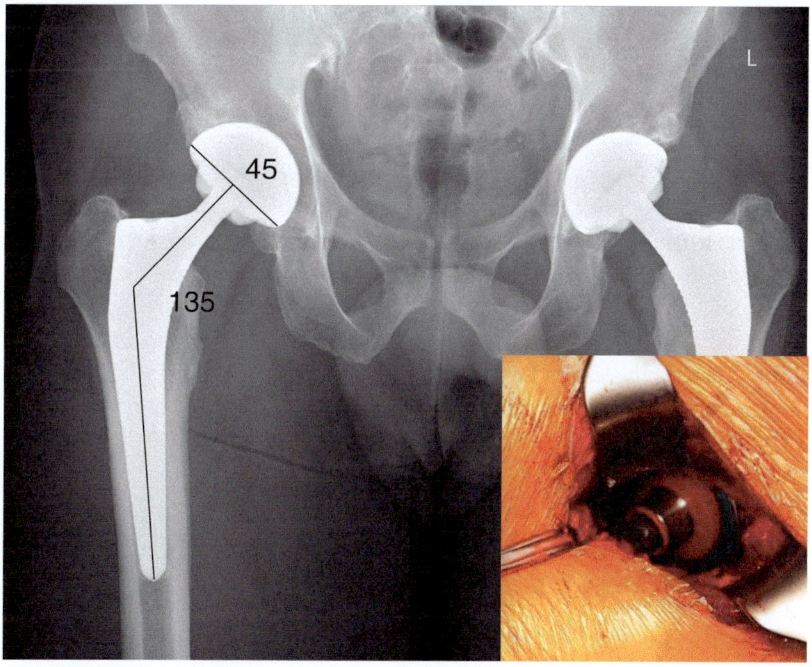

Fig. 29.4 Cup alignment may be estimated by the relation of the trial head equator the rim of the polyethylene using a 135° CCD neck. If the leg is placed in about 15° of flexion (to correct for acetabular anteversion) and 15° of internal rotation (to correct for femoral antetorsion), the equator of the trial head should perfectly align with the rim of the prosthetic liner

In cases of difficult reduction due to high soft tissue tension, the leg might be rather too long or the implant has too much offset or a combination of both. In case of an unstable joint in full extension end external rotation, either the combined anteversion is too high, or the soft tissue tension is too low (leg is too short) causing instability. In case of instability in flexion and internal rotation, the components might be incorrectly positioned. Increasing hip stability by enhancing soft tissue tension and lengthening the leg are not indicated. Here, it can be quite helpful for assessing the alignment of the components. Even in the absence of a C-arm, one can use the 135° trial neck in relation to the acetabular opening, and if they are coplanar or with slight medial opening, then acetabular abduction is not too excessive. This is similar to the FEAR index of the native hip as introduced by Wyatt et al. [2].

In summary, adhering to these principles had allowed for an anatomic reconstruction of offset and leg length in the majority of our patients with a dislocation rate of around 0.3% in 964 patients [3].

Fluoroscopy for LLD and Offset in DAA

Juan C. Suarez

Recreation of leg length is an important component of total hip arthroplasty. There are various described intraoperative techniques of assessing leg length. One of the shortcomings of the posterior or lateral approach to total hip arthroplasty is the inaccuracy of intraoperative leg length assessment. The lateral decubitus position inhibits proper leg length assessment both clinically and radiographically [4]. Hip and knee flexion and extremity adduction prevent accurate clinical assessment. Furthermore, obtaining reliable radiographs with the patient in the lateral position can be cumbersome and unpredictable. One of the main advantages of the anterior approach to total hip arthroplasty is the supine position, which allows for consistent physical and radiographic examination, which aids in leg length assessment.

The most accurate way of assessing intraoperative leg length in DA THA remains controversial [5]. Proponents of the anterior approach using a standard operative table typically utilize physical examination for judgment of leg length. Commonly, the medial malleoli of both lower extremities are used as reference in order to gauge reestablishment of planned leg length. Although such technique has its merits, the relationship of the medial malleoli can be inaccurate for multiple reasons. Patient positioning, pelvic obliquity, knee flexion contractures, knee, and ankle deformities can all affect the relationship of both medial malleoli. Therefore, aiming equal distance on the malleoli may not be a true representation of accurate anatomical lengthening at the hip joint and can lead to unintended clinically relevant leg length discrepancy. Nevertheless, "tableless" DA THA may still allow for facile intraoperative examination of stability and soft tissue tension, which can help when determining leg length changes.

Alternatively, radiographic assessment may provide a more accurate assessment of preoperative leg length discrepancy and actual changes achieved during surgery. Studies have shown improved accuracy in restoration of leg length and offset when utilizing intraoperative fluoroscopy in DA THA [6]. Several methods of evaluating leg length radiographically have been described.

Preoperative templating establishes a proposed plan in order to achieve the intended lengthening. The plan provides information regarding cup placement with intended center of rotation with stem size and height, which in turn determines the femoral neck cut distance from the lesser trochanter and the distance from the tip of the greater trochanter to the shoulder of the prosthesis. Intraoperative execution of plan should approximate the planned lengthening, which can be confirmed intraoperatively with fluoroscopy.

The inferior ischial line or inferior teardrop line and its relationship with specific anatomical locations in the femur, most commonly the superior aspect of the lesser trochanter or tip of the greater trochanter, are commonly used to assess leg length. This technique is limited by X-ray asymmetry and femoral abduction/adduction and

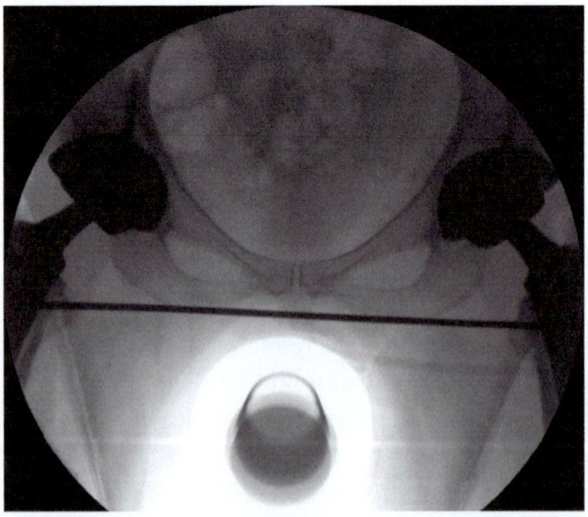

Fig. 29.5 Describes the inferior ischial line and relationship with lesser trochanter as measure of leg length

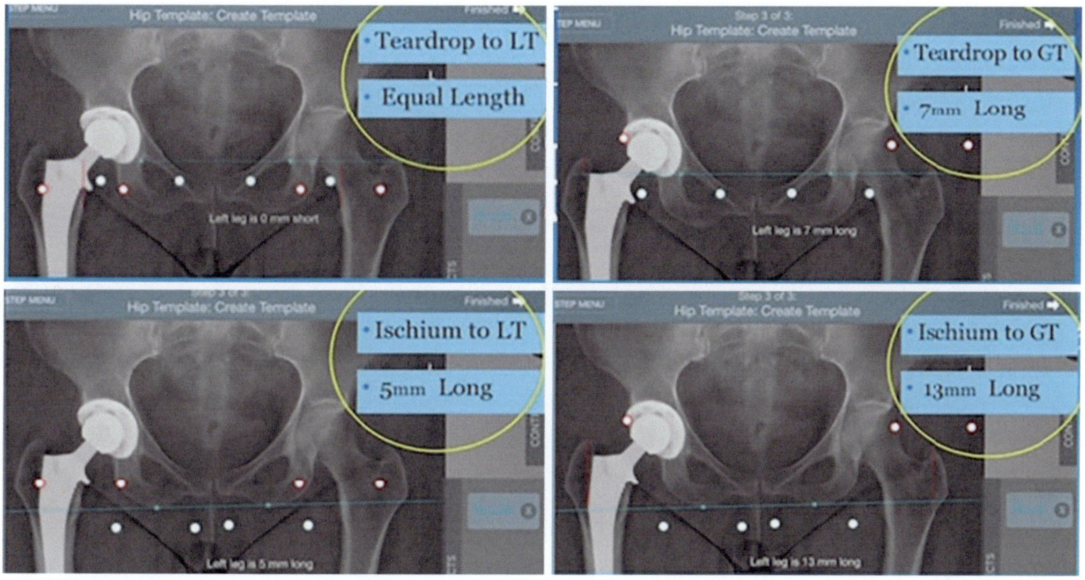

Fig. 29.6 Demonstrates the inconsistency of utilizing the inferior ischial or teardrop line as a measurement of leg length on the same X-ray

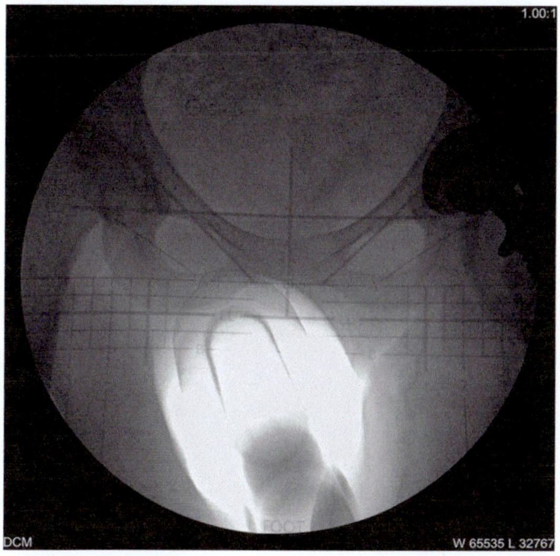

Fig. 29.7 Demonstrates the use of OrthoGrid for leg length assessment utilizing grid lines parallel to the inferior teardrop line and its relationship with the lesser trochanter

rotation differences (Figs. 29.5 and 29.6). However, these relationships can still be employed with success to determine changes from pre-op to post-op. It is important to obtain this measurement at the time of surgery and prior to making bony cuts and compare it to when trail implants are in place. This can help quantify the change from pre-op to post-op. Utilizing this technique solely when the trials are in place can provide erroneous information. Enabling technologies such as OrthoGrid® have been developed to enhance the accuracy of using these relationships when evaluating changes in leg length and offset (Fig. 29.7).

Alternatively, comparing a normal contralateral side with the surgical hip with an overlay technique can provide information on differences in leg length and offset. This technique can provide accurate assessment of both leg length and offset as long as the overlayed images are a mirror image of each other accounting for pelvic rotation and femoral abduction/adduction variations. This technique, popularized by Joel Matta, MD, can be executed by printing the images and superimposing them and assessing the relationships of the femoral outlines [7] (Fig. 29.8). Similarly, an ipsilateral overlay of the presurgical image with one with the trials in place can also be used to assess changes in leg length and offset. Improved accuracy is obtained when both images are as similar. Enabling technologies such as VELYS® digital navigation allow for

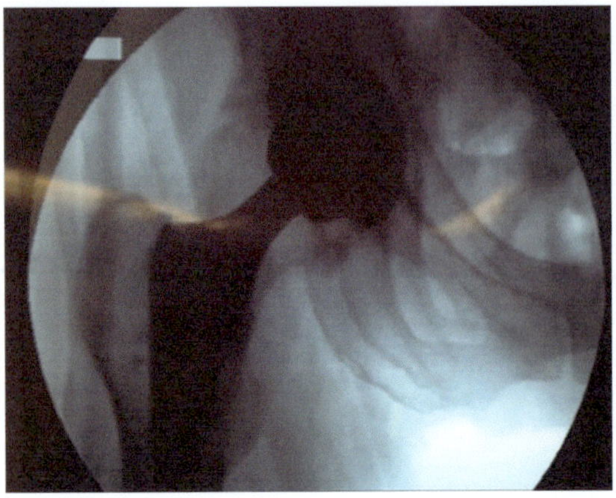

Fig. 29.8 Demonstrates the contralateral overlay technique for assessment of leg length

such ipsilateral overlay and account for differences in femur abduction and adduction (Fig. 29.9).

An advantage of the anterior approach to THA is the supine position, which facilitates the utilization of fluoroscopy. Fluoroscopy has been shown to improve component positioning and leg length and offset reconstruction. Various radiographic methods of assessing intraoperative leg length have been described. Although not without limitations, radiographic techniques with evolving enabling technologies promise improved consistency.

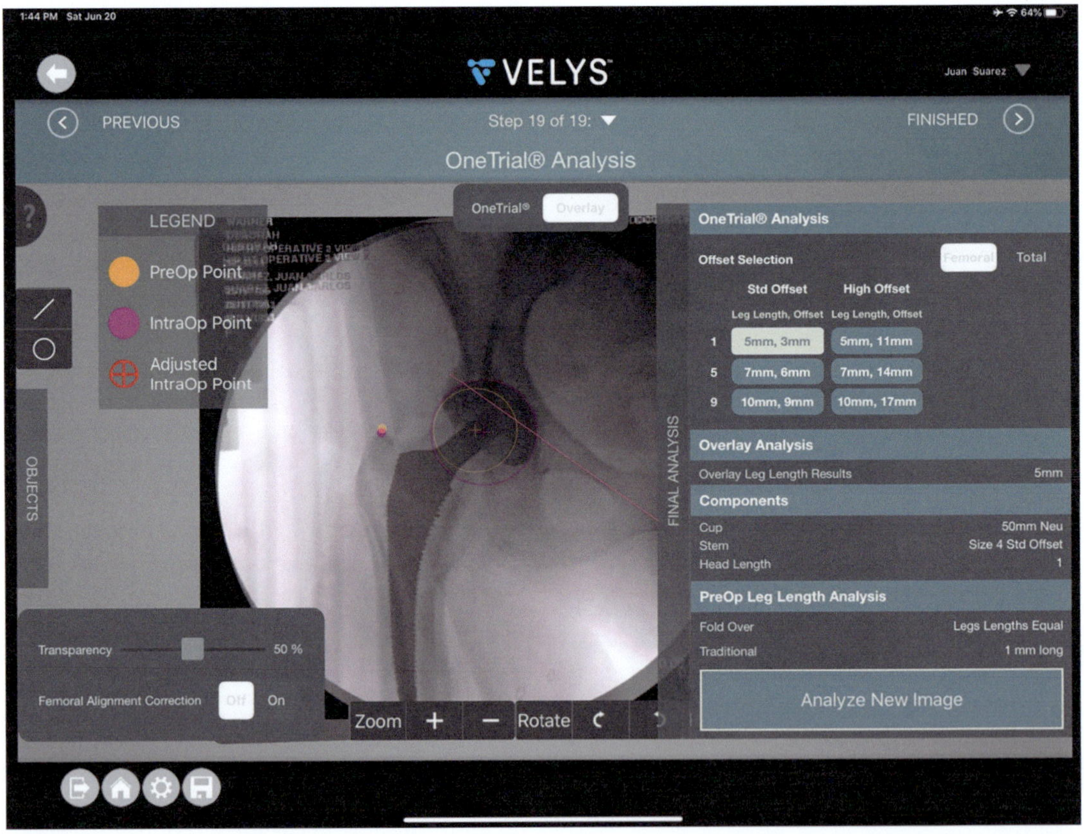

Fig. 29.9 Demonstrates the ipsilateral overlay technique

References

1. Rudiger HA, Fritz B, Impellizzeri FM, Leunig M, Pfirrmann CW, Sutter R. The external obturator footprint as a landmark in total hip arthroplasty through a direct anterior approach: a CT-based analysis. Hip Int. 2019;29(1):96–101.
2. Wyatt M, Weidner J, Pfluger D, Beck M. The Femoro-Epiphyseal Acetabular Roof (FEAR) index: a new measurement associated with instability in borderline hip dysplasia? Clin Orthop Relat Res. 2017;475(3):861–9.
3. Leunig M, Hutmacher JE, Ricciardi BF, Impellizzeri FM, Rudiger HA, Naal FD. Skin crease 'bikini' incision for the direct anterior approach in total hip arthroplasty: a two- to four-year comparative study in 964 patients. Bone Joint J. 2018;100-B(7):853–61.
4. Herisson O, Felden A, Hamadouche M, Anract P, Biau D. Validity and reliability of intraoperative radiographs to assess leg length during total hip arthroplasty: correlation and reproducibility of anatomic distances. J Arthroplast. 2016;31:2784–8.
5. Bingham J, Spangehl M, Hines J, Taunton M, Schwartz A. Does intraoperative fluoroscopy improve limb-length discrepancy and acetabular component positioning during anterior total hip arthroplasty? J Arthroplast. 2018;33:2927–31.
6. Martin J, Masonis J, Mason J. Anatomic total hip component position is more reproducible with the direct anterior approach using intraoperative fluoroscopy. Arthroplasty Today. 2020,6:777–83.
7. Matta J, Shahrdar C, Ferguson T. Single-incision anterior approach for total hip arthroplasty on an orthopedic table. Clin Orthop Relat Res. 2005;441:115–24.

30 Does Pelvic Tilt Change Anything with the Anterior Approach?

Michael J. Taunton and Joel M. Matta

Spinopelvic Alignment

Michael J. Taunton

Spinopelvic alignment, as a risk factor for dislocation, has become a topic of much discussion and investigation [1–3], but the complex evaluation and dynamic nature render it a difficult clinical scenario to interpret clinically. The anterior approaches to the hip have documented decreased risk of instability when compared to the posterior approach by keeping the posterior structures of the hip joint more intact. Additionally, the anterior musculature is not incised, allowing for improved postoperative anterior stability. These factors lead one to ask, when does the spinopelvic alignment matter?

Spinopelvic alignment often leads to impingement of implants or bony structures relative to one another around total hip arthroplasty (THA). Therefore, impingement is the most frequent cause of dislocation itself [4]. In a cohort of 228 patients presenting for primary THA, Brown et al. found that the prevalence of spinopelvic imbalance was 62.3%, the prevalence of decreased spinopelvic motion was 34.2%, and the prevalence of both spinopelvic imbalance and decreased spinopelvic motion was 22% [5]. Additionally, THA stability in the setting of fixed spinopelvic alignment is a particularly sensitive to implant position [6]. In sitting position, dislocators with fixed spinopelvic alignment typically have acetabular components with less functional inclination and less functional anteversion. Given these points, we see that all THA surgeons must remain mindful of implant position and pelvic tilt when performing any THA, regardless of approach.

In order to discuss spinopelvic alignment, we must first define anterior and posterior pelvic tilt. Assessment of spinopelvic alignment is typically performed with the use of at least two lateral spinopelvic radiographs, one in the standing and the other in the seated position [7]. The pelvic tilt is defined as an angle between a horizontal line and a line connecting the upper border of the symphysis with the sacral promontory. In anterior pelvic tilt, the sacrococcygeal junction is cranial to the pubic symphysis resulting in a large pelvic tilt angle (anterior-positive tilt) (Fig. 30.1a). In posterior pelvic tilt, the sacrococcygeal junction goes caudal to the pubic symphysis and results in a smaller pelvic tilt angle (posterior-negative tilt) (Fig. 30.2a).

Anterior stability with extension and external rotation may be of more concern to the anterior-based surgeons. When studied in a biomechanical model, impingement-free external rotation of a THA is decreased in a posterior pelvic tilt-dependent manner. When more than 20° posterior

M. J. Taunton (✉)
Hip & Knee Reconstructive Surgery, Mayo Clinic, Rochester, MN, USA
e-mail: taunton.michael@mayo.edu

J. M. Matta
Steadman Clinic, Vail, CO, USA

J. M. Matta, A. P. Sah (eds.), *Anterior Hip Replacement*,
https://doi.org/10.1007/978-3-030-91896-5_30

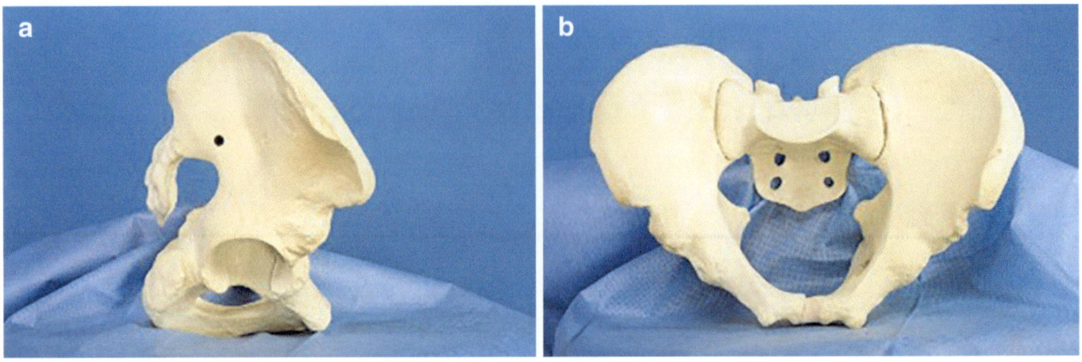

Fig. 30.1 Anterior pelvic tilt, the sacrococcygeal junction, is cranial to the pubic symphysis resulting in a (**a**) larger pelvic tilt angle and a (**b**) positive value for the PSCD

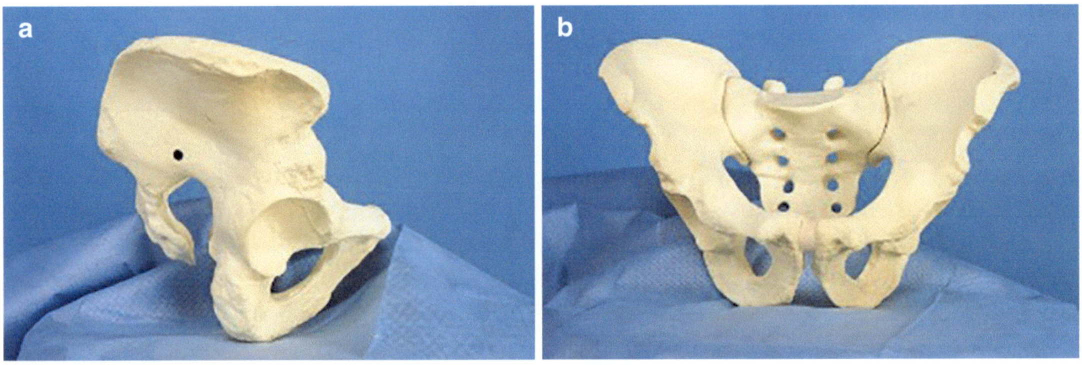

Fig. 30.2 Posterior pelvic tilt, the sacrococcygeal junction, is caudal to the pubic symphysis resulting in a (**a**) smaller pelvic tilt angle and a (**b**) negative value for the PSCD

pelvic tilt is present, cup anteversion of <20° is required to prevent impingement in functional external rotation (30°) [8]. This is important for the anterior-based surgeon. When dealing with patients with posterior pelvic tilt, keeping the acetabular anteversion closer to 10° may be advisable, and certainly, surgeons should check for impingement in external rotation. It is important to note also that there is likely very little change in spinopelvic alignment from preoperatively to postoperatively [9], but release of a flexion contracture will change the overall range of motion.

Alternative methods to ascertain pelvic tilt from an AP pelvis X-ray alone would simplify the process and have been described [10]. One such method utilizes the distance from the pubic symphysis to the sacrococcygeal junction (PSCD), as their anterior to posterior relationship in space allows for estimation of pelvic tilt. Our group found that there is a direct relationship between increasing odds of dislocation and increasing posterior pelvic tilt. We recently found that patients with more posterior pelvic tilt (Fig. 30.2b), and especially those with their pubic symphysis above the sacrococcygeal junction on an AP radiograph (PSCD <0), had had nearly 9 times the odds of dislocation compared to their counterparts. This finding is easy to identify on a commonly reviewed image, and surgeons should be aware of its implications. The complete discussion of each clinical scenario such as flatback deformities and scoliosis is out of the scope of this short perspective, but in no way lessens their importance. Other recent reviews detail comprehensive evaluation strategies for spinopelvic alignment, and I would recommend every THA surgeon review them [3, 7].

In conclusion, spinopelvic alignment is an important clinical factor in performing direct anterior THA as it is in other approaches. Surgeons should take a thorough history and perform a detailed physical exam. If standard radiographs, patient history, or physical examination indicate a possible abnormality in spinopelvic alignment, additional examination is likely warranted. This may lead the surgeon to alter the surgical plan in implant selection and or implant position.

Pelvic Tilt Point Counterpoint

Joel M. Matta

With all the current ongoing discussion and investigation regarding assessment and variations in pelvic tilt, the surgeon may well ask: Am I missing something? Is my patient in for problems because I did not take pelvic tilt into consideration when planning surgery?

The thesis of the following is a follows: Pelvic tilt does not matter! You may ask, "Wow, really?!" Well, I am stretching the truth a little because almost any truth is accompanied by a few exceptions. The real point, however, is that regarding pelvic tilt, some references and authorities are making things way too complicated. In practice, standard thinking and methods go a long way and will cover over 95 percent of cases while ignoring pelvic tilt.

Pelvic tilt is most often defined in relation to the anterior pelvic plane, which is determined by the anterior superior spines and the pubic tubercles which lie just lateral and anterior to the symphysis pubis. It can be measured as the angle between the anterior pelvic plane and the y-axis of the body or between the anterior pelvic plane and the coronal plane. If the plane is oriented at an angle with the ASISs anterior to the pubic tubercles, pelvic tilt is defined as positive in the reverse case with the ASISs posterior to the pubic tubercles the tilt is negative.

Consider two principles: (1) Proper placement of the acetabular component is in relation to the ordinate axes (x, y, and z) of the body or in relation to the body's planes (transverse, coronal, and sagittal) and *not* in relation to the pelvis (anterior pelvic plane or acetabular landmarks), (2) patients who have positional changes (supine, standing, sitting) in pelvic tilt (lumbar spine flexibility) are at less risk of dislocation while patients with fixed pelvic tilt (very stiff or fused lumbar spines) are at a higher risk of dislocation.

Regarding principle (1), the gold standard for measuring acetabular rotational position (inclination and anteversion) that is used as a clinical final assessment and is also used for judgment of methods used to position the acetabulum is a postoperative AP pelvis or AP hip taken with the patient supine. When this X-ray is taken, the X-ray beam is directed perpendicular to the long axis of the patient and perpendicular to the body's coronal plane. In this case, the individual's pelvic plane may be positive or negative or parallel to the coronal plane; however, the pelvic tilt/plane is not a factor in the measurement. Inclination and anteversion are represented by the shape and orientation of the ellipse projected by the acetabular rim irrespective of pelvis orientation. Is this measuring technique correct? I would say yes, because what is important is the acetabular rotational position (ARP) in relation to the body and femur. The motion of the prosthetic hip and lack of impingement depend on the femoral component–cup relationship, not the cup–pelvis relationship (Figs. 30.3a, b and 30.4a, b).

Regarding principle (2), changes in pelvic tilt reduce the motion of the hip joint as clinical hip motion occurs (the angle between the thigh and torso). When an individual with normal functional changes in pelvic tilt sits, pelvic tilt becomes more negative. This tilt change reduces the angle of flexion of the hip joint and thereby the risk of impingement and instability. For the patient with a stiff or fused lumbar spine, the normal pelvic tilt change with sitting cannot occur so the hip joint motion is necessarily greater and the risk of impingement and instability higher.

The takeaway message regarding principle (1) is that different patients will have a baseline positive or negative pelvic tilt that can be represented on preoperative X-rays. These differences, however, do not change the methodology or target

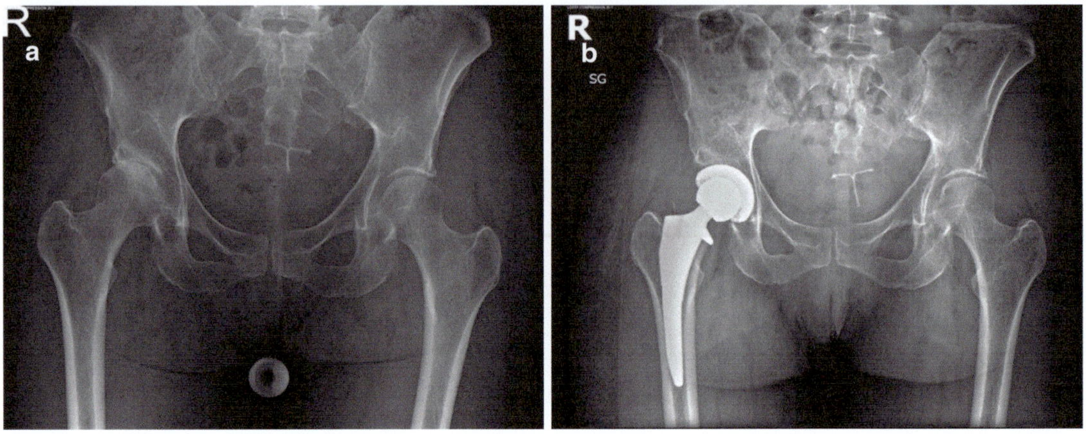

Figs. 30.3 (**a**, **b**) Pre- and postoperative AP pelvis views of a 50-year-old woman with positive pelvic tilt evidenced by AP pelvis appearance: Obturator foramina have low superior–inferior dimension, coccyx proximal to symphysis. Cup placed with supine image view using VELYS® navigation at 43° of inclination and 23° of inclination

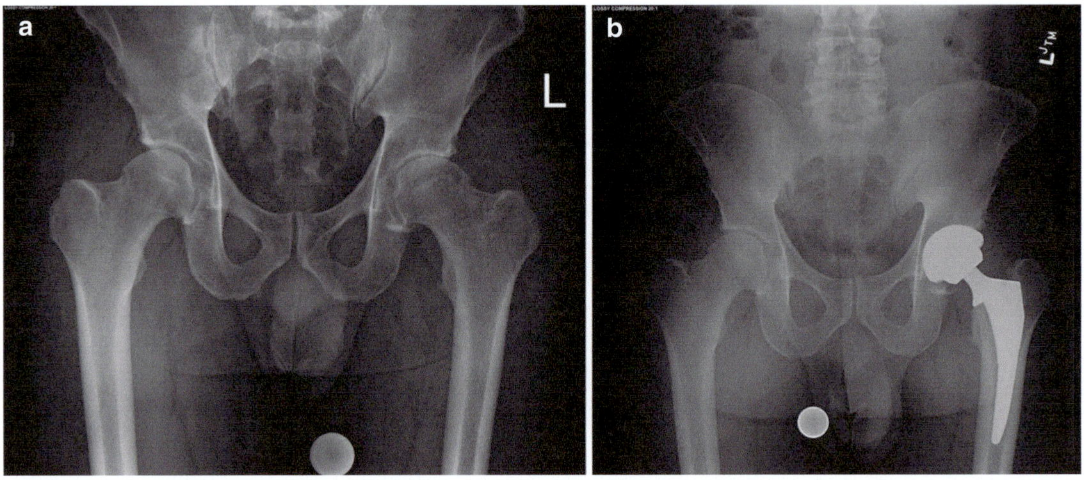

Figs. 30.4 (**a**, **b**) Pre- and postoperative AP pelvis views of a 56-year-old man with negative pelvic tilt evidenced by AP pelvis appearance: Obturator foramina have high superior–inferior dimension, coccyx, and symphysis superimposed. Cup placed with supine image view using VELYS® navigation at 43° of inclination and 23° of anteversion

values for inclination and anteversion. This means essentially, "pelvic tilt doesn't matter."

Also, if preoperative X-rays demonstrate changes in pelvic tilt between standing, supine, and sitting X-rays, the X-rays have demonstrated a normal phenomenon and a beneficial phenomenon. The fact that pelvic tilt changes with patient position indicates expected flexibility in the lumbar spine and does not alter the target value for inclination and anteversion. Normal changes in pelvic tilt "don't matter."

The reader should recognize that there is confusion in terminology regarding a cup's target position. In this chapter and the Ferguson/Matta Chap. 3 on surgical technique and the Matta/Tatka chapter on acetabular positioning, acetabular position is defined as the ARP in relation to the ordinate axes and planes of the body. I would say this is the most widely used definition and simplest to conceptualize and use. On the other hand, some computer guidance systems for acetabular positioning reference cup position in relation to the anterior pelvic plane rather than the body. If the anterior pelvic plane is used as a reference, a patient with positive pelvic tilt will require a cup that has more inclination and anteversion, while the converse is true when placing the cup in relation to a negative tilt pelvis (less inclination and anteversion). To keep things simple and accurate, ignore the pelvic tilt specific to a patient and place the cup in relation to the body.

I began this discussion of "pelvic tilt doesn't matter" by admitting it stretches the truth a little. The exceptions to the rule relate particularly to patients whose pelvic tilt does not change. A lack of change in pelvic tilt is present with very stiff and fused lumbar spines. In this case, the exact degree of pelvic tilt that the patient has does not matter, it is the lack of normal changes in pelvic tilt that increases the risk of impingement and instability. The stiff spine patient has a "smaller window" or range of inclination and anteversion that will be free from impingement and instability. My own practice is to slightly increase inclination and anteversion in the stiff spine patient and consider dual mobility cups.

The anterior approach hip surgeon should also consider that the emphasis on pelvic tilt has primarily come from the posterior approach hip surgeons who I believe, which encounter dislocation problems primarily as a result of inconsistent cup position and surgical sectioning of the external rotators. Focusing on pelvic tilt will not solve these other problems relating to posterior approach.

For anterior approach hip surgeons, will routine multiple preoperative X-rays to assess pelvic tilt and its positional changes positively affect outcomes and be justified in terms of time, cost, and patient radiation? Following the above reasoning and my own patients' incidence of dislocation, I would say no. Currently, using no preoperative measurement of pelvic tilt or its changes, my own incidence of dislocation is between one and two per 1000 hip replacements. The problems I do see are in patients with obviously abnormal spines. Can a prospective evaluation of pre-op assessment of pelvic tilt followed by associated patient-specific acetabular position for all patients reduce this incidence of dislocation? If so, what numbers would be necessary for statistical significance?

My advice for anterior hip surgeons is, for the large majority of patients, to ignore pelvic tilt and place the cup in relation to the body (its axes and planes). This is best done using the C-arm during surgery to target and confirm cup position. For a minority of patients who may have a very stiff lumbar spine, this can be evaluated by standing, supine, and sitting films. If the functional X-rays show no or very limited changes in tilt, this is of concern. On the other hand, if it is known that there is a long spine fusion such as surgically fused L1 to S1 or a case of ankylosing spondylitis, there is no reason to take X-rays to assess for changes in pelvic tilt because pelvic tilt is fixed and cannot change.

How many patients then warrant a pre-op evaluation for pelvic tilt? I would say less than 5%.

References

1. Malkani AL, et al. Total hip arthroplasty in patients with previous lumbar fusion surgery: are there more dislocations and revisions? J Arthroplasty. 2018;33(4):1189–93.
2. McKnight BM, Trasolini NA, Dorr LD. Spinopelvic motion and impingement in total hip arthroplasty. J Arthroplasty. 2019;34(7S):S53–6.
3. Ike H, et al. Spine-pelvis-hip relationship in the functioning of a total hip replacement. J Bone Joint Surg (Am Vol). 2018;100(18):1606–15.
4. Miki H, et al. Detecting cause of dislocation after total hip arthroplasty by patient-specific four-dimensional motion analysis. Clin Biomech. 2013;28(2):182–6.
5. Carender CN, et al. The prevalence of abnormal spinopelvic relationships in patients presenting for primary total hip arthroplasty. Arthroplast Today. 2020;6(3):381–5.

6. Esposito CI, et al. Total hip arthroplasty patients with fixed spinopelvic alignment are at higher risk of hip dislocation. J Arthroplasty. 2018;33(5):1449–54.
7. Luthringer TA, Vigdorchik JM. A preoperative workup of a "hip-spine" total hip arthroplasty patient: a simplified approach to a complex problem. J Arthroplasty. 2019;34(7S):S57–70.
8. Sato T, et al. Effects of posterior pelvic tilt on anterior instability in total hip arthroplasty: a parametric experimental modeling evaluation. Clin Biomech. 2013;28(2):178–81.
9. Blondel B, et al. Pelvic tilt measurement before and after total hip arthroplasty. Orthop Traumatol Surg Res. 2009;95(8):568–72.
10. Tannast M, et al. Estimation of pelvic tilt on anteroposterior X-rays – a comparison of six parameters. Skelet Radiol. 2006;35(3):149–55.

31 Getting Correct Cup Position with the Anterior Approach: Bony Landmarks Versus x-ray Versus Computer Guidance

Michael Nogler, Friedrich Boettner, and Timothy P. Lovell

Bony Landmarks for Cup Position

Michael Nogler and Martin Thaler

One of the specifics of the direct anterior approach is that the surgery is usually performed with the patient in supine position. For surgeons that have learned to do hip arthroplasty this way there is no change. Yet, especially for those who were trained in the posterior approach in a lateral decubitus position having the patient in supine position looks oddly different. The fact that many surgeons who converted to the DAA are posterior trained might be a reason that cup positioning is heavily discussed in the DAA world. Obviously, the position of the acetabulum and its anatomy is the same – no matter how we position the patient. It is just the way the surgeon looks at it that is different. For surgeons that are unfamiliar with the supine position x-ray guidance has been proposed to confirm correct positioning. There is extensive literature that describes how a correct orientation of an intraoperative C-arm shot can be achieved.

In our teaching in Innsbruck we focus more on the understanding of the acetabular anatomy and the pelvic position. It is essential that prior to the surgery, idealy right before we scrub in, the patient's x-ray is carefully studied, and the cup position is templated. In this step it is important to decide the depth of the planned reaming in relationship to the tear drop, which is the bottom of the acetabular fovea. Equally important is to define the location of the inferior border of the cup in relation to the inferior border of the tear drop sign. In the acetabulum this is the transverse ligament. With this information in mind and a template on the x-ray screen throughout the surgery, the surgeon should have a clear concept for the cup placement.

One of the beauties of the supine position is that it is easy to palpate both anterior superior iliac spines and the pubic symphysis. Therefore, the pelvic entrance plane is directly accessible and can be used for cup orientation specifically to guide anteversion. We palpate these landmarks a couple of times during surgery. After dislocation of the hip and after completing the neck osteotomy, it is important to locate the transverse ligament and the bottom of the fovea. This will guide the depth and inclination of the cup. Both landmarks will remain untouched throughout cup implantation. Independent from the templating, the acetabular rim defines the original orientation of the acetabulum in cases with no defects. Even

M. Nogler
Department of Orthopaedic Surgery, Medical University of Innsbruck, Innsbruck, Austria
e-mail: michael.nogler@professor-nogler.at

F. Boettner (✉)
Hospital for Special Surgery, New York, NY, USA
e-mail: boettnerf@hss.edu

T. P. Lovell
Providence Orthopedics & Sports Medicine, Spokane, WA, USA

J. M. Matta, A. P. Sah (eds.), *Anterior Hip Replacement*,
https://doi.org/10.1007/978-3-030-91896-5_31

if the cup position is templated to be different from the natural acetabular orientation, the acetabular rim can serve as reference for the planned cup positioning. While the fovea, the transverse ligament, and the acetabular rim are local landmarks, the pelvic entrance plan serves as reference for the position of the cup impactor for anteversion. The longitudinal axis of the patient is also a reference for the cup inclination and is easy to estimate. If the cup is aligned to all these landmarks one can proceed with implantation. If not, all landmarks need to be re-checked until they align with the desired position targets.

While a C-arm imaging can help with the relationship of the cup to local landmarks we feel that the direct information of the impactor handle's orientation to the pelvic entrance plane and the patient's axis are equaly important. A combination of both will help to get cup positioning right and minimize x-ray exposure. Nonetheless, x-ray can be helpful to confirm cup position.

Navigation and robotics to require usually not readily available hardware. Both authors have used both systems extensively. While navigation focuses primarily on simple 3 D cup placement, robotics does improve 3-D visualization and allows for a more individual cup placement. For both, it is true that they base their cup positioning on 3D data instead of 2D information of standard x-rays. A preoperative CT scan is taken and a volumetric reconstruction of the pelvic is performed. This allows the surgeon to plan the cup position in the three-dimensional space. That is different from what we do with x-ray-based templating and requires some experience but it gives us control over all aspects of cup positioning and bears huge potential for the future in which it, as we hope, allows for a more individual simulation of the patients anatomy as well as position adjustments based on bone quality, bone impingement and spino-pelvic position.

In summary, we think great cup placement can be achieved without x-ray or computer guidance. For surgeons early in their learning curve with the patient in supine position intraoperative x-rays might give a higher level of assurance. Navigation and robotics based on CT scans render the highest precision and execution of the preoperative plan.

Getting Correct Cup Position with x-ray

Anna Jungwirth-Weinberger and
Friedrich Boettner

Optimal cup positioning is important to reduce the risk of dislocation and psoas impingement, as well as avoid excessive plastic wear and implant impingement. A number of different options have been described to determine correct acetabular component positions during anterior total hip arthroplasty.

The safe zone of acetabular component positioning is considered to be an inclination angle of 40° ± 10° and an anteversion angle of 15° ± 10°. Malposition can result in abnormal contact (impingement), increased plastic wear, and dislocation [1]. It can be necessary to adjust these target values based on approach, pelvic tilt or decreased spinopelvic mobility.

Position Based on Anatomic Landmarks

With the patient in a supine position, acetabular component placement can be based on bony landmarks of the anterior pelvic plane. This plane is formed by the anterior superior iliac spines and the pubic tubercles, which can be palpated. However, even a minor failure to correctly identify these anatomic landmarks due to differences in patient anatomy or improper positioning on the operating table can lead to inaccuracies in the final cup alignment [2].

Alternatively, Archbold et al. reported a technique to determine the intraoperative position of the acetabular component based on the transverse acetabular ligament. Utilizing this technique resulted in a low dislocation rate of 0.6% in a consecutive series of 1000 hip arthroplasties [3].

Utilizing C-Arm Imaging

One advantage of the anterior approach is that the supine position of the patient accommodates the use of a C-arm to control component position [4]. Parallax has to be taken into consideration when measuring cup inclination on a 12-inch C-Arm monitor. Boettner and Rueckl recommended adding a correction factor of 5° to the intraoperative C-Arm inclination measurement [5]. This number might vary by C-arm model. In addition, Boettner and Zingg reported on a technique to use the C-arm tilt angle to measure acetabular anteversion [6]. A cup with 40° of inclination, a tilt angle of 30° has a true cup anteversion of 20°. This allows for relatively simple determination of inclination and acetabular component anteversion, and the anteversion measured with this technique was on average 0.2° (range −3.0 to 3.1) greater than the anteversion in a control group measured with CT. 100% of the cups using this technique were in the safe zone, the average inclination was 40.8°, and the average anteversion was 18.4° [7].

Alternatively, software can be used to process the images and compare the operative side to the normal contralateral side based on reference points or restore an AP pelvis image based on multiple intraoperative C-Arm images (Radlink®, El Segundo, CA; Jointpoint® DePuy Orthopaedics, Inc., Warsaw, IN). Utilizing this software improved accuracy and precision of cup positioning with only modest increases in surgical time [8].

Alternatively a grid can be placed on the C-arm that corrects Parallax directly and allow measurement of component alignment on this corrected image (OrthoGrid®, Salt Lake City, UT).

Navigation: Systems

Computer navigation systems consist of a camera, probe, and tracker within the sterile field and a workstation monitor outside of the sterile field. Intraoperatively, the workstation computes the 3D positional relationship between the camera and tracker and provides this information in real-time on the workstation display [9]. The surgeon maps the left and right anterior superior iliac spine and the symphysis pubis; the system's camera safes the location and identifies the pelvic plane based on the position of the tracker antenna on the iliac crest. During acetabular reaming, an additional tracker can be positioned onto the impactor, and anteversion and inclination are shown on the workstation monitor [4]. Comparing the intraoperative position to postoperative radiographs, 93% of radiographic anteversion and inclination measurements were within 10° of the intraoperative measurement [9].

Alternatives to standard navigation systems are systems based on either optical alignment in relation to a reference plane (Intelljoint®, Kitchener ON, Canda) or a small computers within the sterile field that determines cup position based on anatomic landmarks (OrthoAlign®, Aliso Viejo, CA).

Robotic Hip Replacement

Modern robotic hip replacement is based on preoperative CT images. These images are used to create a 3D model of the pelvis that intraoperatively can be used to identify the position of the pelvis based on surface mapping. Using an antenna tracker to determine the position of the pelvis, a robotic arm is positioned in relation to the pelvis during reaming and impaction of the acetabular component (MAKO®, Stryker Howmedica, Kalamazoo, MI). Robotic THA improves accuracy in achieving acetabular component positioning, but is associated with additional radiation exposure [10].

Computer Guidance for Component Positioning

Tim Lovell

Correct acetabular component positioning is known to be one of the most difficult yet critical things to achieve in hip replacement [11]. While supine direct anterior approach has markedly improved our ability to achieve appropriate cup position, including by the use of intraoperative fluoroscopy [12], there is still a need for improvement. Recent studies have shown wide variability in pelvic tilt among patients going from standing to sitting, and this is felt to be a significant contributor to dislocation even among patients with components in the supposed "safe zone" [13]. Using imageless or CT-based robotic-arm-assisted THA to assist in acetabular component positioning is not a new concept, and has been shown to be effective in improving accuracy [14]. A breakthrough in CT-based robotic-arm-assisted THA component positioning has recently been developed allowing individualized component positioning, including taking into account each individual patient's change in pelvic tilt between standing and sitting. This will be discussed in the next few pages.

To help the surgeon optimize component positioning for each patient, a CT scan from the top of the pelvis to the knee joint is obtained preoperatively. Each patient also has a lateral x-ray of the spinopelvic junction taken in a standing and sitting position and the pelvic tilt or sacral slope for each are noted. The CT scan is then reformatted to allow three-dimensional modeling of that specific patient's anatomy. Extremely detailed preoperative planning is then possible for both the acetabular and femoral components, including allowing position changes of each component in all 6° of freedom (Fig. 31.1). Each component can be assessed in the transverse, coronal, and sagittal planes. The amount of bone to be reamed away is also clearly visualized.

The change in that specific patient's pelvic tilt when going from standing to sitting is then incorporated into the model and the surgeon can then see how the acetabular component changes in abduction and anteversion when that individual goes from supine to standing to sitting (Fig. 31.2). The software then allows the surgeon, preoperatively, to put that specific patient's hip through a range of motion with the implants in their planned position and check for areas of component to component and bone to bone impingement (Fig. 31.3). This includes all positions including extension and external rotation AND flexion and internal rotation, again, incorporating that specific patient's change in pelvic tilt between standing and sitting. The surgeon may then modify either component position, size, or even system (i.e., dual mobility) to maximize the impingement-free range of motion in that specific patient with their own individual change in pelvic tilt between standing and sitting.

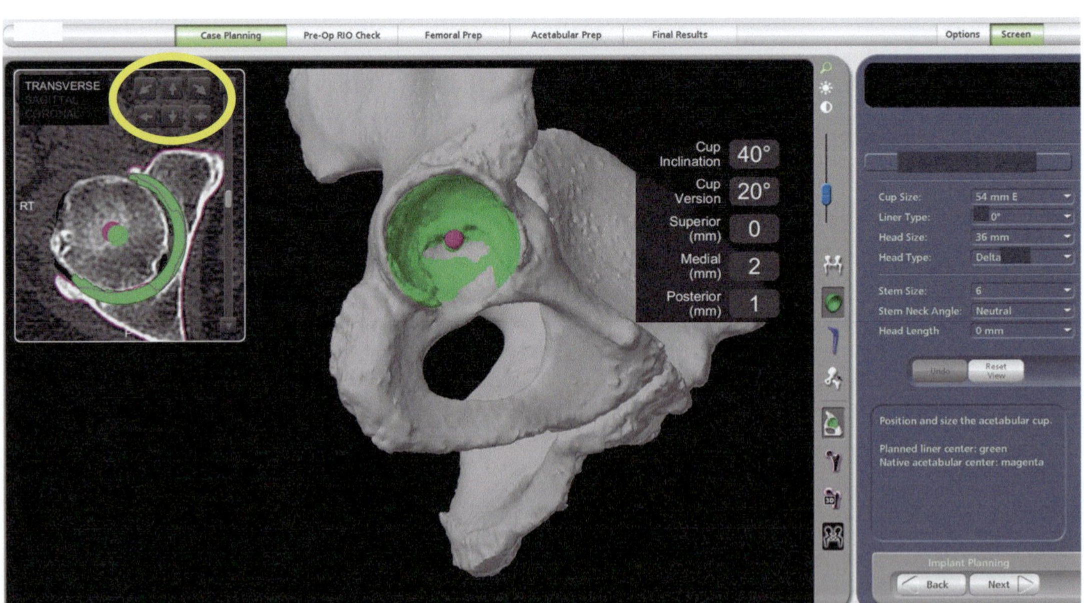

Fig. 31.1 Preoperative planning allowing position change of acetabular component in all 6° of freedom (see arrows inside yellow ellipse)

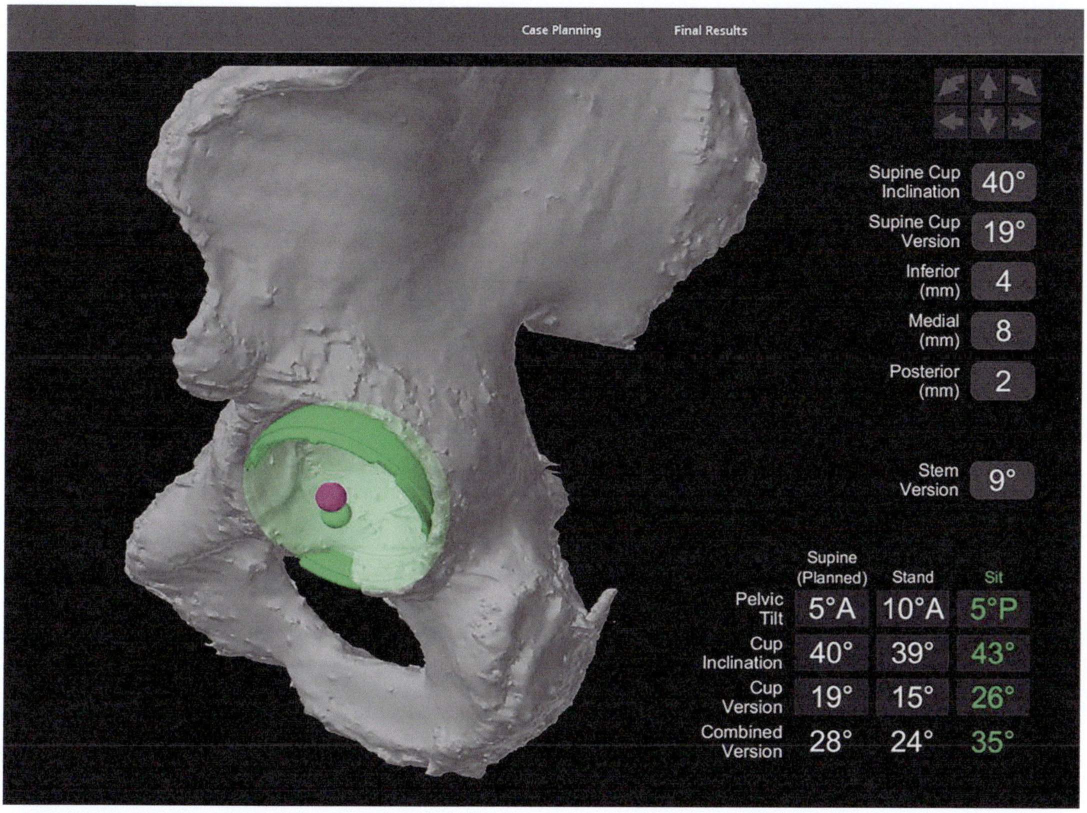

Fig. 31.2 Acetabular component changes in abduction and anteversion when that individual goes from supine to stand to sit

Intraoperatively 3 pins are placed in the contralateral iliac crest and an array is attached to them. A camera sees the array as well as a surgeon-held probe. After exposure, the surgeon touches the tip of the probe to various parts of the pelvis and the femur, and the computer correlates these with the patient-specific CT scan. The preoperatively planned neck cut can then be precisely marked on the femoral neck. Acetabular reaming is assisted by a robotic arm controlled by a haptic boundary that accurately carries out the reaming as per preoperative plan, typically with one reamer. The robotic arm then assists the surgeon in placing the acetabular component in the preoperatively planned position with a very high degree of accuracy [15]. Femoral component anteversion can also be assessed. After reduction hip length and offset can be assessed and compared to that hip preoperatively as well as the contralateral hip (Fig. 31.4).

Robotic-arm-assisted total hip replacement has improved our ability to accurately place an acetabular component in a predetermined position and has been shown to have improved short-term outcomes compared to manual cases [16, 17]. Further studies are needed to determine if this short-term improvement will continue long-term.

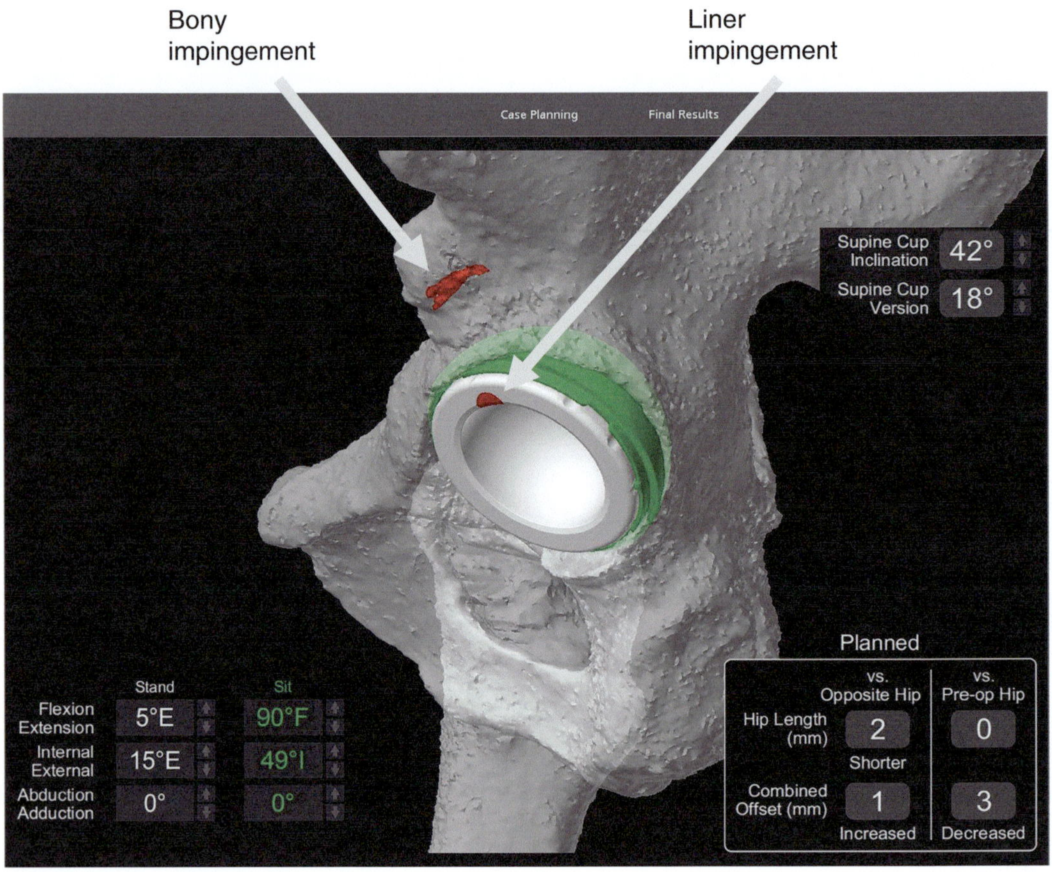

Fig. 31.3 Areas of impingement (seen in red) with flexion (90°) and internal rotation (49°). The femur has been removed for clarity

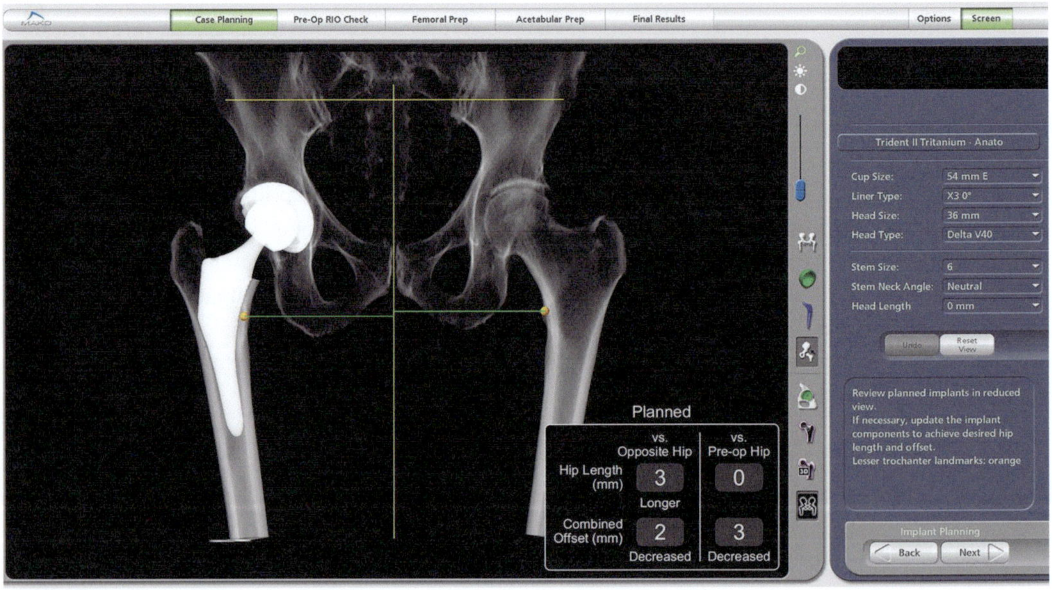

Fig. 31.4 After reduction leg lengths and offset can be checked and compared to that hip preoperatively as well as the contralateral hip

References

1. Herrlin K, Selvik G, Pettersson H, Kesek P, Onnerfält R, Ohlin A. Position, orientation and component interaction in dislocation of the total hip prosthesis. Acta Radiol. 1988;29(4):441–4. PMID: 3408605.
2. Wolf A, DiGioia AM 3rd, Mor AB, Jaramaz B. A kinematic model for calculating cup alignment error during total hip arthroplasty. J Biomech. 2005;38(11):2257–65. https://doi.org/10.1016/j.jbiomech.2004.09.033. Epub 2004 Nov 11. PMID: 16154413.
3. Archbold HA, Mockford B, Molloy D, McConway J, Ogonda L, Beverland D. The transverse acetabular ligament: an aid to orientation of the acetabular component during primary total hip replacement: a preliminary study of 1000 cases investigating postoperative stability. J Bone Joint Surg Br. 2006;88(7):883–6. https://doi.org/10.1302/0301-620X.88B7.17577. PMID: 16798989.
4. Parvizi J, Benson JR, Muir JM. A new mini-navigation tool allows accurate component placement during anterior total hip arthroplasty. Med Devices (Auckl). 2018;11:95–104. https://doi.org/10.2147/MDER.S151835. PMID: 29606894; PMCID: PMC5868583.
5. Rueckl K, Alcaide DJ, Springer B, Rueckl S, Kasparek MF, Boettner F. Intraoperative measurement of cup inclination using fluoroscopy requires a correction factor. Arch Orthop Trauma Surg. 2019;139(11):1511–7. https://doi.org/10.1007/s00402-019-03168-w. Epub 2019 Apr 1. PMID: 30937525.
6. Zingg M, Boudabbous S, Hannouche D, Montet X, Boettner F. Standardized fluoroscopy-based technique to measure intraoperative cup anteversion. J Orthop Res. 2017;35(10):2307–12. https://doi.org/10.1002/jor.23514. Epub 2017 Mar 29. PMID: 28075046.
7. Boettner F, Zingg M, Emara AK, Waldstein W, Faschingbauer M, Kasparek MF. The accuracy of acetabular component position using a novel method to determine anteversion. J Arthroplast. 2017;32(4):1180–5. https://doi.org/10.1016/j.arth.2016.10.004. Epub 2016 Oct 12. PMID: 27839959.
8. Hamilton WG, Parks NL, McDonald JF 3rd, Pfefferle KJ. A prospective, randomized study of surgical positioning software shows improved cup placement in Total hip arthroplasty. Orthopedics. 2019;42(1):42–7. https://doi.org/10.3928/01477447-20190103-02. PMID: 30658003.
9. Bradley MP, Benson JR, Muir JM. Accuracy of acetabular component positioning using computer-assisted navigation in direct anterior total hip arthroplasty. Cureus. 2019;11(4):e4478. https://doi.org/10.7759/cureus.4478. PMID: 31249755; PMCID: PMC6579332.
10. Kayani B, Konan S, Ayuob A, Ayyad S, Haddad FS. The current role of robotics in total hip arthroplasty. EFORT Open Rev. 2019;4(11):618–25. https://doi.org/10.1302/2058-5241.4.180088. PMID: 31754468; PMCID: PMC6851528.
11. Grammatopoulos G, Alvand A, Monk A, Mellon S, Pandit H, Rees J, Gill H, Murray D. Surgeons' accuracy in achieving their desired acetabular component orientation. J Bone Joint Surg. 2016;98(17):e72.
12. Slotkin E, Preetesh P, Suarez J. Accuracy of fluoroscopic guided acetabular component positioning during direct anterior total hip arthroplasty. J Arthroplast. 2015;30(Suppl. 1):102–6.
13. Phan D, Bederman SS, Schwarzkopf R. The influence of sagittal spinal deformity on anteversion of the acetabular component in total hip arthroplasty. Bone Joint J. 2015;97-B:1017–23.
14. Xu K, Li Y, Zhang H, Wang C, Xu Y, Li Z. Computer navigation in total hip arthroplasty: a meta-analysis of randomized controlled trials. Int J Surg. 2014;12:528e533.
15. Nodzo SR, Chang CC, Carroll KM, Barlow BT, Banks SA, Padgett DE, Mayman DJ, Jerabek SA. Intraoperative placement of total hip arthroplasty components with robotic-arm assisted technology correlates with postoperative implant position: a CT-based study. Bone Joint J. 2018;100-B(10):1303–9.
16. Perets I, Mu BH, Mont MA, Rivkin G, Kandel L, Domb BG. Current topics in robotic-assisted total hip arthroplasty: a review. Hip Int. 2020;30(2):118–24.
17. Jerabek S, Cohen R, Levine A, Cruz A, Scholl L. Robotic-assisted total hip arthroplasty yields enhanced surgical and clinical outcomes compared to manual hip arthroplasty using the same implant system. EPiC Series in Health Sciences, vol. 3; 2019, p. 206–9, CAOS 2019. The 19th Annual Meeting of the International Society for Computer Assisted Orthopaedic Surgery.

Stem Choice for Anterior Approach Total Hip Arthroplasty: Surgeon Perspectives

32

Atul F. Kamath, Jonathan Yerasimides, Michael Nogler, William G. Hamilton, Stefan W. Kreuzer, and John L. Masonis

Commentary on Cemented Indications and Technique in Anterior Approach Total Hip Arthroplasty

Atul F. Kamath

The use of cemented arthroplasty is likely underutilized in North America when compared to rates of use elsewhere in the world. The philosophy, technique, and teaching of cemented hip replacement in North America are also not being appropriately transferred to the next generation of orthopedic surgeons in training programs. The proper use and indications for cemented arthroplasty have a continued role in the armamentarium of the hip arthroplasty surgeon, regardless of favored approaches in the primary and revision setting. Rates of femoral loosening and periprosthetic fracture may be mitigated in patients with poor bone quality or elderly patients with the proper use of cemented arthroplasty. While certain critiques of the anterior approach include femoral loosening and/or periprosthetic fracture, this is not due to the surgical approach, but rather the techniques for femoral exposure and training necessary to safely perform this approach. In the same vein, complications may be due not only to a learning curve associated with adoption of any new technique, but in my opinion more related to mismatch of cementless fixation with poorer bone quality.

A. F. Kamath (✉)
CCLCM, CWRU SOM, Hip & Knee Reconstruction, Department of Orthopaedic Surgery, Cleveland Clinic Foundation, Cleveland, OH, USA

Center for Hip Preservation, Orthopaedic and Rheumatologic Institute, Cleveland Clinic, Cleveland, OH, USA

J. Yerasimides
Norton Orthopedic Institute, Louisville, KY, USA

M. Nogler
Department of Orthopaedic Surgery, Medical University of Innsbruck, Innsbruck, Austria
e-mail: michael.nogler@professor-nogler.at

W. G. Hamilton
Anderson Orthopaedic Research Institute, Alexandria, VA, USA

S. W. Kreuzer
INOV8 Orthopedics, Houston, TX, USA
e-mail: skreuzer@inov8hc.com; stefan@inov8hc.com

J. L. Masonis
OrthoCarolina Hip & Knee Center, Atrium Musculoskeletal Institute, Charlotte, NC, USA

J. M. Matta, A. P. Sah (eds.), *Anterior Hip Replacement*,
https://doi.org/10.1007/978-3-030-91896-5_32

In my practice, the use of cemented primary arthroplasty is reserved for those patients with poor bone quality (osteoporosis and/or Dorr C canals) and/or elderly patients (generally older than 75 years of age), certain hip fracture patients indicated for total hip or hemiarthroplasty, selected conversion arthroplasty patients, certain patients with versional mismatch, and/or proximal femoral deformity, select inflammatory arthropathy, and/or previously irradiated/pathologic fields, and reimplantation arthroplasty with history of infection if antibiotic-loaded bone cement is preferred. I must say that the use of a compaction broaching stem with a collar (e.g., DePuy Corail, DePuy Actis stems) has obviated the need for cemented fixation in the vast majority of patients due to the excellent track record, versatility in essentially all bone types, and the bone-friendly/preserving nature of the compaction broaching technique that does not rely on strict cortical fixation as needed with other types of cementless blade/wedge stems. The compaction broaching philosophy necessarily allows for a cancellous mantle, which provides surgical safety with impaction, and a collared stem increased the axial and rotational stability when compared to an equivalent collarless design.

I like cementing through the anterior approach, given the ability to see circumferentially about the mantle about the proximal femur. This allows not only equal cement mantle placement, but also the ability to match version and depth with excellent visualization of the proximal femur mouth. There is also a nice distribution of the cement in the canal, given the relatively vertical orientation of the femur as it is extended, adducted, and externally rotated to draw the proximal femoral mouth into the surgical field.

Meticulous surgical technique is imperative for cementing arthroplasty. Adequate femoral exposure is important for femoral stem trajectory. I like the aim for placement of a cemented femoral stem in neutral or slight valgus (depending on stem geometry), so co-linear axis to the femoral canal is important. Proper femoral exposure also aids in the application of adjunctive cementing techniques, such as pressurization and horse collar (stem seal) use. My femoral technique is independent of approach, and generally includes the following surgical tips and techniques:

- Have all the tools available for cementing, e.g., long-tip irrigator and cement nozzles
- Always alert anesthesia that you are performing the cementing stage of the procedure; I also aim for hypotensive anesthesia in general if safe from a patient perspective
- Note that a femoral stem allows the ability to make final subtle length adjustments by cementing the final stem deeper or more proud; mark depth of broach when trialing; similarly, mark final version of the broach after trialing phase to adjust version accordingly with final stem
- Do not disturb the cancellous mantle; aim for 2–3 mm mantle circumferentially if possible
- Use of a cement restrictor is important
- My preference is epinephrine-soaked sponges to dry the canal, instead of hydrogen peroxide, to avoid theoretical oxygen toxicity
- I prefer to heat the stem (e.g., in a 60 °C normal saline bath), as well as the cement, to improve interdigitation; apply cement in a doughy state
- Place a pediatric suction tube into the canal during the cementation; as you begin to retrograde fill the canal, remove the tube once the tube is not drawing suction
- Use a pressurizer, as well as thumb pressure over the calcar to continue pressurization during each sequential step; you may see fat expressed from the nutrient holes in the proximal femur; maintenance of pressure is important for high-quality cement mantle and to prevent back-bleeding into the interfaces
- I apply some extra cement into the shoulder region of the proximal femur for rotational stability augmentation; this is also a region that is commonly missed with standard cementing techniques
- Do not move or trial the stem till cement is completely hardened; test hardening with a knife blade; approximate hardening time with warm cement is around 7 minutes at 21 °C and humidity 40%

Avenir Complete

Jonathan Yerasimides

My preferred femoral stem is the Zimmer Biomet Avenir Complete™. It is a rectangular cross section, fully coated hydroxyapatite stem. This style of femoral stem has over 30 years of clinical history and has been widely used with anterior approach hip surgeons for over 15 years in the United States. The Avenir Complete™ is a mod ernized version addressing the problems associated with the original such as neck length, distal potting, and lack of collar.

The neck has been shortened to address what was thought to be long on the legacy stem. In addition to shortening the neck, a third offset option was added with a 126.5° coxa vara option. This is one of the key design qualities of this implant for me as an anterior approach hip surgeon. My goal is always to recreate the patient's natural anatomy. There are multiple recent anatomical studies showing average femoral neck-shaft angle to lie between 125° and 127° which begs the question of why haven't our femoral stems changed to correspond to normal anatomy? My opinion is that hip replacement didn't rely on modern technology to reproduce anatomy. We would put in components, examine leg length by external landmarks, feel soft tissue tensions, and close the patient. Anterior approach has changed the way we look at leg length and offset. We spend the time to do fluoroscopic overlays, or have computer and tablet programs designed to show us these parameters within millimeters. Having only two neck options of standard or high offset makes this much more difficult. Having a varus neck angle option simplifies the surgery by allowing me to perform similar neck cuts on the majority of patients and using the neck angle to assist in leg length adjustments. The math is very simple with the standard and high offsets differing 6 mm in horizontal offset throughout all sizes while maintaining the same leg length. The coxa vara and the high offset differ 6 mm in leg length throughout all sizes while maintaining the same offset. By having a coxa vara neck angle in addition to traditional standard and high options, I have the ability to recreate the natural anatomy and biomechanics of the hip.

Fully coated hydroxyapatite femoral stems have a very long history of success dating back decades. Some of the disadvantages of the older versions were problems with overall stem length and distal potting, especially in Dorr type A femoral canals. A distally potted, full coated stem has been a very difficult problem to deal with because the implant isn't loose, but still causes thigh pain. Revising this type of failure is difficult because the implant is well fixed in the most difficult part of the femur to access without osteotomy. This stem was narrowed distally to avoid the problem of distal potting. By beveling the distal lateral border of the stem, it allows the implant to fill proximally before it pots, providing better opportunity for proximal ongrowth and long-term success. The overall length of the stem was shortened as well making it a mid-length femoral stem. I am personally not a proponent of short stems which have become popular with anterior approach hip replacement surgery. They have been popularized to help surgeons prepare the femur easier due to difficulty with exposure. Unfortunately, we are now showing increased incidence of subsidence, loosening, and fracture with short stems compared to standard length stems. My personal experience of over 9000 anterior approach hip replacements parallels the findings of others. I have tried short stems in the past and not been happy with the incidence of failure and revision. I believe in learning good femoral exposure and using standard length implants. This implant was designed by a team of surgeons from all three exposure backgrounds. It was not designed short or specifically for anterior approach, therefore, its been my preferred implant.

The third, and maybe most controversial feature of this implant is the option of collar or collarless. The collar vs. collarless debate has surgeons on both sides that are steadfast in their belief one way or another. My personal preference is an uncemented collared stem. The tapered wedge stem has become the most popular stem design over the past few decades because of its ease in preparation and implantation. The early reports of these stems were from a time in hip replacement where weight-bearing was protected in the early postoperative period. These stems were given time to ongrow before full weight-bearing was allowed. Now we are in a time of immediate weight-bearing and faster recovery times. In my opinion, this is why more recent papers are showing increased incidence of subsidence and early postoperative fractures and failures with these stems compared to other designs. I also saw this in my own practice and therefore switched to a collared implant. Collared stems have been shown to provide better immediate stability than collarless. They can withstand much greater vertical and horizontal forces, preventing subsidence and failure. I disagree with the concept that a stem may need to subside to get stability. A stem should have stability when it leaves the operating room because stability leads to ongrowth which leads to long-term success. For those who prefer collarless however, this stem comes in that option with all sizes and offsets as well.

For the reasons I've outlined above, the Avenir Complete™ from Zimmer Biomet is my preferred femoral stem. The shape and hydroxyapatite coating have excellent results with decades of implantation. Having a coxa vara offset option allows me to reproduce a patient's natural anatomy and simplifies my ability to recreate length and offset. Lastly, I prefer a collared stem to reduce my risk for subsidence and improve the important initial stability needed for long-term success of a total hip replacement.

Stem Choice for Anterior Approach

Martin Thaler and Michael Nogler

General Considerations

For the direct anterior approach (DAA) for total hip arthroplasty (THA), the use of designated instruments is mandatory and the use of dedicated stems is recommended. The broaching trajectory and insertion pathway with the DAA are not always linearly related to the patient body habitus, femoral exposure as well as the patient's proximal femoral anatomy. Especially in muscular male and obese patients, the exposure of the stem might be challenging in inexperienced hands. However, all types of stems can be used for the DAA in primary arthroplasty. Adding proximal releases (e.g., release of the tensor fascia latae muscle (TFL)) provides straight access to the femoral canal enabling the implantation of all stem designs. There is also no approach-related limitation regarding shape of the stem, loading modes that are applied to the reconstruction, stem material or cemented as well as non-cemented stems.

According to the classification by Mont [1], all classified stem types can be used for the DAA. Single wedge stems and double wedge stems, which are usually proximally coated, are frequently used for the DAA.

If a surgeon wants to change approach, we recommend to change implants as well as instruments first to get used to the handling of the new devices. It is after 20–50 procedures with the new implants and instruments that the approach can consequently be changed.

In revision arthroplasty, all types and designs can be implanted through the interval of the DAA. A proximal release of the tensor muscle increases the femoral exposure and provides straight access to the femoral cavity during revision cases. Hence, modular stems, proximal femur replacement, and total femur replacement are feasible with the DAA. Therefore, the tensor is partially released proximal 1 cm distal from its insertion at the anterior superior iliac spine (ASIS) and pulled down by a femoral retractor. This enables straight access to the femoral canal, while the external rotators keep untouched and the femur stays in the same location. At the end of the surgery, the distal part of the partially released tensor muscle can be easily reattached to the proximal part of the tensor with sutures.

In terms of revision, no significant difference is reported in collared femoral stem compared to cementless as well as cemented, collarless femoral stem and long femoral stem compared to short femoral stem [2].

Cemented Stems

Several reports show successful outcomes using the DAA with a cemented conventional length metaphyseal-diaphyseal engaging stem. In addition to that, cemented stems of different lengths did not compromise femoral component positioning. Lastly, the angulated introduction of cemented femoral components did not compromise the quality, extent, or thickness of the cement mantle quality [3, 4].

Stem Designs

Short stems are a valuable option for the DAA, but they are absolutely not mandatory. Short hip stems had been developed with the thought of easier insertion in patients with high BMI or in less invasive procedures. These stems have been shown in the literature to have stable, dependable fixation and equivalent outcomes to standard-length stems [5, 6]. However, there is still a lack of definition: What is really a short and a lack of evidence in the long-term outcome with the use of short stems in THA? Therefore, the authors do not believe that short stems with the DAA are not superior to normal stems used for THA. In addition, most short stems require a very distinct surgical technique to reproduce excellent results, which are comparable to other stems. Using a morphometrically optimized metaphyseal-diaphyseal engaging tapered femoral stem instead of a short stem reduces component malposition and minimizes risk of loosening. Some stem designs, such as anatomically or wedged-shaped stems, confer an advantage during broaching and insertion compared with angular shoulder stems. If the lateral side of the stem is curved or had an obtuse angle, the insertion pathway is easier.

Short Stems

Straight femoral stems with a proximal shoulder are not ideal for the DAA in primary THA. There are rare data reports showing a higher revision rate in straight femoral stems with a proximal shoulder for the DAA and the anterolateral approach compared to the posterior approach [7]. The shape of the femoral stem can be an important factor in inexperienced hands causing malalignment of the femoral component due to poor exposure and broaching of the femoral canal. There might be a tendency to place stems with a prominent lateral shoulder in a slight varus position. To prevent varus alignment, we recommend accurate preoperative templating and to perform an extensive lateral preparation during stem broaching in the area of the greater trochanter with curettes, luer, or rat-tail.

Although, the implantation of a stem with a proximal shoulder for DAA is possible and shows good results, our recommendation is to use a wedge or anatomic type stem without a lateral shoulder.

Stem Length

Stems of all sizes can be implanted with the DAA as mentioned above. However, in primary THA releases of the external rotators, the TFL and stab incisions should be avoided.

Therefore, according to the author's opinion, some design philosophies are more appropriate for the DAA and, from a technical point of view, particular stem designs allow easier broaching, stem insertion, and therefore implant alignment. In addition, muscular damage, e.g., of the TFL can be avoided during broaching and implantation.

Recent reports also show that shorter stems reduce the risk of TFL damage during DAA THA [8]. More damage to the TFL occurred in patients with male sex and increased BMI. The use of a shorter stem can be considered for patients with increased BMI to limit damage to the TFL.

A shorter insertion pathway with shorter stems, not short stems, allows easier positioning of the implant. An estimated length of 15 cm of the stem has shown excellent results.

Commentary: Triple-tapered, Collared, HA-Coated Cementless Stem (Actis, Depuy Synthes)

William G. Hamilton

Given the multitude of products that have good long-term survivorship, choosing the appropriate femoral stem for total hip arthroplasty may seem straightforward. However, using decades old studies that report survivorship from a single center and single surgeon may not be the best measure to gauge a products performance. The "performance" of a stem needs to fulfill a number of criteria, only one of which is survivorship. Other criteria to be considered include ease of insertion, initial stability, resistance to periprosthetic fracture, pattern of osseointegration, and clinical performance including incidence of thigh pain. This commentary will illustrate why I believe the best cementless stem to meet the needs of today's patient is a shorter, dual-tapered, collared, HA-coated stem with a geometry that allows easy implantation from the anterior approach. The Actis stem[1] (Depuy Synthes, Warswaw, IN) is an example of this type of product (Fig. 32.1).

While the exposure of the proximal femur is quite good with the anterior approach, it can be challenging to gain straight access to the femoral canal, making it difficult to implant a longer, straight stem. Therefore, implanting a femoral stem via the anterior approach is facilitated by specific design features. A relatively shorter length stem makes preparation and insertion easier. Relief of the lateral proximal shoulder of the prosthesis also promotes the insertion technique and avoids the need to remove trochanteric bone and lateralize the stem. Also, having a product that allows for implantation with broach only bone preparation will make insertion easier. Other helpful features of the Actis stem include an insertion feature that is angled to improve access for the insertion tool, and broaches that incorporate hybrid teeth. The teeth on the Actis broach system have cutting teeth in the mediolateral (ML) direction, while the teeth in the anteroposterior (AP) plane have compaction teeth to compact rather than remove bone. This can help to preserve the bony envelope surrounding the stem and therefore enhance its rotational stability.

While the shorter design is not unique to this product, the length is short enough to make insertion easier for all patients. Furthermore, the reduced length can help avoid the stem becoming "stuck" within a tight canal. It is well accepted that a mismatch between the metaphyseal and diaphyseal width known as a champagne flute femur (Dorr, type A bone) can lead to the stem gaining fixation in the canal before it fills the metaphysis. If this scenario occurs, a

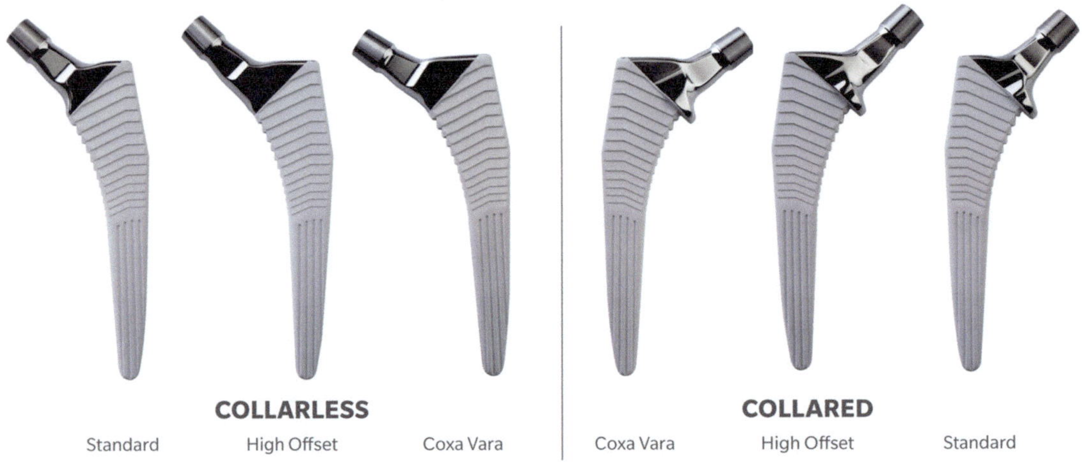

Fig. 32.1 The Actis stem (Depuy Synthes, Warsaw, IN). Triple-tapered, collared, proximally porous-coated, distally grit-blasted, fully HA-coated

[1]**Disclosure**: The Author (WGH) is a consultant and receives royalties from Depuy Synthes on total hip products, including the femoral stem described in this commentary

tapered, semi-flexible reamer can be used to ream the canal to prevent distal fixation and allow upsizing the stem until it gains bony fixation in the metaphysis. The Actis stem is not as short as a "neck sparing" implant, a design that while attractive, may not have the initial stability required to allow full weight-bearing and activities in the immediate postoperative timeframe.

One feature that is important for initial stability is the geometry of the femoral stem. One of the most widely used designs, the flat, parallel-sided, tapered titanium stem, has been used for decades with published high success rates. This stem design is also conducive for use with a modern anterior approach, but some problems have been encountered. Subsidence, failure of ingrowth, and periprosthetic fractures have been reported. Because this design relies on the stem gaining its stability primarily from the ML press fit of the stem, rotational stability of the stem may be suboptimal. A design that in some studies shows improved rotational stability is a dual-tapered stem, which provides fill in both the AP and ML plane. Higher initial stability can improve the rates of ingrowth and reduce the catastrophic complication of early periprosthetic fracture. Both a flat-tapered wedge and a dual taper design CAN be successful, but in my experience the stability conferred by the dual-tapered design is more reliable and leads to more predictable outcomes.

The design feature that may be the most important for initial stability, and the most controversial, is the collar. Historically, tapered cementless stems have been collarless. This was thought to allow the stem to find its position of optimal stability, slightly sinking until the stem locks into place. Advocates for a collarless design argued that a collar would prevent this subtle subsidence and prevent ingrowth. In hindsight, it appears this rationale was not only flawed but opposite of what facilitates stability and ingrowth. As long as the bone is prepared properly with proper broaching technique, the addition of the collar can help to improve initial stability, reduce micromotion, and therefore enhance the rates of osseointegration. Furthermore, allowing the stem to subside can lead to arguably the most morbid of the early complications, a Vancouver-B periprosthetic fracture. The collar can prevent subsidence and reduce the rate of this dreaded complication. Due to the high forces placed on the stem via modern rapid recovery protocols, stems that may have been stable under lower forces decades ago, now are subject to early motion and consequently suboptimal outcomes. Some recent studies have shown the collar to be independently predictive of lower revision rates.

Lastly, the implant surface that allows for osseointegration can also contribute to clinical outcomes. Virtually all cementless implants have an ingrowth surface over the proximal portion of the stem, and the Actis stem is no exception. Titanium sintered beads cover the proximal portion of the stem, providing the primary surface for ingrowth. This stem is also grit blasted over the remaining distal portion of the stem, and this surface allows for bony ongrowth. The entirety of the stem is coated with a clinically proven hydroxyapatite coating to enhance early bony ingrowth. By providing for a more diffuse area of bony attachment to the stem, the weight-bearing forces of the proximal femur can be distributed more physiologically, leading to higher stability, less stress shielding, and potentially less thigh pain.

All of these design features of the Actis stem make solid conceptual sense to promote clinical outcomes and performance. Early use has shown promising indicators that the optimism resulting from these enhanced design features is being realized by clinical performance. It remains to be shown, through well-designed outcome studies and registries whether large-scale usage can deliver the results the designers and engineers expect.

My Perspective on Implant Choice

Stefan W. Kreuzer

During my discussion with my patients, I always discuss three topics. These topics include the benefits of the anterior approach, the proper implant choice for each patient, and reasoning of such choice, and the bearing surface choice that is best suited for each case. The choice of the implant stem is critical in reducing the chance of postoperative complications.

During many years of my practice, I have treated patients from different ages, however there has been a significant increase in the number of younger patients who need total hip replacement. These individuals are typically more active and have higher life expectancy therefore I had to focus on implants more suitable to accommodate for specific lifestyle and expectations of such patients. Specifically, we started to utilize hip resurfacing and neck preserving implants besides ceramic-on-ceramic bearing surfaces for our younger patients.

Initially, my patients had shown interest in hip resurfacing stems, therefore, I started using these implants to perform THA procedures by using direct anterior approach (DAA). I was highly interested to combine the benefits of DAA THA with the added benefits of using resurfacing approach, as it would facilitate maintaining the blood supply to the femoral neck and to reducing the risk of neck necrosis. However, the hip resurfacing was quite challenging to be performed through the anterior approach; thus, I shifted my focus on neck preserving implants. Specifically, we started to use the MiniHip™ (Corin Inc., UK), a hydroxyapatite-coated neck preserving implant. The major benefits of a neck preserving implant are preservation of bone stock, physiological loading of the proximal femur, and maintaining physiological femoral version and femoral offset that is associated with biomechanical advantages [9].

After multiple implanted neck preserving implants, we performed a retrospective review comparing three implant types (Resurfacing, Neck Preserving, and Conventional). While anterior hip replacement patients depicted significant post-operative improvements in all cases regardless of implant choice, we observed significant clinical improvements in patients treated by neck preserving implants compared to conventional [10, 11]. The outcome of these studies along with additional findings in literature further encouraged us to continue using neck preserving stems in the treatment of our patients, particularly those younger ones. Currently, in my practice, we have performed over 2000 cases treated with neck preserving stems and patients have shown excellent clinical outcome.

Despite the aforementioned benefits, surgeons should be cautious when using neck preserving implants in DAA THA as there are some challenges while using these implants and the surgical team should be fully prepared to address them. The first challenge is caused by the retained femoral bone that increases the difficulty of acetabular preparation and exposure compared to cases in which conventional implants are used. To address this issue, I have adjusted my surgical approach by inserting the reamer basket by itself and connecting it to the reamer in situ. The acetabular shell is also placed over the neck into the socket by itself and then it is connected in situ to the cup inserter. These modifications in surgical approach are also being used for cases that are treated with conventional dual taper stems. The second challenge is related to the broaching technique as there is an increased risk of neck fracture in cases with neck preserving stems; therefore, a careful technique of impaction and cutting broaches was developed to further facilitate the technique and avoid neck fractures. Occasionally, a cerclage wire must be placed around the femoral neck resulting in touchdown weight-bearing for the patient for 6 weeks. Last, the inventory of the neck preserving implants is a concern, as there are limited sizes available (currently only seven femoral sizes are available); therefore, this implant choice may not be optimal in patients with extreme anatomical sizes. More specifically, in patients with protrusio acetabuli neck preserving stems may not be an optimal option. To avoid intraoperative complications, we always keep a conventional implant as a backup option if bone quality is sub-optimal, a significant fracture is noted intraoperatively, or femoral offset is increased beyond the planned amount.

To summarize, we use the following steps to choose proper stems. We use a cemented stem in patients 75 years old and older unless in cases who have excellent bone quality. We utilize a conventional dual taper or fully coated

CORAIL-type stem in patience between age of 60 and 75 unless their activity level includes running. Finally, neck preserving stems are used only on patients with younger patients (less than 60 years old) with a BMI less than 35 who plan to be active. The definition of active individuals in this group is the patients who engage in exercises with higher intensity compared to golfing.

Medacta Femoral Stems via the Anterior Approach for Total Hip Arthroplasty

AKA: Femoral Morphology Matching

John L. Masonis

Overview

Many uncemented femoral stems (and a select group of cemented femoral stems) have demonstrated mid to long-term success in total hip arthroplasty (THA) [12–14]. By the chronological nature of their development, these stems were designed for posterior and lateral hip surgical approaches. With the increasing popularity and shift to the anterior approach (AA) for THA, these stems continue to be utilized due to their "track record", but the details of stem design have received some new attention and scrutiny with regard to their utility when using the anterior approach. Subtle stem (and instrument) design changes can carry a significant impact with regard to soft tissue preservation, accuracy of alignment, and prevention of insertional femur fractures. Perhaps more importantly, there has been a recent increase in the literature highlighting two main concerns: (1) increased rate of femoral periprosthetic fracture following cementless femoral fixation in suboptimal bone quality (Dorr type C), and (2) increased rate of aseptic femoral component failure in patients with a high metaphyseal:diaphyseal femoral canal ratio (Dorr type A) [15–17].

Medacta has a long history of femoral component morphologies designed to complement the anterior approach for THA thanks to the clinical research and designs of multiple surgeons including Dr. Frederick Laude (Paris, France). Over the last decade, Medacta has amplified its commitment to the Anterior Approach, and this included the development of multiple femoral stems designed for the approach.

To address the unique demands of each femoral morphology (Dorr Type), Medacta has developed a portfolio that focuses on "morphology matching" of the proximal femur. This system allows the surgeon to utilize femoral stem designs that can replicate the femoral anatomy and provide reliable uncemented fixation.

Dorr Type A Femur

Two main design considerations become relevant in the Dorr Type A femur: Shorter femoral stem design and a rapid tapering geometry into the femoral metaphysis. Medacta's femoral portfolio has three main options in this arena:

1. SMS – the "Short Medacta Stem" provides a trapezoidal cross-sectional geometry and tapers rapidly to avoid meta-diaphyseal fixation. This stem is most useful in the Dorr Type A and B femur.
2. Minimax – this stem shares the concept of proximal fixation and tapers rapidly to avoid metadiaphyseal fixation. The other unique design option for the minimax stem is an anteverted neck. The neck proved 15° of anteversion for left/right stem options.
3. The most bone-conserving Medacta option for the Dorr Type A femur is the neck preserving MPress stem. Based on a long history of neck preserving stems, the MPress stem exploits the high-quality proximal femoral bone in the Dorr Type A femur.

Dorr Type B Femur

Medacta stem option for the Dorr Type B femur includes metaphyseal fixation and metadiaphyseal fixation. Stem options include:

1. Masterloc – the Masterloc is a flat taper stem design that enjoys the robust literature on flat tape (blade) style metaphyseal femoral fixation.
2. Quadra –Quadra system serves as Medacta's "conventional length" primary hip stem. It has a reduced lateral shoulder to assist with insertion via the AA. The Quadra P system is the

latest rendition of the stem and utilizes a proximal plasma spray coating with hydroxyapatite (mectagrip) for enhanced frictional stability and osseointegration Unique to the Quadra system, the cemented Quadra C stem design allows for cemented fixation with a polished tapered stem using the same broach system as is used for the uncemented Quadra H and Quadra P stems. This dual broaching system allows for easy intra-operative conversion from uncemented to cemented femoral fixation.

3. The Medacta AMIS stem was created as a modification of the Quadra specifically for AA THA. The AMIS shares the Quadra proximal cross-sectional geometry, but combines this with a more reduced lateral proximal shoulder and a significantly shorter distal stem design. These features make the AMIS stem very "anterior approach friendly". Holding true to its Quadra heritage, the AMIS stem also has a polished cemented version and has been used for both primary fixation and revision fixation with impaction grafting.

Dorr Type C Femur

Femoral fixation in the Dorr Type C femur has been controversial with proponents of uncemented and cemented fixation. Recent literature has documented a higher periprosthetic fracture rate in the uncemented femoral fixation of Dorr Type C femurs. However, there are many manuscripts documenting successful uncemented fixation in this cohort. Overall, the author prefers cemented fixation in the Dorr Type C Femur due to its reliability and reduced risk of periprosthetic fracture. Specific cases may favor uncemented fixation (i.e., severe pulmonary compromise in which pulmonary fat embolus could be deleterious). For this reason, an uncemented option is available:

1. Quadra C – This stem is a polished tapered design and utilizes a relatively small cement mantle.
2. Quadra P Collared – This stem is the "traditional length" tapered stem design with plasma spray and HA coating (mectagrip). The collared option is a recent addition to the stem design and was created for the Dorr B and Dorr C femurs where additional rotation stability of the stem is helpful in resisting retroversion.

Revision Femoral Options

With the tremendous increase in anterior approach THA, there will undoubtedly be cases requiring revision and also an interest to utilize the internervous/intermuscular benefits of the anterior approach in the revision setting. Medacta has addressed these issues on femoral revision with the development of the M-Vizion femoral revision stem. This bi-body taper fluted modular system covers stem lengths from 180 to 305 mm. Importantly, the instrumentation for this revision stem was developed with the anterior approach in mind. This helps prevent impingement on the ASIS and allows modular femoral preparation.

Summary

Femoral morphology matching has been created to address the demands for primary THA. This has created stem(s) best suited for a particular femoral endosteal anatomy.

No matter how "minor" the changes are when modifying a previously successful implant, clinical follow-up will be imperative to document the success of newer designs.

References

1. Khanuja HS, Vakil JJ, Goddard MS, Mont MA. Cementless femoral fixation in total hip arthroplasty. J Bone Joint Surg Ser A. 2011;93(5):500–9.
2. Panichkul P, Bavonratanavech S, Arirachakaran A, Kongtharvonskul J. Comparative outcomes between collared versus collarless and short versus long stem of direct anterior approach total hip arthroplasty: a systematic review and indirect meta-analysis. Eur J Orthop Surg Traumatol. 2019. https://doi.org/10.1007/s00590-019-02516-1.
3. Siguier T, Siguier M, Brumpt B. Mini-incision anterior approach does not increase dislocation rate: a study of 1037 total hip replacements. Clin Orthop Relat Res. 2004. https://doi.org/10.1097/01.blo.0000136651.21191.9f.
4. Mayr E, Krismer M, Ertl M, et al. Uncompromised quality of the cement mantle in Exeter femoral components implanted through a minimally-invasive direct anterior approach. J Bone Joint Surg Ser B. 2006. https://doi.org/10.1302/0301-620X.88B9.17538.

5. Gustke K. Short stems for total hip arthroplasty: initial experience with the Fitmore™ stem. J Bone Jointt Surg Ser B. 2012. https://doi.org/10.1302/0301-620X.94B11.30677.
6. Molli RG, Lombardi AV, Berend KR, et al. A short tapered stem reduces intraoperative complications in primary total hip arthroplasty. Clin Orthop Related Res. 2012;470(2):450–61.
7. Janssen L, Wijnands KAP, Janssen D, et al. Do stem design and surgical approach influence early aseptic loosening in cementless THA? Clin Orthop Relat Res. 2018. https://doi.org/10.1007/s11999.0000000000000208.
8. Frye BM, Berend KR, Lombardi AV, et al. Do sex and BMI predict or does stem design prevent muscle damage in anterior supine minimally invasive THA? Clin Orthop Relat Res. 2015. https://doi.org/10.1007/s11999-014-3991-1.
9. Rajakulendran K, Field RE. Neck-preserving femoral stems. HSS J® [Internet]. 2012 [cited 2013 Apr 25];8(3):295–303. Available from: http://www.pubmedcentral.nih.gov/articlerender.fcgi?artid=3470665&tool=pmcentrez&rendertype=abstract.
10. Malanka SJK, Dettmer M, Pourmoghaddam A, Veverka M, Kreuzer SW. Comparison of patient-reported outcomes of total hip arthroplasty between a neck-preserving short-stem implant and a conventional neck-sacrificing implant. J Hip Surg. 2019;03(02):078–85.
11. Dettmer M, Pourmoghaddam A, Kreuzer SW. Comparison of patient-reported outcome from neck-preserving, short-stem arthroplasty and resurfacing arthroplasty in younger osteoarthritis patients. Adv Orthop. 2015;2015:1–7.
12. Kim YH, Park JW, Jang YS. Long-term survival (up to 34 years) of retained cementless anatomic femoral stem in patients <50 years old. J Arthroplast. 2021;36(4):1388–92. https://doi.org/10.1016/j.arth.2020.10.055. Epub 2020 Nov 1. PMID: 33223411.
13. Kim YH, Park JW. Long-term outcomes of ultra-short metaphyseal-fitting anatomic cementless femoral stem in total hip arthroplasty with ceramic-on-ceramic articulation for young patients. J Arthroplast. 2019;34(10):2427–33. https://doi.org/10.1016/j.arth.2019.04.036. Epub 2019 Apr 22. PMID: 31200989.
14. Ateschrang A, Weise K, Weller S, Stöckle U, de Zwart P, Ochs BG. Long-term results using the straight tapered femoral cementless hip stem in total hip arthroplasty: a minimum of twenty-year follow-up. J Arthroplast. 2014;29(8):1559–65. https://doi.org/10.1016/j.arth.2014.02.015. Epub 2014 Feb 13. PMID: 24656056.
15. Cidambi KR, Barnett SL, Mallette PR, Patel JJ, Nassif NA, Gorab RS. Impact of femoral stem design on failure after anterior approach total hip arthroplasty. J Arthroplast. 2018;33(3):800–4. https://doi.org/10.1016/j.arth.2017.10.023. Epub 2017 Nov 11. PMID: 29137901.
16. Meneghini RM, Elston AS, Chen AF, Kheir MM, Fehring TK, Springer BD. Direct anterior approach: risk factor for early femoral failure of cementless total hip arthroplasty: a multicenter study. J Bone Joint Surg Am. 2017;99(2):99–105. https://doi.org/10.2106/JBJS.16.00060. PMID: 28099299.
17. Macheras GA, Lepetsos P, Galanakos SP, Papadakis SA, Poultsides LA, Karachalios TS. Early failure of an uncemented femoral stem, as compared to two other stems with similar design, following primary total hip arthroplasty performed with direct anterior approach. Hip Int. 2020;14:1120700020940671. https://doi.org/10.1177/1120700020940671. Epub ahead of print. PMID: 32662662.

Hip Resurfacing Arthroplasty Using the Hueter-Anterior Approach

33

Niall P. McGoldrick and Paul E. Beaulé

Introduction: Evolution of Hip Resurfacing Arthroplasty to Modern-Day Use

Resurfacing arthroplasty has a long history extending as far back as the early to mid-twentieth century. Early efforts including Smith Petersen's mould arthroplasty made of glass and later vitallium, and Wile's stainless-steel femoral component were largely unsuccessful. Later precursors appeared in the 1960s and 1970s including Sir John Charnley's polytetrafluoroethylene (Teflon) and Freeman's metal-on-polyethylene double cup arthroplasties, although the results reported were also disappointing [1].

The 1990s marked a renaissance point in modern hip resurfacing technology with the re-introduction of metal-on-metal bearings. McMinn introduced first the McMinn prosthesis (Corin, Circencester, UK), then the Birmingham Hip Resurfacing (BHR, Smith & Nephew, Tennessee, USA), while the Conserve Plus (MicroPort Orthopaedics, Memphis, Tennessee, USA) was introduced by Harlan Amstutz. Both of these devices remain in clinical use today, and are similar in design philosophy, comprising an uncemented acetabular component coupled with a short-stemmed cemented femoral component which is cemented. Of note, the BHR has hydroxyapatite on its acetabular side with a press-fit, i.e., no mantle between the femoral component and femoral bone, whereas the Conserve Plus has a porous-beaded surface with 1 mm cement mantle [2]. The Conserve Plus has the additional option of an uncemented femoral component. Both implants have been remarkably successful, with high volume resurfacing surgeons reporting 10-year survivorship rates of 96–99% [3–5].

The initial success of these prostheses prompted further metal-on-metal HR devices being introduced to the market, including the widely used Anatomical Surface Replacement (ASR, Depuy (Johnson & Johnson), New Jersey, USA). The ASR, however, performed poorly and was recalled in 2010. With a more sub-hemispherical shell and lower radial clearance than other designs, the resultant edge loading of the ASR articulation produced runaway/edge metal wear and failure of the component [6]. Coupled with a typically larger soft tissue exposure, and concerns regarding adverse reaction to metal particulate debris following the ASR recall, the past decade has seen the orthopaedic community limit the indications for hip resurfacing procedures while limiting its use to high volume centres/surgeons.

N. P. McGoldrick · P. E. Beaulé (✉)
Division of Orthopaedic Surgery, The Ottawa Hospital, University of Ottawa, Ottawa, ON, Canada
e-mail: pbeaule@toh.ca

J. M. Matta, A. P. Sah (eds.), *Anterior Hip Replacement*,
https://doi.org/10.1007/978-3-030-91896-5_33

Nonetheless, hip resurfacing remains an attractive option for the young patient with end-stage osteoarthritis of the hip providing high level of function and high patient satisfaction. Advantages include preservation of femoral bone stock, maintenance of normal hip biomechanics, reduced dislocation risk, reduced femoral stress shielding, and ease of revision surgery [7]. Moreover, it should be noted that in properly selected patients (males less than 60 years of age, minimal acetabular dysplasia) coupled with accurate component placement, modern metal-on-metal resurfacing articulations provides high functional scores with lower dislocation rate than total hip arthroplasty [8]. Having said that, the failure of the ASR highlights the importance of design philosophy and the biomechanics for a well-functioning hip resurfacing arthroplasty. The literature supports the option of hip resurfacing in men younger than 60 years of age, with female gender being a relative contra-indication [9].

Rationale for the Hueter-Anterior Approach

Critical to the success of hip resurfacing arthroplasty is the preservation of the blood supply to the femoral head [10]. Compromise of the vascularity of the head significantly increases the result of osteonecrosis, with subsequent femoral neck fracture and failure of the resurfacing arthroplasty [11]. Although the precise underlying mechanism of neck fracture remains elusive, retrieval analyses and available evidence strongly point to an osteonecrotic event and/or a traumatic insult to the femoral head-neck junction being the likely initiating factor [11, 12]. Moreover, fracture of the femoral neck remains the leading cause of early failure of metal-on-metal resurfacing in the short-term [7, 13]. Of note because of concern for osteonecrosis, the first generation of metal on polyethylene hip resurfacing the majority of the approaches was anterior-based, i.e. hip dislocated anterior through either an extra-capsular trans-trochanteric osteotomy or anterior or lateral approaches [10]. The posterior approach, however, is the most commonly used for the current generation of hip resurfacing, being the most familiar to most arthroplasty surgeons and providing a relatively easy and safe exposure of the femur and acetabulum [14, 15]. However, because the short external rotators of the hip are divided and reflected, there is direct injury to the primary blood supply of the femoral head, i.e. the ascending branch of the medial circumflex femoral artery is ligated. Hence, it has been modified for hip resurfacing to keep a soft tissue envelope around the neck to preserve some of the blood supply [16]. Conversely, the anterolateral approach theoretically avoids this particular complication, at the expense of the release of a significant portion of the hip abductor musculature [17].

Surgeons favouring the posterior approach for hip resurfacing argue that there is minimal increased risk of osteonecrosis because of the so-called intraosseous blood supply to the femoral head [18]. However, research both in animal models and in vivo in the setting of arthritis have debunked this showing the critical importance of the ascending branch of the medial femoral circumflex artery in relation to the extraosseous blood supply of the head as well as the retinacular vessels at the femoral head-neck junction [19–22].

It follows, therefore, that the optimal approach for hip resurfacing would be one that preserves the vascularity of the head, while minimizing trauma to the soft tissue anatomy around the hip. Several studies have confirmed that anterior dislocation of both native and arthritic femoral heads maintains blood supply [20, 21, 23]. In this chapter we present the Hueter-anterior approach to the hip using an orthopaedic positioning table as a safe and effective approach to hip resurfacing. Not only those the Hueter-anterior approach significantly reduces soft tissue trauma through minimal or no muscle detachment, is the only truly "inter-nervous" approach to the hip, facilitates accurate component positioning through the use of intra-operative imaging, and protects the vascularity of the femoral head [14].

Applied Anatomy of the Blood Supply of the Femoral Head

The vascular anatomy of the proximal femur has been well described in anatomy textbooks as well as original scientific articles [24, 25]. The medial femoral circumflex artery (MFCA) is the dominant supply to the weight-bearing portion of the femoral head and the most relevant vessel to the hip surgeon. The medial epiphyseal artery general only supplies the area adjacent to the fovea, while there is limited contribution from the branches of the lateral femoral circumflex artery [26]. In one recent study of ten fresh-frozen cadavers, Dewar et al. demonstrated the marked dominance of the MFCA in terms of blood supply to the femoral head. Following injection of contrast solution, the courses of the MFCA and LFCA, as well as the retinacular arterial supply were comprehensively mapped on quantitative magnetic resonance imaging (MRI) and computed tomography (CT). Subsequent surgical dissection further confirmed the extra-articular, intra-capsular and intra-osseous courses of the vessels. The MFCA was found to supply 82% of the femoral head, with the balance supplied by the LFCA [25]. Moreover, the MFCA was also found to supply much of the femoral neck (67% vs. 33%). The LFCA's main contribution is to the anteroinferior femoral head. Gautier et al. have shown that these vessels enter the femoral head through 3–6 foramina along the posterosuperior neck, at a mean of 6.5 mm from the cartilage margin [24]. The initial course of these intraosseous vessels is a mean of 5.3 mm from the same cartilage margin [24]. The implications are clear for resurfacing in terms of the depth of bone resection. Overzealous reaming of the femoral head risks compromise and damage of these vessels, with ever-increasing chance of osteonecrosis.

Indications for Hip Resurfacing Arthroplasty

Indications

Resurfacing arthroplasty is best indicated in active, healthy male patients younger than 60 years of age, with a diagnosis of osteoarthritis [9]. Although controversial, it is the senior authors view that hip resurfacing also may be indicated in females in select cases. Female patients between the ages of 40 and 50 years old, with function-limiting degenerative disease, and a femoral head size of at least 48 mm have been shown to have comparable outcomes to male patients following resurfacing arthroplasty [27]. However, with the recent introduction of ceramic on ceramic hip resurfacing, a larger proportion of female patients could benefit from a hip resurfacing.

Contraindications

Absolute contraindications to resurfacing of the hip include severe cystic changes in the femoral head or neck, which leave the bone vulnerable to fracture or failure of fixation, patients with underlying renal disease, or history of metal hypersensitivity. Relative contraindications include acetabular and/or femoral dysplasia, which may compromise optimal sizing and positioning of components.

Patient Positioning and Surgical Exposure

Following induction of anaesthesia, the patient is positioned in a supine position on an orthopaedic positioning table. In our institution, we have used the Delacroix Device from Maquet, the Hana® table (Mizuho OSI, USA) and the ROTEX table. Care is taken to ensure bony prominences are protected from injury by applying suitable padding to pressure areas. Slight traction is then applied to the contralateral limb to ensure the pelvis remains level throughout the procedure. Starting 1–2 cm inferior and lateral to the anterior superior iliac spine, a slightly oblique incision is made following the line of fibres of the tensor fascia lata and centred over the greater trochanter, aiming towards the fibular head. The incision is approximately 10–12 cm in length, and usually longer than the typical incision made for a primary total hip replacement. The subcutaneous tissue is carefully incised to expose the blue hue of the underlying tensor muscle. The fascial sheath overlying the tensor is incised in the same line as the skin incision. A fingertip or the blunt end of the scalpel is then passed to atraumatically elevate the muscle off the anterior leaf of fascia. Once correctly mobilized, the fat stripe that defines the interval between the tensor muscle and the rectus femoris should be clearly visualized. A broad cobra retractor is placed laterally, retracting the tensor. The fascia of the rectus femoris is carefully divided, with the ascending branches of the lateral circumflex femoral vessels being visualized. These must be carefully dissected, ligated and divided. Inadvertent division can result in significant bleeding. The rectus is then mobilized and retracted medially. A deeper fascial plane, known as the innominate or Letournel's fascia, is then incised to expose the pre-capsular fat pad overlying the capsule of the hip joint. The fat pad may be mobilized or swept off the capsule using a sponge. This structure can be quite a vascular tissue and use of diathermy to mobilize the fat pad is well advised. Blunt Hohmann's retractors are then positioned along the inferomedial neck of the femur, and superior neck to expose the entire anterior capsule. An anterolateral partial capsulectomy is performed in conjunction with partial elevation of the reflected head of the rectus. The hip joint is now exposed. At this point in the procedure, the labrum is excised as well as anterior rim osteophytes could impede dislocation.

Dislocation of the head of the femur requires a composite movement between surgeon and the un-scrubbed circulating nurse. The operative table is first elevated. A Weber spoon is introduced into the acetabulum without traction by the surgeon and placed on the medial surface of the head. Then the leg is externally rotated as the Weber spoon is levered on the anterior wall of the acetabulum. Once dislocated, the fascia of tensor and rectus is further released. Further release of the avascular inferomedial capsule by diathermy or may scissors completes femoral mobilization. The operative leg is then lowered down to the floor without traction and rotation being unlocked. External rotation through 180 degrees clears the iliac crest and brings the femoral head into the operative field.

Although generally no additional muscle releases are required with this approach, it should be realized that many resurfacing patients are younger active men with a larger more extensive musculature about the hip and pelvis. In those patients with large tensor muscles, a 1–2 cm release of the tensor off its iliac crest origin may be necessary to facilitate exposure of the femoral head.

Femoral Head Preparation

Starting with preparation of the femoral head is essential before exposing the acetabulum as it makes it easier for the surgeon to visualize the cup and retract the femur from blocking access to the acetabulum. A spherometer head gauge is positioned to assess the femoral component size (Fig. 33.1). The head gauges increase in 2 mm increments and correspond to the femoral component size. Accurate sizing is a critical step for several reasons. It guides removal of osteophytes and in some cases underlying cam deformity which is essential for accurate identification of the head-neck axis and therefore component position. Moreover, over-sizing the femoral component requires over reaming the acetabulum to allow for the matching acetabular component. Conversely, under-sizing the femoral component risks notching the neck through excess removal of bone. This increases the possibility of neck fracture post-operatively as well as injury to retinacular vessels running along the neck. In most hip resurfacing systems, the acetabular component is determined by the femoral head size, and usually 6 mm larger in diameter.

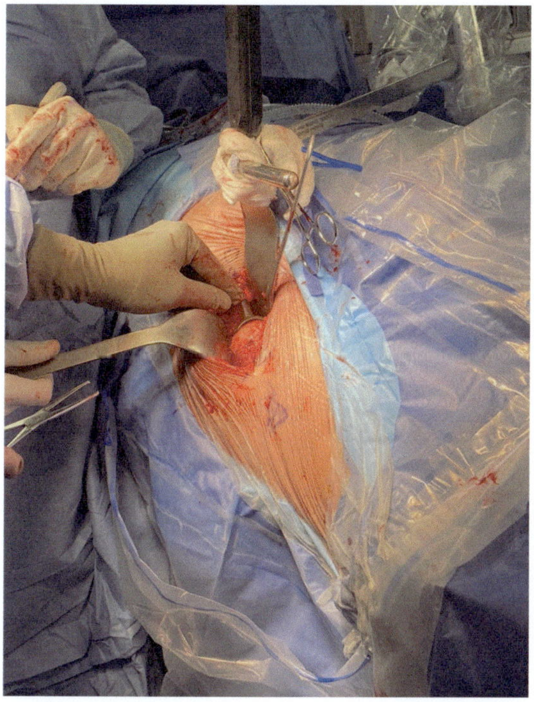

Fig. 33.1 Spherometer head gauge positioned to assess optimal head size

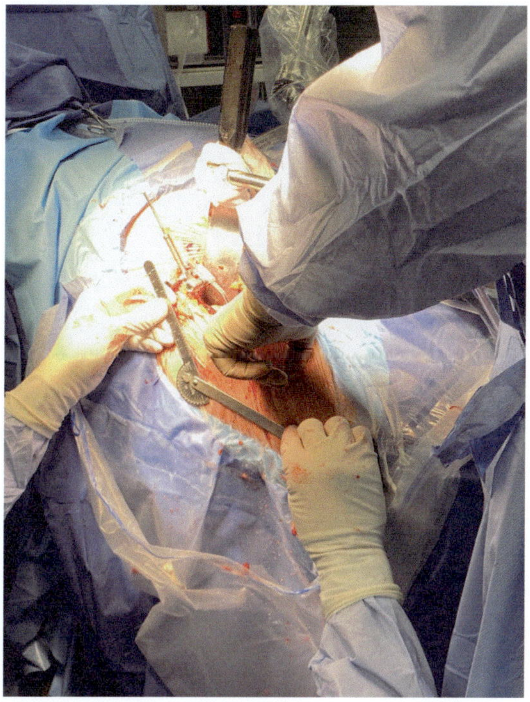

Fig. 33.2 Goniometer positioned to assess neck shaft angle of the planned component

Having determined the appropriate size, a guide-wire is positioned into the mid-part of the neck axis in reference to the infero-medial neck, the so-called Harty's recess [28]. This must be done free-hand since the anterior approach will not facilitate the use of a proprietary jig. As a reference aid, the entry point for the guidewire is approximately 10–15 mm superior to the fovea. If positioned correctly, the femoral component will sit flush against the infero-medial neck, protecting the retinacular vessels and avoiding notching. Once positioned, the planned femoral component neck-shaft angle is calculated using a goniometer (Fig. 33.2). In general, the aim is to place the component within 5–10° valgus of the native neck-shaft angle. In practice, this usually reflects a component neck shaft angle of 140°. Varus malposition is to be avoided.

The femoral head preparation is then completed with the manufacturer's instrumentation which typically consists of cylindrical, followed by a dome cut and chamfer reamers (Fig. 33.3). A trial component is then positioned. Any residual bony ridges or osteophytes should be debrided with a rongeur and/or osteotome to ensure full seating of the component. Caution is advised that only impinging osteophytes are debrided. Overzealous and excessive bone resection with exposure of underlying cancellous bone risks generating a stress riser and potential neck fracture upon weight-bearing. One might consider marking the fully seated position with a sterile surgical marking pen on the neck. This mark may then be used to ensure that the definitive component has been fully seated.

Both cemented and uncemented options exist for the femoral component. Femoral component insertion is completed after acetabular component preparation/insertion. Following reaming, the femoral head should be washed with a pulsatile lavage and thoroughly dried. If a cemented option is selected, depending on the clearance between the implant and reamed femoral bone one can use high viscosity bone cement if 1 mm or more of clearance or low viscosity if a tighter fit. One must be mindful of the risk of over-

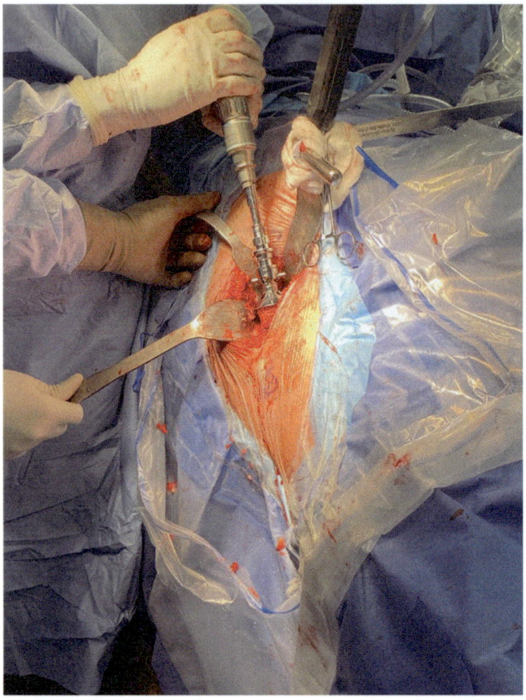

Fig. 33.3 Chamfer cut being made to femoral head after cylindrical and dome cuts

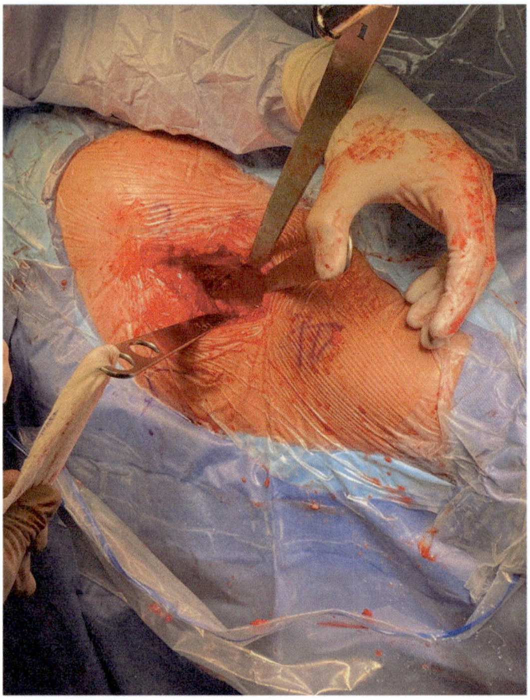

Fig. 33.4 Acetabular exposure

penetration of the cement into the cancellous bone and thermal injury to intraosseous vessels when temperature peaks during the hardening phase.

Acetabular Preparation

Exposure of the acetabulum is achieved by returning the leg to its neutral position and allowing it to fall into external rotation. A curved Hohmann retractor is placed over the anteromedial wall of the acetabulum. It is the senior author's preference to use the SPIDER (Single Port Instrument Delivery Extended Reach) device (TransEnterix, Durham, NC, USA) to hold this retractor, as it more efficiently allows the assistant to retract tissues posteriorly. A straight Hohmann retractor positioned over the posterior wall tensions the medial capsule. Release of this portion of the capsule with diathermy allows the prepared femoral head to be carefully retracted postero-superiorly to sit deep to the abductor musculature (Fig. 33.4).

An offset acetabular reamer is introduced and the acetabulum is prepared in the usual fashion. Acetabular version should be set on the initial ream with reference to osseous anatomy. Particular care should be taken to avoid excessive inclination which may result in point loading and excessive wear, or to leave the cup prominent in respect of the anterior wall, which may irritate the adjacent psoas tendon. The acetabulum is subsequently expanded to the desired size. Removal of each reamer risks injury to adjacent soft tissues. Therefore, the reamer is disengaged in the acetabulum and removed manually. Most implants are designed around a press-fit of the component. In practice, many patients will have hard sclerotic bone which necessitates an over-ream by 1 mm of the component size to facilitate seating of the cup. A trial acetabular component should be impacted to ensure appropriate stabil-

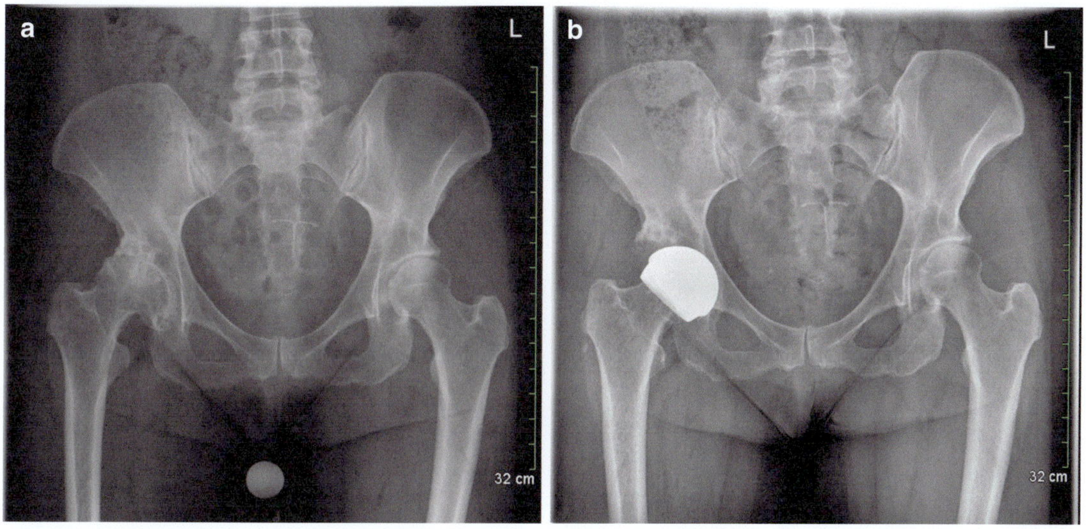

Fig. 33.5 (**a**) Pre-operative radiograph of 45-year-old female with symptomatic osteoarthritis right hip. (**b**) Post-operative radiograph of right hip ceramic-on-ceramic resurfacing arthroplasty

ity of the final component. Given the definitive component is monobloc in nature, one of the technical errors in a surgeon's early learning curve is incomplete seating of the final component. A trick to avoid this error is to use to a sterile marking pen to mark the depth of the trial component in its fully seated position. This further helps guide correct version of the definitive acetabular component. The final component should be placed in 15° anteversion and 40° of inclination. A McGoey punch is used to assess each of the four quadrants of the cup for stability. An intraoperative plain film radiograph may be taken to confirm accuracy of placement, with the supine position of the patient in this approach easily facilitating this. Post-operative x-ray imaging confirms satisfactory positioning of components (Fig. 33.5a,b).

Post-operative Recovery

With modern multimodal analgesia protocols, many hip resurfacing patients can be managed on an out-patient basis. Patients are mobilized early following surgery and allowed weight-bear as tolerated. Prophylaxis against thromboembolic disease is initiated as per local protocol. Return to sport or impact activities may be considered after week 12, which permits time for osseous in-growth of the components.

Clinical Outcomes

Currently, the vast majority of metal-on-metal hip resurfacing devices implanted worldwide are either the hybrid Birmingham Hip Resurfacing (BHR) (Smith & Nephew, Memphis, Tennessee, USA) or the Conserve Plus (MicroPort Orthopaedics, Memphis, Tennessee, USA). The latter system has both hybrid and fully uncemented options. The available recent literature further provides evidence of the mid- to long-term performance of these implants. Ford et al. reported Kaplan-Meier estimates of 5- and 10-year survivorship of the BHR for all cause revision of 97.2% (95% confidence interval [CI] 94.7% to 98.5%) and 93.8% (95% [CI] 88.8% – 96.7%) respectively [29]. In this cohort, mean modified Harris Hip Scores (mHHS) and University of California, Los Angeles (UCLA) significantly improved in the post-operative period ($p < 0.001$). When matched to a cohort of THA, post-operative UCLA scores in the BHR cohort were also superior to THA ($p < 0.001$), while there was a greater likelihood of remaining highly active with BHR (61% compared with 20%; $p < 0.001$).

In 1321 hips, Amstutz reports an overall survivorship at 15 years for all cause revision of the Conserve Plus of 89.4% (95% [CI] 86.8% to 91.4%) [30]. Male patients with idiopathic osteoarthritis fared better than female patients with a 15-year survivorship of 94.5% compared to 82.2% ($p = 0.001$).

Moreover, although total hip arthroplasty has increasingly been used in younger patients, recent reports suggest resurfacing arthroplasty may confer some advantage to this cohort of patients in terms of gait [31, 32]. Wiik et al. have demonstrated that following resurfacing arthroplasty, gait improves to a point that it is almost indistinguishable from healthy controls [31]. Interestingly, the authors did observe that resurfacing patients had weaker push-off strength on uphill walking, which was hypothesized related to the posterior approach and/or release and repair of the gluteus maximus tendon. As there are no known reports of gait analysis after hip resurfacing through an anterior approach, it remains inconclusive whether the same observation of weak push-off strength would also be seen in the anterior approach cohort.

Future Developments

The well-described concerns regarding adverse reaction to metal debris have renewed research interest in alternative bearing combinations for hip resurfacing. In the coming years, it is likely that the choice of bearing in resurfacing arthroplasty will expand, although the long-term clinical outcomes of these novel designs remain to be fully established.

The quality of modern highly crosslinked polyethylene (XLPE) is such that volumetric wear has significantly lessened as a cause for revision in arthroplasty. At mid-term follow-up of 8 years, Pritchett reports a 97% survivorship for a bearing combination of XLPE on a cementless nitride-coated titanium femoral resurfacing head [33]. Further trials into newer resurfacing designs are currently ongoing, including a metal-on-polyethylene hybrid resurfacing, and two trials examining ceramic-on-ceramic bearings [34–36] (Fig. 33.6).

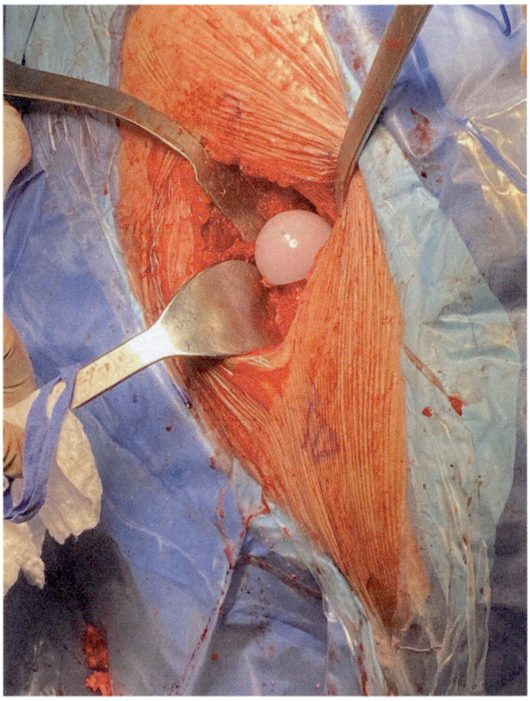

Fig. 33.6 Ceramic femoral component cemented in position

Pearls and Pitfalls

- Hip resurfacing is best indicated in younger active male patients between the ages of 40 and 60 years of age.
- Avoid excessive reaming of the femoral head to protect retinacular vessels entering the head
- Consider the use of a sterile marking pen intra-operatively to guide seating of both acetabular and femoral components.
- Intra-operative imaging is advisable to ensure accurate component position, and easily performed in the supine position.

References

1. Charnley J. Surgery of the hip-joint: present and future developments. Br Med J. 1960;1(5176):821.
2. Beaulé PE, Matar WY, Poitras P, Smit K, May O. 2008 Otto Aufranc Award: component design and technique affect cement penetration in hip resurfacing. Clin Orthop Relat Res. 2009;467(1):84.
3. Mehra A, Berryman F, Matharu GS, Pynsent PB, Isbister ES. Birmingham hip resurfacing: a single surgeon series reported at a minimum of 10 years follow-up. J Arthroplast. 2015;30(7):1160.
4. Matharu GS, McBryde CW, Pynsent WB, Pynsent PB, Treacy RB. The outcome of the Birmingham Hip Resurfacing in patients aged < 50 years up to 14 years post-operatively. Bone Joint J. 2013;95-B(9):1172.
5. Pailhe R, Matharu GS, Sharma A, Pynsent PB, Treacy RB. Survival and functional outcome of the Birmingham Hip Resurfacing system in patients aged 65 and older at up to ten years of follow-up. Int Orthop. 2014;38(6):1139.
6. Langton DJ, Jameson SS, Joyce TJ, Hallab NJ, Natu S, Nargol AV. Early failure of metal-on-metal bearings in hip resurfacing and large-diameter total hip replacement: a consequence of excess wear. J Bone Joint Surg Br. 2010;92(1):38.
7. Shimmin A, Beaulé PE, Campbell P. Metal-on-metal hip resurfacing arthroplasty. J Bone Joint Surg Am. 2008;90(3):637.
8. Lingard EA, Muthumayandi K, Holland JP. Comparison of patient-reported outcomes between hip resurfacing and total hip replacement. J Bone Joint Surg Br. 2009;91(12):1550.
9. Society CA. The Canadian Arthroplasty Society's experience with hip resurfacing arthroplasty. An analysis of 2773 hips. Bone Joint J. 2013;95-B(8):1045.
10. Beaulé PE, Campbell P, Lu Z, Leunig-Ganz K, Beck M, Leunig M, Ganz R. Vascularity of the arthritic femoral head and hip resurfacing. J Bone Joint Surg Am. 2006;88 Suppl 4:85.
11. Campbell P, Beaulé PE, Ebramzadeh E, Le Duff MJ, LeDuff M, De Smet K, Lu Z, Amstutz HC. The John Charnley Award: a study of implant failure in metal-on-metal surface arthroplasties. Clin Orthop Relat Res. 2006;453:35.
12. Zustin J, Sauter G, Morlock MM, Rüther W, Amling M. Association of osteonecrosis and failure of hip resurfacing arthroplasty. Clin Orthop Relat Res. 2010;468(3):756.
13. Della Valle CJ, Nunley RM, Raterman SJ, Barrack RL. Initial American experience with hip resurfacing following FDA approval. Clin Orthop Relat Res. 2009;467(1):72.
14. Benoit B, Gofton W, Beaulé PE. Hueter anterior approach for hip resurfacing: assessment of the learning curve. Orthop Clin North Am. 2009;40(3):357.
15. Jacobs MA, Goytia RN, Bhargava T. Hip resurfacing through an anterolateral approach. Surgical description and early review. J Bone Joint Surg Am. 2008;90 Suppl 3:38.
16. Steffen RT, De Smet KA, Murray DW, Gill HS. A modified posterior approach preserves femoral head oxgenation during hip resurfacing. J Arthroplast. 2011;26(3):404.
17. Martinez Gomez A, Grammatopoulos G, Beaulé PE. Contemporary surgical approaches for hip resurfacing. Ann Joint. 2020;5:9.
18. Freeman MA. Some anatomical and mechanical considerations relevant to the surface replacement of the femoral head. Clin Orthop Relat Res. 1978;134:19.
19. Beaulé PE, Campbell PA, Hoke R, Dorey F. Notching of the femoral neck during resurfacing arthroplasty of the hip: a vascular study. J Bone Joint Surg Br. 2006;88(1):35.
20. Beaulé PE, Campbell P, Shim P. Femoral head blood flow during hip resurfacing. Clin Orthop Relat Res. 2007;456:148.
21. Khan A, Yates P, Lovering A, Bannister GC, Spencer RF. The effect of surgical approach on blood flow to the femoral head during resurfacing. J Bone Joint Surg Br. 2007;89(1):21.
22. Amarasekera HW, Costa ML, Foguet P, Krikler SJ, Prakash U, Griffin DR. The blood flow to the femoral head/neck junction during resurfacing arthroplasty: a comparison of two approaches using Laser Doppler flowmetry. J Bone Joint Surg Br. 2008;90(4):442.
23. Steffen R, O'Rourke K, Gill HS, Murray DW. The anterolateral approach leads to less disruption of the femoral head-neck blood supply than the posterior approach during hip resurfacing. J Bone Joint Surg Br. 2007;89(10):1293.
24. Gautier E, Ganz K, Krügel N, Gill T, Ganz R. Anatomy of the medial femoral circumflex artery and its surgical implications. J Bone Joint Surg Br. 2000;82(5):679.
25. Dewar DC, Lazaro LE, Klinger CE, Sculco PK, Dyke JP, Ni AY, Helfet DL, Lorich DG. The relative contribution of the medial and lateral femoral circumflex arteries to the vascularity of the head and neck of the femur: a quantitative MRI-based assessment. Bone Joint J. 2016;98-B(12):1582.
26. Sevitt S, Thompson RG. The distribution and anastomoses of arteries supplying the head and neck of the femur. J Bone Joint Surg Br. 1965;47:560.
27. Smith AJ, Dieppe P, Howard PW, Blom AW, Wales NJRfEa. Failure rates of metal-on-metal hip resurfacings: analysis of data from the National Joint Registry for England and Wales. Lancet. 1759;380(9855):2012.
28. Harty M. Symposium on surface replacement arthroplasty of the hip. Anatomic considerations. Orthop Clin North Am. 1982;13(4):667.
29. Ford MC, Hellman MD, Kazarian GS, Clohisy JC, Nunley RM, Barrack RL. Five to ten-year results of the Birmingham Hip Resurfacing implant in the U.S.: a Single Institution's Experience. J Bone Joint Surg Am. 2018;100(21):1879.

30. Amstutz HC, Le Duff MJ. The mean ten-year results of metal-on-metal hybrid hip resurfacing arthroplasty. Bone Joint J. 2018;100-B(11):1424.
31. Wiik AV, Lambkin R, Cobb JP. Gait after Birmingham Hip Resurfacing: an age-matched controlled prospective study. Bone Joint J. 2019;101-B(11):1423.
32. Gerhardt DMJM, Mors TGT, Hannink G, Van Susante JLC. Resurfacing hip arthroplasty better preserves a normal gait pattern at increasing walking speeds compared to total hip arthroplasty. Acta Orthop. 2019;90(3):231.
33. Pritchett JW. Hip resurfacing with a highly cross-linked polyethylene acetabular liner and a titanium nitride-coated femoral component. Hip Int. 2018;28(4):422.
34. Treacy RBC, Holland JP, Daniel J, Ziaee H, McMinn DJW. Preliminary report of clinical experience with metal-on-highly-crosslinked-polyethylene hip resurfacing. Bone Joint Res. 2019;8(10):443.
35. Cobb J, Halewood C, Wozencroft R, Logishetty K, Jeffers J, Clarke S. H1 anatomic ceramic hip resurfacing: results of a 20 patient safety study. In: International Society of Technology in Arthroplasty Annual Meeting. London, UK. 2018.
36. De Smet K. New materials for hip resurfacing: why choose ceramic? In: International Society of Technology in Arthroplasty Annual Meeting. London, UK. 2018.

Part VI

Introduction to Part VI

Revision Surgery

As anterior approach for primary THA has risen to prominence, I have heard from AA opponents, "OK, we see that AA primary is possible but what about revision? You will still need an extensile approach like posterior or lateral when revision is necessary." This section will dispel the misconceptions contained in this statement and demonstrate the capabilities as well as advantages of using AA for revision.

For those that have years of experience with posterior or lateral approach for primary and revision THA, it can create a reaction when they are told that the posterior and lateral approaches are not extensile approaches to the hip. These approaches are extensile distal along the femoral shaft but are not extensile proximal for exposure of the innominate bone because proximal access is limited by the course of the superior gluteal nerve. The anterior approach, on the other hand, is the true extensile approach to the hip because it follows the inter-nervous plane and is thereby extensile for exposure of both the innominate bone and femur. Because of this extensile capability, I began use of AA for certain THA revisions at least 10 years before I began AA for primary. For me, therefore, using AA for revision opened the door for AA primary, and then growing command of primary AA furthered indications for revision AA.

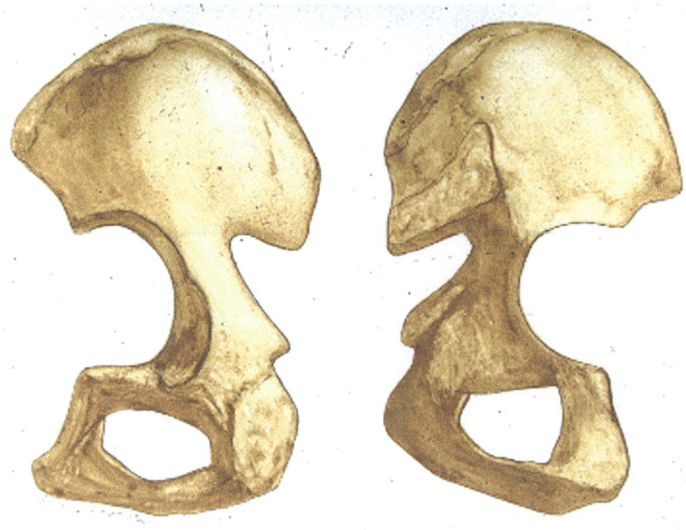

Fig. 1 Artist's conception drawing of common acetabular bone defect requiring revision THA. This defect will appear on an AP pelvis X-ray as a cup protrusion, though it is primarily confined to the anterior column with absence of the anterior wall and a segment of the pelvic brim

It is my opinion that a large number of acetabular bone defects that present with revision are primarily anterior column defects and are often not recognized as such. These bone defects involve the anterior wall and a segment of the pelvic brim (Fig. 1). The posterior approach solution to this is to ignore the defect and endeavor to attach the cup to the remaining posterior, superior, and inferior bone. I believe that the enhanced exposure to the innominate bone with AA will lead to new and better methods and implants for acetabular revision, and this section will represent the beginning of that evolution.

The strongest arguments for using AA for revision is to gain the same advantages that AA for primary THA has over posterior and lateral approaches. Supine position is advantageous for anesthesia, as well as judging cup position and leg length. Acetabular and femoral bony landmarks are also usually compromised with revision surgery, and so capability for accurate C-arm confirmation of cup position, leg length, and offset becomes even more important.

AA has become the first choice for revision for the majority of cases that I do or are done by the authors in this section. A "complete" hip surgeon, however, should be facile with all standard approaches to the hip. This section addresses use of AA for revision; however, specific soft tissue, bone, and implant problems and previous incisions may make AA less ideal than another approach for a specific revision case.

Revision Surgery Exposure Techniques for the Anterior Hip Approach, Including Osteotomies

34

Anthony T. Carter

Important Points

The surgical approach chosen for revision total hip arthroplasty depends on many variables, including anticipated deformities and defects, the surgeon's experience, and prior surgical approaches. The surgeon should be comfortable with all approaches and choose the best one for the patient.

- Clinical/surgical perils – precise preoperative planning is essential to determine anticipated defects.
- Advantages of the DAA include utilizing a true internervous intermuscular plane, limited soft tissue stripping, limited or no hip precautions, and a decreased dislocation rate. The DAA is an extensile approach proximally through a true Smith-Peterson incision with or without an iliac wing osteotomy and is extensile distally with or without an extended trochanteric osteotomy.
- Improved component positioning is possible with supine positioning of the patient and the use of intraoperative fluoroscopy.
- Clinical/surgical pitfalls – the DAA for complex primary and revision surgery has somewhat of a steep learning curve. Surgeon experience should dictate its utilization. It may not be applicable when posterior wall or column acetabular reconstruction is required.

A. T. Carter (✉)
Hampton Roads Orthopaedics & Sports Medicine, Newport News, VA, USA

Exposure

Surgical exposure is a key in total hip arthroplasty, especially with complex primary and revision surgery. A solid understanding of the anatomy allows adequate exposure. Traditionally, posterior approach with or without extended femoral osteotomy has been the workhorse for revision total hip arthroplasty. it is easily adaptable to the primary situation and offers wide exposure of the femur and acetabulum. However, recovery can be delayed due to extensive soft tissue stripping, osteotomy nonunion, and dislocation rates up to 28% [2, 3]. The direct anterior approach for total hip arthroplasty has become well established as a true internervous and intermuscular approach that facilitates accelerated recovery as well as enhanced stability [4–6]. Many surgeons are expanding its application from primary to complex primary and complex revision surgery of both the femur and acetabulum, both on and off a specialized Table [7–11]. The potential advantages and disadvantages are outlined in Table 34.1. The initial dissection remains unchanged (Fig. 34.1) and is extensile both proximally and distally affording wide exposure of the acetabulum, anterior column of the pelvis, the inner and outer tables of the pelvis can be assessed simulta-

J. M. Matta, A. P. Sah (eds.), *Anterior Hip Replacement*,
https://doi.org/10.1007/978-3-030-91896-5_34

neously, as well as extensile exposure of the femur down to the knee (Figs. 34.2 and 34.3). The exposure can be enhanced with osteotomies as required, including iliac wing osteotomy or ASIS slide, and various femoral osteotomies for stem removal including an extended trochanteric osteotomy. Extensile exposure can be required in difficult primary as well conversion surgery from previous orif, acetabular or femoral revision surgery requiring component removal or periprosthetic fractures [12].

Possible Disadvantages of the Anterior Approach for Revision THA

- Difficulty with femoral access requiring proximal extension
- Improper distal extension risks vastus lateralis denervation

Table 34.1 Possible advantages of the anterior approach for revision THA

Lower dislocation rate
Live fluoroscopy use to aid with hardware removal, femoral preparation, limb length and offset restoration, osteotomy planning, and cup position
Supine patient positioning
Lower risk of fracture of the greater trochanter
Decreased rate of VTE
Limited or no hip precautions
Quicker early recovery

- Lateral femoral cutaneous nerve injury
- Difficulty with access to fractures of the trochanter, diaphysis
- Difficulty treating abductor tendon pathology
- Increased operative time
- Increased blood loss
- Increased risk of wound complications

Most surgeries can be accomplished through normal approach with minimal additional releases. By maintaining a true internervous, intermuscular plane to the hip, this approach can be valuable in preserving musculature that has previously been compromised by trauma or surgery, affords protection of the superior gluteal artery and inferior gluteal nerve, and can maintain the posterior capsule in short rotators if possible or not previously compromised (Fig. 34.4).

If necessary the exposure is extensile both proximally and distally, with the extent of the exposure/releases dependent on multiple factors including:

- Previous approach – Anterior or posterior.
- Type and placement of hardware.
- Type and degree of fixation of the stem to be removed, or type of stem to be inserted.
- Fracture pattern.

As with primary DAA, it is important to have a plan and take a step-wise approach with consistent releases, and the skin incision is typically planned

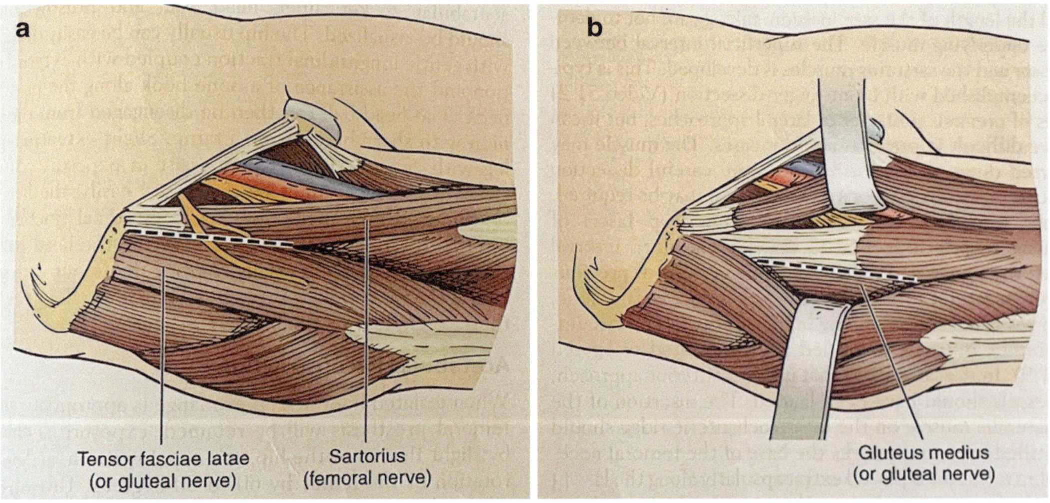

Fig. 34.1 Schematic diagrams of the superficial (**a**) and deep dissection (**b**) intervals utilized for the direct anterior approach

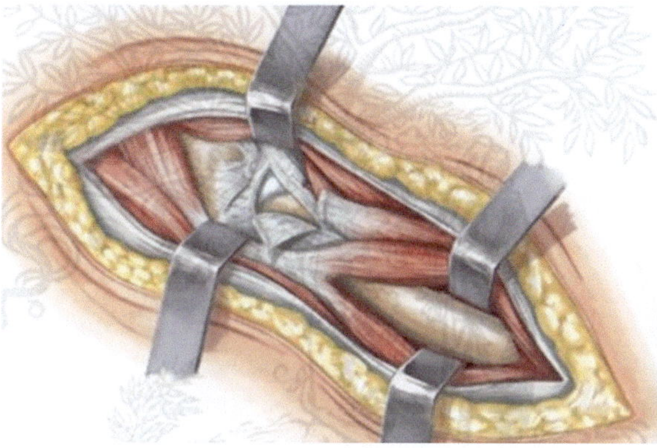

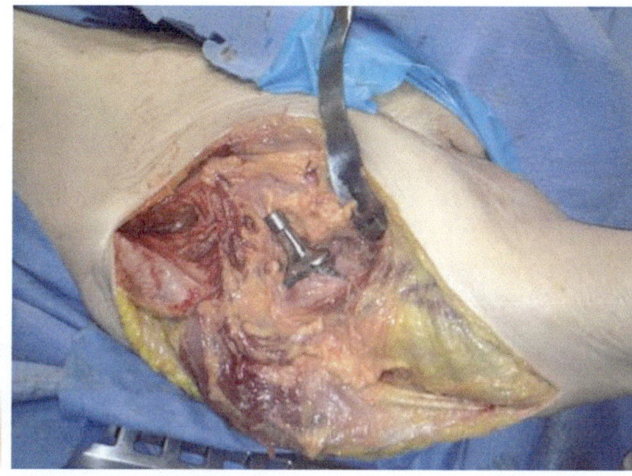

Figs. 34.2 and 34.3 Schematic diagram and cadaveric dissection demonstrating extensive proximal and distal exposure

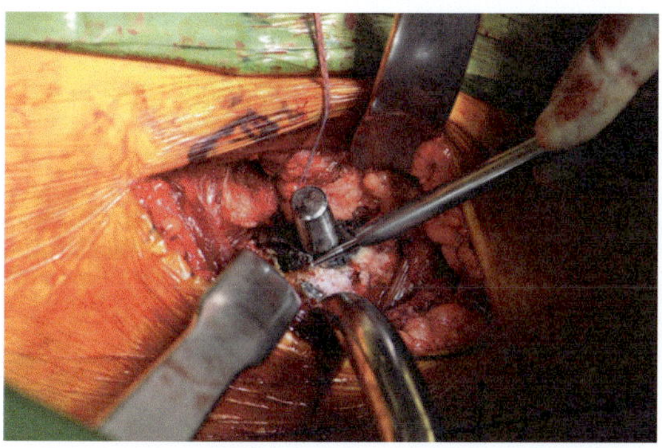

Fig. 34.4 Exposure for stem removal with primary approach and aggressive capsular management. No extension of the primary skin incision was required and no additional muscle releases required

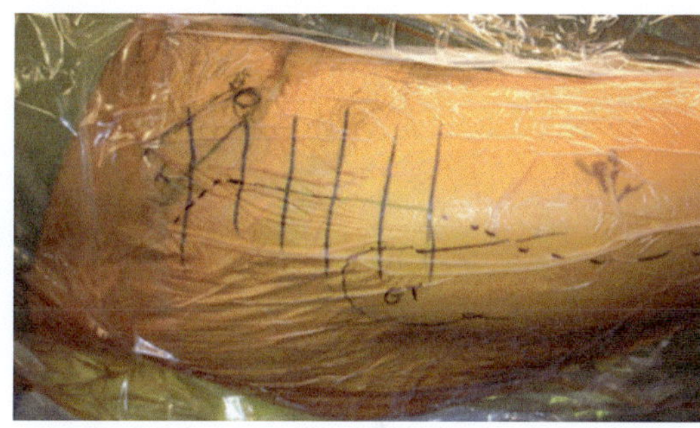

Fig. 34.5 Skin incision sentinel surgery (solid line) and proposed proximal and distal extension as required (dotted line)

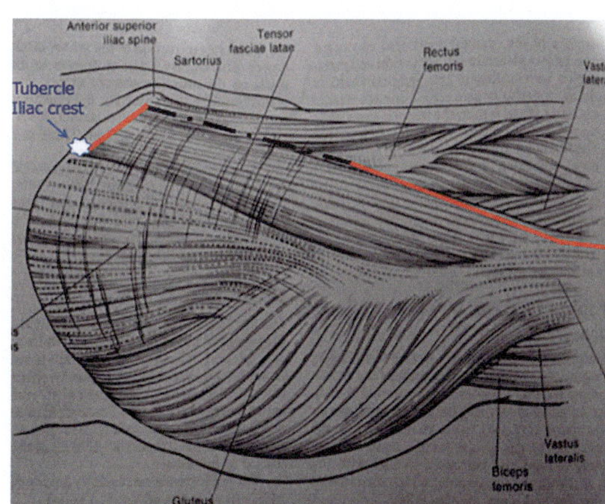

Fig. 34.6 Schematic diagram of potential soft tissue extension

for a more extensile exposure Initially, the superficial interval between the tensorfascia muscle, innervated by the superior gluteal nerve and the sartorius muscle femoral nerve, and the deep interval, is between the tensor or gluteus minimus muscle, the superior gluteal nerve, and the rectus femoris nerve.

Proximally, the skin incision can then be extended to a standard Smith-Peterson approach along the iliac crest and distally the incision can be curved slightly posteriorly and extend down the mid aspect of the femur all the way down to the knee (Figs. 34.5 and 34.6).

If the patient had a previous posterior approach, the initial exposure is essentially the same as the primary direct anterior approach. The tissue planes should be easy to identify and develop. The capsule may be very thickened, even from a previous posterior approach and may need to be debulked or excised. If the patient had a previous direct anterior approach, it is important to re-create the superficial and fascial planes.

The TFL plane may be scarred in and the fascia might not be easily separated from the muscle. This may need to be required utilizing electrocautery to carefully peel the scarred tensor from the overlying fascia (Fig. 34.7).

Initial dislocation is often very difficult due to the contracted capsule and TFL. All fascial bands of the TFL must be released to the leading aspect of the ASIS. Often times a dislocation in situ is required. Longitudinal traction with internal rotation to the leg is applied and the head ball is disengaged from the trunion into the cup (Fig. 34.8a, b). The ball is pushed into the cup while the femur is further externally rotated to disengage the head from the neck.

The soft tissue releases are then titrated concentrating on meticulous and generous release of the capsule to the posterior border of the femur, followed by rotators if present beginning with the obturator internus and then the piriformis. As with a primary approach, release of the often scarred and contracted pubofemoral ligament to the lesser trochanter is important for femoral mobilization, and the thickened superior capsule released completely (Fig. 34.9). An attempt should be made to

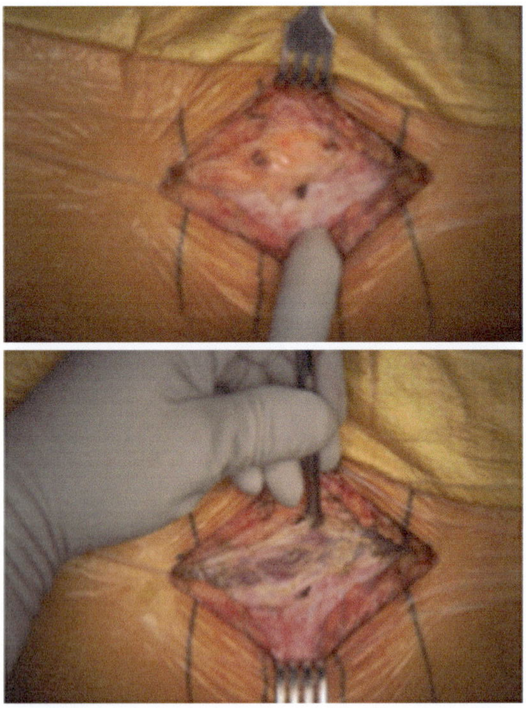

Fig. 34.7 The tensor muscle may be very adherent to the overlying facia, especially if a previous anterior approach was performed. Careful, meticulous release from the facia can prevent damage to the muscle and enhance exposure

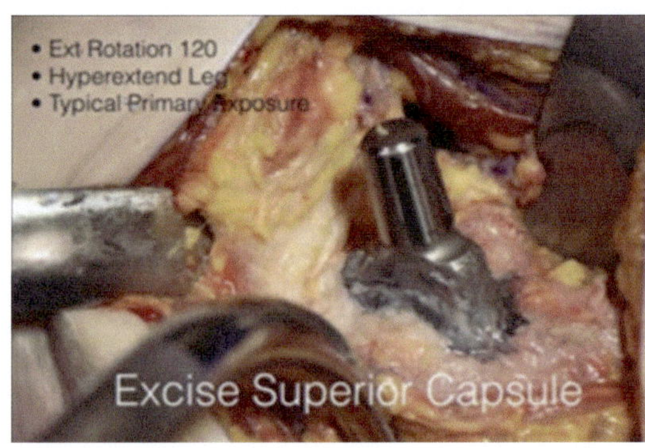

Fig 34.9 The superior capsule is often very thickened, and complete excision is critical to allow proper exposure of the femur

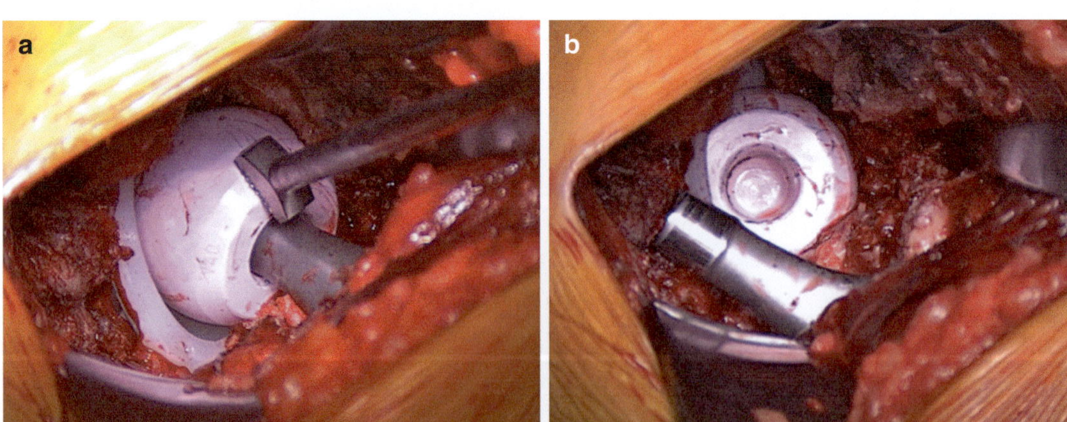

Fig. 34.8 (**a**, **b**) In situ removal of the femoral head can facilitate exposure especially when dislocating the hip is difficult

preserve the rotators if present, but release them as necessary in a step-wise fashion. If additional exposure is required, minimal release of the TFL 1–2 cm off the iliac crest can markedly enhance mobilization of the femur and should be considered if exposure is difficult after complete release of the capsule and rotators (Figs. 33.10, 33.11, 33.12, 33.13, 33.14, and 33.15).

TFL release also allows the femur to relax more posteriorly to allow access to the lateral ilium and acetabulum as necessary for grafting or custom acetabulur components (Fig. 34.16a–d). The femur is typically flexed slightly, externally rotated approx. 80–90 degrees and no traction to allow the neck of the stem to fall behind the acetabulum.

If more extensive exposure is required, completion of a more formal extended ilioinguinal approach could be performed by releasing the TFL completely off the iliac crest to the gluteal ridge tubercle and releasing the leading edge of the gluteus minimus exposing the outer wing of the ilium. Care is taken to protect the neurovascular pedicle of the ascending branch of the lateral femoral circumflex artery(deep branch of the superior gluteal artery) and superior gluteal

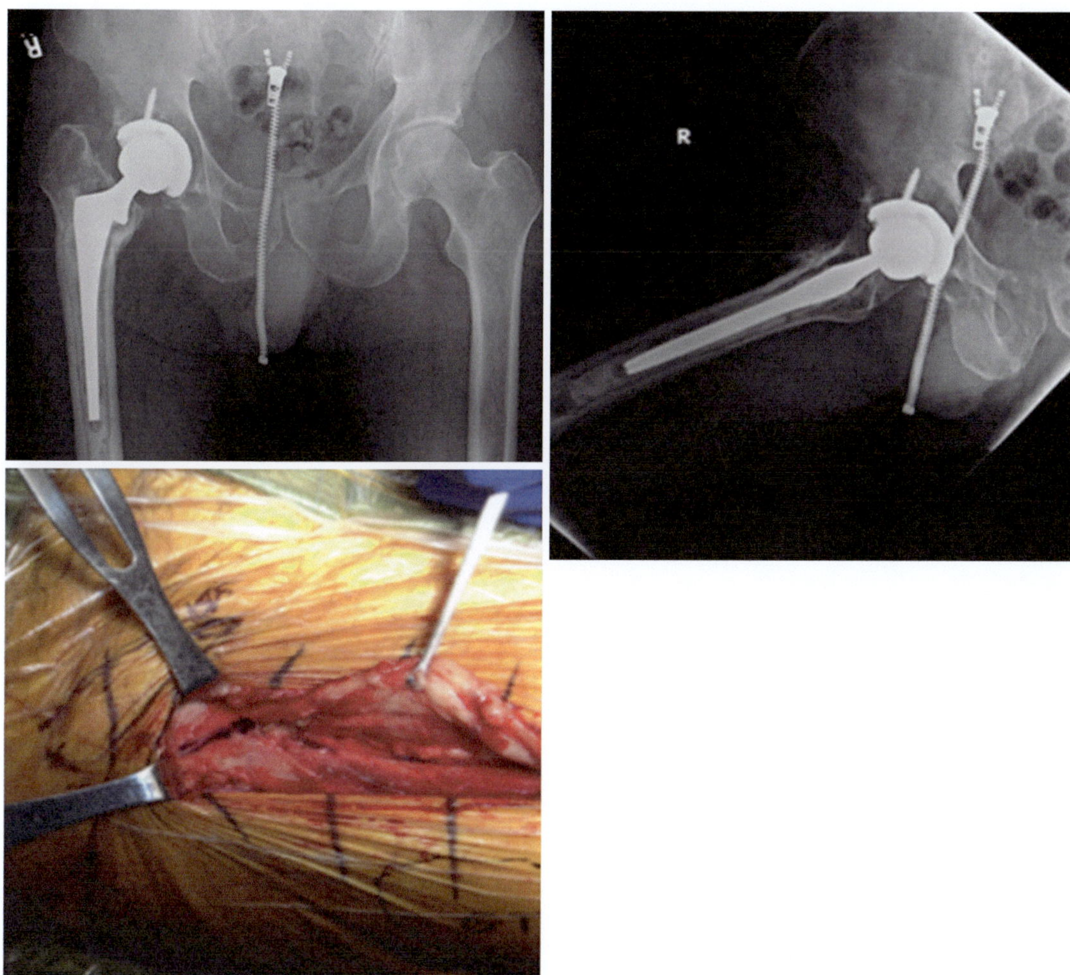

Figs. 34.10, 34.11, 34.12, 34.13, 34.14, and 34.15 Case of a painful loose cemented stem with subsidence. Release of the TFL aided in femoral mobility for stem and cement removal and placement of a long straight stem utilizing otherwise the normal capsular and external rotator releases. No distal extension was required

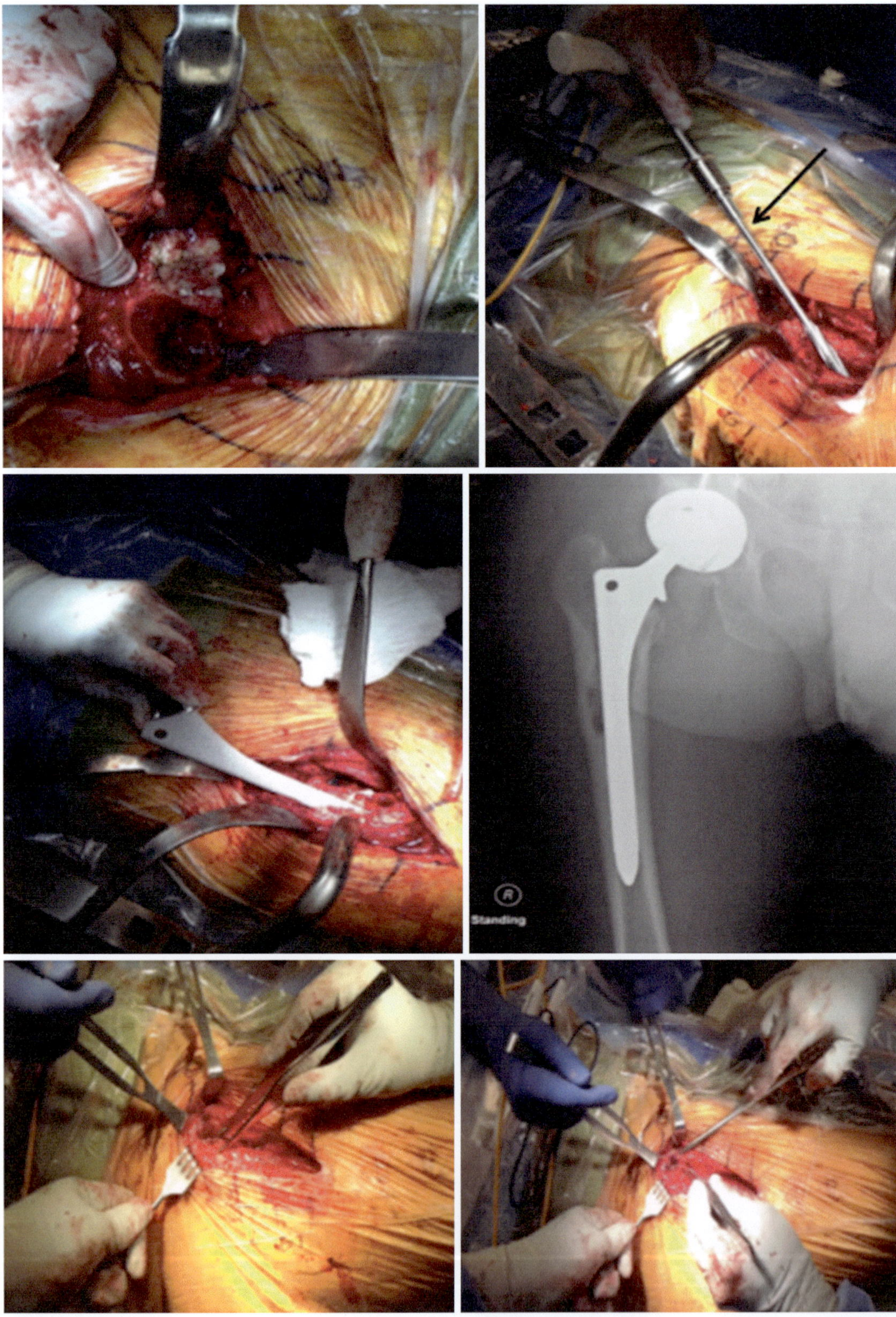

Figs. 34.10, 34.11, 34.12, 34.13, 34.14, and 34.15 (continued)

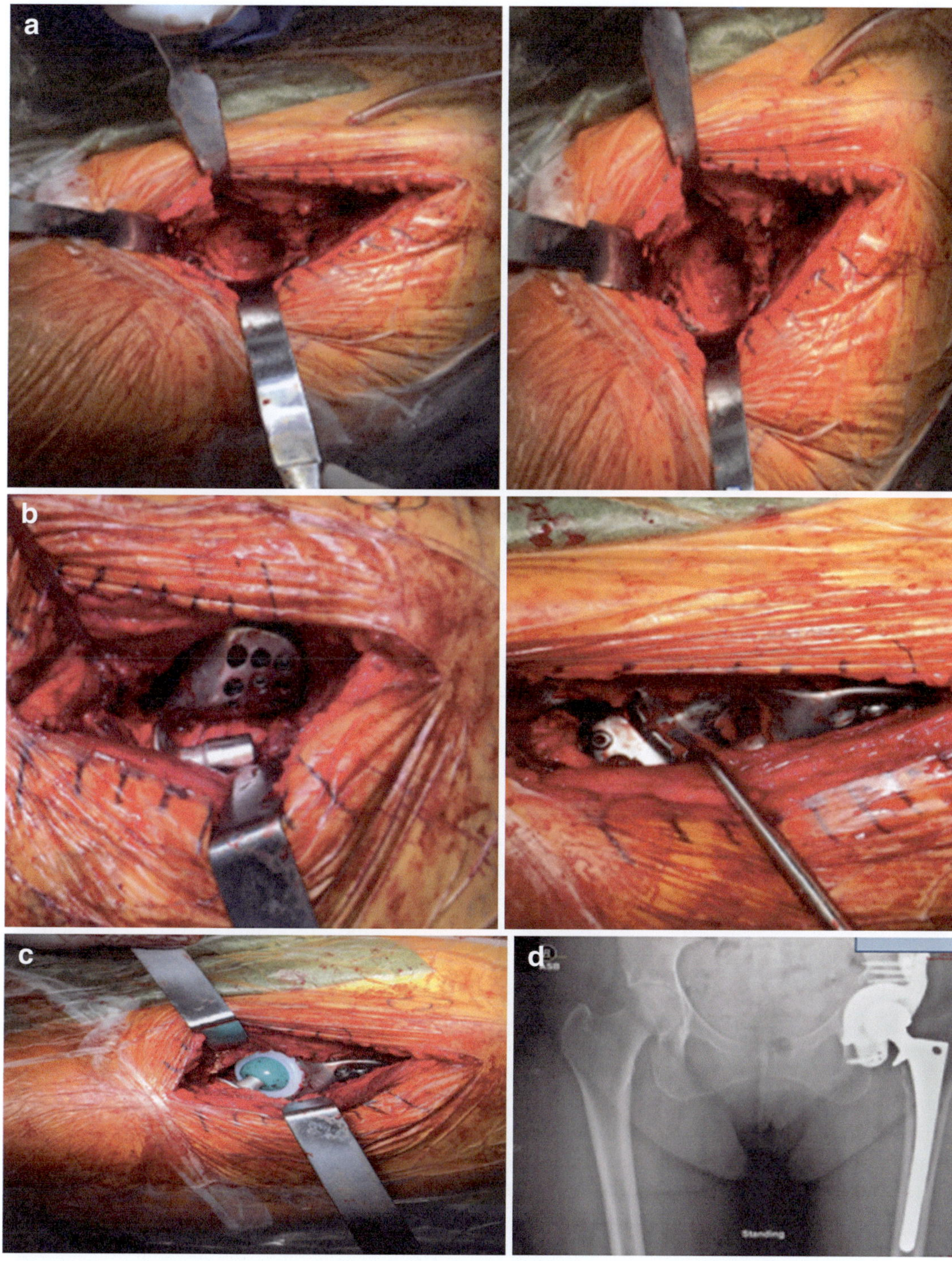

Fig. 34.16 (**a**) Proximal skin extension and release of 2–3 cm of TFL affords wide exposure of the superior acetabulum and iliac wing. Care is taken not to detach the gluteus minimus. (**b**) the femoral neck typically falls behind the posterior rim of acetabulum with slight hip flexion and rotation of approximately 90 degrees. (**c**) custom triflange. (**d**) post op radiograph

nerve which enter the muscle at the level of the junction of the proximal and middle thirds of an axis drawn from the anterior superior iliac spine to the lateral patella. Caution must be taken to preserve the tendinous origin of the TFL for later repair.

If more than a minimal release of the TFL is required, an iliac wing osteotomy can be performed. This affords extensile proximal exposure of the acetabulum and pelvis, as well as tremendous exposure of the femur. It respects the internervous and intermuscular intervals, maintains stability with minimal soft tissue dissection affording limited postoperative precautions, and allows more predictable bone to bone healing. The incision is carried out proximally along the iliac crest, typically extending the incision below the crest to avoid scar irritation from rubbing on clothing (Fig. 34.17). The ASIS is identified, and the incision is extended along the crest from the ASIS posteriorly approximately 4–5 cms. The abdominal oblique musculature is reflected subperiosteally in a medial fashion (Fig. 34.18a, b). The inguinal ligament and sartorius can be tagged and also reflected medially subperiosteally, or alternatively a small wafer osteotomy of the leading edge of the ASIS can be performed, leaving a bony attachment of the Sartorius and inguinal ligament for later repair. This musculature and ligament are tagged and mobilized medically, and dissection is carried out along the internal medial table of the iliac wing with an elevator reflecting the iliacus. The direct head of the rectus can be released if further intrapelvic exposure is necessary of the acetabulum. Drill holes for later repair of the osteotomy are pre-drilled into the iliac crest (2 or 3 drill holes are drilled) beginning about 2 cm posterior to the ASIS and extending posteriorly. Using an oscillating saw, an osteotomy is performed from the inner table approximately 3 cm inferior to the crest between the ASIS and AIIS (Fig. 34.19a, b). This is extended posteriorly and superiorly toward the iliac tubercle, extending for about 5 cm. It can be done in a crescentic or straight fashion. Care should be taken not to perforate the outer table of the ilium and causing damage to the overlying

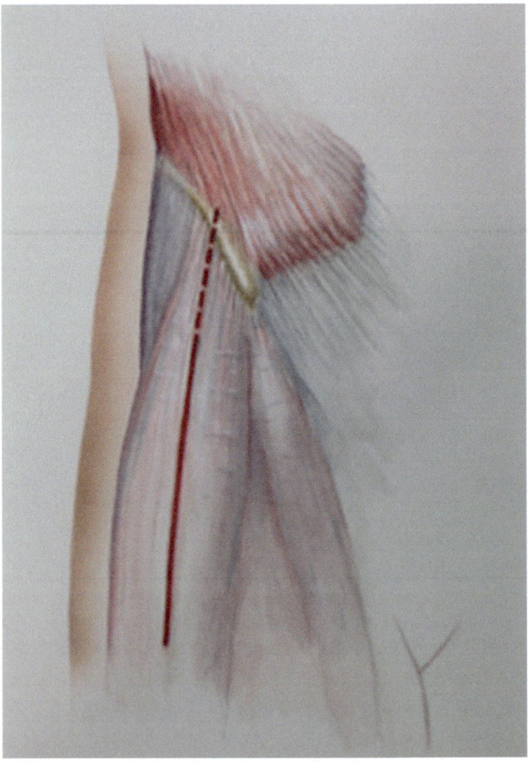

Fig 34.17 Initial skin incision typically is extended proximally. This can be in a straight line or directed posteriorly below the iliac crest to prevent a painful scar

gluteal muscles or the neurovascular bundle. The osteotomy is then completed with a curved osteotome reflecting the iliac wing laterally with the attached TFL (Fig. 34.20). This allows complete release of the tensor muscle without any soft tissue stripping of the abductors and greatly enhances access to the acetabulum, pelvis and proximal femur (Fig. 34.21a, b). The osteotomy should be approximately 5 cm to 8 cm long. The osteotomized fragment is then fixed to the crest with 2 or 3 screws(Fig. 34.22), and the apeneurosis of the abdominal musculature along with the Sartorius and inguinal ligament are reapproximated (Figs. 34.23, 34.24, 34.25, 34.26, 34.27, 34.28, 34.29, and 34.30).

Distal extension of the incision is also easily accomplished, which can further assist with femoral exposure and can be coupled with osteotomies of the femur to aid in exposure for stem removal, distal fixation, or ORIF of periprosthetic

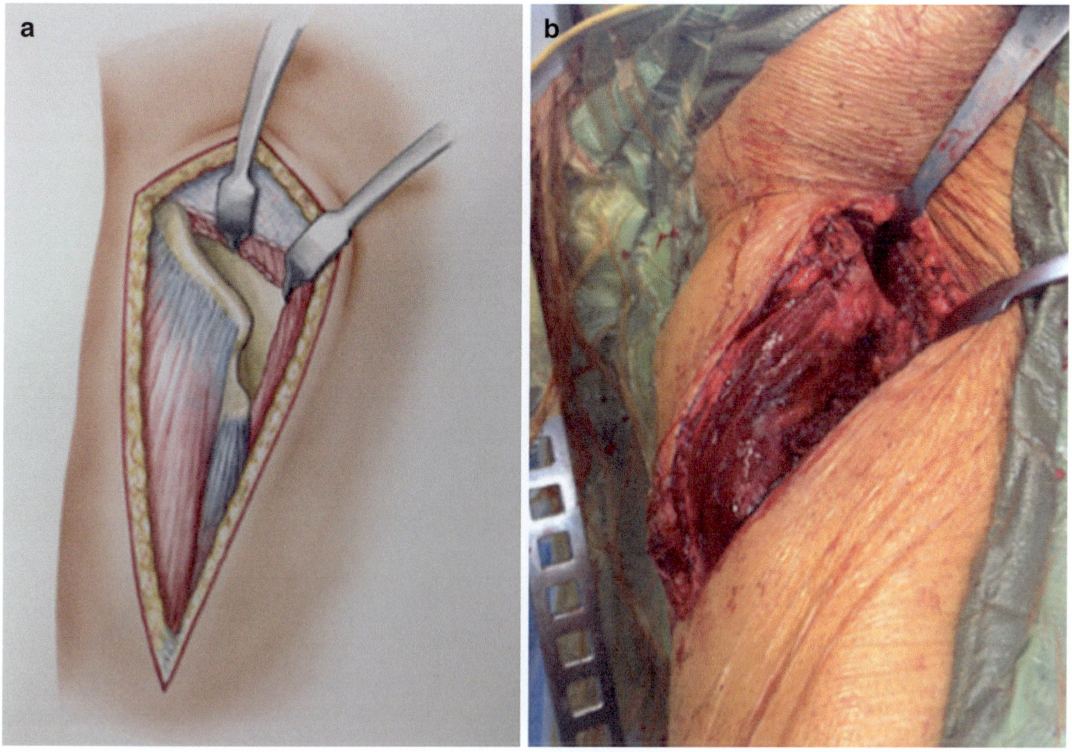

Fig. 34.18 (**a**) Illustration of the subperiosteal reflection of the oblique abdominal musculature from the iliac crest. (**b**) intraoperative photo of reflection of oblique abdominal musculature to access inner wall of ilium

fractures. The distal limb of the extended incision is essentially the same as would be performed for a more commonly used posterior approach (Fig. 34.31).

After distal extension of the skin and subcutaneous tissue, the IT band is identified distal to the tensor (Fig. 34.32a, b). It is incised distally the length of the incision, taking care to keep the muscle belly tensor fascia lata attached to the posterior aspect of the ITB (Fig. 34.33).

The gluteus maximus tendon can be easily identified as a consistent landmark (Fig. 34.34). Distal extension for exposure of the femur at this point can be accomplished through a simple subvastus approach to the femur, carefully elevating the vastus lateralis off the femur (Fig. 34.35).

This allows extensile exposure of the entire femur. Several osteotomies of the femur can be considered to aid in exposure or assist in removal of femoral prosthesis. Any dissection of the proximal femur should respect the neurovascular innervation of the vastus. The femoral nerve innervates the quadriceps at a relatively high level of the femur just distal to the calcar [13] (Fig. 34.36). Any dissection or osteotomy in this area needs to maintain and respect this innervation (Fig. 34.37). One significant advantage of the direct anterior approach is the ability to use fluoroscopy to check for perforations by osteotomes, reamers, or broaches and to define the extent of any planned osteotomy around the femur. Multiple options for osteotomies exist depending on type of stem requiring removal or fixation required including:

- Femorotomy(episiotomy)
- Modified anterior osteotomy
- Distal cortical window
- Extended trochanteric osteotomy(ETO)

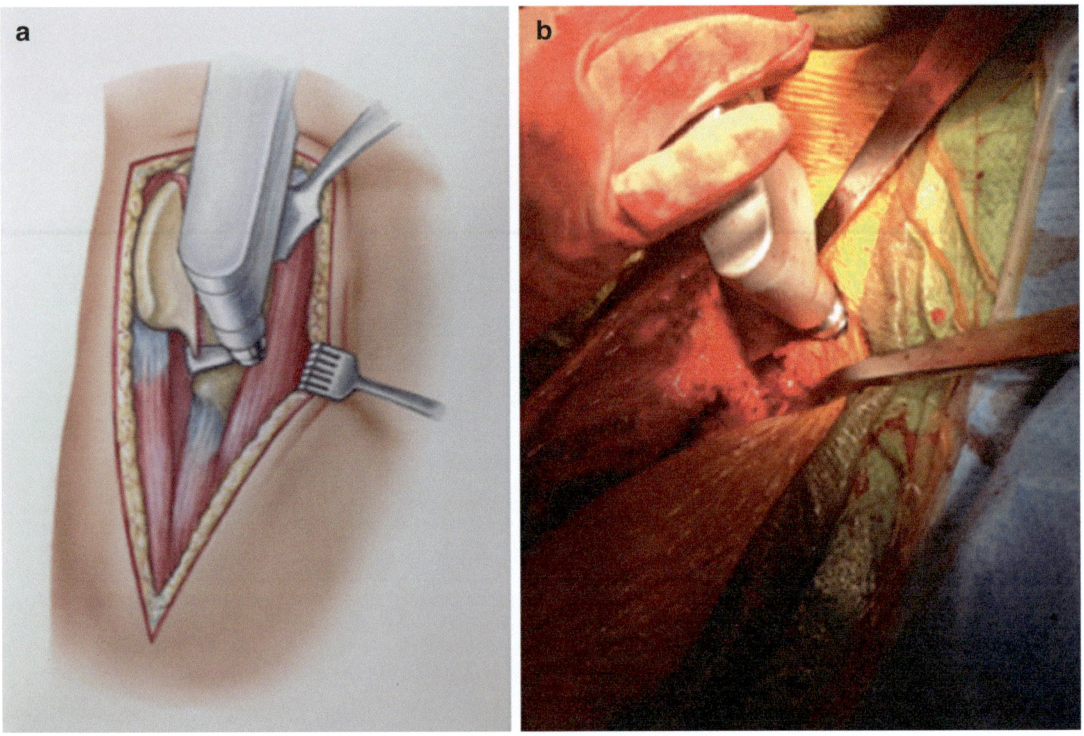

Fig. 34.19 (a, b) Illustration and intraoperative photo of iliac wing osteotomy respectively

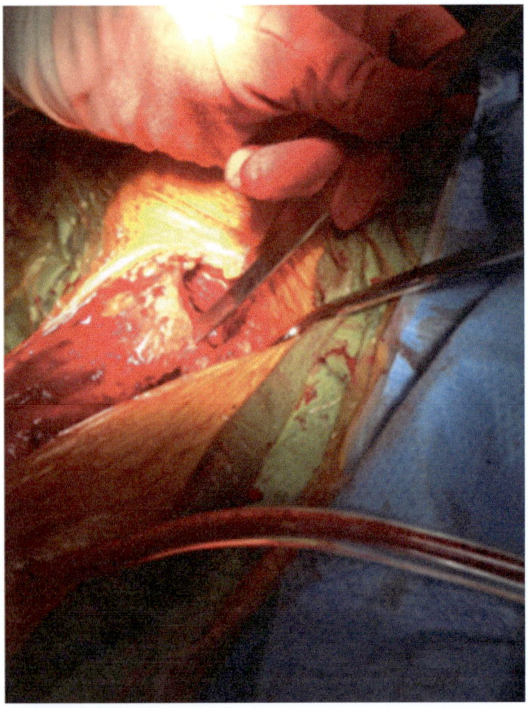

Fig 34.20 Completion of the osteotomy utilizing an osteotome to minimize damage to the abductors

If minimal additional exposure is required such as a proximally fixed blade type stem a simple episiotomy may be utilized. With the leg slightly extended and externally rotated, and respecting the neurovascular innervation of the proximal femur, an episiotomy with a pencil tip high speed bur or microsagittal saw along the medial femur allows access to a well fixed stem, can be bypassed with a long femoral component is easily cabled and does not disrupt the extensor mechanism (Figs. 34.38 and 34.39). This osteotomy yields only 2–3 mm of opening and care must be taken not to completely fracture the femur.

A modified anterior osteotomy can be particularly helpful and has several advantages over a conventional ETO, including easier access from the front, maintenance of the blood supply to the osteotomized fragment, sparing of the trochanter/abductor mechanism and can be easily fixed with cerclage cables. However, direct access to the lateral and distal aspect of the stem is limited. The distal extent of the window can be precisely mea-

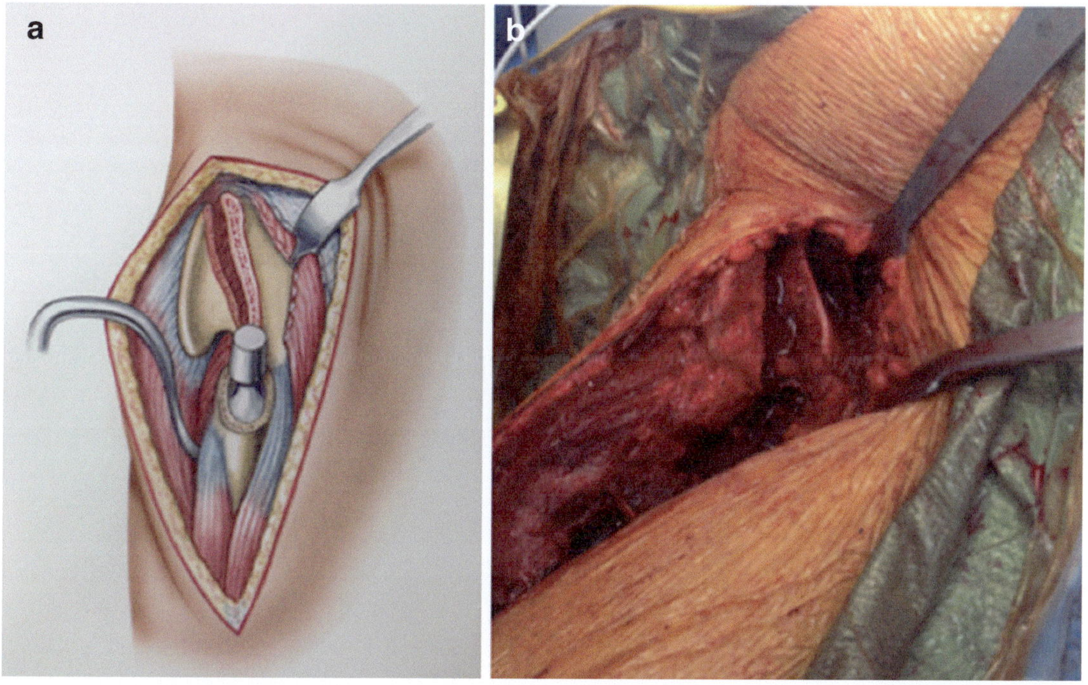

Fig. 34.21 (**a**, **b**) illustration and intraoperative photo of completed osteotomy. With the crest reflected laterally and elevation of the femur, direct linear access to the proximal femur for straight reamers and stems is markedly improved

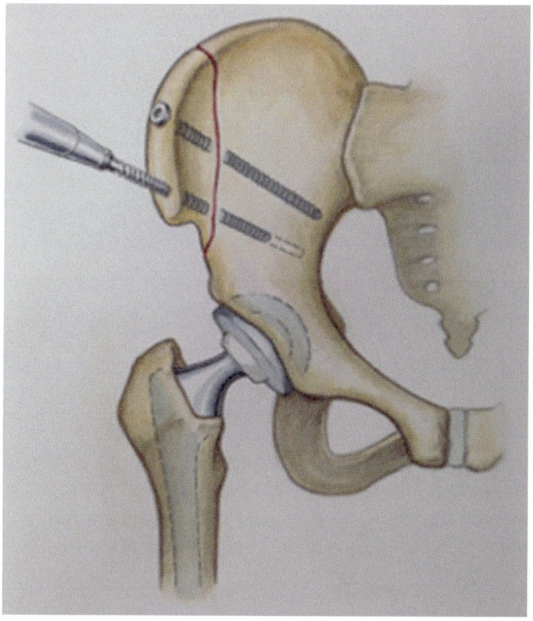

Fig. 34.22 Fixation of the predrilled iliac crest with 2–3 (6.5–7.0) screws

sured using fluoroscopy intraoperatively to allow easy removal of a well-fixed stem (Fig. 34.40a–f).

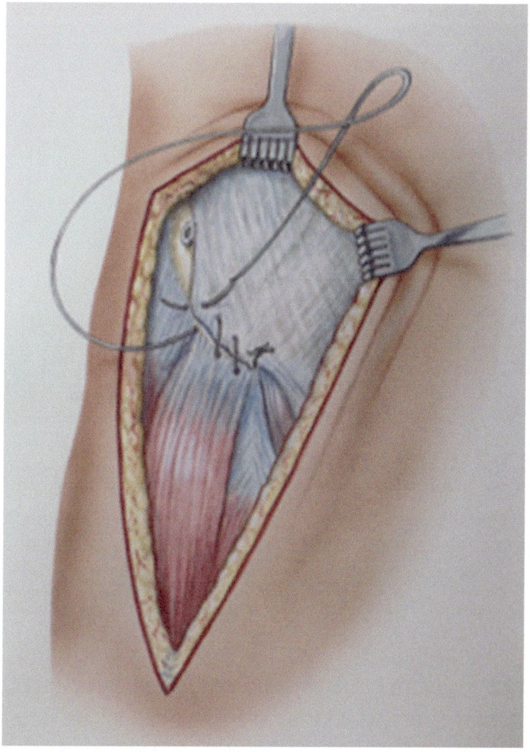

Fig 34.23 Illustration of subperiosteal repair of the aperneurosis

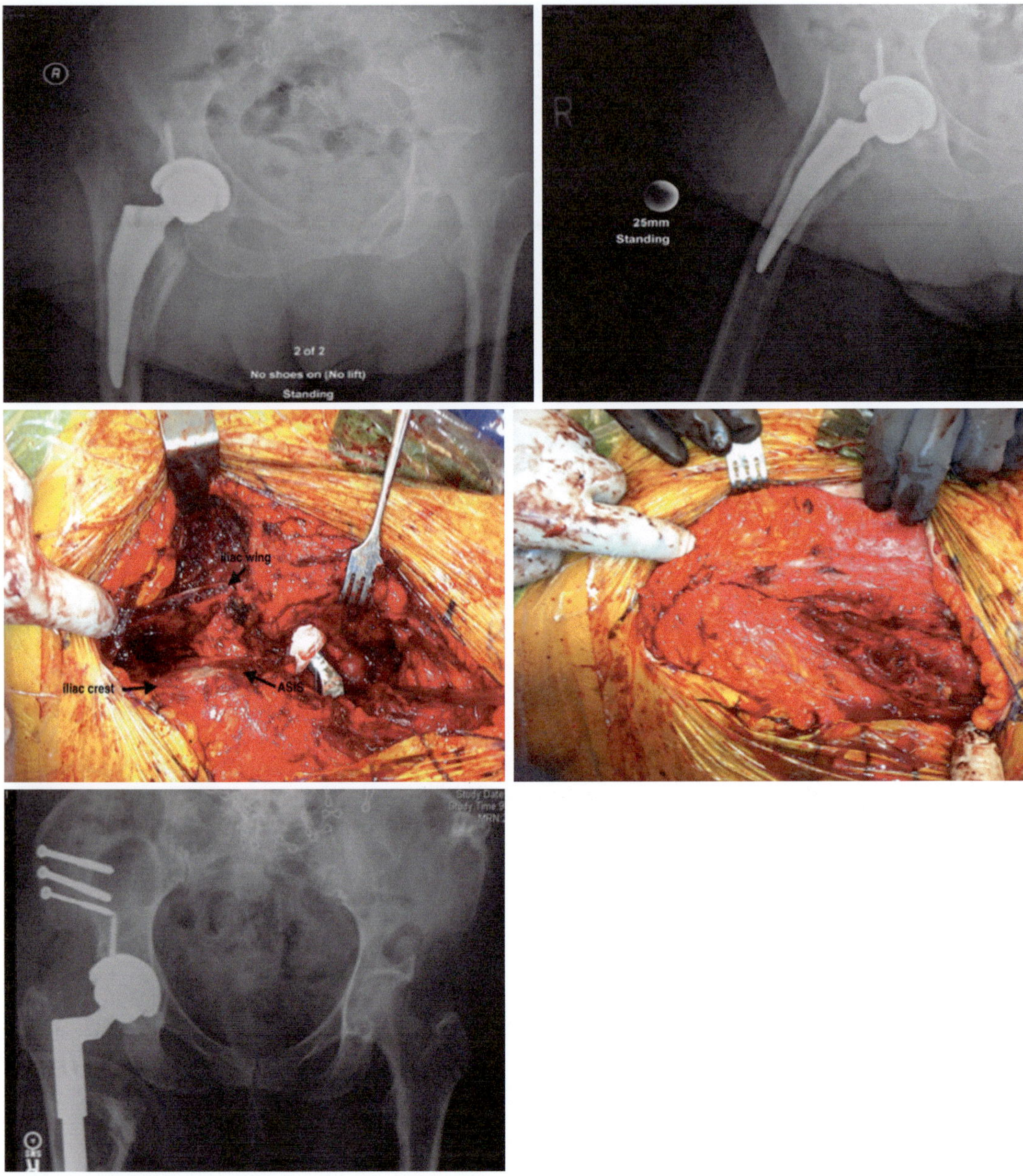

Figs. 34.24, 34.25, 34.26, and 34.27 Use of the iliac wing osteotomy in a 68-year-old female, approximately 10 months status post total hip arthroplasty who sustained a periprosthetic fracture 2 weeks postoperatively treated with benign neglect. She presented to the office with marked shortening, pain with any attempted limited ambulation with a walker. Because of the chronicity of the marked shortening of the femur and the width of her iliac crest, an iliac wing osteotomy was performed with excellent result

Proximally the vastus is split and peeled anteriorly, distally a Subvastus exposure of the lateral femur is performed, and the femur can be osteotomized thru a series of drill holes or with an oscillating saw. Of importance, the osteotomy is completed from a lateral to a medial direction and care taken to maintain the neurovascular insertions to the vastus in the area within 5 cm of the calcar, and care is taken to spare the greater trochanter and abductors (Fig. 34.41).

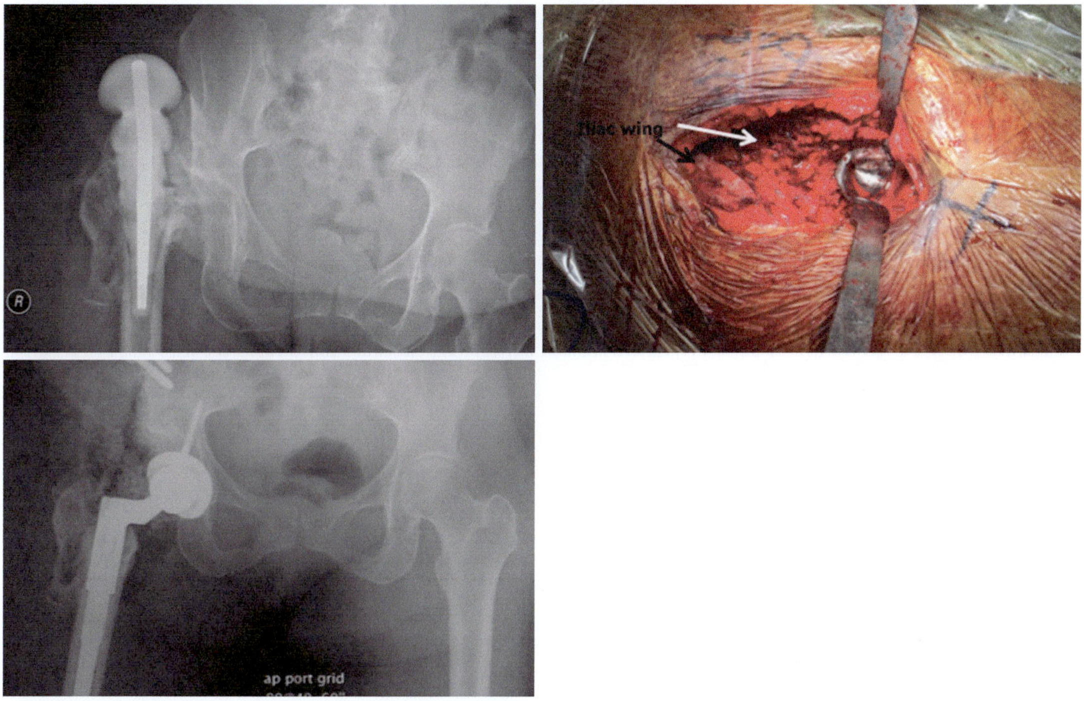

Figs. 34.28, 34.29, and 34.30 A 70-year-old female approximately 9 months status post Prostalac spacer which dislocated 2 weeks after it was placed. She presented to the office from a nursing home complaining of pain, inability to ambulate, and was essentially wheelchair-bound. On exam, her leg was severely shortened and externally fixed at about 65 degrees to 70 degrees of flexion with no rotation and moderately painful with any attempts at range of motion This patient also underwent an iliac wing osteotomy intraoperatively requiring only proximal extension of her incision to allow placement of her components with excellent result

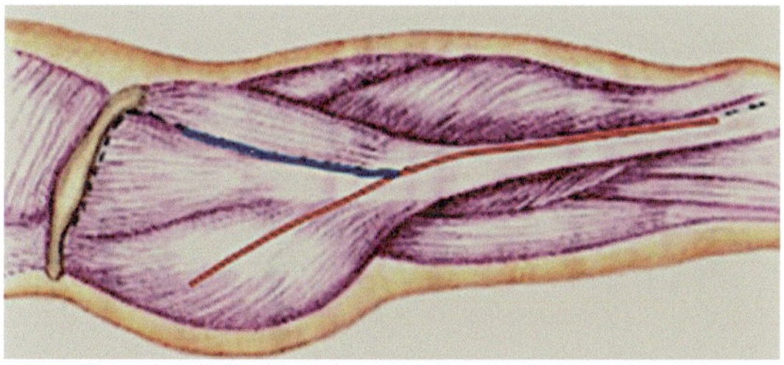

Fig. 34.31 Illustration of distal extension of the approach. The red line represents the commonly used posterior approach, while the blue line depicts the anterior approach. Note that they intersect at the start of the ITB

A distal cortical window can also be helpful in removing a stem that is distally fixed or potted, typically after working the stem proximally with osteotomes and burrs. Fluoroscopy can be used to define the area of the lateral cortical window, which is typically made just distal to the tip of the stem and extending 2 cm to 3 cm proximal to the tip of the stem. A subvastus approach to the femur is made either through extension of the primary incision or through a separate distal incision(Fig. 34.42).

The bony window is typically created with multiple drill holes connected with a high-speed burr and rounded at its edges to prevent any fracture propagation(Fig. 34.43).

Osteotomes or a high-speed burr can assist in removing the distally fixed stem (Fig. 34.44).

A hole can be created in the stem to allow retrograde impaction of the stem out of the canal (Fig. 34.45).

The lateral cortical fragment is easily repaired with simple cerclage cabling (Fig. 34.46).

When more exposure is required to remove a well-fixed stem a direct anterior extended trochanteric osteotomy can be performed. It is a variation of a familiar technique typically performed through a posterior approach. The oste-

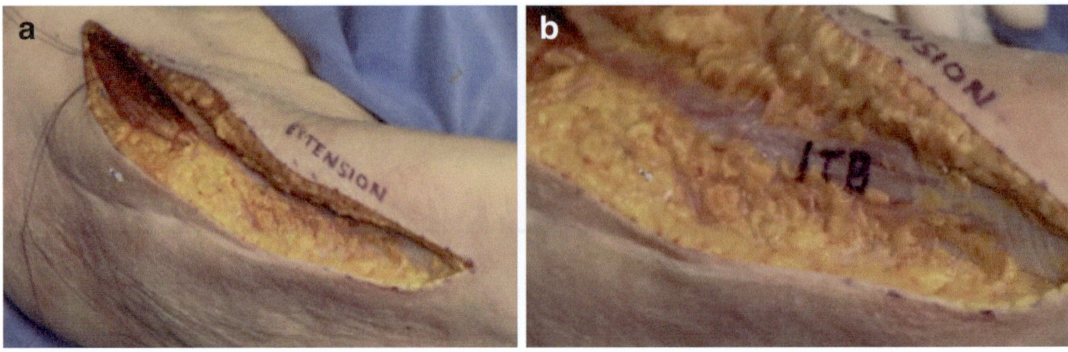

Fig. 34.32 (**a**) Distal extension of the incision is initially directed posterior and then along the midline of the femur. (**b**) Close up of distal extension identifying the ITB (iliotibial band)

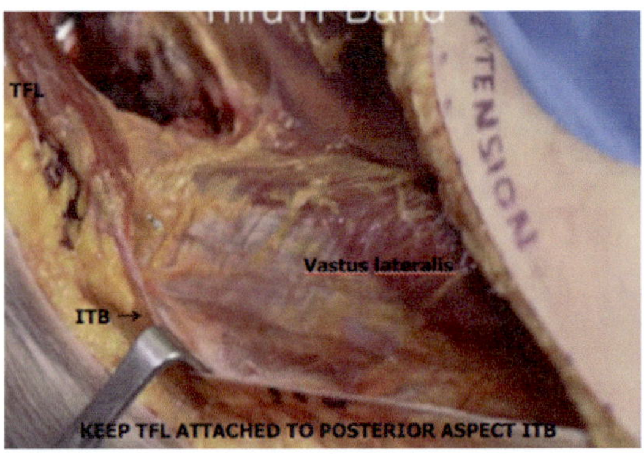

Fig. 34.33 The ITB is split distally, keeping the tensor fascia muscle attached to the posterior band of the ITB. this allows direct exposure to the vastus laterals

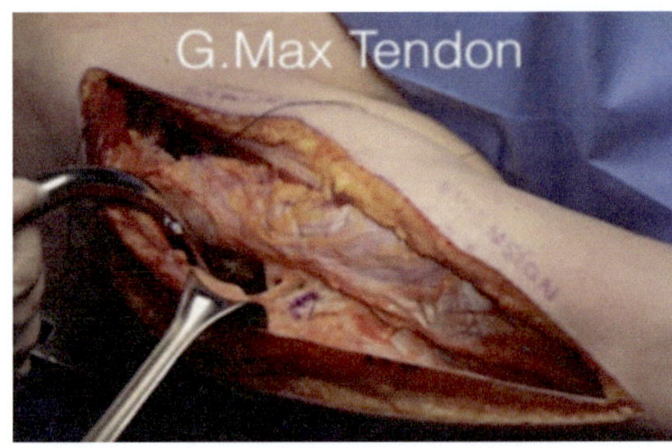

Fig. 34.34 Direct exposure of the lateral femur is possible. The gluteus maximus tendon is a reliable landmark

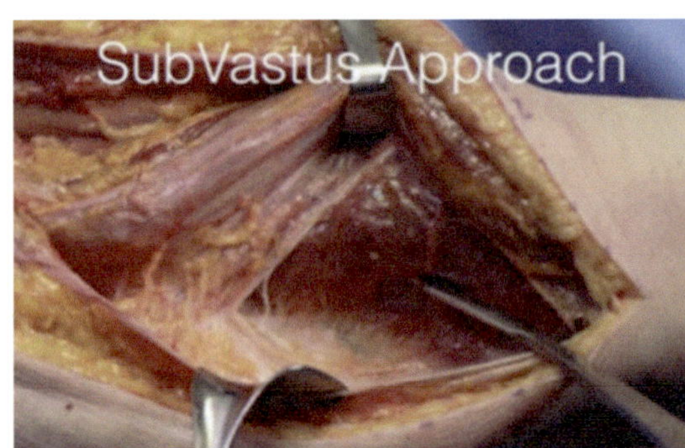

Fig. 34.35 Wide exposure of the entire lateral femur

otomy is performed in an anterior to posterior direction. Initially, the leg in a neutral position or slightly externally rotated for the initial anterior cut. The vastus is split or elevated laterally, an oscillating saw is used to create the anterior cut directed in a posterior direction. The distal limb of the osteotomy can be created with a saw or high-speed burr with the leg in slight internal rotation with a subvastus dissection, curving the anterior and posterior aspects to lessen the chance of fracture propagation. A cerclage cable is placed 1 cm distal to the osteotomy site to prevent fracture during canal preparation. The leg can then be maximally internally rotated for using drill holes or a saw to begin the posterior osteotomy site. The ETO is typically the lateral one-third of the femur, and care should be taken not to create too thin of a fragment which could fracture during mobilization. Completion of the osteotomy is performed with osteotomes carefully in an anterior to posterior direction with the abductors on the posterior fragment of the greater trochanter (Fig. 34.47a–d).

Removal of the stem can then be accomplished. The osteotomy is easily cabled in a standard fashion.

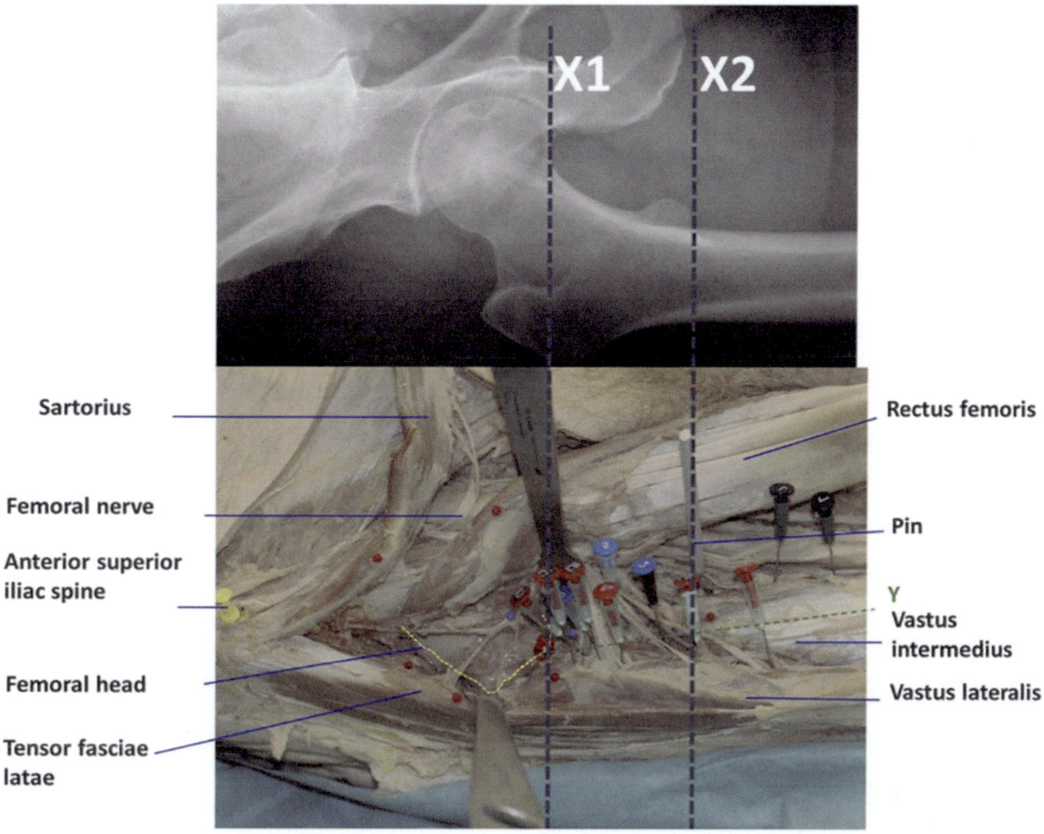

Fig. 34.36 Dissection of the femoral nerve innervations to the vastus lateralis and intermedius arise proximal andmedial. inadvertent trauma to this area, either directly or indirectly as in passage of a cerclage cable could result in a neurovascular injury

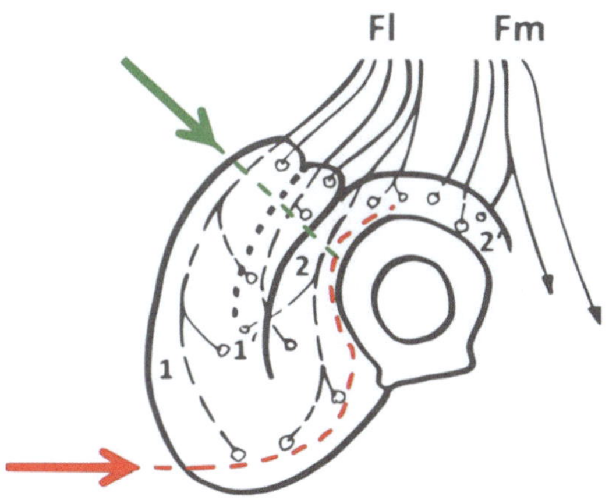

Fig. 34.37 Distal exposure of the vastus lateralis should proceed laterally lifting up the muscle to avoid injury tothe nerves as depicted in red

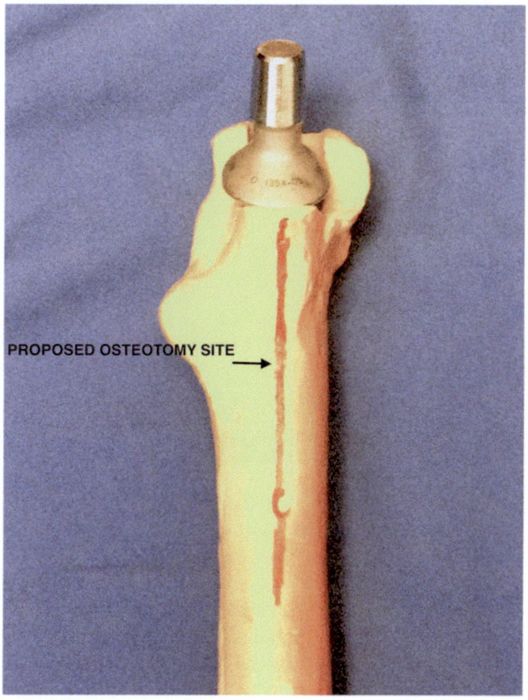

Fig. 34.38 Proposed osteotomy site for episiotomy of the femur to facilitate stem removal

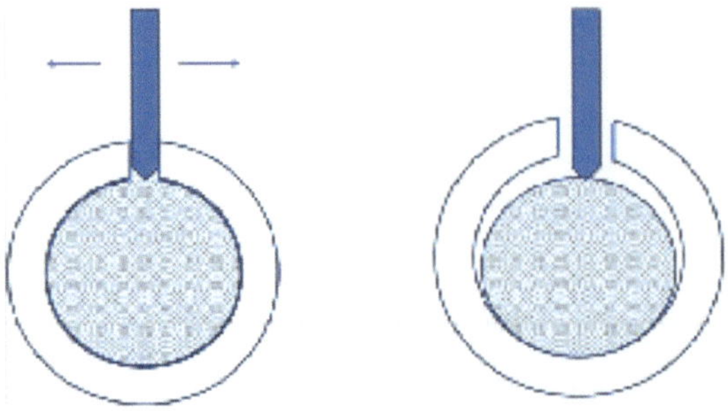

Fig. 34.39 A long, wide osteotome can be used to gently pry the site open, taking care not to create anuncontrolled fracture

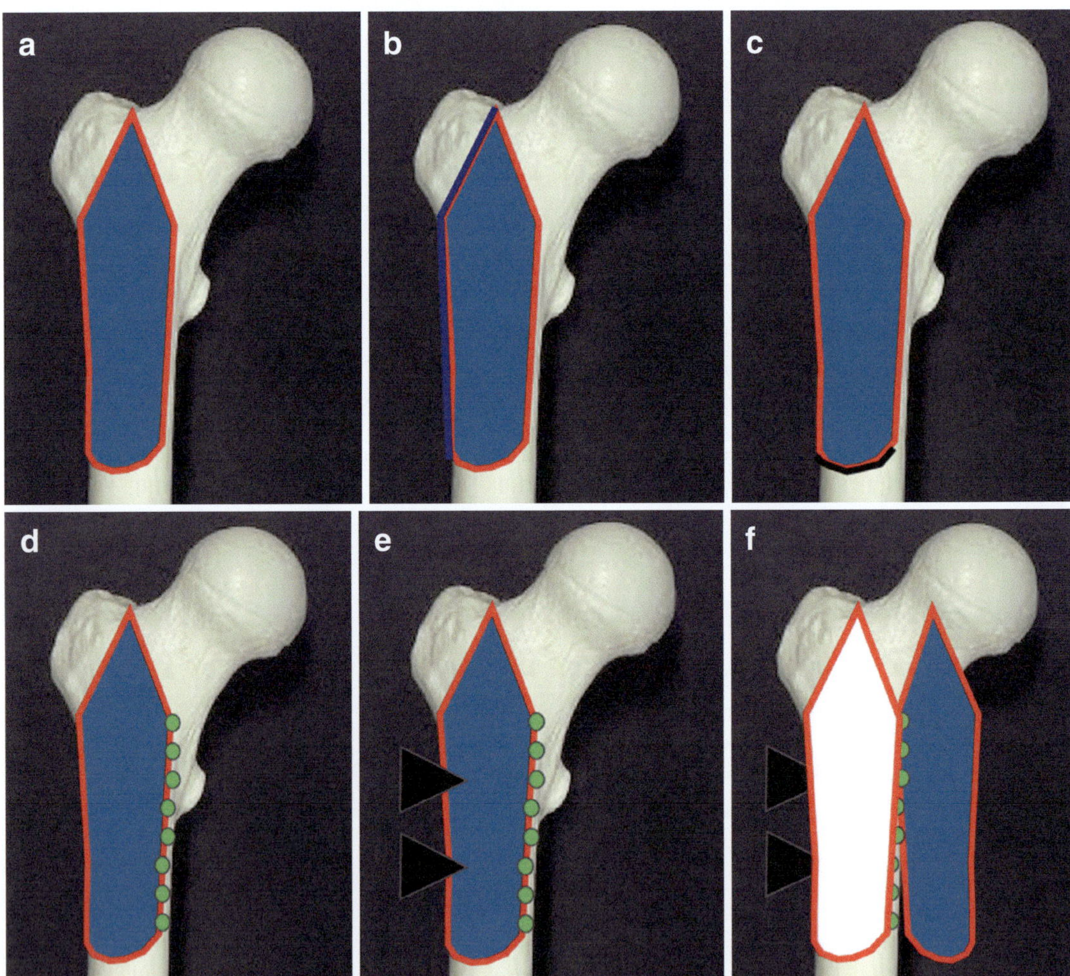

Fig. 34.40 (**a**) The proposed osteotomy site. (**b**) the blue line depicts the initial osteotomy performed with a sagittal saw. The vastus lateralis is peeled anteriorly to expose the anterolateral femur. Care is taken to avoid the greater trochanter, and the fragment should not be so thin that it will easily fracture during mobilization. (**c**) The black line illustrates the inferior cut which is made with a sagittal saw or high-speed burr with rounded edges to prevent fracture propagation. (**d**) With the leg externally rotated 90 degrees, multiple drill holes are made anteromedially, taking care to preserve the neurovascular supply. Care should be taken not to extend the osteotomy too medial to violate the calcar. (**e**) The black arrows indicate the direction of the osteotomes which are directed anteromedially to carefully elevated the anterior fragment. (**f**) The osteotomy is complete, allowing extensile exposure of the prosthesis within the canal while preserving the abductors, calcar and the blood supply of the osteotomized fragment

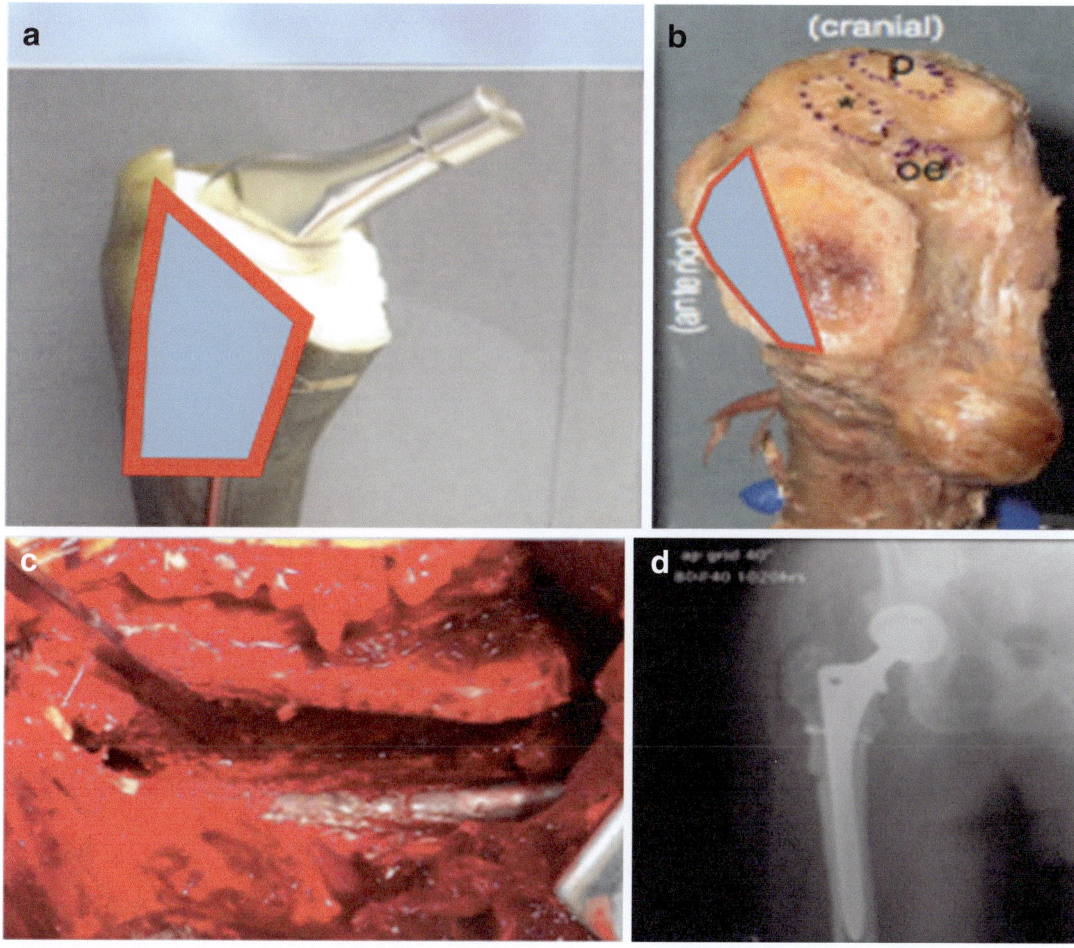

Fig. 34.41 (**a**) Proposed MAO. (**b**) intraoperative photo of elevated anterior ragment with exposed stem. (**c**) note calcar and greater troch spared. Also note thickness of osteotomized fragment. (**d**) post op radiograph with single cerclage cable fixing fragment

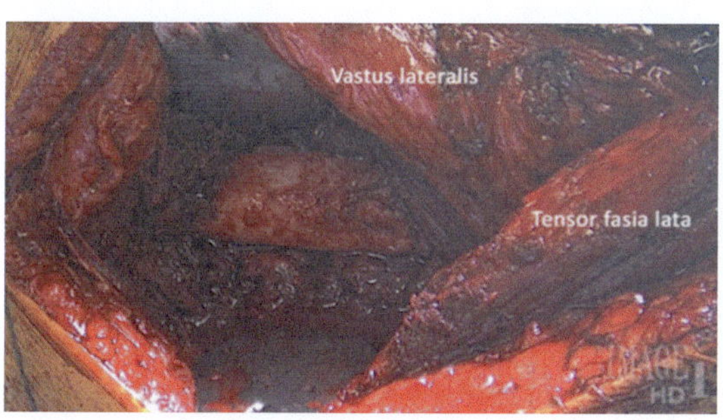

Fig. 34.42 Subvastus approach to the lateral femur via distal extension of incision

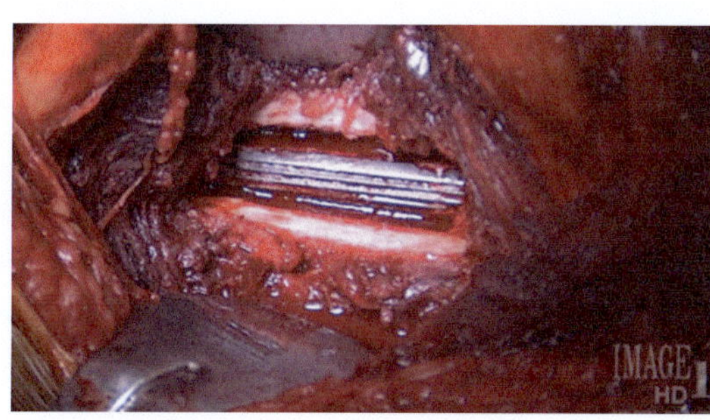

Fig. 34.43 Completed osteotomy with distal stem exposure

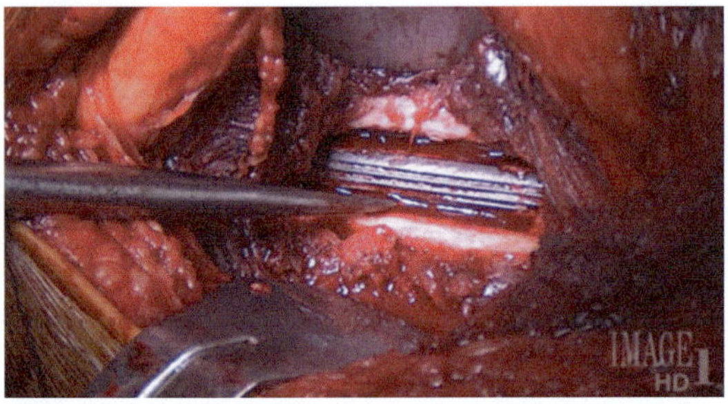

Fig. 34.44 Access to the stem for removal.

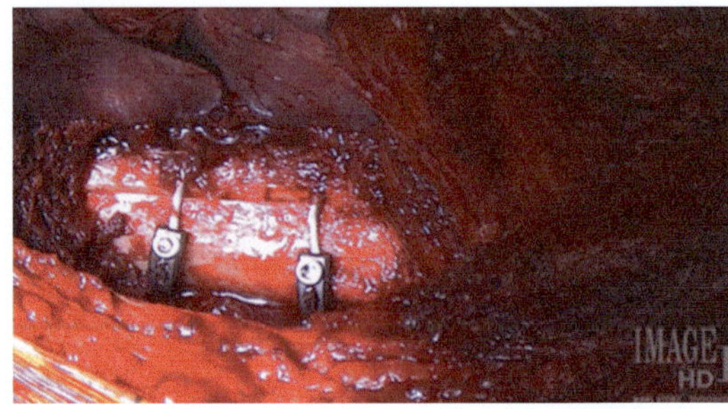

Fig. 34.46 Repair of window with cerclage cable

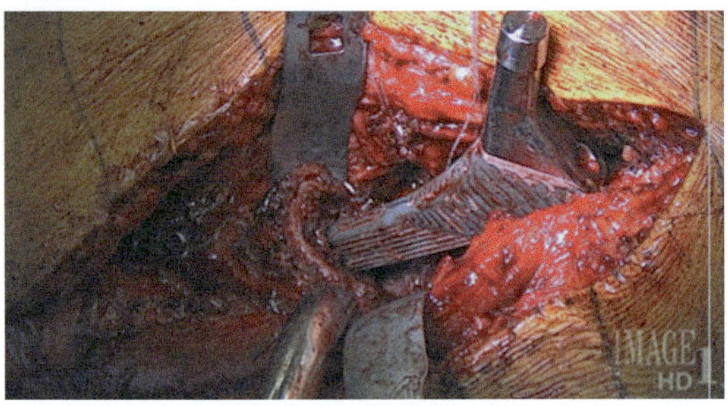

Fig. 34.45 Retrograde extraction of stem

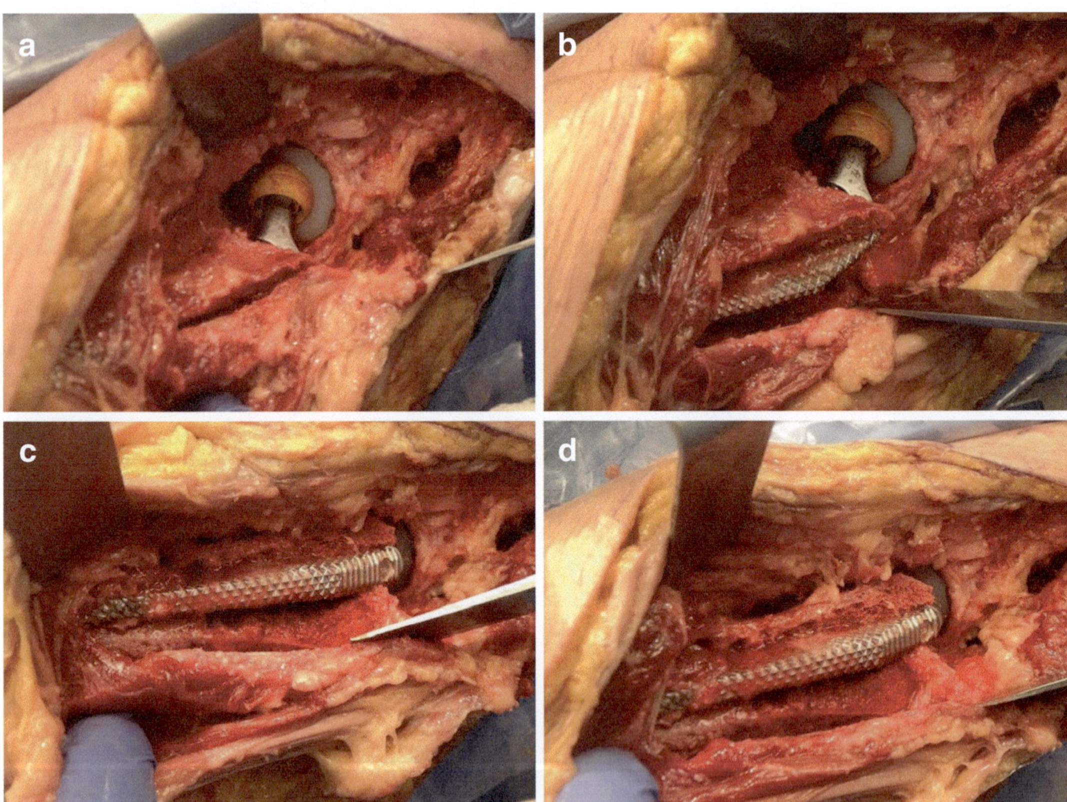

Fig. 34.47 (**a–d**) (**a**) Initial cut directed anterior to posterior after reflection of the vastus, (**b**) osteotomes used to carefully reflect the osteotomy posteriorly. (**c**) the osteotomy fragment should be roughly lateral 1/3 of the femur to prevent fragmentation. (**d**) access to stem for removal

In conclusion, the anterior approach to the tip is extensile both proximally and distally, and can be the preferred method for revision total hip arthroplasty. The majority of releases remain the same without compromising stability. As in with the primary approach, meticulous preparation and methodical stepwise releases done with patience is the key. Osteotomies about the hip can be performed both proximally and distally to aid in exposure and should be used judiciously as needed to obtain the desired result.

References

1. Kurtz S, Ong K, Lau E, et al. Projections of primary and revision hip and knee arthroplasty in the United States from 2005–2030. J Bone Joint Surg Am. 2007;89:780–5.
2. Alberton GM, High WA, Morrey BF. Dislocation after revision total hip arthroplasty: an analysis of risk factors and treatment options. J Bone Joint Surg Am. 2002;84:1788–92.
3. Sporer SM, Paprosky WG. Revision total hip arthroplasty: the limits of fully coated stems. Clin Orthop Relat Res. 2003;417:203–9.
4. Berend KR, Lombardi AV Jr, Seng BE, Adams JB. Enhanced early outcomes with anterior supine intermuscular approach in primary hip arthroplasty. J Bone Joint Surg Am. 2009;91:107–20.
5. Matta JM, Shahrdar C, Ferguson T. Single incision anterior approach for total hip arthroplasty on an orthopaedic table. Clin Orthop Relat Res. 2005;441:115–24.
6. Restrepo C, Parvizi J, Pour AE, Hozack WJ. Prospective randomized study of two surgical approaches for total hip arthroplasty. J Arthroplast. 2010;25:671–9.
7. Mast NH, Laude F. Revision total hip arthroplasty performed through the Hueter interval. J Bone Joint Surg Am. 2011;93 Suppl 2:143–8.
8. Manrique J, Chen AF, Heller S, Hozack WJ. Direct anterior approach for revision total hip arthroplasty. Ann Trans Med. 2014;2:100.
9. Molenaers B, Driesen R, Molenaers G, Corten K. The direct anterior approach for complex primary total hip arthroplasty: the extensile acetabular approach on a regular operating room table. J Arhroplasty. 2017;32:1553–9.
10. York PJ, Smarck CT, Judet T, Mauffrey C. Total Hip arthroplasty via the anterior approach: tip and tricks for primary and revision surgery. Int Orthop. 2016;40(10):2041.
11. Nogler MM, Thaler MR. The direct anterior approach for hip revision: accessing the entire femoral diaphysis without endangering the nerve supply. J Arthroplasty. 2017;32:510.
12. Thaler M, et al. Extension of the direct anterior approach for the treatment of periprosthetic femoral fractures. J Arthroplast. 2019;34(10):2449–53.
13. Grob K, Monahan R, Gilbey H, Yap F, Filgueira L, Kuster M. Distal extension of the direct anterior approach to the hip poses risk to neurovascular structures: an anatomical study. J Bone Jt Surg. 2015;97:126–32.

Complex Femoral Revision Using the Direct Anterior Hip Approach

35

Kris Alden

Introduction

The purpose of this section is to demonstrate the utility of the direct anterior approach (DAA) in the setting of complex femoral revision total hip arthroplasty (RTHA). As the DAA has gained a wider acceptance over the past 15 years, exploring anterior RTHA techniques and instrumentation will enhance its wider adoption. It is the general hope of DAA surgeons that the substantial benefits of the DAA in primary arthroplasty can be translated to the revision arthroplasty population. In particular, techniques employing the DAA can be modified so that extensile femoral exposure can be obtained to treat a number of RTHA challenges including congenital deformity, bone loss, prior hardware placement, stem removal, and periprosthetic fracture. Describing the techniques, and further identifying the potential difficulties to avoid, will facilitate a wider adoption of femoral revision arthroplasty utilizing the DAA. This review describes the indications, surgical anatomy, femoral revision techniques, and complications with DAA in RTHA procedures to illustrate essential components of successful anterior revision surgeries.

K. Alden (✉)
Hinsdale Orthopedics Associates/Illinois Bone and Joint Institute, Hinsdale, IL, USA

Indications

The muscle and tissue sparing, internervous anatomic planes used in the exposure of primary DAA THA, can be applied in the RTHA setting and with successful results [1]. Patients with a large abdominal pannus (usually those of a higher BMI) may present a general challenge due to the abundant overlapping soft tissue, which can result in postoperative wound irritation, superficial infection, and the potential need for wound irrigation and debridement. As with any hip surgical approach, obesity and a large pannus can cause wound issues. However, the potential problems for wound problems and superficial wound infection should be safeguarded more diligently in DAA in comparison to other surgical approaches in the setting of substantial obesity. In addition, anterior revision surgery is not contraindicated in patients whose index hip arthroplasty procedure was performed through a different approach (such as posterior or lateral approaches). The potential advantages, particularly the use of internervous muscular dissection, earlier restoration of gait kinematics can provide enhanced muscle function postoperatively, improved stability of the joint, and expedited recovery following RTHA. Nevertheless, femoral exposure can be more challenging for the surgeon in the RTHA setting than other surgical approaches. The potential difficulty merits the increased effort when considering the improved

J. M. Matta, A. P. Sah (eds.), *Anterior Hip Replacement*,
https://doi.org/10.1007/978-3-030-91896-5_35

recovery and enhanced surgical outcome for the patient. The DAA, through its extensile surgical exposure, affords unparallel access to the femur to allow for revision of the femoral component. However, the initial surgical exposure, femoral releases, proximal femoral osteotomies, and stem insertion may require additional effort and can be substantially different from other RTHA techniques.

Incision and Surgical Approach

If the index arthroplasty was performed through the DAA, then the same incision should be incorporated into the RTHA procedure. If another approach was used then a traditional DAA incision (generally 1 cm distal and 3 cm lateral to the ASIS) can be employed [2]. Dissection through new tissue planes facilitates the ease of access for the RTHA procedure and DAA is not contraindicated when a different approach was utilized in the index arthroplasty. The incision and superficial dissection can be performed distally approximately 10 cm in line with the tensor fascia lata (TFL) with careful preservation of the lateral femoral cutaneous nerve.

Generally developing, finding, and dissecting out the TFL-sartorial interval can be difficult in the RTHA setting when the index procedure was also performed through the DAA due to excessive scar formation and significant adhesions in the primary muscle interval. The DAA superficial surgical plain exploits the interval between the TFL innervated by the superior gluteal nerve (SGN) and the sartorius muscle innervated by the femoral nerve (FN). Once the TFL-sartorial interval is created, the remainder of the dissection is substantially similar to the primary DAA. Deeper proximal DAA dissection utilizes the interval between the gluteus minimus, innervated by the SGN, and the rectus femoris muscle innervated by the FN. Further distal extension of the DAA utilizes deep exposure between the vastus lateralis muscle (FN) and the semimebranosus (sciatic nerve). After the hip capsule is encountered and identified, a standard capsulotomy can be performed. In addition, in the setting of RTHA, after appropriate reflection of the capsule and to facilitate adequate exposure, the redundant and excessive hip capsule often requires extensive debulking. If exposure remains difficult, distal extension of the incision and further exposure can be performed. In addition, using a lateral incision in the mid-sagittal plane of the proximal thigh as described by Kennon et al. [3] can also facilitate exposure to the femur to perform a range of procedures as part of the RTHA procedure. The distal extension of the incision continues down to the mid-sagittal plane including the knee joint and can be additionally utilized to perform a wide range of femoral revision procedures including proximal femoral replacement [4].

Femoral Revision

When performing femoral revision through the DAA, achieving adequate exposure is paramount to prevent complications such as trochanteric fracture or displacement. A soft bump placed under the operative side of the pelvis or the use of a special anterior hip surgical table can facilitate hip extension and thereby promote elevation of the proximal femur sufficiently to afford access to the proximal femur. As in a primary DAA THA, appropriate releases and adduction, extension, and sufficient external rotation of the femur will afford access to the proximal femur so that any stem can be utilized in the RTHA setting. Distal extension of the incision and splitting of the vastus lateralis will allow for femoral exposure to perform cabling, open reduction-internal fixation, or an extended trochanteric osteotomy (ETO) [5] as needed to effect stem removal. Less invasive techniques such as an anterior cortical window have been developed to facilitate femoral stem removal without performing an ETO [6].

Hip Dislocation and Femoral Head Removal

Two generally recognized techniques exist for femoral head extraction in RTHA. With a smaller femoral head, dislocation with traction and external

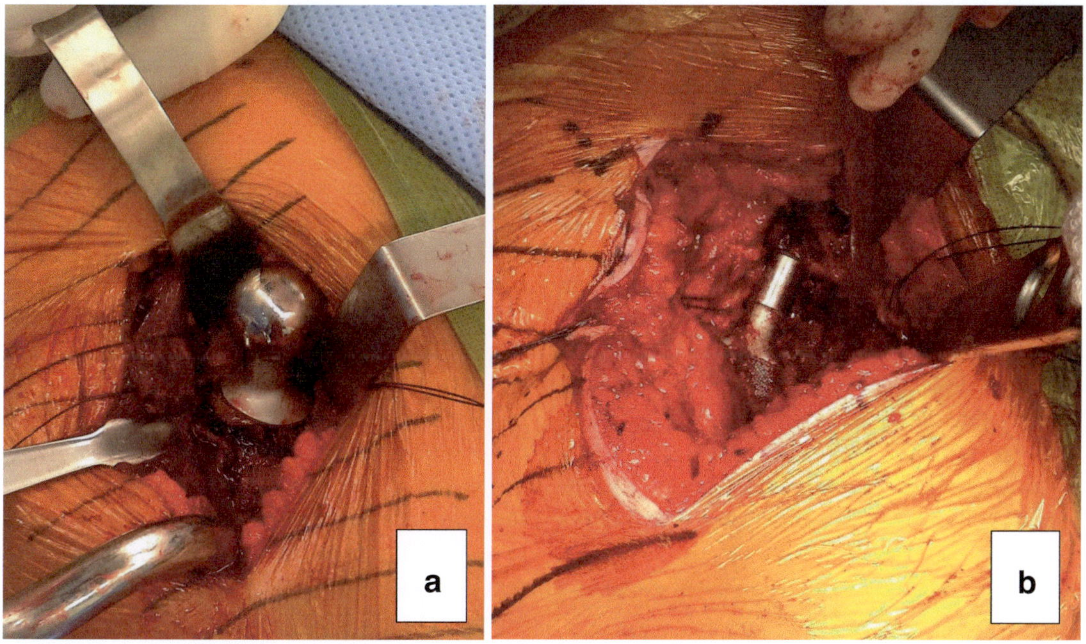

Fig. 35.1 (**a**) Dislocation of femoral component with head intact, and (**b**) subsequent disimpaction of the femoral head from the trunnion during a DAA RTHA procedure

rotation with a bone hook placed around the trunnion can be performed. Following dislocation, the femur is placed in extension and adduction to allow femoral head removal using a bone tamp to disimpact the head from the trunnion (see Fig. 35.1).

With larger femoral heads or in the case of a more difficult exposure, a second technique is more practical. Prior to dislocation, traction is applied to the femur to provide space within the head-acetabular construct. With slight internal rotation of the hip, a bone tamp can dislodge the femoral head from the trunnion and allow sufficient space to provide extraction. Leaving the femoral head in situ allows for additional space to provide for dislocation of the femoral component. Following this, removal of the femoral head from the acetabular liner can be performed.

Soft Tissue Releases for Femoral Revision DAA Exposure

Following external rotation of 90 degrees and extension of the dislocated hip, the posterior soft tissue can be released to facilitate femoral elevation and further exposure as required. The posterior capsule is generally hypertrophic from the prior arthroplasty and hinders proximal femoral elevation. Sequential releasing of the posterior capsule and related ligamentous structures provides access to the proximal femur and decreases the risk of trochanteric fracture. The following soft tissue releases should be performed in a stepwise fashion: posterior ischiofemoral ligament, superior iliofemoral ligament, anterior/inferior pubofemoral ligament, and conjoined tendon (obturator internus and gemelli). Finally, in cases with more difficult exposure (i.e., severe deformity, muscular patients, or those with a wide pelvis) access to the femur can be limited. In those patients and additionally when there is a need for femoral canal reaming, and/or implantation of a longer modular stem, often releasing the proximal 3–4 cm of the TFL from the iliac crest can provide much needed exposure of the proximal femur. Release of 3–4 cm of the TFL within the tendinous portion of the TFL directly off the iliac crest allows for tendinous repair with interrupted sutures and further diminishes the risk of muscle damage during the RTHA procedure.

Stem Removal

Once access to the proximal femur is achieved, a series of instruments can be employed for stem removal including a pencil tip high speed burr and application of flexible thin osteotomes to break the bone/implant interface. Careful removal of bone from the shoulder of the implant is often required to allow for extraction of the stem even if the stem is known to be loose. Additionally, removing offending bone from the shoulder of the femoral implant will decrease the propensity for trochanteric fracture during stem removal (see Fig. 35.2). Once the proximal femur is free and the stem is sufficiently loose, an extraction device can be applied to the trunnion to effect stem removal.

Femoral Osteotomies

Femoral osteotomies such as an ETO can be a necessary technique to remove a well-fixed hydroxyapatite-coated implant or fully porous-coated stem particularly in the setting of infection and assist in femoral exposure and thereby implant removal. The value of an osteotomy lies in the reproducible healing of bone-to-bone anastomoses assuming vascularity to the involved area has been preserved. However, the use of the ETO technique despite being repaired with cables is not absent potential complications including intraoperative femoral fracture [7], abductor insufficiency [8], trochanteric fracture [9], and postoperative stem loosening [10]. Therefore, less bone disruptive techniques have been developed to diminish the risk of postoperative complications [11]. Utilizing a standard ETO in the setting of the DAA for revision arthroplasty can often be difficult due to access and repair techniques. The transfemoral (Wagner) osteotomy [12] has been utilized to afford intramedullary access using an anteriorly based osteotomy in a variety of settings including removal of a fully porous stem and correction of severe anterior bowing of the femur. The Wagner osteotomy differs in both direction and size. The

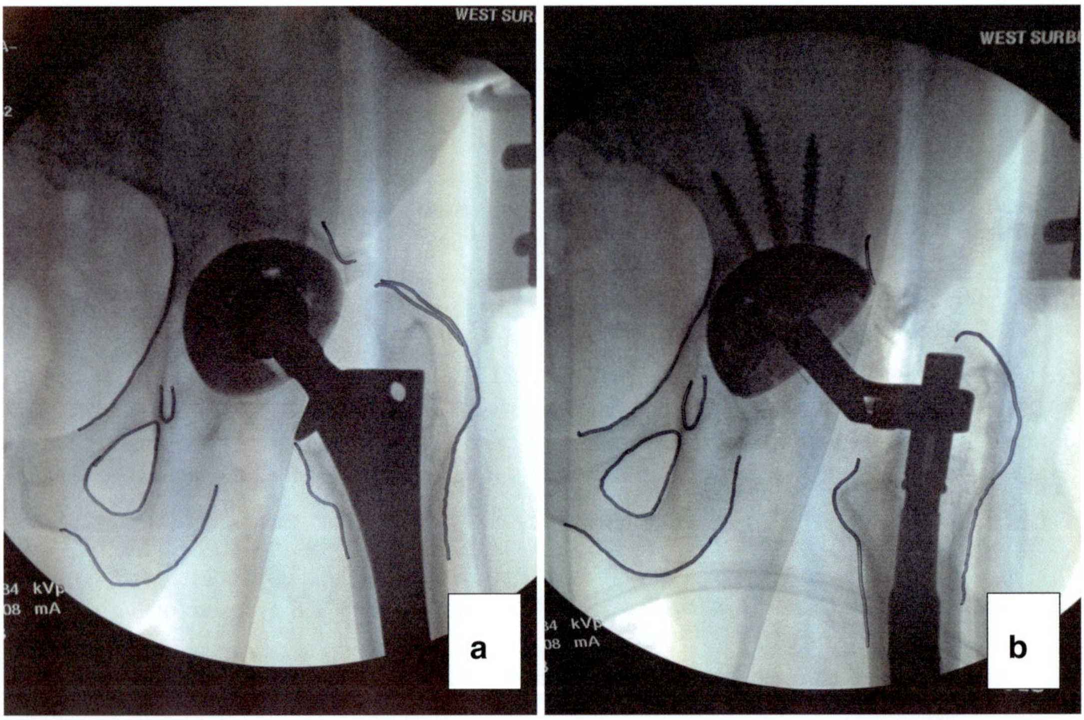

Fig. 35.2 (**a**) Preoperative fluoroscopy outlining landmarks prior to revision of loose cup and stem, and (**b**) fluoroscopy image of subsequent cup revision and trial of proximal body of modular femoral revision to assess leg length and offset restoration

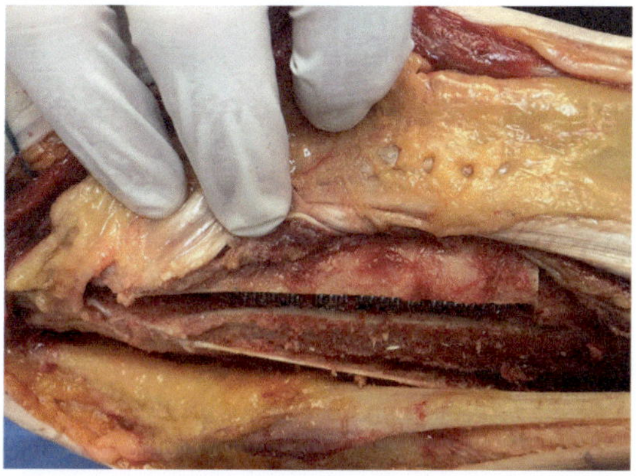

Fig. 35.3 Cadaveric dissection of a laterally based Wagner transfemoral osteotomy demonstrating reflection of the anterolateral 1/3 of the proximal femur to access the femoral stem for implant removal

osteotomy is performed in the sagittal plane [13] incorporating the anterolateral one-third of the proximal femur with the femoral fragment reflected anteriorly. The length and thereby location of the transverse cut of any osteotomy (ETO or transfemoral) is based on the length of the implant and is at the discretion of the operating surgeon. Union rates in the transfemoral osteotomy are 95–100% in several studies [14–17]. Surgeons who utilize trochanteric osteotomies, irrespective of the technique, should be cognizant of the innervation of the gluteal and vastus muscle groups by remaining anterior or lateral for access to the desired osteotomy site of the proximal femur (Fig. 35.3).

Post-osteotomy, several trochanteric fixation techniques are available and include cable fixation, cable plate systems, and non-metallic polymer cable systems. They share the common benefits as well as drawback including fixation failure leading to nonunion, and particularly with bulky plate systems can often result in painful hardware that often requires hardware removal. Despite these potential limitations, a trochanteric osteotomy is exceptionally useful for femoral exposure in the RTHA setting. In the DAA setting, safeguarding the obturator internus and piriformis intact affords a stabilizing force against the gluteus muscles and prevents anterolateral migration. For this reason, and the high rate of union, application of cable-plate systems can be avoided over the greater trochanter. Repair of the ETO is typically performed following the revision femoral implantation.

Window and femoral episiotomies have been described at various sites in the proximal femur to aid in removal of cement, access to a broken implant, or additional disruption of an ingrown porous femoral component. These episiotomies are best completed with a microsagittal saw to reduce the risk of fracture propagation and further bone loss. In the case of window episiotomy, the reduced fragment with its muscular attachments intact can be restored and secured using standard cable fixation. Similarly, repair of the femoral episiotomy can be performed using cerclage wires or cables.

Implant Selection

RTHA femoral implant choice is determined primarily on bone loss, quality of bone remaining, degree of deformity, and indication for revision. Femoral bone loss as a result of osteolysis, stress shielding, infection, or prior revision should direct the choice of implant rather than the approach. There are multiple classification systems to guide surgeons on the best options to manage varying degrees of bone loss in and around the femur [18, 19]. Direct access to the femoral canal can typically be afforded by using the techniques described above and implant choice should not be predicated on the surgical approach to the hip. Preoperative planning is essential to assess the type and degree of proximal femoral deficiency, leg length differences, and determine the size and type of implant that is required to bypass the deficient bone. Using simple x-rays can often help guide decisions on implant choices, and rarely would computed tomography (CT) be required. The use of magnetic resonance imaging (MRI) can be implemented in the case of concerns about metal-on-metal articulation, soft tissue integrity, and evaluation of the abductor musculature. The overriding goals of implant choice include preservation of the remaining femoral bone stock, restoration of hip joint biomechanics, stability of the revision prosthesis, and leg length equality. Implant choices can vary and include in some cases a primary component, cemented stem fixation, impaction grafting, and monoblock or modular diaphyseal engaging stems. Modular, tapered, fluted stems have several advantages in the setting of more significant bone loss [20–22]. These stems incorporate distal (i.e., diaphyseal) femoral engagement, fixation that bypasses significant proximal femoral bone loss, and the ability to vary the proximal body to optimize leg length, offset, and hip stability. The successful use of these stems require precise diaphyseal cortical tapered reaming and therefore appropriate femoral exposure is needed. The appropriate stepwise surgical releases of the proximal femur are essential to avoid contact with the iliac crest and protect the TFL musculature from intraoperative damage. Therefore, release of the TFL tendon as outlined above can easily facilitate the use of diaphyseal reamers and placement of 190 mm (or greater) stems.

Intraoperative Fluoroscopy

Trial reduction for the assessment of hip stability, and the restoration of leg length and hip offset can be easily performed using intraoperative imaging such as fluoroscopy. This modality reduces the risk of leg length inequality by direct assessment as well as dislocation by appropriately restoring offset.

References

1. Mast NH, Laude F. Revision Total hip arthroplasty performed through the Hueter interval. J Bone Joint Surg Am. 2011;93(Suppl 2):143–8.
2. Bender B, Nogler M, Hozack WJ. Direct anterior approach for total hip arthroplasty. Orthop Clin North Am. 2009;40:321–8.
3. Kennon R, Keggi J, Zatorski LE, et al. Anterior approach for total hip arthroplasty: beyond the minimally invasive technique. J Bone Joint Surg Am. 2004;86-A Suppl 2:91–7.
4. Manson TT, Moskal JT. Proximal femoral replacement using the direct anterior approach to the hip. Instr Course Lect. 2020;69:53–66.
5. Younger TI, Bradford MS, Magnus RE, Paprosky WG. Extended proximal femoral osteotomy. A new technique for femoral revision arthroplasty. J Arthroplast. 1995;10(3):329–38.
6. Park CH, Yeom J, Park JW, Won SH, Lee YK, Koo KH. Anterior cortical window technique instead of extended trochanteric osteotomy in revision total hip arthroplasty: a minimum 10-year follow-up. Clin Orthop Surg. 2019;11(4):396–402.
7. Mardones R, Gonzalez C, Cabanela ME, Trousdale RT, Berry DJ. Extended femoral osteotomy for revision of hip arthroplasty: results and complications. J Arthroplast. 2005;20(1):79–83.
8. Huffman GR, Ries MD. Combined vertical and horizontal cable fixation of an extended trochanteric osteotomy site. J Bone Joint Surg Am. 2003;85(2):273–7.
9. Charity J, Tsiridis E, Gusmao D, Bauze A, Timperley J, Gie G. Extended trochanteric osteotomy followed by cemented impaction allografting in revision hip arthroplasty. J Arthroplast. 2013;28(1):154–60.
10. MacDonald SJ, Cole C, Guerin J, Rorabeck CH, Bourne RB, McCalden RW. Extended trochanteric osteotomy via the direct lateral approach in revision hip arthroplasty. Clin Orthop Relat Res. 2003;417:210–6.
11. Kim YM, Lim ST, Yoo JJ, Kim HJ. Removal of a well-fixed cementless femoral stem using a microsagittal saw. J Arthroplasty. 2003;18(4):511–2.
12. Wagner H. [Revision prosthesis for the hip joint in severe bone loss]. Orthopade. 1987; 16(4):295–300.
13. Werner SD, Satterly T, Skakun W, Jacofsky DJ. The transfemoral approach to revision total hip arthroplasty. In: Callaghan JJ, Rosenberg AG, Rubhas HE, Clohisy JC, Beaule PE, Della Valle CJ, editors. The adult hip: hip arthroplasty surgery, vol. 2. 3rd ed. Ch 105. Philadelphia, PA: Wolturs Kluwer; 2016. p. 1268–74.
14. Fink B, Grossmann A, Schubring S, Schulz MS, Fuerst M. A modified transfemoral approach using modular cementless revision stems. Clin Orthop Relat Res. 2007;462:105–14.
15. de Menezes DFA, Le Béguec P, Sieber H-P, Goldschild M. Stem and osteotomy length are critical for success of the transfemoral approach and cementless stem revision. Clin Orthop Relat Res. 2012;470:883–8.
16. Nozawa M, Shitoto K, Mastuda K, Maezawa K, Yasuma M, Kurosawa H. Transfemoral approach for revision total hip arthroplasty. Arch Orthop Trauma Surg. 2002;122:288–90.
17. Fink B, Oremek D. The transfemoral approach for removal of well-fixed femoral stems in 2-stage septic hip revision. J Arthroplasty. 2016;31:1065–71.

18. D'Antonio J, McCarthy JC, Bargar WL, Borden LS, Cappelo WN, Collis DK, Steinberg ME, Wedge JH. Classification of femoral abnormalities in total hip arthroplasty. Clin Orthop Relat Res. 1999;296:133–9.
19. Valle CJ, Paprosky WG. Classification and an algorithmic approach to the reconstruction of femoral deficiency in revision total hip arthroplasty. J Bone Joint Surg Am. 2003;85-A Suppl 4:1–6.
20. Kwong LM, Miller AJ, Lubinus P. A modular distal fixation option for proximal bone loss in revision total hip arthroplasty: a 2- to 6-year follow-up study. J Arthroplast. 2003;18:94–7.
21. McCarthy JC, Lee JA. Complex revision total hip arthroplasty with modular stems at a mean of 14 years. Clin Orthop Relat Res. 2007;465:166–9.
22. Paprosky WG, Aribindi R. Hip replacement: treatment of femoral bone loss using distal bypass fixation. Instr Course Lect. 2000;49:119–30.

36 Femoral Revision Total Hip Arthroplasty Using the Direct Anterior (Hueter) Approach

Frédéric Laude
and Maria-Roxana Viamont-Guerra

Introduction

The number of revisions THA tends to increase annually, probably due to the ageing of the population and the performance of THAs in younger and more active patients [1–3]. Revision THA is deemed a technically demanding procedure, therefore it is crucial to select the most suitable surgical technique which allows soft tissue and bone stock preservation as much as possible [4].

Most surgeons are familiar with the posterior or lateral approaches for revision THA; however, the direct anterior approach (DAA), also known as Hueter approach, can be a successful alternative to perform revision THA as well. Although the DAA has been considered more challenging than the two other approaches, it is a less invasive and anatomically preserving technique [5–7]. Sparing muscular tissues is a valuable advantage.

Concerning the bone stock preservation, there is no consensus on the ideal stem design features to use in revision THA. Long stems are traditionally used for revision THA, especially those with distal fixation, because they provide stability in femurs with poor proximal bone stock [8–10]. However, they increase the risk of intraoperative femoral fracture, distal femoral loading, proximal stress shielding, and stem fracture [11–15], all of which could reduce bone stock in case of future revisions. Aiming to avoid these adverse complications, as well as to preserve the diaphyseal bone stock and proximal femoral loading in order to restore metaphyseal bone stock, some surgeons have started to use primary stems in revision THAs, with satisfactory outcomes [11, 16–23]. In the interest of preserving soft tissue and bone as much as possible, the main purposes of this chapter are:

1. To describe the surgical technique for femoral revision THA through the DAA and describe its extension when needed
2. To report the senior surgeon's experience on femoral revision THA through the DAA using primary stems, shorter than those removed

Surgical Technique

To perform revision THA through DAA, it is important to have experience in this approach, an efficient and trained team, and also suitable instruments.

F. Laude (✉)
Clinique du sport, Paris, France

M.-R. Viamont-Guerra
Hip Surgery Unit, Hospital Israelita Albert Einstein, São Paulo, SP, Brazil

J. M. Matta, A. P. Sah (eds.), *Anterior Hip Replacement*,
https://doi.org/10.1007/978-3-030-91896-5_36

Patient's Positioning

The patient is positioned supine on an orthopaedic traction table, which can provide operative assistance by facilitating femur exposure and the use of intraoperative fluoroscopy, as well as ensuring the need of no more than one scrub assistant.

Antiseptic preparation is performed from the inferior costal margin to the level of the ipsilateral knee, allowing proximal and distal surgical extension if necessary. The sterile fields are draped as usual.

Incision and Surgical Approach

If the primary THA was performed through another approach, the revision THA through the DAA will try to avoid that previously compromised soft tissues suffer another surgical trauma. The incision is made over the belly of the tensor fascia lata (TFL) muscle, starting from a point located approximately 2 cm distally and 2 cm laterally to the anterior superior iliac spine (ASIS), and running obliquely for approximately 10 cm (Fig. 36.1).

If a Hueter incision was performed previously, the same one must be used. In these cases, excessive scar tissue may be present; therefore, special care must be taken in order to identify the correct superficial muscle interval (between TFL and sartorius) and not to damage the lateral femoral cutaneous nerve (LFCN). A small autostatic retractor tensioning the soft tissue is very useful for finding the good plane.

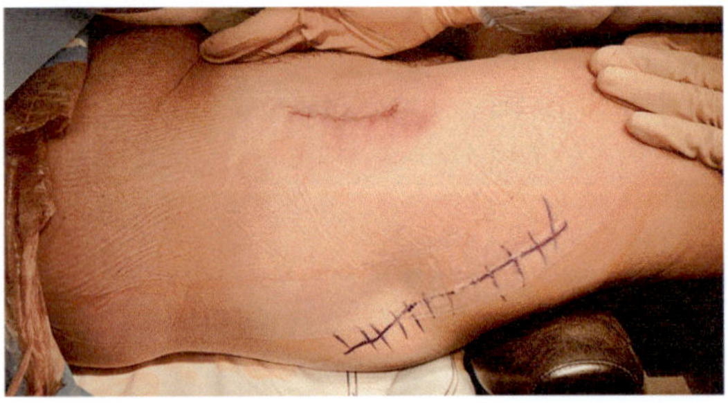

Fig. 36.1 Anterior incision for revision with DAA. The previous posterior approach is marked in blue

The TFL fascia is split slightly lateral to the true interval and in line with muscle fibres, aiming to protect LFCN fibres. Next, the muscle belly is released from the fascia by slipping the surgeon's finger in this space proximally and distally, as far as possible. The TFL muscle belly is mobilized laterally and held by an autostatic retractor. At this point, rectus femoris muscle belly is visualized, its anterior fascia is opened laterally, and its muscle belly is pushed medially by means of the autostatic retractor. Usually, the lateral femoral circumflex vessels can be seen ligated due to previous THA through DAA.

In revision THA, routinely the tendinous indirect head of the rectus femoris muscle is sectioned. This helps to better expose the superolateral surface of the ilium and anterior aspect of the acetabular rim, which is used as an osseous landmark.

The capsule is exposed, then an anterior capsulotomy is performed and, if needed, the lateral and posterior capsule is progressively released. The gradual capsular release is important because additional mobilization, especially external rotation, of the femur may be required during the surgery to access the acetabulum and expose the femoral canal properly. We usually do little or no release for a primary stem, but in case of revision surgery, the release is often more extensive. The femur needs to be easily mobilized in order not to break it, particularly, the greater trochanter. Insufficient capsular release is the most common reason for poor visualization of structures and femoral fracture.

Prosthetic Femoral Head Removal

The prosthetic femoral head must be removed at the beginning of the procedure. A traction table is a helpful tool for this procedure. A slight traction is applied to the operated limb, creating a space between prosthetic head and liner. The head is hammered in its inferior portion towards the liner until it is loosened and drops into the liner. Then, hip external rotation helps to retrieve the prosthetic head of the liner.

Femoral Revision

Femoral Stem Removal

While acetabulum exposure is relatively simple in DAA, femoral exposure may be more difficult and delicate.

If the stem is loose and easy to remove, there is no need to consider complex strategies, but care must be taken with the greater trochanter. As many stems have a prominent shoulder, this part of the stem can force and cause a fracture of the greater trochanter while the stem is being removed. This fracture is not severe because all muscle attachments in the greater trochanter remain intact after a DAA and the fragment will not tend to move. This is in contrast to a posterior approach, where the greater trochanter fragment tends to move forward if not fixed, and to a transgluteal approach, where it tends to move backwards. In the DAA, this fracture can even be left without osteosynthesis fixation. This is already done in our practice if it happens in a primary THA, and it is not very different in revision procedures.

However, to avoid this kind of problem, it is preferable to thoroughly clean the external surface over the stem shoulder before removing it. There is often a slightly sclerotic bone at this level, and it must be removed with a rongeur, a curette or a gouge chisel. If the stem is cemented, again, do not hesitate to start removing the cement to create sufficient space. The stem can be removed using a conventional femoral stem extractor, but we tend to prefer the system developed by Dr. Fabian Kalberer (Kantonsspital Winterthur, Switzerland) and Medacta International (Castel San Pietro, Switzerland), which is very suitable for the DAA (Fig. 36.2).

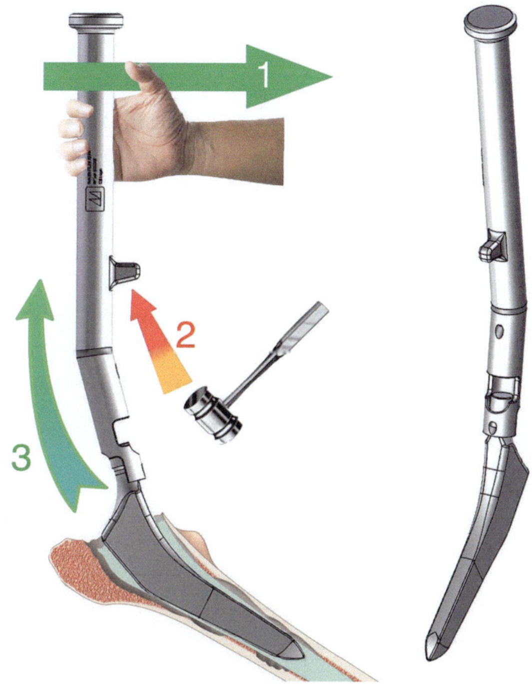

Fig. 36.2 The Kalberer stem extractor. The surgeon pulls the upper part of the extractor (arrow 1) and hammer hit the distal specific part (arrow 2) trying to always place the stem far away from the GT (arrow 3) in order to minimize the risk of GT fracture

If the stem is retroverted, which is not so rare, this can be problematic, because placing the extractor on the femoral neck becomes impossible or very difficult. As the neck is always in excessive internal rotation, by forcing the stem extractor positioning, this will only result in creating a femoral spiral fracture. If there is any doubt about the stem version in the preoperative assessment, we feel that a CT scan is necessary to measure it.

The extraction of a properly integrated cementless stem can be difficult and problematic with any approach, and it is not uncommon that the surgeon performs a femorotomy in certain cases. It is clear that this can be even more complex through the DAA, and a surgeon who is not experienced in this area must reflect carefully before performing it! Personally, we are less and less hesitant to operate complex cases through DAA, but 30 years of experience allow us to know the limits of this surgery. Revision of a well-fixed femoral stem through DAA may require partial or more complex femorotomies. We will describe two techniques that we have developed that do not really require an extension of the approach. If well executed, both are atraumatic and do not damage the surrounding soft tissues.

Less Invasive Femorotomies

The first technique is known as "bicycle technique"in reference to the fixation of the seatpost on a regular bike (**d**). A simple medial longitudinal osteotomy is made on the calcar, in the axis of the prosthetic neck, using a narrow oscillating saw and a long osteotome (Fig. 36.3a,b).

This technique may require additional distal exposure, avoiding damage to the vastus lateralis vessels and nerves, which are below the lesser trochanter. In the majority of cases, it is sufficient to simply take off and slide under the vastus lateralis for 5–7 cm. It is not useful to place the lower limb in extension, because anterior soft tissues will be under increased tension and may be damaged. The lower limb should simply be placed in full external rotation and no extension with the orthopaedic traction table. To make the procedure even safer, the person handling the table should be asked to push the femur towards the iliac crest. This gives the possibility to work on the upper 7–8 cm of the femur without increasing the size of the incision.

This longitudinal osteotomy of 3–7 cm on the upper part of the femur gives a certain flexibility to the bone and will allow thin and long osteotomes to be passed on each side of the implant to mobilize it and finally extract it. Only at this time, it is necessary to position the hip in extension, with the leg back on the ground.

After removing the stem, one or two 3.5 mm cortical lag screws are used to firmly close the medial femorotomy at the level of the lesser trochanter (Fig. 36.3c). It is quite possible to use a cerclage wire if the bone quality is not suitable for screw fixation.

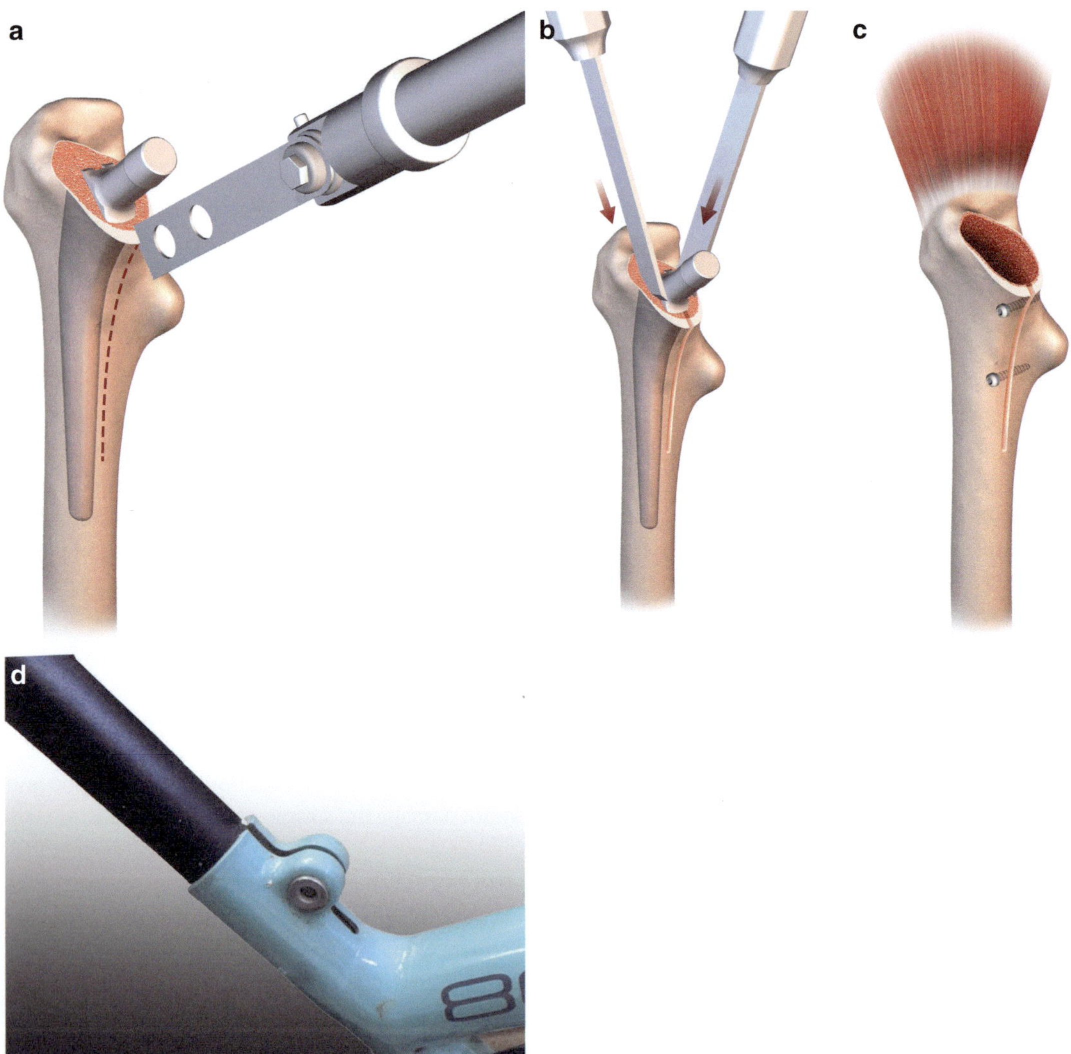

Fig. 36.3 The technique of the bicycle: a medial longitudinal femorotomy is done in the calcar, along the femoral shaft (**a**). Long and narrow chisels are used to mobilize the stem (**b**). Then, if the bone thickness is good, one or 2 cortical screws can be used to fix the osteotomy (**c**). The fixation mechanism of a bicycle seat post, from where comes the name of this technique (**d**)

The other technical solution consists of an osteotomy of the greater trochanter (trochanterotomy from the inside), which can be performed through the inner part of the hip after its dislocation in external rotation and extension. The osteotomy is done with an oscillating saw and finished with a curved chisel. It starts laterally to the stem shoulder, at the junction level of the femoral neck and greater trochanter. Ideally, a chevron osteotomy should be performed (Fig. 36.4a), as

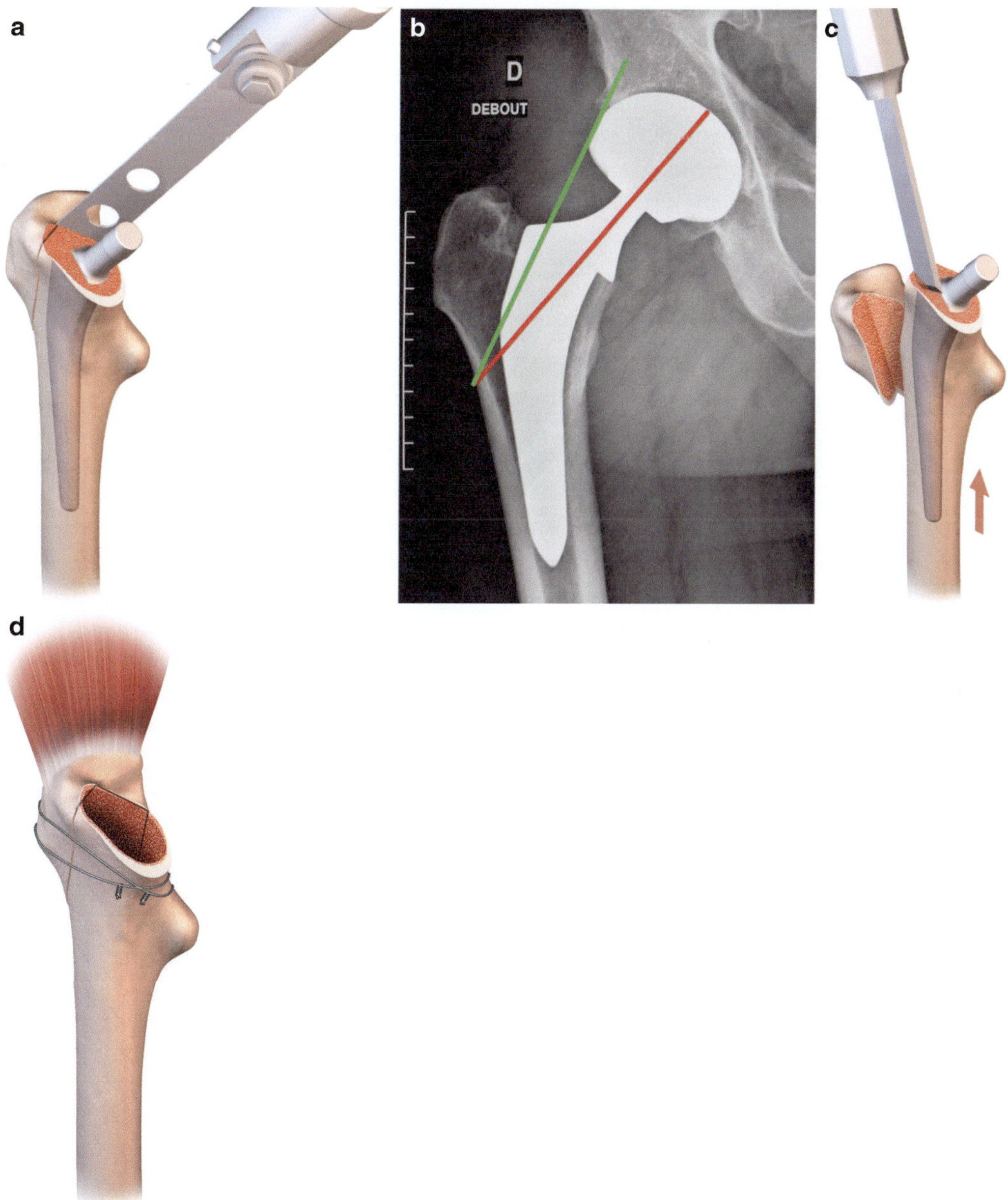

Fig. 36.4 A chevron osteotomy is started through the anterior approach (**a**). The leg is extended. The osteotomy line must be as vertical as possible. The femoral neck of the stem can be used to define the perfect angle on the preop X-ray (**b**). The traction table is used to push the femoral shaft outside the incision (**c**). The foot can even be removed from the extension table to really help the manoeuvres. At the end of the procedure the osteotomy can be left unfixed but for antalgic reason, it is preferable to stabilize the GT with one or 2 cerclages (**d**)

it allows simple bone repositioning at the end of surgery and improves the postoperative stability. It is also essential to make an osteotomy line as vertical as possible, because the more vertical is the line, the easier the osteosynthesis and consolidation will be (Fig. 36.4b). A line that is too horizontal can lead to non-union. A curved chisel can be used to continue the cut distally beyond the vastus ridge, as far as possible on the femoral shaft, and the cut does not even need to be completed in order to keep a hinge at the lower part of the greater trochanter. The main advantage of this greater trochanter osteotomy is that gluteal and vastus lateralis muscles remain unharmed and attached to the greater trochanter, leading to vascularization preservation and increasing final stability.

By detaching the greater trochanter, the femoral shaft can be easily mobilized, improving the stem exposition and removal (Fig. 36.4c). This trochanterotomy from the inside makes possible the mobilization of the femur in a very impressive way, and if the leg is detached from the extension table, we will have a perfect view of the femoral canal. Using this artifice, it is possible to place a long stem and to extract distal cement fragments in case of infection, for example.

As the soft tissues surrounding the greater trochanter are intact, its antero-posterior movements will be prevented and it will not tend to mobilize afterwards. Therefore, at the end of the procedure the surgeon has the choice of not fixing the trochanterotomy, since the fragment simply returns to the right place and consolidates easily. However, fixation using one or two cerclage wires to stabilize it, for analgesic purposes, can be performed at the end of the surgery (Fig. 36.4d).

Distal Approach Extension

In complex cases, the first and second techniques can be combined (Fig. 36.5). But if a large anterior femoral flap needs to be detached to remove a distally well-fixed femoral stem, an extended trochanteric osteotomy (ETO) should be performed. For this purpose, it is necessary to extend the incision downwards.

The DAA can be extended distally by lengthening the skin incision towards the lateral midline of the thigh (Fig. 36.6a). By placing the lower limb in abduction, we will reduce the tension on the fascia lata and give ourselves a better view. The fascia lata is split in its anterior third as far as necessary for femoral exposure. Subsequently, the vastus lateralis muscle can be elevated off its intermuscular septum from posterior to anterior or split in line with its fibres depending on the surgeon's preference and the amount of femur requiring exposure. It is also advisable to apply rotations. Internal rotation gives access to the posterior part of the vastus lateralis. Caution must be taken with the perforating vessels that supply vastus lateralis and they must be ligated to minimize bleeding (Fig. 36.6b).

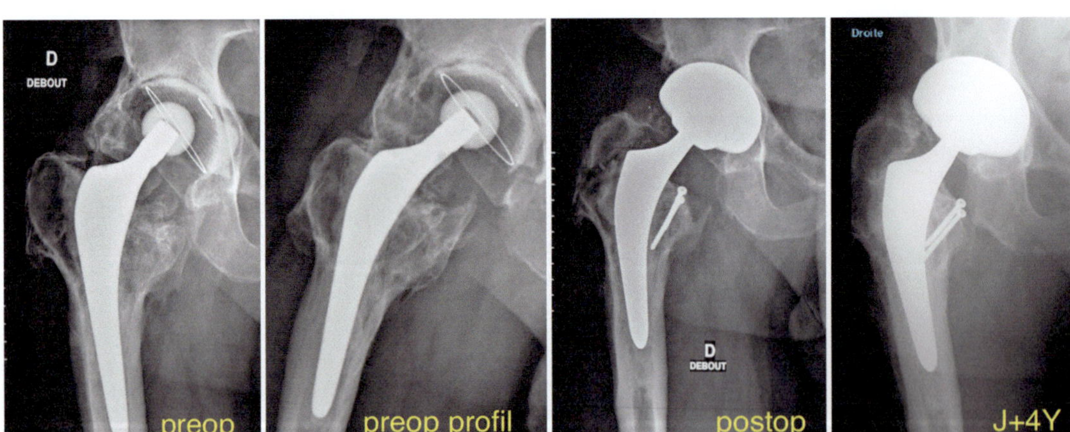

Fig. 36.5 Loose cup but the prosthetic femur was placed with more than 15° of retroversion. To remove the stem an inside trochanterotomy was mandatory. We also use the bicycle technique to extract the stem. Both techniques in difficult cases can be associated

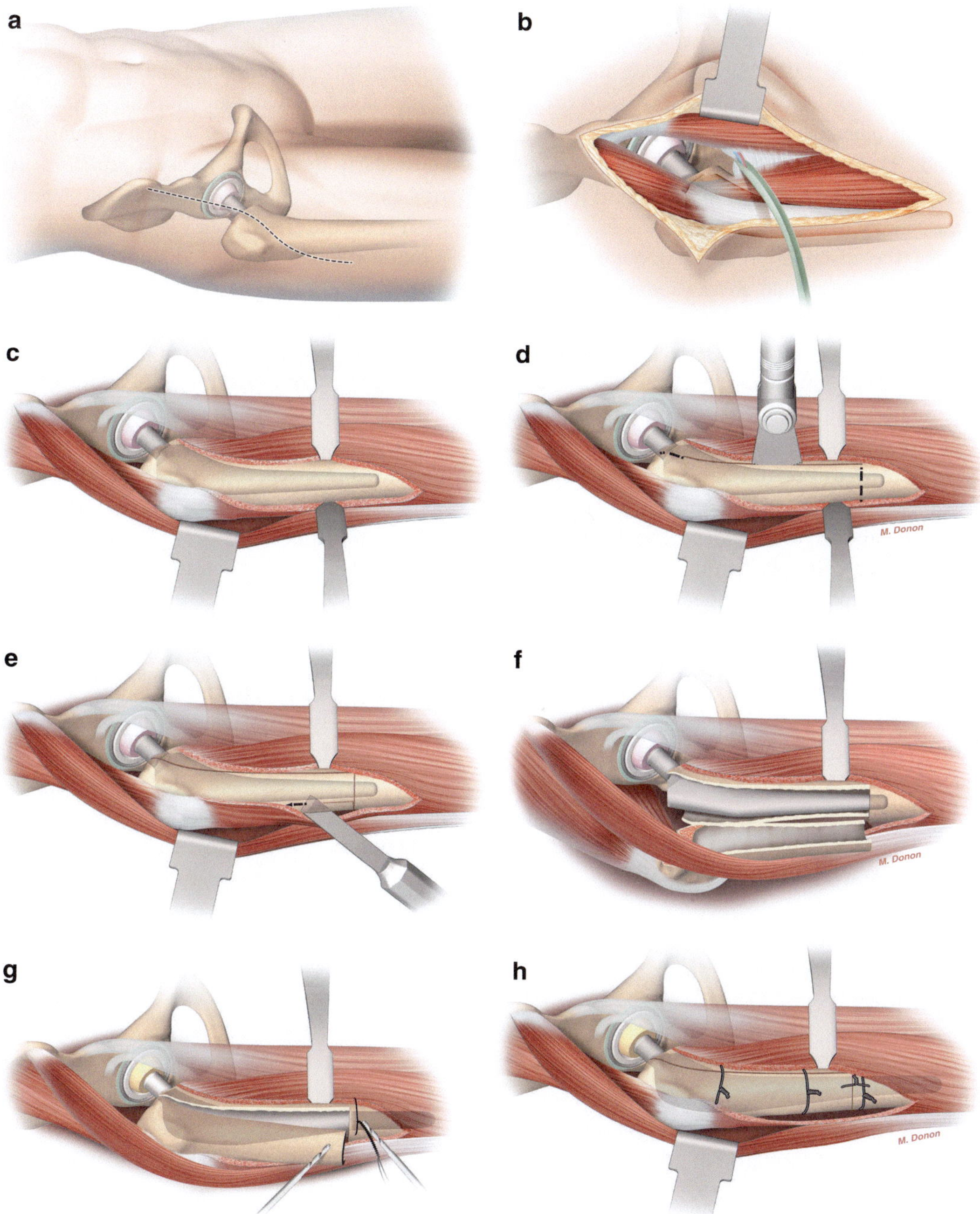

Fig. 36.6 Incision is extended as necessary in the direction of lateral midline of the tight (**a**). It is important to see and protect the vessels and the nerves of the vastus lateralis (**b**). Detaching the vastus lateralis from the lateral and anterior part of the femur preserves the vascularization of the muscle. The muscle is pushed inward (**c**). The first anterior cut is done with an oscillating saw (**d**). The posterior cut is done with a long and narrow chisel to preserve the muscle insertion (**e**). The osteotomy is opened, preserving a posterior hinge (**f**). The stem is removed, a prophylactic cerclage wire is placed distally to the osteotomy level and a new long stem can be inserted (**g**). Tensioning the soft tissue with the traction table and using fluoroscopy control may be helpful to adjust the length and offset. The ETO is fixed with 2 or 3 cerclages (**h**)

An alternative and more traditional distal exposure of the femur can be performed by making a separate lateral approach along the posterior palpable border of the femur. A skin bridge of 5–7 cm between the two incisions is recommended. The exposure is carried distally and splits the fascia lata, similar to a standard femoral lateral approach.

Since the distal approach extension is performed, the vastus lateralis is reflected off the femur for at least 10 cm, exposing its lateral and anterior cortices (Fig. 36.6c). The length of the ETO should be preoperatively planned according to the underlying stem (Fig. 36.6d,e). The lines of the osteotomy are drawn using a marker, and a saw is used to cut the antero-lateral femoral cortical vertically and horizontally. Then, using a drill bit, aligned multiple perforations in the postero-lateral femoral cortical are performed, serving as a posterior hinge. Osteotomes are placed in the anterolateral cut, allowing the fragment to be levered and opened in the anterior-posterior direction (Fig. 36.6f). This exposes the anterior, lateral and posterior sides of the stem. It is important to maintain an intact muscular sleeve attached to the greater trochanter and diaphyseal femoral fragment. After removing the stem and inserting another one, the ETO must be fixed with cerclage wires (Fig. 36.6g–h).

Evolution of Stem Revision Techniques

The implants in THA have developed considerably in the last 20 years. Aiming to not damage the bone stock, the bearing surfaces and stem designs have substantially improved. The new polyethylene and ceramic bearing surfaces are more resistant, causing less osteolysis, minimal wear and debris. At the same time, primary stems have been shortened and are granting satisfactory results [24–28]. Therefore, we have found it to be particularly interesting to use a primary stem, shorter than the one removed, in our anterior revision procedures.

When a standard cemented stem is extracted, the majority of surgeons remove all the cement mantle, the plug and the distal bone formation when present, thus risking to create a false trajectory, perforation, or a femur fracture. However, if we use a primary stem that is shorter than the one removed, it is not necessary to remove the plug or distal bone formation, reducing these risky steps. This simplifies the procedure and diminishes the risk of complications.

After cleaning the intramedullary femoral canal, a careful bone stock evaluation must be done and we have two options:

1. In cases with minimal bone defects and a good bone quality, uncemented short stems can be used for revision, since they achieve sufficient primary stability (press fit) and metaphyseal fixation (Fig. 36.7a–d).
2. In cases with extensive bone defects, proximal femoral deformities or poor bone quality, it is possible to envisage reconstruction with impacted bone grafts and to cement a shorter stem than the one removed leaving the plug and the distal cement. This reconstruction technique consists of impacting morselized bone grafts in the intramedullary femoral canal, which improves its inner quality and allows a better imbrication of the cement that is subsequently introduced (Figs. 36.8a–g).

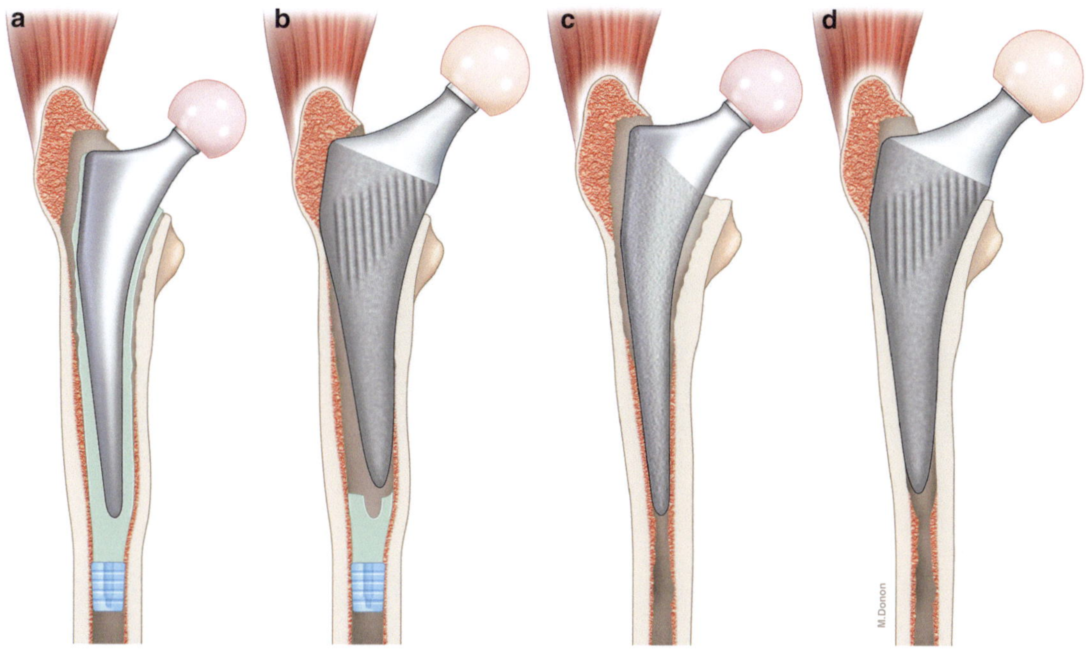

Fig. 36.7 A loose cemented stem is removed (**a**). The inside trochanterotomy or the bicycle technic can be used if needed. The bone quality is satisfactory to implant a stable cementless primary stem, shorter than the one removed. The distal cement and the plug do not need to be removed (**b**). A loose cementless stem is removed (**c**). The remaining bone has also good quality and a stable cementless primary stem, shorter than the one removed, is implanted. No need to fight to remove a bony pedestal to pass a longer stem (**c**, **d**)

Some Surgical Experience

Between 2010 and 2017, the senior surgeon performed revision THA through DAA (AMIS®, Anterior Minimally Invasive Surgery), using shorter stems than those removed, in 45 hips (42 patients). This cohort was composed of 24 women (26 hips) and 18 men (19 hips), aged 64.5 ± 9.5 years and with a BMI of 25.1 ± 4.0 kg/m^2. The reasons for revision THA were aseptic loosening in 37 hips (82%), periprosthetic joint infection in 4 hips (9%), periprosthetic fracture in 2 hips (4%) and instability in 2 hips (4%).

Twenty-two hips (49%) had isolated stem revision, while 23 hips (51%) had cup and stem revision. Previous stem fixation was cemented in 23 hips (51%) and uncemented in 22 hips (49%). To help in stem extraction, 3 cases needed adjuvant procedures: 2 femorotomies (4%) and 1 greater trochanter osteotomy combined with the "bicycle technique". Regarding the stems, 24 hips (53%) were revised with primary cemented stems and impaction bone grafting technique using the polished AMIStem® (Medacta International, Switzerland) while 21 hips (47%) were revised with primary uncemented stems using the fully hydroxyapatite-coated AMIStem® (7 hips, 16%) or MiniMax® (14 hips, 31%) (Medacta International, Switzerland) (Fig. 36.9).

During revision THA, morselized bone grafts were used in all cemented stems (24 hips, 100%), and in some uncemented stems (10 hips, 47%) when any small remaining gaps between the stem and the host bone were present.

Regarding rehabilitation, patients were authorized to walk with crutches in partial weight-bearing for 3–6 weeks, before walking unaided. All patients received low-molecular-weight heparin for 3–6 weeks as routine thromboprophylaxis.

Amongst the 45 hips (42 patients), 4 hips (4 patients) were lost to follow-up. One hip (1 patient) had a stem re-revision after 13 months

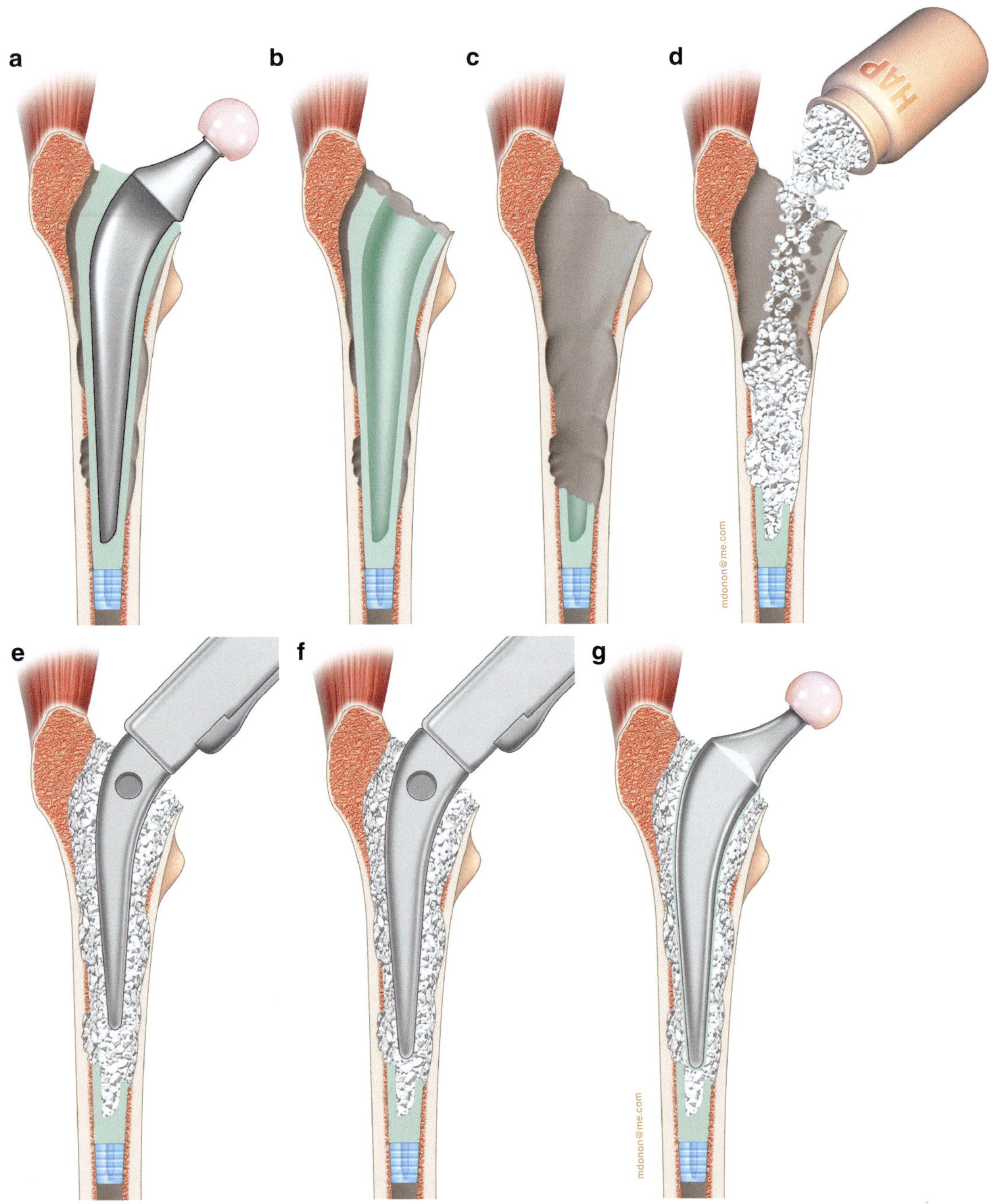

Fig. 36.8 The loose cemented stem is removed (**a**, **b**). If the bone quality does not allow the implantation of a cementless primary stem, a reconstruction with impaction bone grafting and cemented stem is the solution. There is no need to remove the distal plug or the distal cement if they are well fixed (**c**). The morselized bone graft is impacted in the femoral canal gradually (**d–f**) and the new cemented primary stem, shorter than the one removed, is implanted (**d–g**)

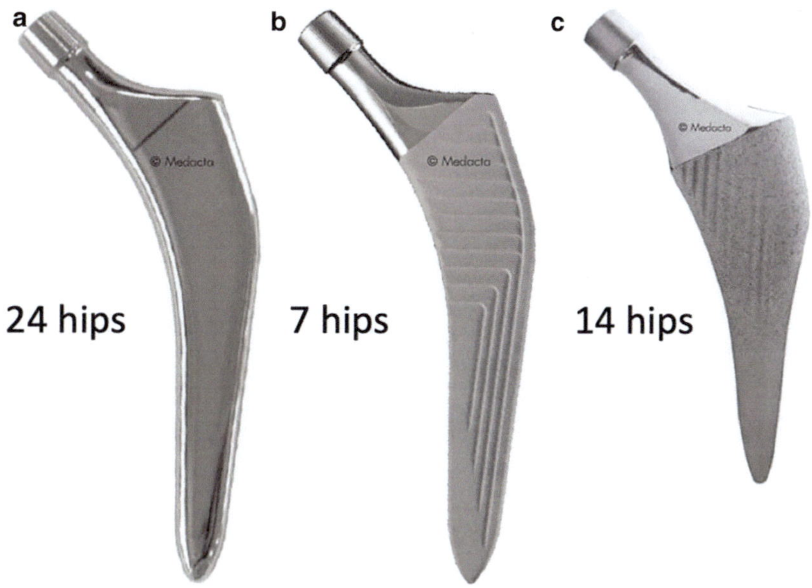

Fig. 36.9 Stems used for revision THA through DAA. (**a**) The polished AMIStem®. (**b**) The fully hydroxyapatite-coated AMIStem-P®. (C) The fully Titanium plasma-sprayed (MectaGrip®) and hydroxyapatite-coated MiniMax®

due to stem loosening, which was associated with an intraoperative calcar crack not fixed during first revision, and another hip (1 patient) had a reoperation to exchange the femoral head after 1 month to treat limb length discrepancy.

Intraoperative complications were observed in 5 hips (5 patients): 1 small femoral calcar crack, fixed with orthoCord wire; 3 femoral fractures, 2 of which were fixed with cerclage wire only, and 1 of which was fixed with a trochanteric plate, screws and cerclage wire; 1 greater trochanter non-displaced fracture was left untreated. Postoperative complications, treated without stem re-revision, were noted in 3 hips (3 patients): 1 transitory neuropraxia of the LFCN, and 2 cases of dislocation, undergoing closed reduction.

The final cohort of 40 hips (40 patients) was assessed at 3.5 ± 1.9 years (range, 1.1–8.1). Their modified Harris Hip Score (mHHS) improved from 50.9 ± 12.7 to 87.9 ± 16.0, with 28 patients (30 hips, 75%) claiming to be very satisfied after the revision THA (Table 36.1). The only patient who had a stem re-revision was evaluated at 2 years and had a mHHS of 100.

Concerning the post-revision THA radiographic assessment, bone remodelling was observed in 4 hips, cortical hypertrophy in 3 hips, subsidence <2 mm in 4 hips and subsidence <4 mm in 1 hip. In the cemented stems, 1 hip had a distal cement fracture, while radiolucent lines <2 mm thick were observed, in less than 4 Gruen zones, at the bone-cement interface in 3 hips and at the cement-stem interface in 3 hips. In the uncemented stems, 1 hip had progressive stress shielding, but all stems were well osteointegrated. Grade I heterotopic ossification was seen in 6 hips and grade II was seen in 1 hip. There were no signs of osteolysis, loosening, or fractures at final follow-up (Figs. 36.10a–c, 36.11 and 36.12).

Table 36.1 Clinical outcomes for the final cohort

	Final Cohort (n = 40 hips)			Cemented stem RTHA (n = 20 hips)			Uncemented stem RTHA (n = 20 hips)			
	Mean ± SD	Median	Range	Mean ± SD	Median	Range	Mean ± SD	Median	Range	*p-value*
Follow-up (years)	3.5 ± 1.9	2.6	(1.1 – 8.1)	4.0 ± 2.1	3.8	(1.2–8.1)	2.9 ± 1.4	2.4	(1.1 – 6.5)	*0.204*
mHHS										
Pre-revision	50.9 ± 12.7	51	(32–81)	46.5 ± 11.8	45	(32–68)	55.2 ± 12.3	57	(33–81)	*0.035*
Post-revision	87.9 ± 16.0	94	(33–100)	87.0 ± 18.6	94	(33–100)	88.8 ± 13.3	96	(52–100)	*0.912*
Net improvement	37.0 ± 19.0	39	(−21–65)	40.5 ± 21.9	47	(−21–65)	33.5 ± 15.3	32	(3–61)	*0.070*
Post-revision satisfaction										
Very satisfied	30 (75.0%)			15 (75.0%)			15 (75.0%)			
Satisfied	8 (20.0%)			4 (20.0%)			4 (20.0%)			
Disappointed	2 (5.0%)			1 (5.0%)			1 (5.0%)			

Abbreviations: *RTHA* revision total hip arthroplasty, *mHHS* modified Harris hip score, *SD* standard deviation
Comparison between cemented and uncemented RTHA

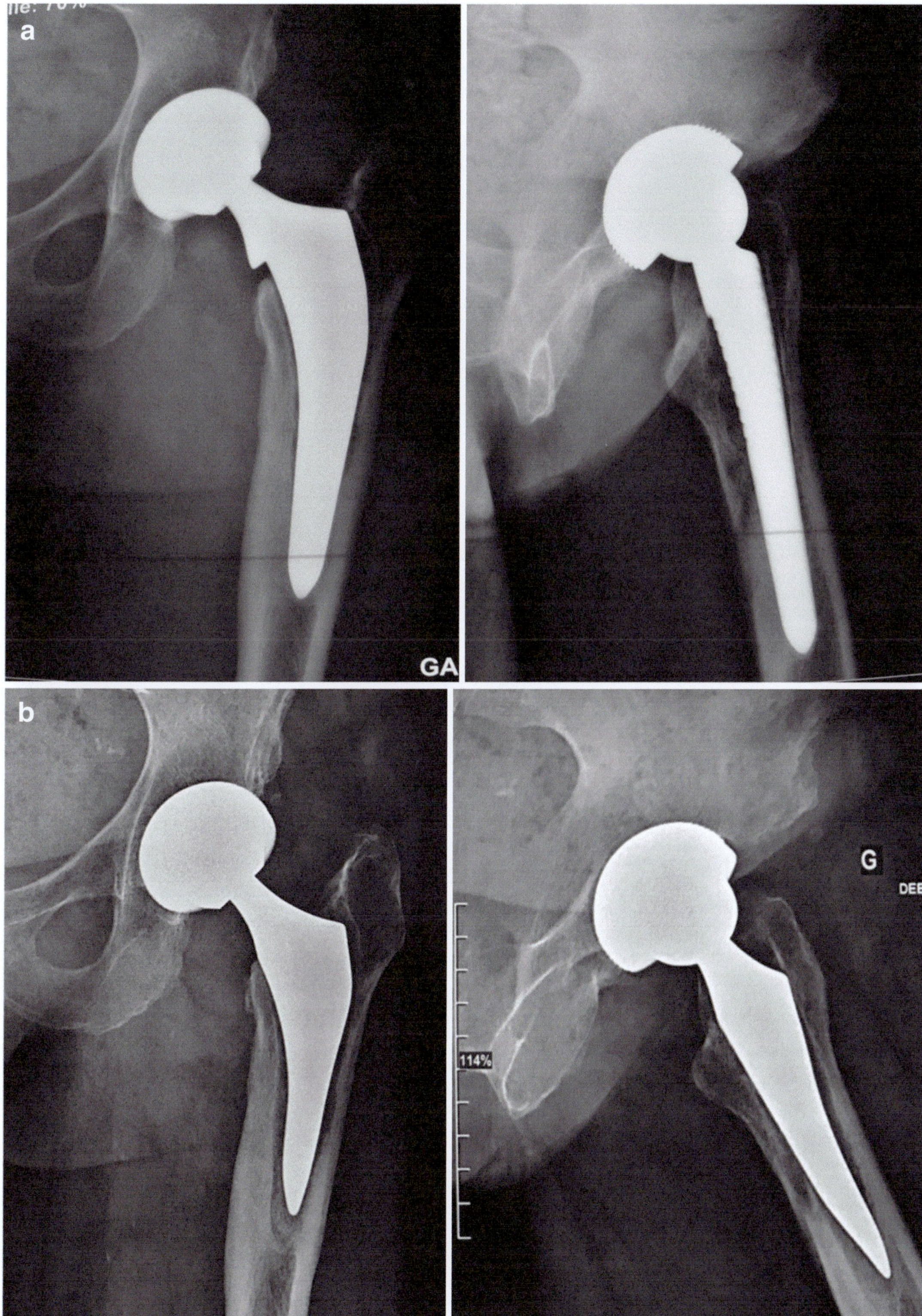

Fig. 36.10 Preoperative (**a**), 2 months postoperative (**b**), and 2 years postoperative (**c**) radiographs of the left hip (Paprosky II) underwent revision THA through DAA using shorter stem than the one removed

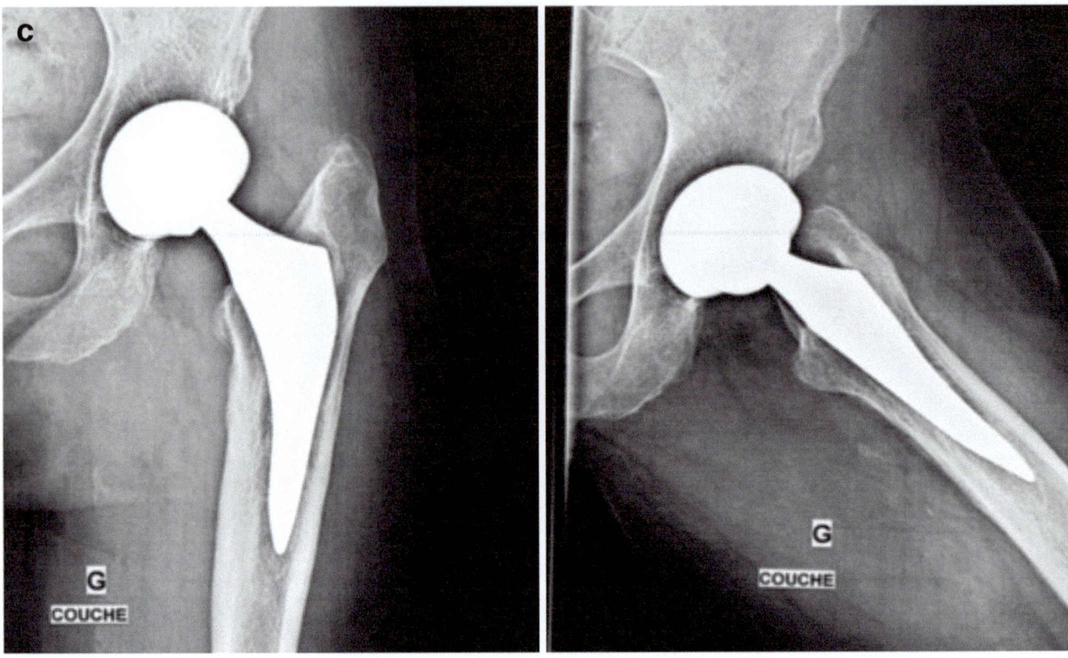

Fig. 36.10 (continued)

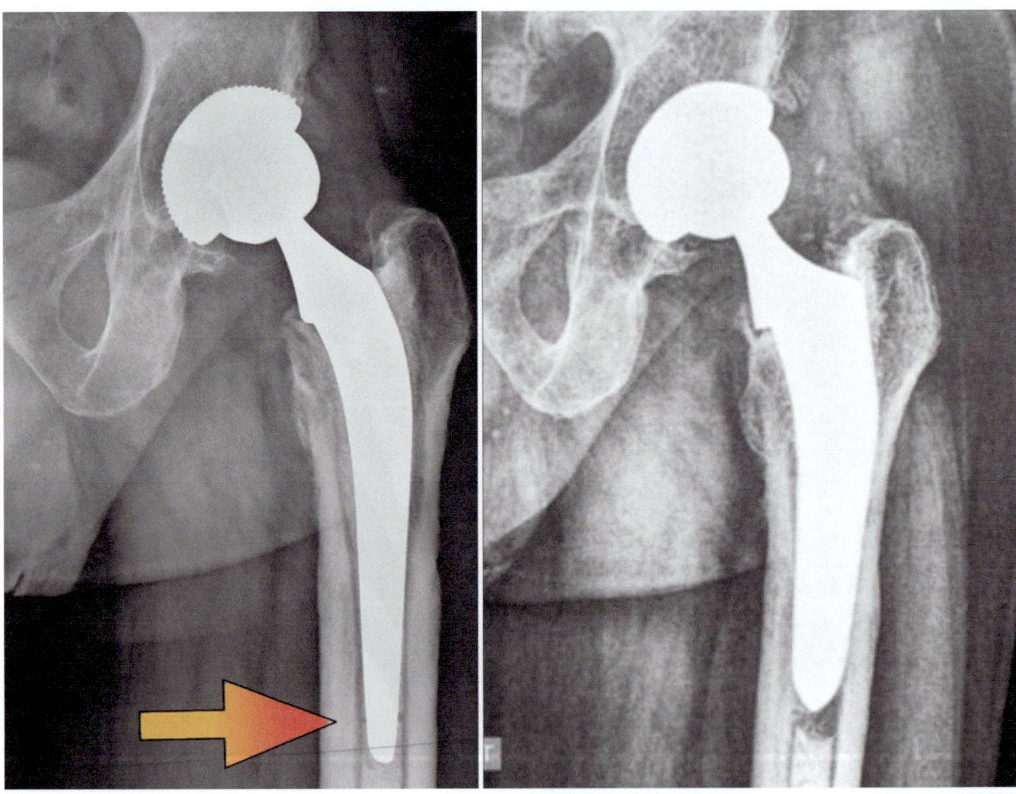

Fig. 36.11 Preoperative (**a**), 2 months postoperative (**b**), and 5 years postoperative (**c**) radiographs of the left hip (Paprosky II) underwent revision THA through DAA using shorter stem than the one removed. The distal cement of the previous stem did not need to be removed using this technique

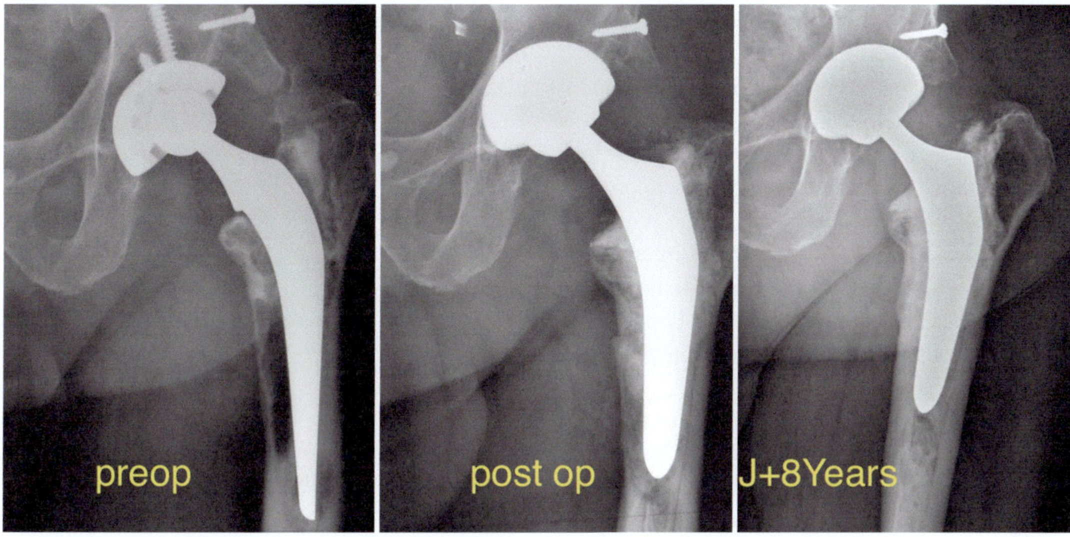

Fig. 36.12 Preoperative (**a**), one-month postoperative (**b**), and 8 years postoperative (**c**) radiographs of the left hip (Paprosky III A) underwent revision THA through DAA using shorter stem than the one removed. The femoral reconstruction used impacted bone grafts and cementation

Discussion

The DAA for THA has a long tradition in Paris. For surgeons, students of Letournel or Robert Judet, the Hueter's approach has always been the "gold standard" for hip arthroplasties. Since the development of minimally invasive techniques, the DAA is once again being performed and far beyond Paris.

In the USA, the DAA has been used by some surgeons. Keggi and Kennon [29] have already presented a large series of revision THA through DAA without a traction table. Their series was the first to publish revision THA through DAA. The main technical difference with our series is that we systematically use an orthopaedic traction table. Some surgeons have shown that the traction table is not a necessary element for performing THA through DAA [30–33]. This may be true for primary THA, but in cases of revision THA, the traction table seems to be indispensable in order to position the lower limb correctly to facilitate exposure. Moreover, in cases of revision, the traction table decreases the surgical time and the work of the assistant is greatly simplified. The more experience we acquire with an orthopaedic traction table, the more useful it becomes, especially when a perioperative difficulty arises.

Regarding the bone stock preservation in revision THA, the use of primary stems has resulted in satisfactory outcomes and has become a more attractive practice [11, 16–23]. Furthermore, its use is more suitable, particularly through DAA, and it is even better if shorter primary stems than those removed are used, because the surgeon does not need to be aggressive with distal bone management and plug removal.

Concerning soft tissue preservation, the DAA offers some advantages over the others, such as reduction of pain, recovery time, and dislocation rates [15–22], mainly because it is a minimally invasive approach, which preserves the inter-nervous and inter-muscular planes [23]. Primary THA performed through the DAA has proven to grant excellent outcomes [24–26]. For an isolated liner change or revision of a resurfacing failure, the surgical exposure remains similar to a primary arthroplasty and the post-operative recovery remains comparable too, so we consider it very fast. Additionally, acetabular cup revision through the DAA also presented satisfactory results [27–29]. However, there is little evidence regarding outcomes of femoral revision through the DAA [29].

In cases of revisions of the femoral component requiring a longer revision stem, this approach is not recommended, especially if the surgeon does not have enough experience with this approach. Nowadays, we are able to manage complex cases, but we also believe that the surgeon who has a good experience in the posterior approach for revision THA should probably continue in this way, especially if he does not have a large revision volume.

In cases of significant retroversion of the femoral implant, it is very important to be aware that it may be impossible to extract it without performing a trochanterotomy, and therefore, before considering a DAA, a preoperative CT scan should be assessed. If the retroversion is greater than 15 degrees, the choice of approach should be discussed.

Femoral bone grafting can be performed by the DAA if the bone defect is grade II or grade III in the Paprosky classification. Grade IV bone loss is a contraindication for this approach, while grade III should be discussed case-by-case.

With experience, we are becoming more and more confident in our technique and currently most of our revisions are performed using DAA and shorter stems, even if the patient has had a posterior approach initially.

Conclusions

Despite the fact that THA through DAA is not yet widely incorporated into hip surgeons' routines, its popularity is increasing thanks to the well-known advantages regarding the faster functional recovery and rehabilitation. Through this chapter, our aim has been to provide tips and tricks with respect to this surgical technique for revision THA through DAA, including the extensile approach, which may be used in some cases. Moreover, we noted satisfactory outcomes of this technique in the senior surgeon's experience, particularly using shorter stems than those removed. It is of utmost importance for the surgeon to gather enough experience in DAA before choosing to incorporate revision THA through DAA in his/her own practice.

References

1. Kurtz S, Ong K, Lau E, Mowat F, Halpern M. Projections of primary and revision hip and knee arthroplasty in the United States from 2005 to 2030. J Bone Joint Surg Am. 2007;89(4):780–5.
2. National Joint Registry for England W, Northern Ireland and the Isle of Man. 15th Annual Report. In. 2018.
3. Australian Orthopaedic Association National Joint Replacement Registry. Annual Report: Hip, Knee & Shoulder Arthroplasty. In. 2019.
4. Kerboull L. Selecting the surgical approach for revision total hip arthroplasty. Orthop Traumatol Surg Res. 2015;101(1 Suppl):S171–8.
5. Mast NH, Laude F. Revision total hip arthroplasty performed through the Hueter interval. J Bone Joint Surg Am. 2011;93 Suppl 2:143–8.
6. Manrique J, Chen AF, Heller S, Hozack WJ. Direct anterior approach for revision total hip arthroplasty. Ann Transl Med. 2014;2(10):100.
7. Goldberg TD, Torres A, Molli R. Femoral component revisions in direct anterior approach. EC Orthopaedics. 2016;4(3):518–26.
8. Gabor JA, Padilla JA, Feng JE, Schnaser E, Lutes WB, Park KJ, et al. Short-term outcomes with the REDAPT monolithic, tapered, fluted, grit-blasted, forged titanium revision femoral stem. Bone Joint J. 2020;102-b(2):191–7.
9. Ngu AWT, Rowan FE, Carli AV, Haddad FS. Single 3 degrees tapered fluted femoral stems demonstrate low subsidence at mid-term follow-up in severe bony deficiency. Ann Transl Med. 2019;7(23):725.
10. Herry Y, Viste A, Bothorel H, Desmarchelier R, Fessy MH. Long-term survivorship of a monoblock long cementless stem in revision total hip arthroplasty. Int Orthop. 2019;43(10):2279–84.
11. Cavagnaro L, Formica M, Basso M, Zanirato A, Divano S, Felli L. Femoral revision with primary cementless stems: a systematic review of the literature. Musculoskelet Surg. 2018;102(1):1–9.
12. Bugbee WD, Culpepper WJ 2nd, Engh CA Jr, Engh CA Sr. Long-term clinical consequences of stress-shielding after total hip arthroplasty without cement. J Bone Joint Surg Am. 1997;79(7):1007–12.
13. Busch CA, Charles MN, Haydon CM, Bourne RB, Rorabeck CH, Macdonald SJ, et al. Fractures of distally-fixed femoral stems after revision arthroplasty. J Bone Joint Surg Br. 2005;87(10):1333–6.
14. Krishnamurthy AB, MacDonald SJ, Paprosky WG. 5- to 13-year follow-up study on cementless femo-

ral components in revision surgery. J Arthroplast. 1997;12(8):839–47.
15. MacDonald SJ, Rosenzweig S, Guerin JS, McCalden RW, Bohm ER, Bourne RB, et al. Proximally versus fully porous-coated femoral stems: a multicenter randomized trial. Clin Orthop Relat Res. 2010;468(2):424–32.
16. Stigbrand H, Ullmark G. A 3- to 18-year follow-up of revision total hip arthroplasty with impacted bone allografts and cemented Lubinus SP II stem. Clinical, radiographic, and survivorship analysis with comparison to the literature. J Arthroplast. 2017;32(9):2810–4.
17. Petrie MJ, Harrison TP, Buckley SC, Gordon A, Kerry RM, Hamer AJ. Stay short or go long? Can a standard cemented femoral prosthesis be used at second-stage Total hip arthroplasty revision for infection following an extended trochanteric osteotomy? J Arthroplast. 2017;32(7):2226–30.
18. Gastaud O, Cambas PM, Tabutin J. Femoral revision with a primary cementless stem. Orthop Traumatol Surg Res. 2016;102(2):149–53.
19. Tetreault MW, Shukla SK, Yi PH, Sporer SM, Della Valle CJ. Are short fully coated stems adequate for "simple" femoral revisions? Clin Orthop Relat Res. 2014;472(2):577–83.
20. Pinaroli A, Lavoie F, Cartillier JC, Neyret P, Selmi TA. Conservative femoral stem revision: avoiding therapeutic escalation. J Arthroplast. 2009;24(3):365–73.
21. Howie DW, Wimhurst JA, McGee MA, Carbone TA, Badaruddin BS. Revision total hip replacement using cemented collarless double-taper femoral components. J Bone Joint Surg Br. 2007;89(7):879–86.
22. Kelly SJ, Incavo SJ, Beynnon B. The use of a hydroxyapatite-coated primary stem in revision total hip arthroplasty. J Arthroplast. 2006;21(1):64–71.
23. Khanuja HS, Issa K, Naziri Q, Banerjee S, Delanois RE, Mont MA. Results of a tapered proximally-coated primary cementless stem for revision hip surgery. J Arthroplast. 2014;29(1):225–8.
24. Jia F, Guo B, Xu F, Hou Y, Tang X, Huang L. A comparison of clinical, radiographic and surgical outcomes of total hip arthroplasty between direct anterior and posterior approaches: a systematic review and meta-analysis. Hip Int. 2019;29(6):584–96.
25. Wang Z, Hou JZ, Wu CH, Zhou YJ, Gu XM, Wang HH, et al. A systematic review and meta-analysis of direct anterior approach versus posterior approach in total hip arthroplasty. J Orthop Surg Res. 2018;13(1):229.
26. Rodriguez JA, Deshmukh AJ, Rathod PA, Greiz ML, Deshmane PP, Hepinstall MS, et al. Does the direct anterior approach in THA offer faster rehabilitation and comparable safety to the posterior approach? Clin Orthop Relat Res. 2014;472(2):455–63.
27. Sariali E, Leonard P, Mamoudy P. Dislocation after total hip arthroplasty using Hueter anterior approach. J Arthroplast. 2008;23(2):266–72.
28. Siguier T, Siguier M, Brumpt B. Mini-incision anterior approach does not increase dislocation rate: a study of 1037 total hip replacements. Clin Orthop Relat Res. 2004;426:164–73.
29. Kennon R, Keggi J, Zatorski LE, Keggi KJ. Anterior approach for total hip arthroplasty: beyond the minimally invasive technique. J Bone Joint Surg Am. 2004;86-A Suppl 2:91–7.
30. Bender B, Nogler M, Hozack WJ. Direct anterior approach for total hip arthroplasty. Orthop Clin North Am. 2009;40(3):321–8.
31. Lovell TP. Single-incision direct anterior approach for total hip arthroplasty using a standard operating table. J Arthroplast. 2008;23(7 Suppl):64–8.
32. Rachbauer F, Kain MS, Leunig M. The history of the anterior approach to the hip. Orthop Clin North Am. 2009;40(3):311–20.
33. Seng BE, Berend KR, Ajluni AF, Lombardi AV. Anterior-supine minimally invasive total hip arthroplasty: defining the learning curve. Orthop Clin North Am. 2009;40(3):343–50.

37 Complex Acetabular Reconstruction Using the Direct Anterior Approach

Jonathan Yerasimides and Daniel March

Acetabular Defects (Paprosky & AAOS Classifications)

Complex acetabular reconstruction presents one of the greatest technical challenges in the field of arthroplasty, as loss of bone stock and column support can make achieving stable component fixation difficult. Historically, polyethylene wear following total hip arthroplasty led to osteolysis and generated aseptic loosening of the acetabular component with large associated bone defects. Acetabular defects can also be caused by fracture (traumatic or insufficiency), infection, oncogenic processes, or be iatrogenic due to over reaming or prior oncogenic resection. They can also present in the native hip due to developmental dysplasia of the hip, avascular necrosis, or inflammatory arthritis.

As with all complex cases, thorough preoperative planning is critical to help guide the surgeon's choice of technique and implants. In the setting of acetabular deficiencies, the two most widely accepted classification systems that provided detailed defect descriptions and help guide treatment are those of Paprosky et al. and the American Academy of Orthopaedic Surgeons (AAOS) [1, 2]. Larger defects, classified as Paprosky 3A and 3B or AAOS Type III and IV, particularly those involving pelvic discontinuity, tend to create the greatest reconstructive challenges. Pelvic discontinuity is a rarer type of defect, involving complete dissociation of the superior and inferior hemipelvis and representing only 0.9–2.1% of revision THA cases [3]. Matching the appropriate construct to a given pattern of acetabular deficiency is necessary for success.

Treatment Options

The last 15 years have seen a steady increase in the use of the direct anterior approach (DAA) with the theoretical advantages of using an internervous and intermuscular plane and minimizing muscle damage, thus improving patient recovery and outcomes. In studies comparing DAA to a posterior approach, DAA patients have been found to have less postoperative pain and require less pain medication during their hospital stay [4], were able to ambulate farther [4], had a shorter hospital stay [4, 5], and were more likely to meet goals for discharge home [6]. When compared to an anterolateral approach, studies have found DAA patients demonstrate improved ambulation and single-leg support at 6–12 weeks postoperatively [7]. Compared to a mini-posterior approach, DAA patients were also able to ambulate earlier without assistive devices [8]. Given these advantages to DAA in the primary setting, surgeons becoming more comfortable with the

J. Yerasimides (✉) · D. March
Norton Orthopedic Institute, Louisville, KY, USA

J. M. Matta, A. P. Sah (eds.), *Anterior Hip Replacement*,
https://doi.org/10.1007/978-3-030-91896-5_37

approach have expanded indications to include complex primary and revision surgeries. Surgeon experience and a growing body of literature support the ability to successfully manage even the most complex cases through the anterior approach.

Many treatment options for acetabular reconstruction in the setting of bony defects have been described in the literature. An incomplete list includes bone impaction grafting; structural allografts; non-cemented hemispherical cups, including highly porous cups such as Trabecular Metal™ (Zimmer Biomet, Warsaw, IN); jumbo cups; pelvic distraction; porous metal augments; antiprotrusio cages; cup-cage constructs; bilobed and oblong cups; and custom-made triflange acetabular components (CTACs) [9–15]. The majority of publications describing these techniques are small case series providing low levels of evidence, and even large systematic reviews typically include only a few hundred total cases [3, 15]. As management has evolved over the past 3 decades and outcomes have been compared among these various techniques, some options, such as bilobed and oblong cups, have fallen out of favor and are now of mostly historical interest. A full description of all of these techniques and related research is beyond the scope of this chapter. We will instead focus on a smaller number of constructs with good clinical track records, emphasizing how they can be successfully performed via an anterior approach.

Augments

Given some of the problems associated with structural allograft, porous metal augments have become an increasingly popular tool for filling bone defects in acetabular revision. Porous metal offers several advantages: a high coefficient of friction that provides a "scratch fit" to assist with initial stability; a modulus of elasticity similar to bone; and the highly porous internal structure mimics that of cancellous bone to permit biologic fixation through extensive bony in-growth.

This implant type was initially popularized in the form of the Trabecular Metal™ Acetabular Revision System (Zimmer Inc., Warsaw, IN), with components made from tantalum. Other companies have since created their own highly porous metal constructs through advanced manufacturing processes such as 3D printing of titanium. Among United States-based companies, these materials include Gription® TF (DePuy Synthes, Warsaw, IN), Tritanium (Stryker, Mahwah, NJ), CONCELOC (Smith & Nephew, Memphis, TN), and OsseoTi® (Zimmer Biomet, Warsaw, IN). While these highly porous materials are now used in newer acetabular shell designs, acetabular augments made from many of these materials are also available.

The recommended surgical technique for porous metal augments typically calls for securing the augments with screws to solid host bone stock in such a way that the augment closely abuts the acetabular cup. The augment and cup can then be unitized with bone cement, conferring additional stability while awaiting bony in-growth. Their use in large acetabular defects (Paprosky 3A and 3B, AAOS 3 and 4) has been explored with good short-term to medium-term results [16–19].

In a review of 4 studies including a total of 125 revision THAs classified as having large defects, a construct consisting of one or more tantalum augments and a hemispherical, uncemented shell yielded a 2.4% rate of radiographic loosening and only 3 cases requiring further revision for loosening [15]. Dislocation occurred in 10 hips, infection in 5, nerve palsies in 3, and 19 hips (15.2%) underwent reoperation for any reason [15]. The most common reason for reoperation was liner revision secondary to instability [15], leading some surgeons to select elevated rim or constrained liners in most patients [18].

Another series of 38 patients with Paprosky Type 3 defects treated with Trabecular Metal™ shells with 1 or more augments revealed a 3-year Kaplan-Meier survival rate of 92.1% with the endpoint being revision for any cause, and a survival rate of 94.7% when the endpoint was revision for aseptic loosening [20]. These rates of revision for aseptic loosening are among the best for reviews comparing different constructs in the setting of large acetabular defects or pelvic discontinuity [3, 15].

Anterior Column Reconstruction with Inner Table Augment

A novel technique for addressing anterior column deficiency via an extended direct anterior approach using trabecular metal augments placed on the inner table of the pelvis was originally described by the senior author of this chapter [21]. Anterior column deficiency is an uncommon but challenging problem that can occur in the setting of severe hip dysplasia, acetabular fracture, oncogenic resection, infection, or secondary to acetabular component migration following total hip arthroplasty. Although favorable results have been obtained performing complex acetabular reconstruction using jumbo cups, cup-cage constructs, and custom triflange acetabular components, these generally rely heavily on posterior column structures for stability, bridging the ilium and ischium to compensate for loss of anterior column support. If the major bony deficiency is anterior, large portions of the cup may be left unsupported, leaving the construct at increased risk of failed ingrowth and loosening. The anterior approach offers the ability to access the inner table of the pelvis along with the anterior column and wall of the acetabulum. Access to these structures is important for reconstruction of Paprosky 3B ("up and in") acetabular defects.

The approach is through the interval described by Smith-Peterson with the incision extended proximally to the anterior superior iliac spine (ASIS), then curved lateral to follow the iliac crest [22]. The distal portion of the dissection is the same as it would be for a primary total hip replacement. The fascia lata is opened and blunt dissection is performed through the interval between tensor fascia lata (TFL) and sartorius, extending proximally to the ASIS while staying in this interval. Electrocautery is used to release the origin of the abdominal muscles, making sure to leave a cuff of tissue on the iliac crest for repair and closure.

A Cobb elevator is used to elevate the iliacus from the inner table of the pelvis. The displaced cup will be present on the inner table and limits the ability to elevate the iliacus to the pelvic brim. It is important not to attempt to dissect over the top of the displaced cup as the external iliac vessels are in close proximity, and may be tented over the cup. Some surgeons elect to have the external iliac vein stented prior to revision surgery in order to protect it during this portion of the case. After the cup is encountered, a sponge can be packed into this window for hemostasis while the rest of the dissection is performed.

The dissection is carried around the ASIS, releasing the sartorius and inguinal ligament, connecting the proximal dissection to the interval previously developed between TFL and sartorius/rectus femoris. Dissection is now carried down the anterior border of the pelvis towards the anterior inferior iliac spine (AIIS). In order to gain exposure, the direct head of the rectus femoris is released from the AIIS at this point. Typically, in Paprosky 3B defects, the anterior wall of the acetabulum is missing medial to the AIIS along with the anterior column and the quadrilateral surface of the acetabulum.

At this point the femur needs to be addressed in order to achieve enough mobility to remove the femoral head and start removing the cup. Because the defect typically involves severe protrusio, the femur must be circumferentially released to allow enough traction to remove the cup and gain leg length. A complete anterior capsulectomy needs to be performed and it is critically important to release the entire medial side of the proximal femur until the lesser trochanter can be easily palpated. The lateral capsule needs to be removed and the entire inside of the greater trochanter should be skeletonized of all scar and remaining capsule. It is helpful at this point to bend the tip of the electrocautery and release as much of the posterior capsule as possible from the femur.

If the defect has been present for a long time, the iliopsoas can be released as well, as it will be shortened and extremely tight. Once the femur is mobile enough, traction can be applied and the femoral head removed. In the senior author's experience, the trunnion can be very difficult to work around, and removal of the stem is always preferred if possible. If stem removal is not an option, the trunnion should be placed lateral and posterior to the acetabulum with the femur externally rotated 90 degrees. If surgery is being performed "on-table," traction should be released at this phase.

Once the femoral component has been removed or the trunnion placed posterior to the acetabulum, the cup can be accessed from both proximally (inner table) and distally (outer table). Careful placement of a sharp Hohmann retractor in the superior pubic ramus and another into the iliac wing proximal to the displaced cup will aid in the exposure. Again, it is not advisable to place retractors or attempt dissection over the top of the displaced cup due to the proximity of the external iliac vessels. Hip flexion at this point can help relax the iliopsoas if it has not already been released. Now the cup and any screws can be removed with access both above and below the loose component.

With all implants removed, the remaining bone stock is assessed with a sharp Hohmann retractor placed into the superior pubic ramus medially and a blunt Cobra placed around the posterior wall. In Paprosky 3B defects, the posterior wall and column will be retained, but typically less than 40% of host bone is available and over half of the acetabular rim is missing. The anterior half of the acetabulum and quadrilateral surface are missing. Anterior to posterior fixation is unobtainable due to loss of the entire anterior acetabulum. Reaming is performed under direct visualization until 2-point fixation is obtained between the ischium and the superior lateral acetabulum. The senior author typically reams for a 2 mm press-fit. Depending on the operative setup, fluoroscopy can also be utilized to assess cup position and orientation. The initial scratch fit should be adequate to allow for insertion handle removal without displacing the cup.

Screws are then placed into the posterior wall and column. At least one inferior screw oriented in the direction of the ischial spine should be placed. Screw placement into the ischium itself is usually difficult, as most off-the-shelf cups do not have screw holes peripheral enough to allow this. Now that fixation has been obtained into the posterior wall and column, the anterior defect should be addressed, as the cup will fail through this anterior defect without augmentation.

A trial column buttress augment can be placed on the inner table of the pelvis to assess the ideal position of the implant. The senior author's preferred implant for this application is the Zimmer Biomet Trabecular Metal™ Column Buttress Augment. A Left Posterior/Right Anterior implant is used for a right hip construct and a Right Posterior/ Left Anterior implant for a left hip construct. A high-speed burr is used to contour the inner table to create a footprint for the augment, allowing it to sit nearly flush against the cup. The augment should ideally be in contact with the cup, but typically the components will not fit together perfectly congruent. The augment is fixed to the inner table of the pelvis with screws and cement is placed between the augment and cup to unitize the construct.

A liner can be gently impacted and the head and stem are revised as needed. During closure, the sartorius and inguinal ligament are repaired to the ASIS using nonabsorbable suture through a drill hole and the abdominal muscles repaired to the iliac crest. A deep drain should be used. Patients are toe-touch weight-bearing for 8 weeks and no braces are applied. An example case is depicted in Fig. 37.1.

Spanyer et al. [21] described 5 patients who underwent revision THA with anterior column augmentation with inner table augments using the described technique. Clinical outcomes were good to excellent for all patients, all of whom were satisfied with their ultimate result. One patient out of 5 developed recurrent instability necessitating revision to a constrained liner at 4 months post-revision.

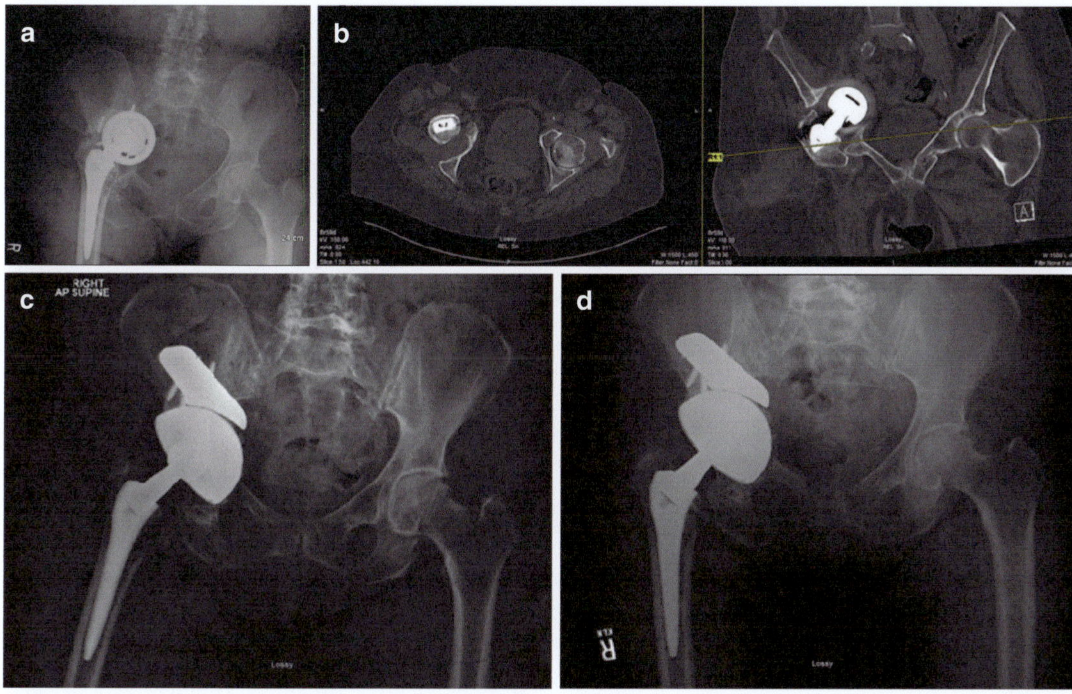

Fig. 37.1 82-year-old female with a history of primary right THA via a posterior approach with later acetabular revision 13 and 7 years prior to presentation to our clinic, respectively. Complaints were of 2 months of increasing groin pain and noticeable shortening of her right leg. Plain films in clinic are shown in (**a**) A CT scan obtained the same day to evaluate her acetabular defect is shown in (**b**), demonstrating severe anterior column deficiency with relatively intact posterior column. Her deficiency was addressed via acetabular component revision with a jumbo cup (74 mm) and an anterior column augment placed on the inner table of the pelvis. The femoral stem did not need to be fully revised for exposure, as the modular neck and head were removed and revised. Immediate post-op film (**c**) and 6-week post-op film (**d**) demonstrate stable position of the construct during a period of restricted weight-bearing to permit bony ingrowth

Cup-Cage Constructs and Custom Triflange Acetabular Components

In cases where there are severe acetabular deficiencies that cannot be reconstructed with jumbo cups or augments, the anterior approach offers excellent exposure for both cup-cage constructs and custom triflange acetabular components. Access to the ischium and lateral ilium can be obtained with minimal extension of the approach. Since the exposure is similar for both, they are grouped together here even though indications may differ between the two constructs.

The cup-cage was developed for acetabular defects where a hemispherical shell and screws alone were deemed to provide inadequate fixation. The construct involves the initial placement of a hemispherical shell, with an ilioischial antiprotrusio cage then being placed over the cup and secured with screws. A polyethylene liner is then cemented into the cup-cage. The technique was originally described using a full cage, with the ischial flange inserted into the body of the ischium, and this demonstrated excellent mid-term results compared to traditional reconstruction cages [23, 24]. However, concerns related to the technical challenges of ischial flange insertion, including iatrogenic fracture and sciatic nerve injury from ischial dissection, led to the development of the half cup-cage modification. This involves cutting the cage in half transversely with a metal cutting burr, removing the ischial flange, and retaining the superior portion and iliac flange. In a retrospective review of 57 patients treated with full and half cup-cage reconstruction of defects ranging in severity from

Paprosky 2B through 3B, both constructs proved highly successful with similar survivorship at a minimum of 2 years follow up [25].

Custom triflange acetabular components (CTACs) have become an increasingly popular solution for reconstruction of large acetabular defects with or without pelvic discontinuity. A thin-cut computed tomography scan of the pelvis with 3D reconstruction is first obtained to assess the acetabular defect and establish the basis for design of the custom implant. The surgeon is able to specify the location and orientation of the acetabular cup, position of the flanges, and the location, number, and direction of screws. The backside of the implant is typically surfaced with hydroxyapatite or porous coatings to facilitate osseointegration. Systematic reviews and meta-analyses of constructs for large acetabular defects have found CTACs to have low mechanical failures rates and high survivability of 90–95% [3, 15, 26].

For either construct, a standard anterior approach is made to the hip between the interval of the TFL and sartorius. Extension of the standard DAA skin incision both distally on the thigh and proximally along the iliac crest will be necessary for adequate exposure. The dissection should be carried all the way proximal to the ASIS. Release 1–2 cm of the origin of the TFL at the iliac crest, leaving a cuff of tissue on the crest for repair at the end of the case. Expose the anterior hip capsule and perform a capsulectomy or capsulotomy, per the surgeon's preference. Next, perform extensive debridement and thinning of the thick, scarred anterior capsule; a superficial layer of capsule may be preserved, but deeper layers must be resected for exposure and mobilization of the femur. The lateral capsule should be almost fully excised for femoral mobility and exposure of the superior and lateral acetabulum and ilium. It is also extremely important to perform a complete release of the anterior and medial capsule from the femur. The femur will not be able to fall posterior and lateral to the acetabulum if the anterior and medial capsule is not properly released.

Before dislocation, release all tissue inside the greater trochanter until it is skeletonized. It is not necessary to release the posterior femur, but inadequate release of the scar and capsule inside the greater trochanter will lead to inadequate femoral mobility and difficulty exposing the acetabulum. At this point, dislocate the hip and remove the femoral head. Externally rotate the leg 90 degrees and place the trunnion lateral and posterior to the acetabulum, releasing traction if operating "on table." A retractor can be placed in front of the trunnion and behind the posterior wall to depress the stem further from the acetabulum for additional exposure. If stem revision is indicated or convenient, performing a complete femur release and explanting the stem will provide still better exposure at this phase. The cup can be removed with the standard Explant® Acetabular Cup Removal System (Zimmer Biomet, Warsaw, IN) or a comparable curved osteotome to minimize bone loss. The use of modified offset handled systems has been described, but the standard straight handle of the Explant® works well through the anterior approach.

If the preoperative plan was for cup-cage with a Trabecular Metal™ cup, have a metal cutting drill bit available to create holes for screws to be placed through the cup. Ream for a 2 mm press-fit and impact the cup into a position maximizing host bone contact. The polyethylene will be cemented in later, so it is not critical to get the cup in ideal orientation with respect to inclination and anteversion. Once the cup has been positioned, drill holes where good fixation into host bone will be obtained. An inferior screw placed into the ischium makes a critical contribution to the fixation and the Trabecular Metal™ cup allows for very peripheral screw placement.

Whether a full or half cup-cage is chosen, exposure must next be performed for placement of the iliac flange. Using a Cobb, elevate the gluteus minimus and medius from the lateral ilium from anterior to posterior until enough bone is cleared to accommodate the iliac flange. A malleable trial cage can be placed to assess when enough bone has been exposed. This trial also helps to dictate the contour needed on the actual implant to fit the remaining host bone. If performing a half cup-cage, the ischial flange should now be removed using a metal cutting burr.

Contour the cage based on the trial and place into the cup with the iliac flange against the lateral ilium. Screws are placed into the lateral ilium and through the cage and cup to unitize the construct. A polyethylene liner can then be cemented into the cup in any position desired.

If using a full cage, the ischium must next be identified; it can be easily palpated with a finger inferior and posterior to the acetabulum. A Cobb elevator can be used to clear the top 1–2 cm of the ischium for orientation, but great care should be taken as not to injure the nearby sciatic nerve. For this reason, it is preferred to insert the ischial flange into the body of the ischium rather than place it laterally and affix it with screws. With one finger on the ischium for orientation, a drill can be used to establish a start point where the ischial flange will be inserted. Use a depth gauge as a feeler to confirm the ischial anatomy and orientation. Next, an osteotome is used to create a slot for the ischial flange. Insert the ischial flange, then impact the cage into the cup until the iliac flange is seated against the lateral ilium. Placing screws through the dome of the cage and cup will also help fully seat the cage. Finally, insert screws through the iliac flange to fix it to the bone. Inferior screws can be used as well, but are not absolutely necessary due to the ischial flange. A liner is cemented into the cage in an appropriate position.

If the preoperative decision was made for CTAC, then the ischium and superior pubic ramus need to be identified and cleared for the ischial flange and the pubic screw. The initial exposure for the iliac flange is the same as described above for the full cup-cage, although the ischium must be more fully cleared to make room to lay the flange laterally onto the bone. The root of the superior pubic ramus must be identified and exposed with careful placement of a Hohmann retractor anterior to the pubic ramus. The acetabulum is gently reamed to expose bleeding cancellous bone. However, care must be taken to minimize bone removal, as the implant has been specifically designed to fit the remaining bone stock.

The implant must be positioned correctly, with particular attention paid to flexion and extension, so as to align the ischial and iliac flanges along with the screw hole oriented for fixation into the superior pubic ramus. All scar tissue needs to be removed to ensure congruent bone contact of the implant, and a high-speed burr can be helpful to contour down any bony prominences that interfere with the fit. Once the implant is firmly seated, the ischial screws are placed first. It is advisable to place all the screws in the ischium first as the bone is poor and lysis is typically present. “Home run” screws are next placed through the cup, and then the iliac flange is secured. The iliac flange accommodates the largest number of screws, and these generally have excellent purchase. If the pubic screw hole is still aligned with the superior pubic ramus after all other screws are in position, that screw may be placed. Since the triflange has a standard cup locking mechanism, the liner is then impacted and remaining revision of the stem and head can be performed.

The only difference in closure compared to a primary DAA THA is repair of the TFL at its origin. This is facilitated by leaving a cuff of tissue for repair on the lateral ilium during exposure, and absorbable suture can be used. A deep surgical drain is recommended for all complex acetabular revisions. Toe-touch weight-bearing is maintained for 8–12 weeks and no braces are applied.

Pelvic Discontinuity and Pelvic Distraction

Pelvic discontinuity remains one of the most difficult pathologies for the hip arthroplasty surgeon to manage. These cases are invariably challenging, but fortunately do not represent a large percentage of acetabular revisions. Each case is unique and should be treated only by experienced surgeons specializing in revision hip replacement. Two of the most common techniques for addressing pelvic discontinuity are custom triflange acetabular components (CTACs) and pelvic distraction technique. Both have shown a less than 5% failure rate in the literature [3]. The technique for CTAC is described in the previous section of this chapter.

Pelvic distraction technique, first described in the literature in 2012, has shown excellent results using off-the-shelf components without the need for custom implants [27]. As long as the posterior wall and column do not require augmentation, the anterior approach offers the exposure needed for pelvic distraction. In many cases these are Paprosky 3B defects and the anterior approach offers the additional ability to augment the anterior column.

A standard incision is made just lateral to the ASIS. An extensile incision, as described previously in the chapter, may be used for anterior column reconstruction if needed. Once the cup has been removed, the discontinuity is confirmed by stressing the ischiopubic segment of the acetabulum. Soft tissue should be debrided to expose host bone, but the acetabular nonunion should not be taken down. The fibrous tissue of the nonunion will provide the needed tension and stability for the revision acetabular component. The acetabulum is then reamed back to bleeding bone.

If there are no defects requiring augmentation and an appropriately sized cup is able to span the defect with adequate bone contact, then a cup can be inserted with a 6–8 mm press-fit. This can be accomplished by engaging the cup into the ischiopubic segment of the acetabulum first, then while the cup is being inserted, applying translational force downward in an attempt to distract the acetabular nonunion. An alternative method utilizes a Jungbluth clamp and screws placed in the ischium and superior to the acetabulum. The clamp will allow distraction as the cup is inserted and, once released, the tension of the distraction provides initial stability.

If larger defects are present, then one or two augments may be used. These are placed in the posterior inferior and/or anterior superior regions of the acetabulum. The cup is then positioned between the augments, and components are unitized with cement. Figure 37.2 demonstrates such a case of pelvic discontinuity, with a defect that was too large to be spanned by even the largest cup (80 mm) in the senior author's preferred acetabular system.

Harrington Technique

A rarely used but potentially useful construct drawn from the oncology literature is the Harrington procedure for acetabular reconstruction. First described by Dr. Kevin Harrington, for whom the eponymous procedure is named, in 1981, this has traditionally been used in the setting of acetabular metastatic disease with severe bone destruction [28]. The original procedure involved the insertion of threaded pins from the acetabular dome retrograde into the iliac wing, which were then cemented together with an acetabular support ring into which a polyethylene cup was cemented. Other surgeons have modified the technique over the years; later publications describe the use of screws or Steinmann pins inserted antegrade into the columns of the remaining acetabulum, sometimes incorporating reconstruction cages into the construct with a cemented cup [29, 30]. Whatever hardware is chosen, the metal acts as rebar, strengthening the cement mantle and transferring the mechanical load to intact bone. This should be considered a salvage procedure and be reserved for low-demand patients, but remains a technique that the revision hip surgeon might keep in their armamentarium for severe defects in poor hosts.

When performing this technique via an anterior approach, the dissection and exposure are the same as described earlier for anterior column reconstruction with an inner table augment. The reason for the extensile Smith-Peterson approach is to have access to the inner table of the pelvis as well as iliac crest for placement of Steinmann pins or screws. After removal of the cup, the remaining lytic bone and soft tissue are debrided back to normal bone. Pins or screws are then placed from the iliac crest into and ideally across the defect. The senior author prefers cannulated screws for their comparative ease of use, as seen in Fig. 37.3. Plan the placement of hardware to allow room for the new cup. It is helpful to have the cup opened and provisionally positioned in the acetabulum to make sure the hardware is not interfering with good placement. In cases of pelvic discontinuity, a screw placed from the inner table of the pelvis into the posterior column can effectively stabilize the

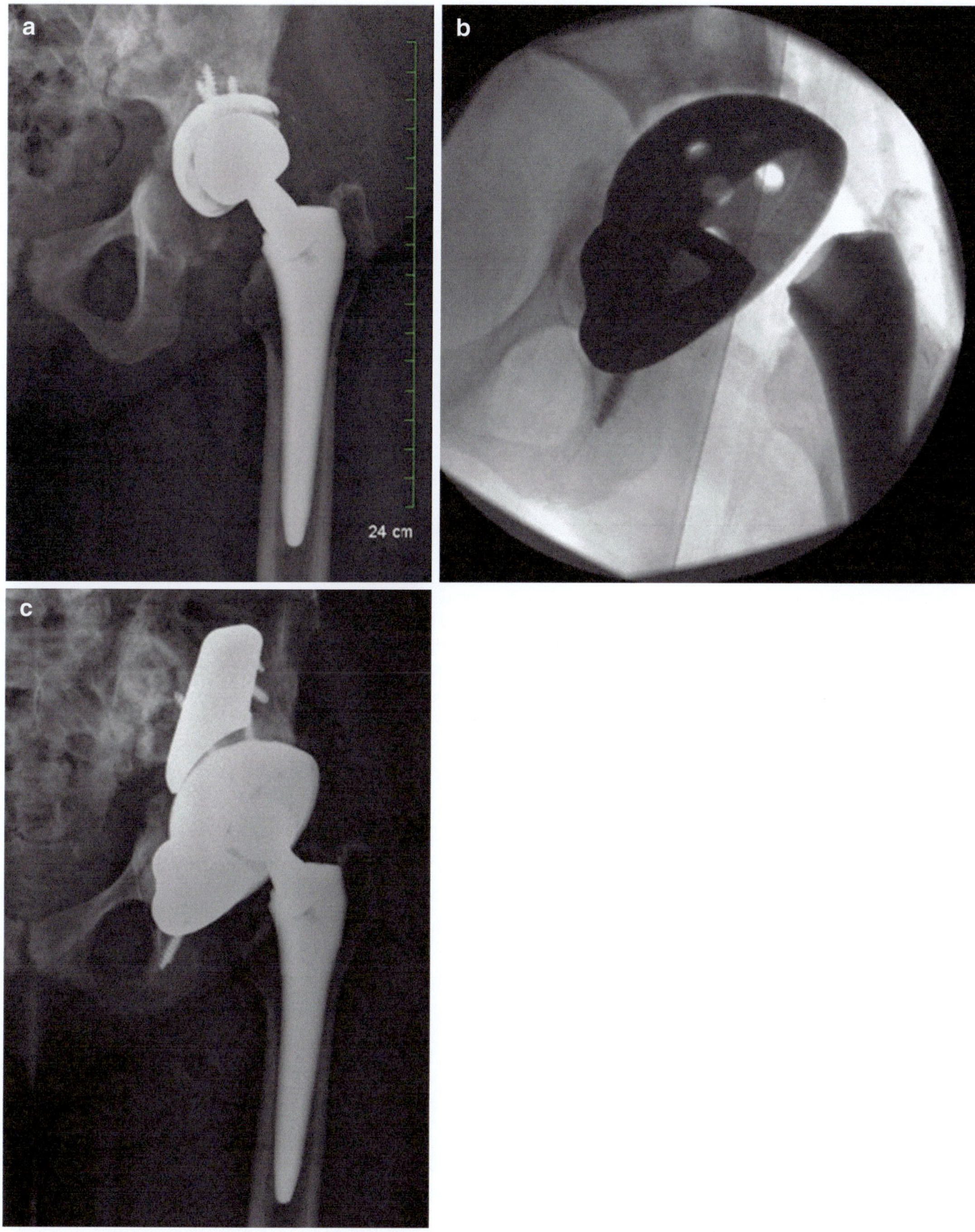

Fig. 37.2 67-year-old female with a history of prior left THA acetabular revision presenting with pain and recurrent acetabular loosening. A plain film from clinic in (**a**) shows a loose cup with a Paprosky 3A defect and a transverse acetabular fracture nonunion indicating associated pelvic discontinuity. A tantalum augment was first secured to the ischiopubic segment with a screw, then distraction technique was used during placement of a 76 mm cup, as seen in the intraoperative fluoroscopic image in (**b**). A concomitant anterior column defect was reconstructed with an inner table buttress augment and both augments were unitized to the cup with cement. A postoperative plain film is seen in (**c**). The patient was kept toe-touch weight-bearing for 8 weeks and returned to painless ambulation

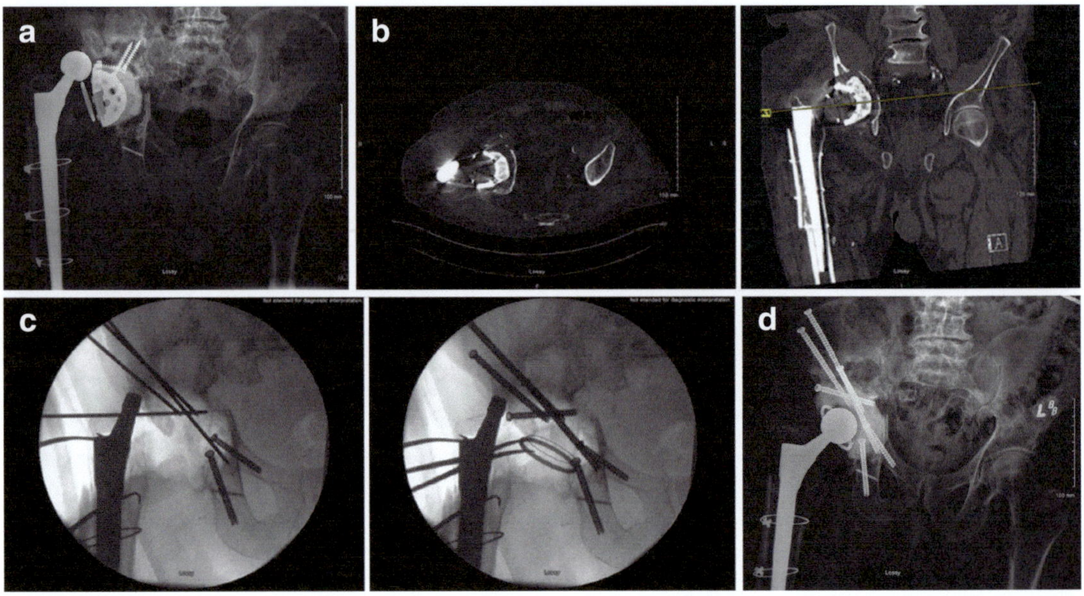

Fig. 37.3 87-year-old male with a history of a right THA for metastatic melanoma and had been previously revised for both infection and periprosthetic femur fracture, who had ultimately been converted to a constrained liner for recurrent instability 4 years prior to presentation. A plain film taken upon presentation to the ED in (**a**) shows a posterolateral dislocation with failure of the constrained liner and loosening of the flanged, cemented cup; screws had previously been placed into the ilium as rebar in an effort to improve fixation of the cement mantle. CT cuts in the axial and coronal planes in (**b**) demonstrate severely deficient bone stock around the loose cup. Intraoperative fluoroscopic images in (**c**) show the use of guidewires to control cannulated screw placement and then provisionally checking the position of the all-polyethylene constrained cup prior to cementation. The patient was made weight-bearing as tolerated and the post-operative film is shown in (**d**)

fracture. Screws can also be placed directly into the ischium and superior pubic ramus, leaving enough of the head and proximal end proud to interdigitate with the cement.

The liner is cemented in an appropriate position, making sure to place cement into all defects and around all pins or screws. This unitizes the hardware and, if screws are used, makes them functionally fixed angle to provide even more stability. The goal of this construct is not biological healing, but immediate stability in a low-demand host to facilitate early mobility. Patients are therefore permitted to be full weight-bearing after surgery.

Conclusion

With proper technique, even the most complex acetabular pathology can be effectively managed through an anterior approach. Success requires that the revision hip surgeon properly diagnose the deficiency being addressed, engage in thorough preoperative planning and construct selection, and understand the exposure modifications necessary to complete the reconstruction. The authors hope this chapter will prove helpful to anterior hip surgeons seeking to expand the utility of the anterior approach in the revision setting.

Avenir Complete

My preferred femoral stem is the Zimmer Biomet Avenir Complete™. It is a rectangular cross section, fully coated hydroxyapatite stem. This style of femoral stem has over 30 years of clinical history and has been widely used with anterior approach hip surgeons for over 15 years in the United States. The Avenir Complete™ is a modernized version addressing the problems associated with the original such as neck length, distal potting, and lack of collar.

The neck has been shortened to address what was thought to be long on the legacy stem. In addition to shortening the neck, a third offset option was added with a 126.5 degree coxa vara option. This is one of the key design qualities of this implant for me as an anterior approach hip surgeon. My goal is always to recreate the patient's natural anatomy. There are multiple recent anatomical studies showing average femoral neck-shaft angle to lie between 125 and 127 degrees which begs the question of why haven't our femoral stems changed to correspond to normal anatomy? My opinion is that hip replacement didn't rely on modern technology to reproduce anatomy. We would put in components, examine leg length by external landmarks, feel soft tissue tensions and close the patient. Anterior approach has changed the way we look at leg length and offset. We spend the time to do fluoroscopic overlays, or have computer and tablet programs designed to show us these parameters within millimeters. Having only two neck options of standard or high offset makes this much more difficult. Having a varus neck angle option simplifies the surgery by allowing me to perform similar neck cuts on the majority of patients and using the neck angle to assist in leg length adjustments. The math is very simple with the standard and high offsets differing 6 mm in horizontal offset throughout all sizes while maintaining the same leg length. The coxa vara and the high offset differ 6 mm in leg length throughout all sizes while maintaining the same offset. By having a coxa vara neck angle in addition to traditional standard and high options, I have the ability to recreate the natural anatomy and biomechanics of the hip.

Fully coated hydroxyapatite femoral stems have a very long history of success dating back decades. Some of the disadvantages of the older versions were problems with overall stem length and distal potting, especially in Dorr type A femoral canals. A distally potted, full coated stem has been a very difficult problem to deal with because the implant isn't loose, but still causes thigh pain. Revising this type of failure is difficult because the implant is well fixed in the most difficult part of the femur to access without osteotomy. This stem was narrowed distally to avoid the problem of distal potting. By beveling the distal lateral border of the stem, it allows the implant to fill proximally before it pots, providing better opportunity for proximal on-growth and long-term success. The overall length of the stem was shortened as well making it a mid-length femoral stem. I am personally not a proponent of short stems which have become popular with anterior approach hip replacement surgery. They have been popularized to help surgeons prepare the femur easier due to difficulty with exposure. Unfortunately, we are now showing increased incidence of subsidence, loosening and fracture with short stems compared to standard length stems. My personal experience of over 9000 anterior approach hip replacements parallels the findings of others. I have tried short stems in the past and not been happy with the incidence of failure and revision. I believe in learning good femoral exposure and using standard length implants. This implant was designed by a team of surgeons from all three exposure backgrounds. It was not designed short or specifically for anterior approach, therefore, its been my preferred implant.

The third, and maybe most controversial feature of this implant is the option of collar or collarless. The collar vs. collarless debate has surgeons on both sides that are steadfast in their belief one way or another. My personal preference is an uncemented collared stem. The tapered wedge stem has become the most popular stem design over the past few decades because of its ease in preparation and implantation. The early reports of these stems were from a time in hip replacement where weight-bearing was protected in the early postoperative period. These stems were given time to on-grow before full weight-bearing was allowed. Now we are in a time of immediate weight-bearing and faster recovery times. In my opinion, this is why more recent papers are showing increased incidence of subsidence and early postoperative fractures and failures with these stems compared to other designs. I also saw this in my own practice and therefore switched to a collared implant. Collared stems have been shown to provide better immediate stability than collarless. They can withstand much greater vertical and horizontal forces, preventing subsidence and failure. I disagree with the concept that a stem may need to subside to get stability. A stem should have stability when it leaves the operating room because stability leads to on-growth which leads to long-term success. For those who prefer collarless however, this stem comes in that option with all sizes and offsets as well.

For the reasons I've outlined above, the Avenir Complete™ from Zimmer Biomet is my preferred femoral stem. The shape and hydroxyapatite coating have excellent results with decades of implantation. Having a coxa vara offset option allows me to reproduce a patient's natural anatomy and simplifies my ability to recreate length and offset. Lastly, I prefer a collared stem to reduce my risk for subsidence and improve the important initial stability needed for long-term success of a total hip replacement.

References

1. Paprosky WG, Perona PG, Lawrence JM. Acetabular defect classification and surgical reconstruction in revision arthroplasty. A 6-year follow-up evaluation. J Arthroplast. 1994;9:33–44.
2. D'Antonio JA, Capello WN, Borden LS, Bargar WL, Bierbaum BF, Boettcher WG, Steinberg ME, Stulberg SD, Wedge JH. Classification and management of acetabular abnormalities in total hip arthroplasty. Clin Orthop Relat Res. 1989;243:126–37.
3. Malahias M-A, Qian-Li M, Gu A, Ward SE, Alexiades MM, Sculco PK. Outcomes of acetabular reconstructions for the management of chronic pelvic discontinuity: a systematic review. J Arthroplast. 2020;35:1145–53.
4. Barrett WP, Turner SE, Leopold JP. Prospective randomized study of direct anterior vs postero-lateral approach for total hip arthroplasty. J Arthroplast. 2013;28:1634.
5. Martin CT, Pugely AJ, Gao Y, Clark CR. A comparison of hospital length of stay and short term morbidity between the anterior and posterior approaches to total hip arthroplasty. J Arthroplast. 2013;28(5):849.
6. Connolly P, Kamath AF. Direct anterior total hip arthroplasty: comparative outcomes and contemporary results. World J Orthop. 2016;7(2):94.
7. Mayr E, Nogler M, Benedetti MG, et al. A prospective randomized assessment of earlier functional recovery in THA patients by minimally invasive direct anterior approach: a gait analysis study. Clin Biomech. 2009;24(10):812.
8. Nakata K, Nishikawa M, Yamamoto K, Hiroto S, oshikawa H. A clinical comparative study of the direct anterior with mini-posterior approach: two consecutive series. J Arthroplast. 2009;24(5):698.
9. Blumenfeld TJ. Implant choices, technique, and results in revision acetabular surgery: a review. Hip Int. 2012;22(3):235–47.
10. Chen AF, Hozack WJ. Component selection in revision total hip arthroplasty. Orthop Clin North Am. 2014;45(3):275–86.
11. Issack PS, Nousiainen M, Beksac B, Helfet DL, Sculco TP, Buly RL. Acetabular component revision in total hip arthroplasty. Part II: management of major bone loss and pelvic discontinuity. Am J Orthop. 2009;38(11):550–6.
12. Jain S, Grogan RJ, Giannoudis PV. Options for managing severe acetabular bone loss in revision hip arthroplasty. A systematic review. Hip Int. 2014;24(2):109–22.
13. Sheth NP, Nelson CL, Springer BD, Fehring TK, Paprosky WG. Acetabular bone loss in revision total hip arthroplasty: evaluation and management. J Am Acad Orthop Surg. 2013;21(3):128–39.
14. Villanueva M, Rios-Luna A, Pereiro De Lamo J, Fahandez-Saddi H, Bostrom MP. A review of the treatment of pelvic discontinuity. HSS J. 2008;4(2):128–37.
15. Baauw M, van Hooff ML, Spruit M. Current construct options for revision of large actebular defects. A systematic review. JBJS Reviews. 2016;4(11):e2.
16. Del Gaizo DJ, Kancherla V, Sporer SM, Paprosky WG. Tantalum augments for Paprosky IIIA defects remain stable at midterm followup. Clin Orthop Relat Res. 2012;470(2):395–401.
17. Flecher X, Sporer S, Paprosky W. Management of severe bone loss in acetabular revision using a Trabecular Metal shell. J Arthroplast. 2008;23(7):949–55.
18. Lingaraj K, Teo YH, Bergman N. The management of severe acetabular bone defects in revision hip arthroplasty using modular porous metal components. J Bone Joint Surg Br. 2009;91(12):1555–60.
19. Weeden SH, Schmidt RH. The use of tantalum porous metal implants for Paprosky 3A and 3B defects. J Arthroplasty. 2007;22(6)(Suppl 2):151–5.
20. O'Neill CJ, Creedon SB, Brennan SA, O'Mahony FJ, Lynham RS, Guerin S, Gul R, Harty JA. Acetabular revision using trabecular metal augments for Paprosky type 3 defects. J Arthroplast. 2018;33:823–8.
21. Spanyer JM, Beaumont CM, Yerasimides JG. The extended direct anterior approach for column augmentation in the deficient pelvis: a novel surgical technique, and case series report. J Arthroplast. 2017;32:515–9.
22. Smith-Peterson MN. Approach to an exposure of the hip joint for mold arthroplasty. J Bone Joint Surg Am. 1949;31A(1):40.
23. Aboighasemian M, Tangsaraporn S, Drexler M, Barbuto R, Backstein D, Safir O, Kuzyk P, Gross A. The challenge of pelvic discontinuity: cup-cage

reconstruction does better than conventional cages in mid-term. Bone Joint J. 2014;96-B(2):195–200.

24. Amenabar T, Rahman WA, Hetaimish BM, Kuzyk PR, Safir OA, Gross AE. Promising mid-term results with a cup-cage construct for large acetabular defects and pelvic discontinuity. Clin Orthop Relat Res. 2016;474(2):408–14.
25. Sculco PK, Ledford CK, Hanssen AD, Abdel MP, Lewallen DG. The evolution of the cup-cage technique for major acetabular defects. Full and half cup-cage reconstruction. J Bone Joint Surg Am. 2017;99:1104–10.
26. Szczepanski JR, Perriman DM, Smith PN. Surgical treatment of pelvic discontinuity – a systematic review and meta-analysis. JBJS Rev. 2019;7(9):e4.
27. Sporer SM, Bottros JJ, Hulst JB, Kancherla VK, Moric M, Paprosky WG. Acetabular distraction: an alternative for severe defects with chronic pelvic discontinuity? Clin Orthop Relat Res. 2012;470:3156–63.
28. Harrington KD. The management of acetabular insufficiency secondary to metastatic malignant disease. J Bone Joint Surg Am. 1981;63-A:653–64.
29. Tillman RM, Myers GJC, Abudu AT, Carter SR, Grimer RJ. The three-pin modified 'Harrington' procedure for advanced metastatic destruction of the acetabulum. J Bone Joint Surg Br. 2008;90-B:84–7.
30. Faisham WI, Muslim DAJ, Bhavaraju VMK, Nawaz AH, Zulmi W. Modified Harrington procedure for acetabular insufficiency due to metastatic malignant disease. Malays Orthop J. 2009;3(1):36–41.

Treatment of Acute and Late Infections Using the Direct Anterior Approach

38

Martin Thaler and Michael Nogler

General

Periprosthetic joint infection (PJI) is a rare but serious complication after total hip replacement. The consequences for the patient are serious and may lead to lifelong impairments for the patient. In many cases, the patient has to deal with the sequelae of the complication for a longer period. This devastating complication is associated with increases in the total number of hospitalizations, duration of hospitalization, total number of operations, total hospital costs, total outpatient visits and has also substantial economic consequences for the patient as well as the health care system [1]. In contrast to revisions for aseptic loosening, septic revisions are characterized by greater use of hospital and physician resources. Treating infected total hip arthroplasties (THAs) can be challenging. The aim of treating an infected hip is limb salvage as well as the preservation of joint function. The incidence of infection following primary THA ranges from 1% to 3% [2]. Scattered data found a higher infection rate in DAA compared to non-DAA approaches [3]. Several studies report the same or lower infection rate with the DAA compared to other surgical approaches to the hip [4, 5]. In our opinion, the infection rate with the DAA is the same compared to other approaches to the hip, such as the posterior approach, the direct lateral approach, or the anterolateral approach. The proceedings of the International Consensus Meeting on Periprosthetic Joint Infection meeting also stated that there is strong evidence that surgical approach in primary THA does not affect the incidence of subsequent PJIs [6].

Many authors distinguish between superficial and deep infection in total hip arthroplasty. A superficial infection can be defined as any wound separation which requires additional treatment beyond the standard wound care, or that leads to a return of the patient to the operating room for a wound revision. So-called deep infections are subfascial or within the artificial hip joint and require revision arthroplasty.

Regarding the treatment of PJI, there should be no approach-related adaption of established treatment algorithm. Hence, the treatment protocol of THA performed through the DAA does not differ from other approaches.

M. Thaler
Helios Klinikum München West, Arthroplasty Center, München, Germany
e-mail: martin.thaler@i-med.ac.at

M. Nogler (✉)
Department of Orthopaedic Surgery, Medical University of Innsbruck, Innsbruck, Austria
e-mail: michael.nogler@professor-nogler.at

J. M. Matta, A. P. Sah (eds.), *Anterior Hip Replacement*,
https://doi.org/10.1007/978-3-030-91896-5_38

Treatment Algorithm for Periprosthetic Joint Infections After DAA

Definition of Terms

After the initial occurrences of symptoms, the following stages can be defined (Table 38.1):

Early-onset Infection occurs 4 weeks or less after the surgery, the reason for occurring symptoms implements an intraoperative contamination.

Delayed Infection occurs up to 2 years after THA, the reason for occurring symptoms may implement an intraoperative contamination is probable.

Late-onset Infection occurs 2 years after the surgery, the reason for occurring symptoms may implement a hematogenous spread.

The symptoms can be distinguished into the following three categories (Table 38.2):

Acute Onset of symptoms are SASIRS (Sudden Acute Systemic Inflammatory Syndromes).

Chronic Onset of symptoms and signs of infection are without SASIRS such as fistulae or reddening.

Table 38.1 Classification of infection according to the time interval after surgery

Early onset	<4 weeks	Intraop. contamination
Delayed	Up to 2 years	Intraop. contamination probable
Late onset	>2 years	Hematogenous spread

Table 38.2 Classification of infection according to the symptoms

Acute	SSIRS (Sudden Acute Systemic Inflammatory Response Syndrome)
Chronic	Signs of infection without SSIRS, e.g. fistula, reddening
Subclinical	Loosening or joint effusion without clinical signs of infection or proof of infection

Subclinical Meaning that the loosening or joint effusion occur without clinical signs of or proof of infection.

Considering these criteria, probable combinations such as an acute early infection, acute delayed infection and acute late infection as well as a chronic delayed infection, chronic late infection and subclinical late infection can be concluded.

Persistent Wound Drainage (PWD) and Superficial Wound Dehiscence or Healing Problems

Wound dehiscence or healing problems are defined as a separation of the edges of a surgical wound. It may just be the surface layer or the entire wound. A PWD is defined as an area of persisting drainage greater than 2 × 2 cm on the incision over 72 hours postoperatively [7]. Drainage can be caused by hematoma, seroma, fat or necrosis [8].

General Considerations

Superficial wound dehiscence or healing problems occur more frequently and require more reoperations for wound dehiscence in patients with a BMI >35 compared to other patient cohorts [9]. Some authors report that severely obese patients have a higher risk of infection after the DAA for THA. They postulate that the relatively thin lateral-anterior skin on the thigh, the overlying pannus and the adjacent genitalia as potential contributors increase the risk of infection [10]. A threshold with a BMI >35 was reported for patients to have a higher risk for PJI. Therefore, careful skin preparation before the surgery with respect to the pannus and the inguinal crease should be performed before the surgery. Latest data shows that a bikini incision type DAA for obese patients might be a promising alternative to reduce skin healing problems. Although inconclusive data has been published, closed incision negative pressure in selected patients after THA might be a therapy option. However, further research is needed to determine whether closed incision negative pressure is more advantageous in high-risk patients undergoing THA. Moreover, crucial for these findings is to define a comprehensive patient population which profits from closed incision negative pressure therapy as well as to evaluate the economic results in THA [11].

However, it is well-known that obesity increases the perioperative risks for all types of total joint arthroplasty [12]. The systemic effects of obesity with a known immune system dysfunction are responsible for the significant increase in infection rates in patients with high BMIs regardless of the surgical approach [13]. As obesity becomes an epidemic worldwide, complications associated with increased BMI will continue to rise. Despite obesity our ageing population is likely to have other chronic diseases such as diabetes, cardiovascular diseases, or rheumatoid arthritis, which increase the risk of surgical wound complications and infections [14]. Total joint arthroplasty (TJA) for patients with post-traumatic arthritis of the hip or knee carries higher risks of developing PJI. The incidence is markedly higher in patients with previous surgeries and retained implants [6].

Technical Considerations with the DAA

Training, education, the use of dedicated instruments as well as implants in THA are essential and even more important in the DAA. The correct location of the skin incision, adequate hemostasis and short operating times can significantly reduce the risk of PWD, wound healing problems and infection. Postoperative wound healing problems can be reduced by the use of curved instruments and wound protecting tools during the surgery. These additional measures reduce the load on the edges of the skin and therefore can be protective against wound healing problems.

These protective measures and variables are not reflected by some studies, which report a higher incidence of wound healing problems or PJI with the DAA [3]. Several studies report the same or lower infection rate with the DAA compared to other surgical approaches to the hip [5]. For primary DAA THA, the skin incision varies from 6 to 10 cm. We recommend to perform a skin incision of approximately 10 cm in obese patients in order to avoid too much load on the edges of the skin incision. In addition, careful follow up of these patients is recommended. The proceedings of the International Consensus Meeting on Periprosthetic Joint Infection meeting also stated that there is strong evidence that a surgical approach in primary THA does not affect the incidence of subsequent PJIs [6].

Diagnosis of the Infection After THA

According to the Philadelphia consensus [15] meeting, we use the following criteria for the definition of PJI after THA:

Major Criteria

There are two major criteria, which lead to the diagnosis that the patient is infected: first, if a patient is tested positive twice for the same organism and second, if there is evident sinus tract is communicating with the hip joint.

Minor Criteria

The minor criteria can be divided into two major categories, which then can be further specified as well as classified by a point system. First category is the serum, whereby ESR and D-Dimer are only useful during a chronic course. The points for CRP or D-Dimer to be given are two or one, respectively.

The second category is the synovial one, whereby there are five subcategories. Three points are to be given, if the leucocyte count is above 3000, the leucocyte esterase test is positive twice, or the alpha defensin test is positive, showing a value of above 1.0.

The second subcategory is PMN (neutrophil share) and, if its count is 70% or higher, two points are to be given. In subcategory three, two points are to be given, if a positive culture is detected, if the histology is positive, which is subcategory four, three points are to be given. As a last subcategory, three points are to be given, if there is an intraoperative purulent aspect.

Depending on the count, the diagnose is "infected" if six or above, "unclear" if three up to five or "not infected" if below three points.

Diagnosis

In general, there is no perfect test, examination or finding to proof as well as to exclude a PJI in THA. Therefore, a combination of clinical evaluation, imaging, serologic tests as well as aspirate tests and biopsies needs to be established for confirming the diagnosis of PJI. However, the combination of clinical findings in accordance with the Philadelphia consensus meeting classification should be used in order to define a PJI.

Clinical Findings

Clinical findings show a high variation and there is no sign which shows high sensitivity and high specificity. Pain in the hip joint is the most sensitive finding with low specificity. This finding justifies the further evaluation to rule out a PJI. More helpful are the detection of a sinus tract, purulence in the artificial joint, or the presence of abscesses. Fever can occur in acute infections, but might be not a good indicator for late or chronic infections. Periarticular inflammation, such as effusion, swelling, warmth, and erythema, are sometimes very difficult to detect in a hip joint. There are few evidences that reduced range of motion or any kind of joint dysfunction in the hip is an indicator for a PJI. All findings mentioned in this abstract are subjective evaluations, which may have more significance in the hands of experienced arthroplasty surgeons. No specific clinical findings can be defined with patients and a PJI after DAA THA.

Laboratory Tests

There is no perfect diagnostic tool to exclude or proof an infection. Erythrocyte sedimentation rate (ESR) and C-reactive protein (CRP) cannot be used to rule out an infection. In cases of slow-growing organism, ESR and CRP might be negative. However, high levels of ESR and CRP might be an indicator for PJI.

Radiographic Findings

In general, radiographic findings are of limited value in diagnosing PJI. Aspetic loosening can occur especially in culture-negative infections, but it is the most common reason for revisions of THA as well.

Aspiration of the Hip Joint

Aspiration of the hip joint is one of the most important steps in diagnosing a PJI in patients suspected of having an infected hip joint. Pre-interventional oral or intravenous antibiotics have to be considered in planning of the aspiration and evaluation of the joint fluid. Concomitant anticoagulation medication is not a contraindication for aspiration in an emergency scenario. Numerous studies have shown that there is no significant increase in complications including bleeding or infection related to the hip joint aspiration in patients taking anticoagulation [16]. We do not recommend injecting normal saline or other sterile fluids into the hip joint in cases of dry aspirations of the hip joint. The aspirated fluid should be microbiologically analyzed. If the joint aspiration was performed under antibiotic therapy for any reason, polymerase chain reaction (PCR) might be an option. However, a limitation of PCR is that the identification of bacterial DNA does not necessarily confirm the presence of living bacteria in the hip joint (Fig. 38.1) [17].

The reported incidence of culture-negative PJIs ranges from 5% to 42% [18]. Therefore, repeated diagnostic protocols can be provided for

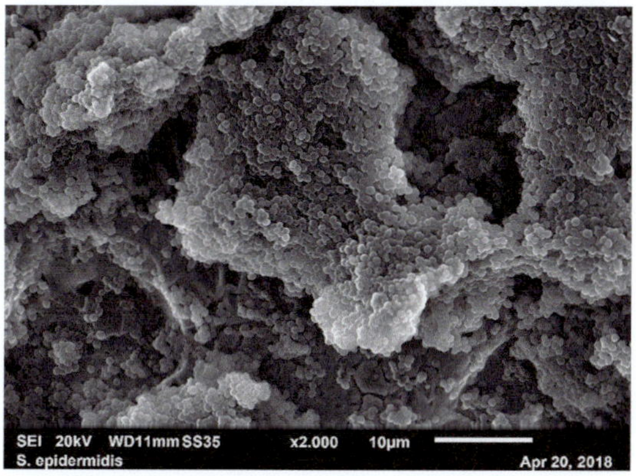

Fig. 38.1 Electron microscope picture showing biofilm with *Staphylococcus epidermidis*

further work up. If a joint aspiration does not provide a proof of infection, repeated aspiration is possible including the use of PCR and other next-generation infection tests. Should the second aspiration of the joint be negative as well but there is still a suspected infection, an arthroscopic or open sample collection can be performed. In this scenario, at least 5 tissue samples should be collected. In addition to that, a histological analysis of the periprosthetic tissue should be conducted.

Therapy of PJI After DAA THA

Our standard approach for primary and revision THA is the DAA interval, which is also used in patients who are referred to other institutions and had another approach for THA elsewhere.

Persistent Wound Drainage (PWD) or Wound Healing Problems After THA

Wound dehiscence and PWD can be treated non-operatively and operatively. Non-operative treatment includes the modification of venous thromboembolism, nutritional supplementation and dressing measures like negative pressure wound therapy. We do not recommend restrictions on range of motion.

Technical Considerations in PWD and Wound Dehiscence with the DAA

The indications for surgical intervention after PWD and wound healing problems can be considered if non-operatives measures are not successful. An indication of surgical intervention for PWS is a persistent wound drainage for more than 7 days after initiation of non-operative treatment.

If the fascia of the tensor muscle is intact and there is no evidence of deep infection, we perform a superficial wound washout. If PWD continues for more than 7 days after THA or implementing the nonoperative measures and there is a superficial wound dehiscence with a perforated fascia of the tensor muscle, we perform, an operative intervention. In these scenarios, we perform irrigation and debridement, synovectomy and head as well as liner exchange. The procedure is described in the next pages.

Dedicated Instruments for DAA

In our opinion, it is mandatory to use dedicated instruments for DAA. Without sufficient training and use of these instruments, a DAA THA should not be performed. Most of the specialized instruments designed for DAA have offset options to avoid too much load on the skin and to enable the possibility to "work around the corner". Many surgeons advocate the use of offset reamer, broaches, cup impactor, and stem inserter for the DAA in order to reduce the risk of wound healing problems and to reduce their skin incision without compromising the correct position of the implants.

Closed Incision Negative Pressure Therapy

Although inconclusive data has been published, closed incision negative pressure in selected patients after THA might be a therapy option. However, further research is needed to determine whether closed incision negative pressure is more advantageous in high-risk patients undergoing THA. Crucial for these findings is also to define a comprehensive patient population, which profits from closed incision negative pressure therapy as well as to evaluate the economic results in THA [11].

Dressings

The majority of surgeons use occlusive dressings, which must be kept clean and dry. If there is no drainage, it may be changed after 7 days. The patient is allowed to shower 72 hours after surgery. If the bandage becomes dirty or wet, it is recommended to replace it with a clean bandage. To take a bath or go swimming is not allowed until the incision is completely healed.

Therapy of Patients with Confirmed Acute Infection of the THA

Early postoperative infection and acute hematogenous infection should be treated identically as long as the onset of symptoms is <4 weeks, the implants are well-fixed, and no fistula to the joint exists [6]. The identification of the microorganism is desirable, but should not postpone the surgical intervention if there is a clinically evident infection of the THA.

In case of a confirmed acute infection of a THA, an exchange of all the modular components during DAIR (Debridement, Antibiotics and Implant Retention) should take place within 48 hours after the patient was referred to an orthopaedic surgeon. An exchange of all modular components during DAIR reduces the risk of PJI recurrence. DAIR with replacement of all modular components has a similar ability to eradicate infection, similar morbidity and complication rates compared with two-stage revisions for the treatment of acute PJI [19]. According to our guidelines, the repeat DAIR with replacement of all modular components is not indicated. Hence, there is a drop down of the eradication rate to 70% after repeat DAIR is reported and the removal of the prosthesis is indicated. However, repeat DAIR patients have a similar implant survivorship similar to primary THA. Patients with higher American Association of Anesthesiologists (ASA) scores have a higher risk of treatment failure. The underlying organism may influence the outcome and decision to perform DAIR. Following these strict diagnostic and therapeutic criteria in patients with suspected periprosthetic joint infection, DAIR and replacement of all modular components can lead to high rates of success in eradicating the infection [20].

General Considerations: Replacement of Modular Components and DAIR

We recommend that 6–9 L of irrigation solution, including saline or antiseptic solution for DAIR of acute PJI. Replacement of all modular components and DAIR are very effective in early PJI (less than 4–6 weeks), where the greater success in the eradication of infection was seen [19].

Replacement of Modular Components

THA Modular parts to be replaced are the femoral head, socket liner, and the locking screw.

Tumour prosthesis or revision prosthesis All modular parts including the femoral head, socket liner, locking screw and the modular neck should be replaced.

Megaprosthesis, Tumor Prosthesis, Modular Stems

The effectiveness of DAIR is not conclusive because of the lack of comparative data between the available treatment options. Due to the limited evidence, no clear recommendation to suggest superiority of any of the available treatments can be done. The treatment decision must be made case-by-case in considering the underlying medical conditions, infection history, organism characteristics and surgical history of the patient [6].

Technical Considerations with the DAA

The best advantage in performing DAIR of the prosthesis is seen in early postoperative PJI and acute hematogenous PJI, defined as symptoms existing for no longer than 4 weeks, and if the implant is stable. If the patient has a primary DAA approach, the same skin incision can be used for this procedure. In most cases, no proximal or distal extension for standard implants has to be performed. When the hip is exposed, instability including soft-tissue laxity and impingement of components, bone and soft tissues should be assessed. We recommend the use of a bone hook on the taper of the stem to dislocate the hip anteriorly. External rotation, adduction and hyperextension of the operated leg provide good exposure for the removal of the femoral head. Following this, the patient's legs can be hyperextended to hide the taper of the stem lateral and posterior to the acetabulum, which enables enough exposure for the liner exchange. Meticulous debridement and removal of all infected or suspicious soft tissue should be part of every revision arthroplasty in the management of PJIs. We then performed a series of trial reductions, with the use of various offset and lipped unconstrained trial polyethylene liners and trial modular heads in an effort to improve stability. With each trial reduction, the range of motion until dislocation was assessed. Although the risk of dislocation in DAA is low, using a larger femoral head or utilizing a constrained or dual-mobility liner to mitigate hip, instability can be considered.

Therapy of Patients with Confirmed Chronic Infection of the THA

In cases of chronic infection of a THA, either one-stage or two-stage revision arthroplasty should be performed. Aggressive debridement and 6–9 L of irrigation solution, including saline or antiseptic solution, are mandatory for both procedures. All foreign material including cement, cables and screws should be removed during either one- or two-stage procedures. Heterotopic ossifications as a potential source for re-infection should be removed as well. However, there may be rare cases of PJIs when removal of all hardware may lead to marked morbidity and precludes opportunity for future reconstruction. In these rare situations, some hardware may be retained.

Functional outcomes, PROMS (Patient Reported Outcome Measures) and eradication of infection are reported to be similar comparing these two techniques. The main advantages of a one-stage exchange arthroplasty are the decrease in surgical morbidity, mortality and earlier functional return. The identification of the microorganism causing infection is necessary to select the surgical method in cases of chronic infection. The only exception to perform DAIR and replacement of all modular components in a chronic infection is on an urgent base in case of a sepsis, when the patient has to be medically optimized prior to one- or two-stage exchange procedure.

General Considerations: One-Stage Versus Two-Stage Revision Arthroplasty

A one-stage change of the prosthesis can be conducted in case of a known microorganism with known resistances. A two-stage change of the prosthesis is recommended in case of a systemic sepsis, extensive comorbidities, infection with resistant organisms, culture-negative infections, the causative organism, and its susceptibility are not known, failure of a previous one-staged procedure, poor soft tissue coverage, fistula, and if a radical debridement of infected tissue including bones or soft tissue is not possible (e.g. perforated acetabulum). Patients with active septic arthritis or chronic osteomyelitis of the hip or knee may be best treated with a two-stage arthroplasty. The lack of local antimicrobial treatment, missing proper bone stock, culture-negative PJI, damage of soft tissue where closure of the joint is not possible, non-availability of appropriate antibiotics during the surgery and the presence of systemic sepsis are relative contraindications for one-stage revision arthroplasty [21–23]. The main benefits of one stage revisions arthroplasty are a single surgical procedure, a shorter period of antibiotic treatment, and reduced costs.

After resection arthroplasty with explantation of the implants and debridement in one-stage procedures, the skin should be closed. Then, all surgical fields and instruments should be changed before re-implantation in order to reduce the bioburden and to improve the outcome after the one-stage procedure. Due to their general conditions, not all patients will tolerate such a long surgery, which should be considered when deciding to perform either one-stage or two-stage revisions.

In case of two-stage procedures, the first surgery involves the removal of the infected implants, surgical debridement and implantation of a spacer. The second procedure consists of surgical debridement and re-implantation of a new prosthesis. An advantage of two-stage revisions is that the spacers can be exchanged in cases of persisted infection.

Spacers

Various types of spacers have been described and include static or articulating, handmade, custom-moulded or preformed spacers. Regarding the use of articulating versus non-articulating spacers in two-stage revision arthroplasty, articulating spacers should be preferred, as they provide better range of motion and have less functional limitations. However, in rare cases of severe bone loss or deficient hip abductor mechanism, non-articulating spacers can be considered. We always tend to use articulating spacers, even in massive bone loss (Fig. 38.2), as articulating hip spacers help improve patient function and clinical outcomes by ensuring early mobilization and restoration of the joint function. Antibiotics added to the spacer cement spacer during resection arthroplasty can be tailored towards the causative organism and its sensitivity. Broad-spectrum antibiotics can be applied in general or in cases of culture-negative PJI. The function of the spacers is to deliver a high dose of antibiotics to the hip joint, to restore the joint height and to reduce shortening and contracture due to scar tissue and fibrosis. We frequently use custom-made articulating spacers (Fig. 38.3) [24]).

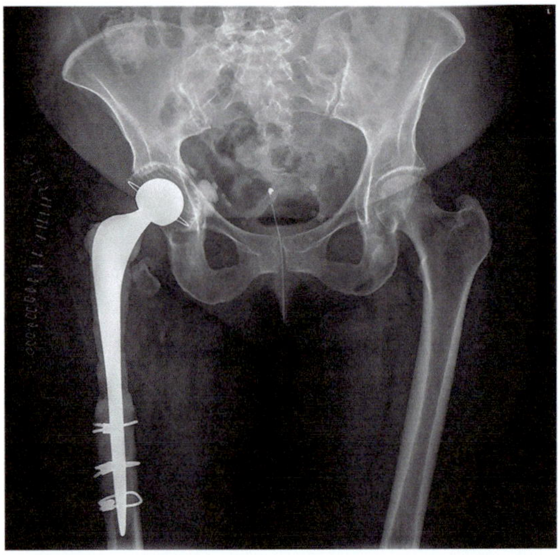

Fig. 38.2 Showing massive bone loss in a patient after first-stage revision resection arthroplasty. X-ray showing the patient with a custom-made spacer

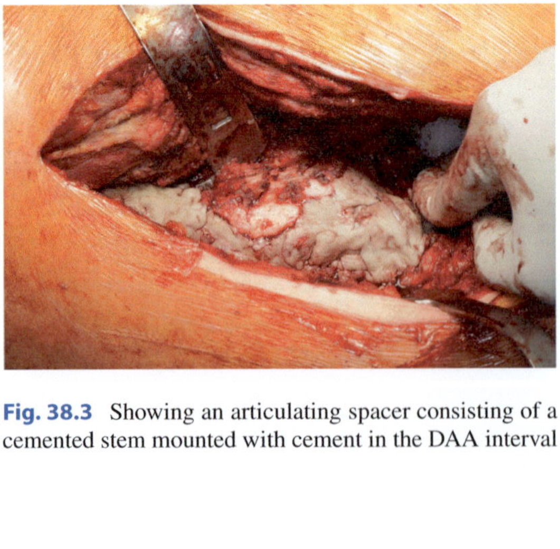

Fig. 38.3 Showing an articulating spacer consisting of a cemented stem mounted with cement in the DAA interval

Timing of Re-implantation in Two-Stage Revisions

The optimal timing for reimplantation of a two-stage exchange arthroplasty of the hip has not been exactly defined yet. We never perform an antibiotic holiday and re-aspiration of the joint fluid before re-implantation. The current evidence does not support the idea of a drug holiday prior to re-implantation. The diagnostic accuracy of joint aspiration prior to re-implantation is unclear and definite thresholds are missing. However, aspiration is a low-cost and simple application which can carried out in an outpatient clinic and therefore can be performed before re-implantation in selected cases.

Several studies report that the optimal timing for the second-stage procedure is between 3 and 11 weeks with comparable eradication rates of infection [25]. A short interval for patients should be considered, if possible, to reduce mortality, morbidity, limited mobilization and inconvenience associated with spacers. If the two-stage revision is performed earlier, faster mobilization, shorter hospital stay, less contraction, and easier surgical dissection can be observed [26]. The exact time point of re-implantation should be decided individually in a multidisciplinary approach. Reimplantation may be performed when the treating medical team feels that the infection is under control. A trend and decline in CRP and ESR is welcomed but in some certain cases, reimplantation may be performed despite abnormal levels of ESR and CRP. Thus, timing of re-implantation should consider resolution of clinical signs of infection and down-trend in the serological markers.

We try to perform the re-implantation as fast as possible with a minimum of a 3 weeks interval if the criteria mentioned above are fulfilled. A fast track re-implantation, 2–3 weeks after explanation can be performed if the bacteria is known, sensitive to antibiotics and the patient has a good soft tissue coverage and is immunocompetent. Most re-implantations in our department are performed after an interval of 6 weeks. We perform an interim cement spacer exchange and repeated irrigation and debridement in the presence of persistent infection instead of re-implantation.

Technical Considerations with the DAA

Few published data reports about the results of one or two-stage revision arthroplasty with the DAA. We published our clinical results about treating periprosthetic joint infections in 49 patients in a two stage revision arthroplasty using the DAA recently. Clinical results, PROMS, eradication rate of infection, and complication rate were comparable with other approaches. Therefore, we believe the DAA can be used safely as a standard operative approach for one- and two-stage revision procedures [24]. For a surgeon generation who were mainly taught in the DAA, and are most familiar with the DAA as their primary approach, revision arthroplasty through the same interval can be recommended. Training, education and the use of dedicated instruments are even more essential and important in revision THA performed through the DAA.

General Considerations with the DAA

The authors of this chapter perform in 90% of cases two-stage revision arthroplasties with the DAA and in 10% one-stage revision arthroplasties with the DAA with regard to the strict criteria mentioned above. Training, education, the use of dedicated instruments as well as implants in THA are essential and even more important in the treatment of infected THA patients with the DAA. The correct location of the skin incision is more crucial in revision DAA than in primary. According to our protocol, there are three exceptions not to use the DAA as approach for one- or two-stage revision arthroplasties:

1. A draining sinus from another approach
2. The need to remove a posterior acetabular plate

3. The need to remove a custom-made implant, which was implanted through another approach

We also perform one- or two-stage revision arthroplasties if the patient had another approach for primary or revision THA elsewhere. All patients receive perioperative intravenous administration of antibiotics. If there was any active draining sinus, the sinus has to be excised. We recommend to perform an aggressive debridement and 6–9 L of irrigation solution during any septic revisions. Multiple (5–6) tissue and fluid samples should be obtained and sent for aerobic and anaerobic culture. Sonication can be performed for all implants.

Approach

The skin incision for revisions starts 2 cm lateral and 2 cm distal to the ASIS, like the primary DAA approach. The incision can be extended distally and proximally. In bigger hip socket revisions, the DAA interval can be extended to the level of the ASIS in order to perform a tensor release. We recommend to carry out this release and not to release the external rotators if possible. If needed, about one-third of the tensor fascia latae (TFL) muscle can be released 1–2 cm distally to his origin at the ASIS. This TFL release is situated within the tendon structure's area of the tensor muscle and facilitates refixating. This extension of the approach offers direct access to the ilium and enables fixation or removal of plates and screws, or the explantation as well as re-implantation of reconstruction cages and augments.

Simple femur revisions can be carried out without any approach extension. Depending on the indicators of the intraoperative situs, proximal and distal extension of the approach can be performed. A proximal extension of the skin incision up to the level of the ASIS can be carried out as described above. Here, the femoral exposure can be significantly improved by a tensor release. Thus, a direct access to the femur is possible after the TFL release (Fig. 38.4). Once more, the author recommends not to release the external rotators if possible, in order to enable a better postoperative function for the patient. Moreover, a distal expansion of the DAA interval can be carried out if additionally a periprosthetic fracture has to be treated [27], if a window needs to be chiselled for cement removal, or if a component cannot be explanted endofemoral and a Wagner transfemoral osteotomy or an extended trochanteric osteotomy has to be performed [28]. For the distal extension and to maintain access to the femoral diaphysis, the skin incision needs to be extended. Due to protection of the lateral cutaneous femoral nerve, branches of the femoral nerve, and cosmetic reasons, we prefer to bend the lat-

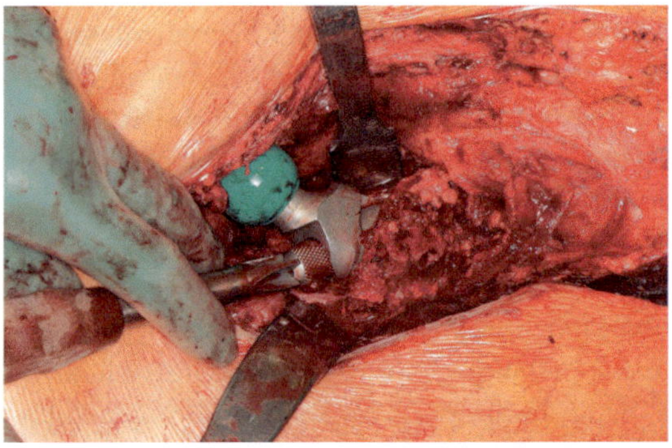

Fig. 38.4 Direct access to a modular stem after a TFL release

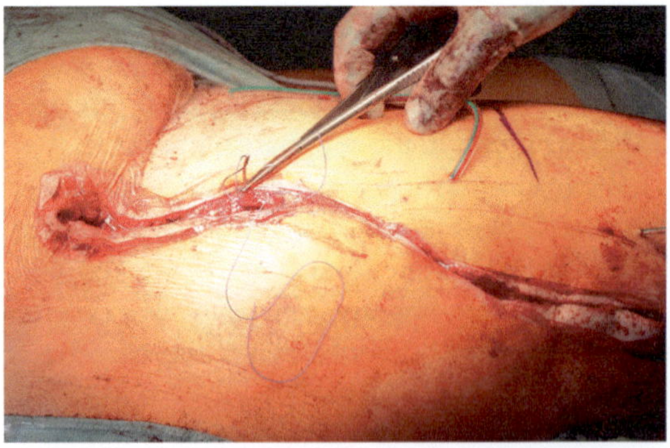

Fig. 38.5 Distal extension of the DAA with the "Lazy-S" extension

eral incision of the most distal point to the original DAA access and to shape a "Lazy-S" form (Fig. 38.5). First, the anterior flange of the TFL is identified. On this level, the iliotibial tract connects typically with the thinner fascia of the quadriceps muscles. We split this fascia longitudinally as far as distally needed.

Then the fascia with the TFL and the complete iliotibial tract can now be bluntly mobilized from the vastus lateralis musculus, which lies underneath. As known from a direct lateral access to the femoral diaphysis, the posterior flange of the musculus vastus lateralis can now be exposed. The further surgical steps do not differ from the direct lateral access to the femoral diaphysis used for fracture treatment.

The Femur

We recommend to explant the femoral component first. This manoeuvre provides better access and exposure to the acetabular cup. External rotation, adduction and hyperextension of the operated leg provide good exposure for the removal of the femoral head as well as for explantation and re-implantation of the femoral component can be carried out (Fig. 38.6). In order to relax the rectus muscle, we also recommend not to bend the knee. An additional relaxation of the tensor can be achieved by flexing the OR table (Fig. 38.7). Flexion of the knee joint leads to contraction of the rectus muscle and consequently to a deepening of the proximal femur, disabling a good exposure of the femoral cana.

The Cup

We recommend to perform the cup implantation first, if a re-implant of the components is required.

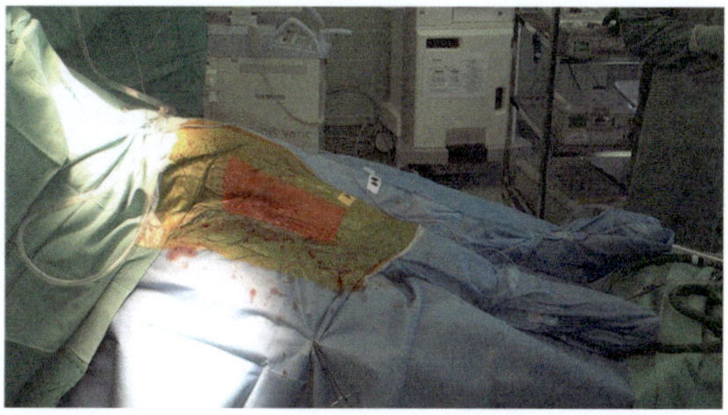

Fig. 38.6 Patient's leg is placed in hyperextension to provide good exposure for the removal of the femoral head as well as for explantation and re-implantation of the femoral component

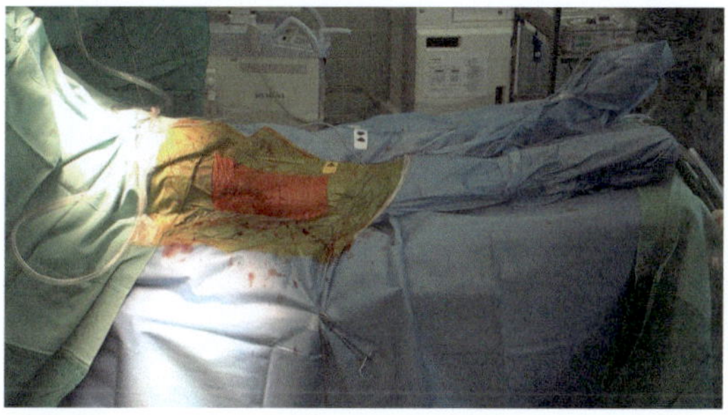

Fig. 38.7 Patient's leg is placed in flexion to relax the rectus muscle

With hyperextension, 20° of adduction of both legs and placement of dedicated retractors good exposure of the cup can be provided. A retractor placed beneath the cup provides the possibility of pushing the femur down, which enables direct access to the cup.

Arthroscopy

Arthroscopic surgery has no role in the treatment of acute or chronic PJI of the knee or hip. In selected cases arthroscopic surgery can be performed as a diagnostic procedure to collect samples for further microbiological or pathological analysis.

References

1. Bozic KJ, Ries MD. The impact of infection after total hip arthroplasty on hospital and surgeon resource utilization. J Bone Jt Surg Ser A. 2005;87(8):1746–51. https://doi.org/10.2106/JBJS.D.02937.
2. Hanssen AD, Osmon DR, Nelson CL. Prevention of deep periprosthetic joint infection. Instr Course Lect. 1997;46:555–67.
3. Aggarwal VK, Weintraub S, Klock J, et al. 2019 Frank Stinchfield Award: a comparison of prosthetic joint infection rates between direct anterior and non-anterior approach total hip arthroplasty. Bone Joint J. 2019;101-B(6_Supple_B):2–8.
4. Purcell RL, Parks NL, Cody JP, Hamilton WG. Comparison of wound complications and deep infections with direct anterior and posterior approaches in obese hip arthroplasty patients. J Arthroplast. 2018;33(1):220–3. https://doi.org/10.1016/j.arth.2017.07.047.
5. Sutphen SA, Berend KR, Morris MJ, Lombardi AV. 2018Direct anterior approach has lower deep infection frequency than less invasive direct lateral approach in primary total hip arthroplasty21. J Surg Orthop Adv. 2018;27(1):21–4. https://doi.org/10.3113/jsoa.2018.0021.
6. Schwarz EM, Parvizi J, Gehrke T, et al. 2018 international consensus meeting on musculoskeletal infection: research priorities from the general assembly questions. J Orthop Res. 2019;
7. Parvizi J, Gehrke T, Chen AF. Proceedings of the international consensus on periprosthetic joint infection. Bone Joint J. 2013;2014:S2–3. https://doi.org/10.1302/0301-620X.95B11.33135.
8. Jaberi FM, Parvizi J, Haytmanek CT, et al. Procrastination of wound drainage and malnutrition affect the outcome of joint arthroplasty. Clin Orthop Relat Res. 2008;466:1368–71.
9. Purcell RL, Parks NL, Gargiulo JM, Hamilton WG. Severely obese patients have a higher risk of infection after direct anterior approach total hip arthroplasty. J Arthroplast. 2016;31(9 Suppl):162–5. https://doi.org/10.1016/j.arth.2016.03.037.
10. Watts CD, Houdek MT, Wagner ER, et al. High risk of wound complications following direct anterior total hip arthroplasty in obese patients. J Arthroplast. 2015;30(12):2296. https://doi.org/10.1016/j.arth.2015.06.016.
11. Redfern RE, Cameron-Ruetz C, O'Drobinak SK, et al. Closed incision negative pressure therapy effects on postoperative infection and surgical site complication after total hip and knee arthroplasty. J Arthroplast. 2017;32(11):3333–9. https://doi.org/10.1016/j.arth.2017.06.019.
12. Murgatroyd SE, Frampton CMA, Wright MS. The effect of body mass index on outcome in total hip arthroplasty: early analysis from the New Zealand Joint Registry. J Arthroplast. 2014;29(10):1884. https://doi.org/10.1016/j.arth.2014.05.024.
13. Belmont PJ, Goodman GP, Hamilton W, et al. Morbidity and mortality in the thirty-day period following total hip arthroplasty: risk factors and incidence. J Arthroplast. 2014;29(10):2025. https://doi.org/10.1016/j.arth.2014.05.015.
14. Zmistowski B, Restrepo C, Kahl LK, et al. Incidence and reasons for nonrevision reoperation after total knee arthroplasty. Clin Orthop Relat Res. 2011;469:138–45.
15. Amanatullah D, Dennis D, Oltra EG, et al. Hip and knee section, diagnosis, definitions: proceedings of international consensus on orthopedic infections. J Arthroplast. 2019;34:329.
16. Foremny GB, Pretell-Mazzini J, Jose J, Subhawong TK. Risk of bleeding associated with interventional musculoskeletal radiology procedures. A comprehensive review of the literature. Skelet Radiol. 2015;44:619–27.
17. Bereza P, et al. Comparison of cultures and 16S rRNA sequencing for identification of bacteria in two-stage revision arthroplasties: preliminary report. BMC Musculoskelet Disord. 2016;17:138.
18. Ibrahim MS, Twaij H, Haddad FS. Two-stage revision for the culture-negative infected total hip arthroplasty: a comparative study. Bone Joint J. 2018;100-B:3–8. https://doi.org/10.1302/0301-620X.100B1.BJJ-2017-0626.R1.
19. Grammatopoulos G, Bolduc ME, Atkins BL, et al. Functional outcome of debridement, antibiotics and implant retention in periprosthetic joint infection involving the hip. Bone Joint J. 2017;99-B(5):614–22. https://doi.org/10.1302/0301-620X.99B5.BJJ-2016-0562.R2.
20. Sendi P, Lötscher PO, Kessler B, et al. Debridement and implant retention in the management of hip periprosthetic joint infection outcomes following guided and rapid treatment at a single centre. Bone Joint J. 2017;99-B(3):330–6. https://doi.org/10.1302/0301-620X.99B3.
21. Nagra NS, Hamilton TW, Ganatra S, et al. One-stage versus two-stage exchange arthroplasty for infected total knee arthroplasty: a systematic review. Knee Surg Sport Traumatol Arthrosc. 2016;24:3106–14.
22. Leonard HAC, Liddle AD, Burke Ó, et al. Single- or two-stage revision for infected total hip arthroplasty? A systematic review of the literature. Clin Orthop Relat Res. 2014;472:1036–42.
23. Gehrke T, Zahar A, Kendoff D. One-stage exchange: it all began here. Bone Joint J. 2013;95-B(11):77–83. https://doi.org/10.1302/0301-620X.95B11.32646.
24. Thaler M, Lechner R, Dammerer D, et al. The direct anterior approach: treating periprosthetic joint infection of the hip using two-stage revision arthroplasty. Arch Orthop Trauma Surg. 2020;140(2):255–62. https://doi.org/10.1007/s00402-019-03317-1.
25. Vielgut I, Sadoghi P, Wolf M, et al. Two-stage revision of prosthetic hip joint infections using antibiotic-loaded cement spacers: when is the best time to perform the second stage? Int Orthop. 2015;39(9):1731–6. https://doi.org/10.1007/s00264-015-2751-5.

26. Winkler T, Stuhlert MGW, Lieb E, et al. Outcome of short versus long interval in two-stage exchange for periprosthetic joint infection: a prospective cohort study. Arch Orthop Trauma Surg. 2019;139(3):295–303. https://doi.org/10.1007/s00402-018-3052-4.
27. Thaler M, Dammerer D, Krismer M, et al. Extension of the direct anterior approach for the treatment of periprosthetic femoral fractures. J Arthroplast. 2019;34(10):2449–53. https://doi.org/10.1016/j.arth.2019.05.015.
28. Nogler MM, Thaler MR. The direct anterior approach for hip revision: accessing the entire femoral diaphysis without endangering the nerve supply. J Arthroplast. 2017;32(2):510–4. https://doi.org/10.1016/j.arth.2016.07.044.

Part VII

Introduction to Part VII

Future Directions in Technique and Technology

Though it is impossible to predict the future, it does not stop us from trying and anticipating. I think that there will be a growing role of devices and technology. The purpose and potential benefit of this is to eliminate, as much as possible, the ill effects from the surgeon variable. At this time, there can be wide variation in results because of variation from surgeon to surgeon as well as variations in results of surgeries performed by an individual surgeon. A potential solution can be more standardized methods plus facilitating devices and technologies.

Commercial aviation has seen a dramatic improvement in its safety record with automated aircraft technologies and standardized procedures. On the other hand, there has been recent aviation accidents when the automation failed or did the wrong thing, and the pilot was unable to effectively take over control by "hand flying" the aircraft. It is postulated that reliance on aircraft automation may be leading to degeneration of pilot "stick and rudder" hand flying skills.

The future of AA will see advances that will lead to better outcomes facilitated by devices and technology, but can we do this without a degeneration of our "hand flying" skills and resultant unfortunate outcomes?

Navigation Technologies for the Anterior Approach in Total Hip Arthroplasty

39

John Jay Perry and Andrew J. Cooper

As many clinicians know, hip arthroplasty is a very successful surgical intervention to improve the function and satisfaction of those with hip pathologies. While surgeon experience and skill can certainly maximize successful outcomes, outliers can exist across the spectrum of surgeon acumen and approaches. This success can be tempered by functional issues related to implant position including cup position, proper leg length, and offset restoration. The importance of cup position for successful outcome during hip arthroplasty has been well studied. Safe zones of acetabular cup position have been described in several studies. Lewinnek et al. determined a safe zone as 30° to 50° of abduction and 5° to 25° of anteversion noting increased dislocation rates outside these zones [1]. Barrack et al. determined the safe zone to be 35° to 50° abduction and 10° to 30° of anteversion to mitigate dislocation [2]. Despite surgeon familiarity with these safe zones reliably attaining them during total hip arthroplasty is less than assured.

Interestingly, surgeon experience has been found to not always assure cup and stem position by visual intraoperative estimation during standard and minimally invasive approaches [3, 4]. Callahan et al. reported experienced surgeons using visual clues alone in 1823 cups studied only half were found to be within the combined target zones of 30° to 45° abduction and 5° to 25° anteversion [4]. Implant positioning can also influence complications such as dislocation [1, 2, 5–7], accelerated bearing surface wear and reduced implant longevity [5, 8–12], impingement with resultant limited range of motion [13], and even catastrophic failure [14–16].

Computer-assisted orthopedic surgery technologies in total hip arthroplasty have been developed to assist the surgeon in optimizing implant positioning and promoting improved patient satisfaction and outcomes. The introduction of intraoperative fluoroscopy was a significant advancement in total hip arthroplasty, enabling guidance of implant placement. Fluoroscopy can be used to facilitate decision making and provide real-time qualitative information on implant positioning including estimation of comparative leg length and offset. Beamer et al. have found fluoroscopy to improve the odds of placing the cup into the surgeon's safe zone abduction 30° to 45° and anteversion of 5° to 25° using different approaches during primary, conversion, and revision total hip arthroplasty [17].

The supine position in direct anterior approach allows surgeons to adopt fluoroscopy into their workflow. Intraoperative fluoroscopy is a readily available, affordable, and facile enabling technology in direct anterior approach and predated the

J. J. Perry
Perry Orthopedics, Melbourne, FL, USA
e-mail: jperry1014@aol.com

A. J. Cooper (✉)
Orthopaedic Associates of West Florida, Clearwater, FL, USA
e-mail: acooper@floridaortho.com

J. M. Matta, A. P. Sah (eds.), *Anterior Hip Replacement*,
https://doi.org/10.1007/978-3-030-91896-5_39

computer-assisted orthopedic surgery systems of today. J. Martin et al. compared anatomic component positioning in 100 patients using posterior approach without fluoroscopy to 100 direct anterior approach patients with fluoroscopy [18]. Direct anterior approach provided more accurate restoration of leg length, femoral offset, and total offset than imageless posterior approach. Direct anterior approach also provided more ideal cup abduction and anteversion than posterior approach [18].

Rathod et al. compared direct anterior approach with fluoroscopy to posterior approach without fluoroscopy including those cases considered during the learning curve of direct anterior approach [19]. They reported reduced variances in cup inclination and anteversion were significantly lower than the direct anterior approach group with target inclination and anteversion achieved more reliably (98% and 97% respectively) compared to the posterior approach group (86% and 77% respectively). Even during the learning curve of direct anterior approach, target inclination was attained in 95% and anteversion 91% of cases reviewed [19]. While fluoroscopy was readily accepted as a qualitative tool into the direct anterior approach surgeon's workflow, it lacked granular, quantitative data for optimizing intraoperative decision making. The need for more quantitative data delivery systems around the readily available fluoroscopy left opportunities for innovation in total hip arthroplasty.

Computer-assisted orthopedic surgery has rapidly expanded over the past three decades to include four basic technologies (Fig. 39.1):

- Computer-assisted preoperative planning
- Computer-assisted navigation
- Robotics
- Patient-specific surgical templates

Many of proprietary systems available today incorporate two or more of these technologies to minimize inaccuracies while attempting to optimize efficiency during hip arthroplasty. Navigation platforms typically incorporate computer-assisted preoperative planning into their workflows whereas robotics require computer-assisted preoperative planning and navigation to direct the action of the robotic device.

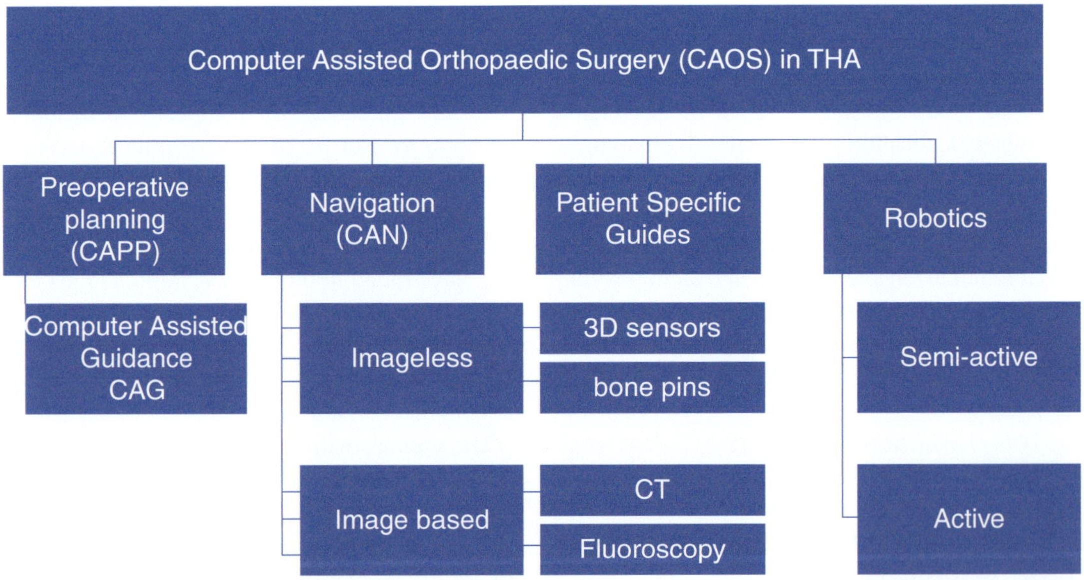

Fig. 39.1 Computer-assisted orthopedic surgery (CAOS) in total hip arthroplasty comprises four basic technologies

Computer-Assisted Preoperative Planning

Preoperative planning with acetate film has long been supplanted by digital and computer-assisted preoperative planning. Most arthroplasty surgeons are versed in the many computer-assisted preoperative planning platforms. These platforms allowed more capable computer-assisted guidance technologies to evolve. Computer-assisted guidance aims to augment fluoroscopy providing more detailed and robust qualitative guidance experience for the surgeon. In general terms, guidance is providing information aimed at resolving a problem or question and maybe considered more qualitative in nature. Conversely, navigation requires detailed quantitative information to afford an objective. Preoperative planning allows guidance, as does intraoperative fluoroscopy, but typically lack the accurate data computer-assisted navigation systems provide.

Computer-Assisted Navigation

Computer-assisted navigation for hip arthroplasty developed in the 1990s with advancements in three-dimensional sensor technology. In general terms, navigation is considered a process of accurately ascertaining position and then planning to execute a planned route. Prior to computer-assisted navigation, acquiring accurate acetabular and femoral positions for implant placement lacked quantitative data in millimeters and degrees. Computer-assisted navigation technologies germinated and evolved quickly in the early 2000s to help address the quantitative deficiencies with conventional visual, mechanical, and fluoroscopic techniques. Computer-assisted navigation systems strived to allow surgeons to accurately plan and place implants to the level of millimeters and degrees not previously attainable with conventional techniques and mitigate the potential for radiographic outliers.

Computer-assisted navigation and computer-assisted guidance systems are considered passive technologies which provide information to guide surgeon decisions and actions using conventional tools. Computer-assisted navigation and computer-assisted guidance do not physically control the surgeon's actions as robotic systems do. Computer-assisted navigation systems are typically image-based or imageless in the way the surgeon acquires the data for intraoperative decision making. Image-based systems rely on either preoperative computed tomography (CT) scans or intraoperative fluoroscopic images. Image-based systems may be considered noninvasive, taking indirect measurements of the relevant bony anatomy (Fig. 39.2).

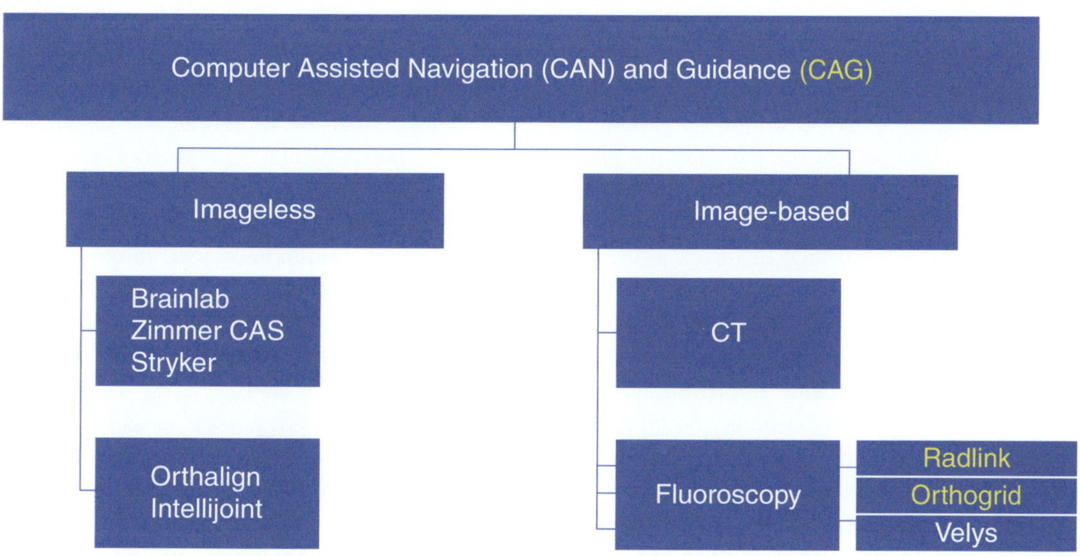

Fig. 39.2 Computer-assisted navigation and guidance systems

Image-based systems may be considered more favorable to surgeons as they take indirect radiographic measurements instead of direct measurements from reference arrays requiring placement of invasive anatomical reference pins in the pelvis and femur. The amount of time it takes to register the bony anatomy using either imageless or image-based computer-assisted navigation systems seems highly variable between technologies and may impose significant learning curves for the surgical team.

Imageless Navigation

Imageless navigation systems first on the market, such as Zimmer Computer-Assisted Surgery (CAS) (Zimmer Biomet, Warsaw, IN), Stryker OrthoMap Navigation (Stryker, Kalamazoo, MI, USA), and BrainLab Navigation (BrainLab, Munich, Germany) required drilling of pins into the pelvis and sometimes femur, to place passive optical trackers which are monitored by the three-dimensional active optic tracker station near the operative field. Accurate registration of acetabular and femoral landmarks are recorded with an optically tracked probe. The registration of landmarks and stability of the anatomic trackers is of the paramount importance in accuracy and success of these procedures. Cup position, notably inclination and anteversion, as well and changes in leg length and often offset, are displayed in real-time to the surgeon with these imageless systems.

The value of these technologies would be based on the accuracy of the data and the precision and efficiency of the input of the registration steps. With careful registration, data could be reliable, providing real-time feedback to the surgeon to make data-driven decisions on implant position and functional metrics. Continual advancements in computers, optics, and tracker technology hope to provide improved accuracy and efficiency over older systems. Some imageless computer-assisted navigation systems are universal with any implants, and some had to be used for optimal data capture with a specific implant company. With the infrequency of intra-operative imaging being used in approaches like posterolateral, lateral, and anterolateral when the patient is placed in the lateral decubitus position, the appeal of this data was to compliment the standard techniques which relied heavily on surgeon experience and skill. Surgeons and approaches which found fluoroscopy cumbersome were the beneficiaries of imageless navigation system development. These systems reinforced the desire to minimize the use of ionizing radiation for certain approaches and surgeons.

The efficacy and accuracy of imageless computer-assisted navigation systems to reduce outliers and improve implant position, including cup position and leg length discrepancy, when compared to standard techniques has been reported [20–22]. While in general, these systems are effective, accurate, and reliable when registration is realized they rarely improve efficiency and reduce operative times [21]. To the contrary, Kruezer et al. reported minor operative time reductions with imageless computer-assisted navigation versus conventional direct anterior approach theorizing the supine positioning allows a less cumbersome registration process than lateral positioned approaches [23]. Despite these radiographic, safety, and potential efficiencies benefits, significant improvements in clinical outcomes have yet to be realized for imageless computer-assisted navigation systems [20, 21].

The navigation systems were somewhat agnostic to the approach and could be used for anterior approach as well as the more common approaches when these products were introduced. As the percentage of anterior approach total hip arthroplasty cases increased, these products become more frequently used in settings which were less common on their initial release. With anterior approach, some advantages to registration were seen, as the anterior superior iliac spine (ASIS), for example, access to both sides was more readily available.

Certain cup analytics, such as defining cup position off of the anterior pelvic plane, became easier with patients in the supine position. These registration points could be done as well on the lateral decubitus position, but often needed to be registered prior to this positioning. This could create a workflow disruption, as some level of sterility was needed as the pins would need to be drilled into the pelvis for this portion of the registration prior to final positioning. Often, surgeons would forgo this registration and the applicable data when using this technology in the lateral decubitus position and would register functional plane of the pelvis.

The advantage of the registration of both ASIS during supine positioning was partly offset by the disadvantage of having the pelvic tracker on the ilium during femoral preparation. During anterior approach surgery, femoral exposure and broaching would often compete with the same real estate as the tracker on the same side of the ilium. Any distortion of the pins in the pelvis during femoral preparation would cause error in data, most notably leg length and offset. Smaller trackers with the newer navigation systems would help this problem somewhat as well as placing the tracker on the contralateral ilium. This could provide some workflow challenges, but navigation systems are successfully used in anterior approach total hip arthroplasty.

The adoption of this technology among surgeons was based on the upside of the data output of the navigation system versus the downside of potential time to the case, change in surgeon workflow, and most often large cost to the hospital system for the additional capital, software, and disposable costs. Additional navigation systems, such as Intellijoint HIP ® (Intellijoint Surgical, Inc., Kitchener, ON, Canada) (Fig. 39.3) and HipAlign® (OrthAlign, Inc., Aliso Viejo, CA, USA) attempted to address some of the cost concerns, portability, and potentially improved ease of use. Although these systems still required registration steps and pins to be drilled for data, they attempted to appeal to a larger user population by addressing some of the concerns of the initial product offerings.

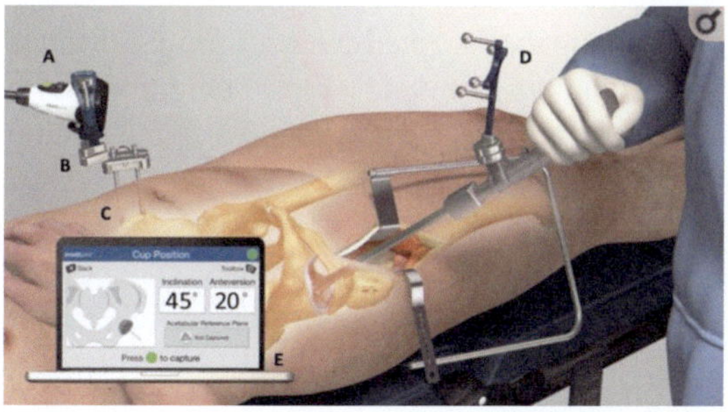

Fig. 39.3 Intellijoint HIP mini navigation system as depicted in Bradley et al. [24]

Image-Based Navigation

Image-based navigation systems have evolved in parallel to the imageless systems. Similarly, to imageless systems, image-based navigation has advantages and disadvantages. Image-based systems in orthopedic surgery are comprised of volumetric imaging including magnetic resonance imaging (MRI), CT, and even new ultrasound technologies and nonvolumetric imaging like two-dimensional and three-dimensional fluoroscopy. CT-based and two-dimensional fluoroscopic-based systems have been the focus of most imaged-based navigation systems in total hip arthroplasty. CT and fluoroscopic platforms expose the patient to ionizing radiation whereas the use of fluoroscopy alone exposes the surgeon, patient, and surgical team. The exposure to surgeon and patient during direct anterior arthroplasty has been recently studied [25–27].

McNabb et al. reported fluoroscopy use during direct anterior hip arthroplasty does not pose undue radiation exposure risk to the patient or surgeon [25]. Curtin et al. reported during a direct anterior approach using fluoroscopy the total radiation exposure was nearly identical to previous published values for a screening mammography (3 m Gy) and four times less than a standard chest CT (13 m Gy) [26]. They concluded while it is difficult to ascertain the exact patient-absorbed radiation, their data suggest a one-time exposure during the approach is likely negligible. Pomeroy et al. concluded a surgeon would need to perform greater than 300,000 direct anterior approach total hip arthroplasty to exceed the 800 m Gy cataract threshold dose but leaving the decision to use protective glasses to surgeon discretion [27].

Increasing surgical time is a concern for patients and surgeons alike. The use of many technologies requiring data acquisition increases surgical times for the advantage of more accurate surgical execution and improved patient outcome. A comparative study by Hube et al. reported both CT and fluoroscopy-based systems increased surgical time over manual techniques with CT-based requiring significant preoperative planning with less intraoperative time and fluoroscopic-based requiring no preoperative planning but more intraoperative time for setup and analysis [28]. Both technologies provided similar accuracy in the mean variation of postoperative abduction angle with preoperative planning. CT-based systems had the advantage of three-dimensional feedback on landmarks but required time-consuming preoperative planning. Hube et al. concluded fluoroscopy-based method may be utilized for routine cases with normal anatomy and lesser deformities while there may be advantages to utilizing CT-based methods for complex deformities [28].

CT-based navigation was first used by Digiola et al. in 1998 to improve accuracy of acetabular component placement in total hip arthroplasty [29]. CT-based navigation yields improved accuracy over conventionally placed acetabular components while also being effective in both anterior and posterior approaches [30, 31]. Sugano et al. in a long-term follow-up study found reduced dislocation and impingement related mechanical complications resulting in revision of cementless total hip arthroplasty and ceramic bearing surfaces [31]. Barriers to CT-based navigation have included time-consuming CT preoperative planning, increased time, cost, and logistical planning with the added radiation exposure [32].

Fluoroscopy-based navigation is a recent evolution in computer-assisted navigation. Historically, invasive navigation systems were infrequently used with anterior approach due to the prevalence of fluoroscopy adoption. More commonly, surgeons performing anterior approach total hip arthroplasty would use fluoroscopy to provide qualitative implant positioning data. The accuracy and need for fluoroscopy during direct anterior approach has been questioned by some authors [33] yet embraced by others [17]. Fluoroscopic images and their interpretation can be affected by patient size, positioning, and C-arm position. The initial setup of the C-arm and stable supine patient positioning is helpful to aid interpretation throughout the case as pelvic motion can confound decision making. Shah et al. reported intraoperative pelvic motion occurred during 86.4% (19/22) direct anterior approach total hip arthroplasty starting in a neutral position trending toward extension by cup impaction [34]. Rolling of the pelvis was also reported. They noted the predicted change in cup version of ≥5° due to changes in pelvic position was seen in 32% (7/22) patients. Shah concluded, "although minor, changes in pelvic position do occur during supine total hip arthroplasty which may affect acetabular orientation" [34].

A learning curve is typical for new adopters of fluoroscopic-assisted direct anterior approach total hip arthroplasty as complications decline with experience [35]. Difficulties with interpreting x-ray and fluoroscopic images led to even the most experienced pelvic surgeon like Jeff Mast, to described interpretation as "the misery of x-rays". X-ray images are shadows which can be distorted leading to misinterpretation, hence the misery for the orthopedic surgeons.

Jang et al. reported the accuracy of perceived cup anteversion and inclination to minor variations in C-arm tilt angles [36]. They noted with just 10° of caudal or cephalad C-arm tilt led to a 9° and 10° error and perceived cup anteversion and inclination respectively. James et al. found total hip arthroplasty relying on routine intraoperative fluoroscopic anteroposterior pelvic imaging utilizing the accepted coccyx to pubis distance resulted in 95% (39/41) hips being placed in unrecognized excess anteversion and inclination due to imaging the pelvis in extension [37]. They recommended positioning the C-arm so the size and shape of the obturator foramen matches the standing preoperative anteroposterior pelvis x-ray. James goes on to explain, "this technique will allow for the native standing pelvic tilt to be accounted for intraoperatively and will result in the least variation in intraoperative and postoperative standing acetabular component orientation" [37]. The dichotomy of opinions and concerns left opportunities to improve the guidance capabilities of fluoroscopy and spurred the need for more quantitative data acquisition to augment and aid in true surgical navigation of total hip arthroplasty.

At the time of writing this chapter, VELYS™ Hip Navigation (DePuy Synthes © West Chester, PA, USA) is the only navigation system using fluoroscopy during anterior approach hip arthroplasty surgery. Other technologies use the images to provide surgeon feedback on implant positioning and leg length and offset include OrthoGrid Hip (OrthoGrid Systems, Inc., Salt Lake City, UT, USA) and Radlink (Radlink, Inc., El Segundo, CA, USA). Surgeons would also use other techniques, not technology, to help interpret the images for feedback. These techniques have been described as printing out overlays, using measurement tools, and guide rods. The success of these techniques has not been widely described and are presumed to depend on the user experience in understanding their limitations. Additional description will follow on these technologies assimilate with fluoroscopy making them more relevant for anterior approach hip arthroplasty surgery.

OrthoGrid

OrthoGrid Hip is an intraoperative surgical application designed specifically for direct approach total hip arthroplasty. The technology may be best known for its ability to correct fluoroscopic distortion, which can easily go unrecognized. Image intensified C-arms, common in many operating rooms around the world, are subject to fluoroscopic distortion primarily as a result of electromagnetic interference. When unaccounted for, distortion may affect the interpretation of component positioning during direct approach total hip arthroplasty, resulting in limb-length discrepancies and undesirable patient outcomes" [38]. Figure 39.4 demonstrates OrthoGrid Hip distortion correction technology enabling more accurate image guidance during direct approach total hip arthroplasty (Fig. 39.4).

Along with distortion correction, OrthoGrid Hip provides key tools and templates that enable surgeons to objectively assess and accurately evaluate component positioning and restoration of hip mechanics, such as cup inclination, hip offset, and leg length. In a study comparing direct approach total hip arthroplastys performed using fluoroscopy with and without the use of OrthoGrid, acetabular inclination, limb length restoration, and hip offset restoration were all improved with the use of OrthoGrid [39]. A different study comparing the analog OrthoGrid Drone system to the digital system concluded that the OrthoGrid Hip digital gridding system "demonstrated an efficient method for consistent and accurate cup positioning and restoration of hip symmetry following direct approach total hip arthroplasty," and showed lower overall surgical and fluoroscopy times compared to the analog system [40].

Radlink

Radlink was the first Picture Archive and Communication System (PACS) system to market provided data for the surgeon using intraoperative imaging. The company leveraged imaging being captured from flat plate technology as well as from a fluoroscopy C-arm, making the technology applicable for both supine and in the lateral decubitus position. The software/hardware company provided meaningful data for hip arthroplasty surgery, including guidance for cup position, leg length, and offset. The system has a tower and monitor allowing implant representatives and surgeons preoperative planning and intraoperative guidance. Radlink provides an intraoperative cup position ellipse for qualitative inclination and abduction estimates (Fig. 39.5).

Hamilton et al. utilized Radlink's cup positioning ellipse and reported improved accuracy and precision of cup placement [41]. The system allowed the surgeon to target a preselected ellipse with 40° abduction and 20° anteversion

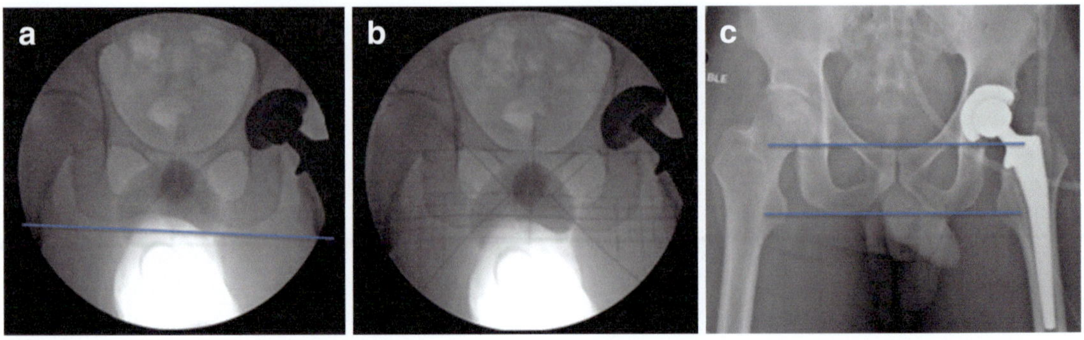

Fig. 39.4 (**a**) Distortion makes operative extremity appear short, (**b**) with distortion correction, the limb lengths are very close, and (**c**) this is confirmed on post-operative imaging

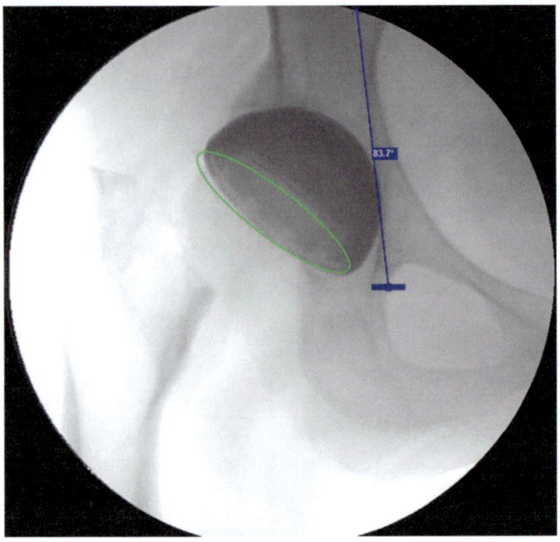

Fig. 39.5 Radlink anteversion and inclination ellipse

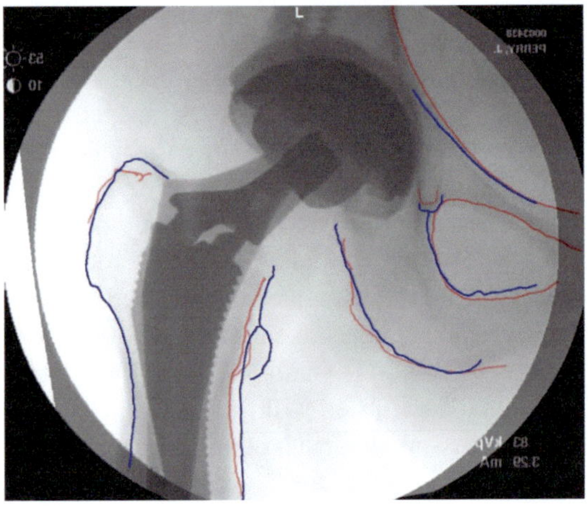

Fig. 39.6 Radlink digital overlay of intraoperative trials and contralateral hip anatomy

during cup impaction was measured for accuracy with postoperative radiographs. The mean abduction angle was 40.4° (range 32.7° to 51.1°) for the computer-guided group and 42.3° (range 33.7° to 51.1°) for the fluoroscopic group. The computer-guided cups were significantly closer to the predetermined targeted abduction angle of 40 ° ($P < 0.001$). They reported a modest increase in surgical and fluoroscopy times over their routine fluoroscopy alone techniques. Surgical time for the impaction of the cup increased from 4:58 minutes with fluoroscopy alone to 7:04 minutes with the computer-assisted guidance group ($P < 0.001$). Fluoroscopic times were increased slightly from 11.1 seconds to 12.9 with the guidance system ($P < 0.001$). Hamilton noted, "although both groups showed accurate and precise placement, and on-screen guide to assist with positioning may help a less experienced surgeon even more" [41].

The system also provides an overlay analysis which is a colored digital outline of the pelvic anatomy similar to the manual fluoroscopic printer acetate overlay technique direct anterior approach surgeons are historically familiar with (Fig. 39.6). Radlink's digital overlay technology allows the surgeon to appreciate relative resultant pelvic anatomies throughout the procedure. The technology helps guide surgeons in selecting the implant size and morphology after reduction of trial implants and allows comparison to both ipsilateral and contralateral hips.

At completion of the surgery and before wound closure, the surgeon can take five overlapping fluoroscopic spot images across the pelvis. The software then digitally stitches these images together providing the surgeon a panoramic view of the entirety of the pelvic anatomy analogous to taking an intraoperative low anterior-posterior (AP) pelvis flat plate x-ray (Fig. 39.7). The system is agnostic for implant vendors.

VELYS Hip Navigation

Described as the first and currently only technology described as fluoroscopic guided navigation for hip arthroplasty, VELYS Hip Navigation, formally JointPoint, incorporates images acquired during surgery and provides data on cup position, leg length, and offset. There are some notable differences to the aforementioned imageless navigation systems in this chapter.

The VELYS Hip Navigation system is noninvasive, as no pins are required to be placed in the pelvis and/or femur. Additionally, the registration steps are often performed by a consultant not in the surgical field. The technology is primarily software-based, as it runs on computers communicating with the fluoroscopic C-arm. This allows the surgical field to remain clear of excess tools and instruments. Both qualitative and quantitative data are displayed on a touch screen monitor (Fig. 39.8). Most computer-assisted guidance, computer-assisted navigation, and robotic systems have a monitor for surgeons to preoperatively plan and make intraoperative changes to surgical plan. Navigation and robotics allow for quantitative assessments using millimeters and degrees.

The monitor allows the industry representative and surgeon to manipulate and make measurements from the preoperative pelvic radiographs for templating and later fluoroscopic images obtained before, during, and after surgery (Fig. 39.9).

The leg length and offset data provided in VHN is displayed in a chart called OneTrial™ (DePuy Synthes Orthopaedics, Inc., Palm Beach Gardens, FL, USA) (Fig. 39.10). The purpose of this chart is to allow the surgeon to not only see the current leg length and offset situation with the

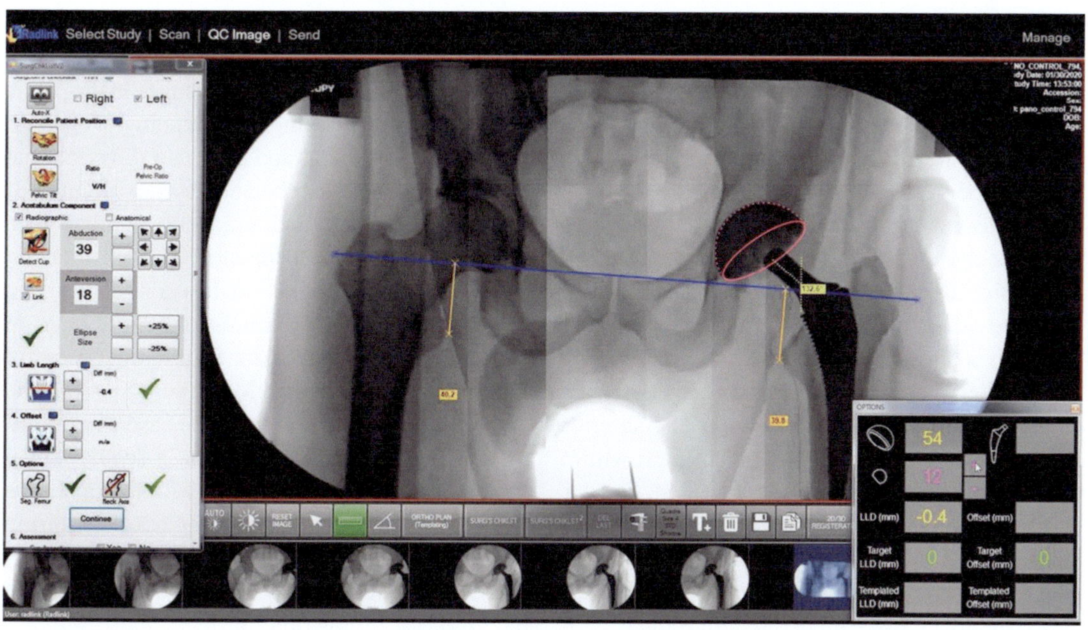

Fig. 39.7 Radlink Panoramic digitally stitched image allows a surgeon to appreciate the full pelvic anatomy prior to wound closure

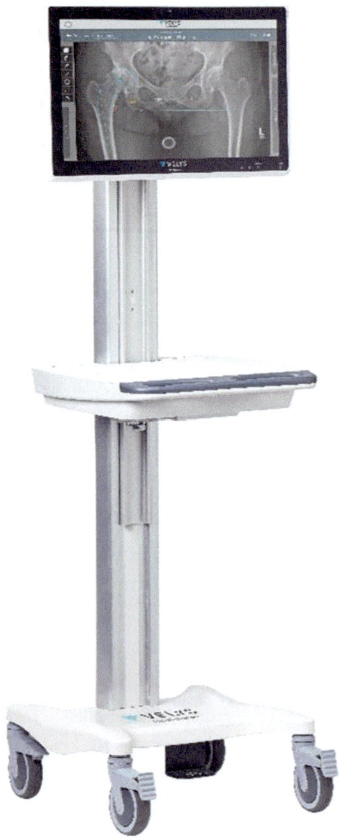

Fig. 39.8 VELYS Hip Navigation system tower with touchscreen monitor

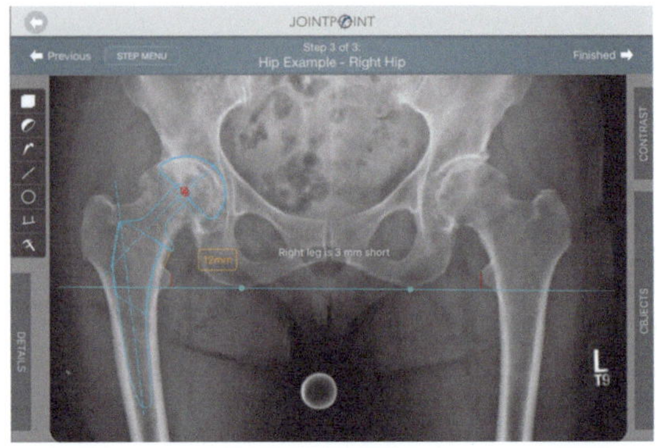

Fig. 39.9 VELYS Hip Navigation system is similar to other computer-assisted guidance and robotic systems which provide computer-assisted preoperative planning

construct being trialed, but the leg length and offset change associated with other modular constructs specific to the stem being utilized. This requires the software to understand the options specific to the applicable stems used, as well as the geometry of the stem and how it would affect the trialing options. With the anterior approach, many surgeons find repetitive trialing, especially when on a special table, to be time-consuming and cumbersome. This technology was designed to address some specific concerns of the anterior approach and was a result of the large growth in this type of surgery.

Fluoroscopy use during anterior approach has been described as potentially time inefficient as well as introducing radiation exposure to the surgical personnel and patient. Accurate interpretation of intraoperative images often requires significant amount of imaging time to address some of the variables affecting data conclusions. VELYS Hip Navigation uses the registration steps to address these variables, potentially reducing the need for repetitive imaging [42].

The importance of cup position for successful outcome during hip arthroplasty has been well studied previously. VELYS Hip Navigation uses a mathematically based ellipse to address cup anteversion and inclination with the use of fluoroscopy. Accurate cup data requires the user to analyze the acetabular component while the pelvis is level. Furthermore, the current technology does not yet account for functional changes in the pelvis that occur during sitting and standing. These tilt changes in the caudal and cephalad direction that occur functionally can be addressed with intraoperative fluoroscopy and preoperative images to assess cup position outside the supine position.

VELYS Hip Navigation has a focus on leg length and offset data in a user-friendly chart to help improve this important feature of successful hip arthroplasty surgery. Many surgeons felt the anterior approach could limit the ease of examining the hip for tension while on a special table, direct anterior approach tables with the operative extremity secured in a traction boot, requiring more emphasis on the imaging for this information. Without technology, existing techniques can be time-consuming and/or inaccurate. VELYS Hip Navigation had a primary focus on providing

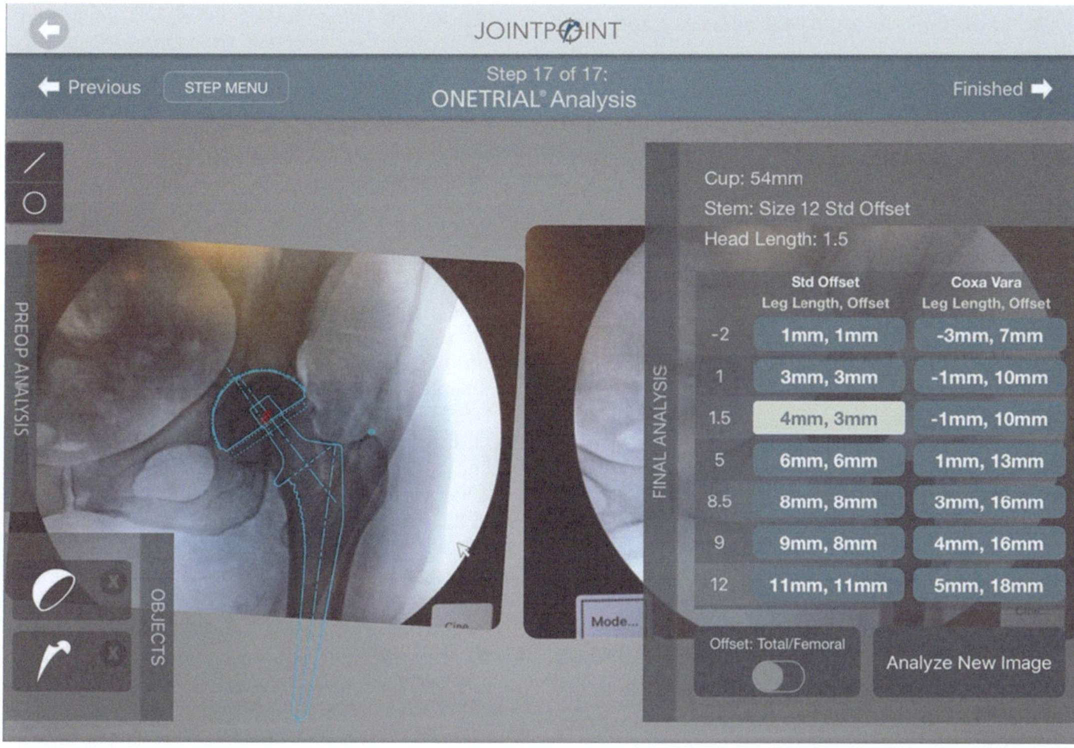

Fig. 39.10 The VELYS Hip Navigation system facilitates intraoperative navigation by calculating leg length and offset of different implant morphologies available to the surgeon to recreate the patient's specific anatomy while allowing comparison to the contralateral hip. Using OneTrial™ technology the surgeon can select the optimal final implant size and geometry from the first trial reduction of the stable broach, neck, and head construct

not only cup data, but leg length and offset data by comparing two images.

Future studies are required to better determine if VELYS Hip Navigation reduces outliers or improves outcomes over traditional techniques. Since VELYS Hip Navigation requires two images for cup position, and two images for leg length and offset, there is a potential for most surgeons to find a reduction in image requirements. Like other navigation systems studied with the posterior approach, data has shown to reduce outliers in cup position, leg length, and offset. Better functional outcomes will have to be researched to compare VELYS Hip Navigation to standard techniques to determine how much of a benefit it can have for patients. Furthermore, reduction in operating room time, fluoroscopy use and radiation exposure, by using VELYS Hip Navigation versus traditional techniques will likely continue to be described.

The previously discussed navigation and guidance technologies help fulfill a need for improved accuracy, precision, and reliability when implanting total hip arthroplasty components previously relied on confoundable human visual and tactile clues. Routine use of anatomical landmarks and mechanical alignment guides have been found to have varied reliability in assuring optimal cup positioning [43–45]. Most computer-assisted systems have been successful in improving cup positioning over conventional surgeon acumen but report the detriment of increased surgical time. Cost, portability, and reduced workflow efficiencies have been a concern for many of these technologies and allowed opportunities for new innovations.

Like most evolving, enabling technologies, costs decline, portability improve, and workflow efficiencies rise as technologies advance and surgical teams acquire experience with these systems. Studies on improved accuracy and precision in determining leg length and offset with these systems have been limited to date. Likewise, despite the radiographic, safety, and potential efficiency benefits, of computer-assisted systems significant improvements in clinical outcomes have yet to be realized. To date, the ideal combined cup angles for any patient's hip arthroplasty is unknown. Established radiologic safe zones reflect a static pelvis and uniform anatomies which are contrary to a dynamic reality. It is now appreciated pelvic and spine anatomy represent a dynamic relationship called spinopelvic mobility which can change from supine, standing, and sitting positions [46–48]. Spinopelvic alignment, balance, and mobility maybe an under-appreciated and misunderstood cause for complications like dislocation [49–51]. It follows to mitigate dynamic problems like dislocation, impingement, wear, and breakage a surgeon must account for the variability in each patient's fixed anatomy and spinopelvic mobility to target their optimal functional implant positions.

As computer-assisted guidance and navigation technologies evolve they will no doubt be an integral tool in elucidating, documenting, and understanding dynamic relationships of spinopelvic anatomy and patient-specific differences and promote accurate, reliable targeting of each patient's optimal, functional implant position mitigating potential adverse outcomes after total hip arthroplasty.

References

1. Lewinnek GE, Lewis JL, Tarr RI, Compere CL, Zimmerman JR. Dislocations after total hip-replacement arthroplasties. J Bone Joint Surg Am. 1978 Mar 1;60(2):217–20.
2. Barrack RL. Dislocation after total hip arthroplasty: implant design and orientation. J Am Acad Orthop Surg. 2003;11(2):89–99.
3. Woerner M, Sendtner E, Springorum R, Craiovan B, Worlicek M, Renkawitz T, Grifka J, Weber M. Visual intraoperative estimation of cup and stem position is not reliable in minimally invasive hip arthroplasty. Acta Orthop. 2016;87(3):225–30.
4. Callanan MC, Jarrett B, Bragdon CR, Zurakowski D, Rubash HE, Freiberg AA, Malchau H. The John Charnley Award: risk factors for cup malpositioning: quality improvement through a joint registry at a tertiary hospital. Clin Orthop Relat Res. 2011;469(2):319–29.
5. Kennedy JG, Rogers WB, Soffe KE, Sullivan RJ, Griffen DG, Sheehan LJ. Effect of acetabular component orientation on recurrent dislocation, pelvic osteolysis, polyethylene wear, and component migration. J Arthroplast. 1998;13(5):530–4.
6. Pierchon F, Pasquier G, Cotten A, Fontaine C, Clarisse J, Duquennoy A. Causes of dislocation of total hip arthroplasty. CT study of component alignment. J Bone Joint Surg. British volume. 1994;76(1):45–8.
7. McCollum DE, Gray WJ. Dislocation after total hip arthroplasty. Causes and prevention. Clin Orthop Relat Res. 1990;1(261):159–70.
8. Del Schutte JH, Lipman AJ, Bannar SM, Livermore JT, Ilstrup D, Morrey BF. Effects of acetabular abduction on cup wear rates in total hip arthroplasty. J Arthroplast. 1998;13(6):621–6.
9. Collaborative AT. I, Bhandari M, Matta JM, Dodgin D, Clark C, Kregor P, Bradley G, Little L. Outcomes following the single-incision anterior approach to total hip arthroplasty: a multicenter observational study. Orthop Clin North Am. 40(3):329–42.
10. Nick JL, Constant AB, John AG. Acetabular polyethylene wear and acetabular inclination and femoral offset. Clin Orthop Relat Res. 2009;467:2895–900.
11. Hart AJ, Ilo K, Underwood R, Cann P, Henckel J, Lewis A, Cobb J, Skinner J. The relationship between the angle of version and rate of wear of retrieved metal-on-metal resurfacings: a prospective, CT-based study. J Bone Joint Surg. British volume. 2011;93(3):315–20.
12. De Haan R, Pattyn C, Gill HS, Murray DW, Campbell PA, De Smet K. Correlation between inclination of the acetabular component and metal ion levels in metal-on-metal hip resurfacing replacement. J Bone Joint Surg. British volume. 2008;90(10):1291–7.
13. D'Lima DD, Chen PC, Colwell CW Jr. Optimizing acetabular component position to minimize impingement and reduce contact stress. J Bone Joint Surg. 2001;83(2):S87–91.
14. Barrett MO, Van Citters DW, Hamilton WG. Mechanical failure of marathon cross-linked polyethylene acetabular liner after total hip arthroplasty. Am J Orthop. 2011;40(10):523.
15. Tower SS, Currier JH, Currier BH, Lyford KA, Van Citters DW, Mayor MB. Rim cracking of the cross-linked longevity polyethylene acetabular liner after total hip arthroplasty. J Bone Joint Surg. 2007;89(10):2212–7.
16. Waewsawangwong W, Goodman SB. Unexpected failure of highly cross-linked polyethylene acetabular liner. J Arthroplast. 2012;27(2):323–e1.
17. Beamer BS, Morgan JH, Barr C, Weaver MJ, Vrahas MS. Does fluoroscopy improve acetabular component placement in total hip arthroplasty? Clin Orthop Relat Res. 2014;472(12):3953–62.
18. Martin JR, Masonis JL, Mason JB. Anatomic total hip component position is more reproducible with the

direct anterior approach using intraoperative fluoroscopy. Arthroplasty Today. 2020;6(4):777–83.
19. Rathod PA, Bhalla S, Deshmukh AJ, Rodriguez JA. Does fluoroscopy with anterior hip arthroplasty decrease acetabular cup variability compared with a nonguided posterior approach? Clin Orthop Relat Res. 2014;472(6):1877–85.
20. Confalonieri N, Manzotti A, Montironi F, Pullen C. Leg length discrepancy, dislocation rate, and offset in total hip replacement using a short modular stem: navigation vs conventional free hand. Orthopedics. 2008;31(10):35.
21. Renkawitz T, Weber M, Springorum HR, Sendtner E, Woerner M, Ulm K, Weber T, Grifka J. Impingement-free range of movement, acetabular component cover and early clinical results comparing 'femur-first' navigation and 'conventional' minimally invasive total hip arthroplasty: a randomized controlled trial. Bone Joint J. 2015;97(7):890–8.
22. Liu Z, Gao Y, Cai L. Imageless navigation versus traditional method in total hip arthroplasty: a meta-analysis. Int J Surg. 2015;21:122–7.
23. Kreuzer S, Leffers K. Direct anterior approach to total hip arthroplasty using computer navigation. Bull NYU Hosp Jt Dis. 2011;69(1):S52.
24. Bradley MP, Benson JR, Muir JM. Accuracy of acetabular component positioning using computer-assisted navigation in direct anterior total hip arthroplasty. Cureus. 2019;11(4)
25. McNabb DC, Jennings JM, Levy DL, Miner TM, Yang CC, Kim RH. Direct anterior hip replacement does not pose undue radiation exposure risk to the patient or surgeon. J Bone Joint Surg. 2017;99(23):2020–5.
26. Curtin BM, Armstrong LC, Bucker BT, Odum SM, Jiranek WA. Patient radiation exposure during fluoro-assisted direct anterior approach total hip arthroplasty. J Arthroplast. 2016;31(6):1218–21.
27. Pomeroy CL, Mason JB, Fehring TK, Masonis JL, Curtin BM. Radiation exposure during fluoro-assisted direct anterior total hip arthroplasty. J Arthroplast. 2016;31(8):1742–5.
28. Hube R, Birke A, Hein W, Klima S. CT-based and fluoroscopy-based navigation for cup implantation in total hip arthroplasty. Surg Technol Int. 2003;11:275–80.
29. Digioia AM 3rd, Jaramaz B, Plakseychuk AY, Moody JE Jr, Nikou C, Labarca RS, Levison TJ, Picard F. Comparison of a mechanical acetabular alignment guide with computer placement of the socket. J Arthroplast. 2002;17:359–64.
30. Sugano N. Comparison of mini-incision total hip arthroplasty through an anterior approach and a posterior approach using navigation. Orthop Clin N Am. 2009;40:365–70.
31. Sugano N, Takao M, Sakai T, Nishii T, Miki H. Does CT-based navigation improve the long-term survival in ceramic-on-ceramic total hip arthroplasty? Clin Orthop Relat Res. 2012;470(11):3054–9.
32. Sugano N. Computer-assisted orthopaedic surgery and robotic surgery in total hip arthroplasty. Clin Orthop Surg. 2013;5(1):1–9.
33. Bingham JS, Spangehl MJ, Hines JT, Taunton MJ, Schwartz AJ. Does intraoperative fluoroscopy improve limb-length discrepancy and acetabular component positioning during direct anterior total hip arthroplasty? J Arthroplast. 2018;33(9):2927–31.
34. Shah SM, Walter WL, Ngo J. Is the pelvis stable during supine total hip arthroplasty? Acta Orthop Belg. 2017;83(1):81–6.
35. Hartford JM, Bellino MJ. The learning curve for the direct anterior approach for total hip arthroplasty: a single surgeon's first 500 cases. Hip Int. 2017;27(5):483–8.
36. Jang ES, Lin JD, Shah RP, Geller JA, Cooper HJ. The effect of c-arm tilt on accuracy of intraoperative fluoroscopy in assessing acetabular component position during direct anterior approach for hip arthroplasty. J Orthop. 2018;15(2):447–9.
37. James CR, Peterson BE, Crim JR, Cook JL, Crist BD. The use of fluoroscopy during direct anterior hip arthroplasty: powerful or misleading? J Arthroplast. 2018;33(6):1775–9.
38. Carlson VR, Elliott IS, DeKeyser GJ, Pelt CE, Anderson LA, Gililland JM. Are we being fooled by fluoroscopy? Distortion may affect limb-length measurements in direct anterior total hip arthroplasty. J Arthroplast. 2020;
39. Gililland JM, Anderson LA, Boffeli SL, Pelt CE, Peters CL, Kubiak EN. A fluoroscopic grid in supine total hip arthroplasty: improving cup position, limb length, and hip offset. J Arthroplast. 2012;27(8):111–6.
40. Thorne TJ, Nishioka ST, Andrews SN, Mathews KA, Nakasone CK. Comparison of component placement accuracy using two intraoperative fluoroscopic grid technologies during direct anterior total hip arthroplasty. J Arthroplast. 2020;35(12):3601–6.
41. Hamilton WG, Parks NL, McDonald JF, Pfefferle KJ. A prospective, randomized study of surgical positioning software shows improved cup placement in total hip arthroplasty. Orthopedics. 2019;42(1):42–7.
42. Goodell PB, Kokubun B, Kollmorgen R. Computer navigation vs. Conventional Overlay Methods in DA THA: A Single surgeon Experience. Poster presented at: Peer Reviewed. Peerless Insight. The 30th AAHKS Annual Meeting. 2020, Nov 5–8. Dallas, Texas, USA.
43. Minoda Y, Ohzono K, Aihara M, Umeda N, Tomita M, Hayakawa K. Are acetabular component alignment guides for total hip arthroplasty accurate? J Arthroplast. 2010;25(6):986–9.
44. Kanoh T, Hasegawa Y, Masui T, Yamaguchi J, Kawabe K, Ishiguro N. Accurate acetabular component orientation after total hip arthroplasty using an acetabular alignment guide. J Arthroplast. 2010;25(1):81–6.
45. Maeda Y, Sugano N, Nakamura N, Hamawaki M. The accuracy of a mechanical cup alignment guide in total hip arthroplasty (THA) through direct anterior and

posterior approaches measured with CT-based navigation. J Arthroplast. 2015;30(9):1561–4.
46. Tiberi JV III, Antoci V, Malchau H, Rubash HE, Freiberg AA, Kwon YM. What is the fate of total hip arthroplasty (THA) acetabular component orientation when evaluated in the standing position? J Arthroplast. 2015;30(9):1555–60.
47. Kanawade V, Dorr LD, Wan Z. Predictability of acetabular component angular change with postural shift from standing to sitting position. J Bone Joint Surg. 2014;96(12):978–86.
48. Lum ZC, Coury JG, Cohen JL, Dorr LD. The current knowledge on spinopelvic mobility. J Arthroplast. 2018;33(1):291–6.
49. DelSole EM, Vigdorchik JM, Schwarzkopf R, Errico TJ, Buckland AJ. Total hip arthroplasty in the spinal deformity population: does degree of sagittal deformity affect rates of safe zone placement, instability, or revision? J Arthroplast. 2017;32(6):1910–7.
50. Esposito CI, Carroll KM, Sculco PK, Padgett DE, Jerabek SA, Mayman DJ. Total hip arthroplasty patients with fixed spinopelvic alignment are at higher risk of hip dislocation. J Arthroplast. 2018;33(5):1449–54.
51. Sultan AA, Khlopas A, Piuzzi NS, Chughtai M, Sodhi N, Mont MA. The impact of spino-pelvic alignment on total hip arthroplasty outcomes: a critical analysis of current evidence. J Arthroplast. 2018;33(5):1606–16.

Robotic Total Hip Replacement with Direct Anterior Approach

40

Stefan W. Kreuzer and Amir Pourmoghaddam

Introduction

Total hip arthroplasty (THA) is the ultimate treatment approach for patients particularly with end-stage hip osteoarthritis (OA). This treatment has an outstanding long-term survivorship such as more than 95% over 10 years and more than 80% after 25 years. The number of cases treating with THA is significantly increasing and despite the successful outcome of THA some patients report dissatisfaction from the surgery due to post-operative complications such as early revisions. Therefore, identifying factors affecting the outcome of the THA is a crucial step in reducing the number of unsatisfied patients. Early research has indicated that proper femoral and acetabular component positioning is a critical factor to prevent major and common THA postoperative complications. These complications may include hip dislocations, poor biomechanical performance, and leg length discrepancy. In addition, these complications may manifest undesired symptoms such as trochanteric bursitis, iliopsoas tendonitis, and rectus tendinitis that require further intervention to alleviate. Surgeons struggle with achieving appropriate acetabular component placement as patients' anatomical structure of spine and hip and lumbo-pelvic kinematic plays a significant role in targeting such optimal placement.

The idea and implementation of automation and computer integration in THAs has been an inevitable process in the advancements of these surgeries. The application of robotics in general surgery is very common [1]. The idea behind this application is to reduce soft tissue injury and improve postoperative clinical outcomes [1]. William Bargar and Howard Paul introduced robotic hip arthroplasty in 1992 [2]. The application of robotic technology in THA has been gaining popularity to reduce the potential human errors during surgery resulting in higher precision in implant position compared to conventional THA [3, 4]. As restoring hip biomechanics can improve postoperative functional outcome and implant survival, the application of robotic surgery has certain advantages over the manual approach [5–7]. Proper anteversion and inclination is achieved in less than 47% of THA cases that are conducted manually as the target acetabular component positioning is hard to achieve. In addition, surgeons with low number of cases are more prone to mispositioning of the implant components outside the safe range [7–10].

S. W. Kreuzer (✉)
INOV8 Orthopedics, Houston, TX, USA
e-mail: skreuzer@inov8hc.com

A. Pourmoghaddam
Memorial Bone & Joint Research Foundation
Orthopaedic Research Houston Texas,
Houston, TX, USA

J. M. Matta, A. P. Sah (eds.), *Anterior Hip Replacement*,
https://doi.org/10.1007/978-3-030-91896-5_40

Computer Assistive Devices/ Navigation Systems

The application of navigation systems has been a revolutionary innovation to use computer-assisted surgery (CAS) to improve component placement accuracy. Even though CAS and robotic surgery might be interchangeably used there is a distinguishable difference between the application of CAS/navigation versus the robotic surgery in THA cases. CAS are based on two different technologies, imageless and image-based. The main purpose of using CAS is to obtain patient-specific anatomical information that can be used to plan for an optimal component placement. Robotic technologies use CAS to further control the implementation of such plans by restraining the surgeons motor movements and facilitating proper execution of the preoperative surgical plans [1, 2]. The level of automation classifies surgical robots into three distinct categories.

Passive Systems

In these systems surgeon has complete control over movements of the robot and the robot acts as a guiding mechanism while the surgeon prepares the bone.

Semi-active

These robots are equipped with mechanisms to provide the surgeon with haptic, visual, or auditory feedback while the surgeon has the capability to manipulate the cutting tools. The feedback provided by the robots is based on identifying the deviation of actual cut versus the pre-planned special constraints. Mako Robotic System (Stryker Corporation, Kalamazoo, MI, USA) is an FDA-approved semi-active robotic system that provides haptic feedback to the surgeon during the surgery.

Active Robots

These robots have been developed to follow more advanced algorithms and can execute some tasks previously only performed by the surgeon. For example, these robots can perform some bone cuts without any intervention or guidance from the surgeon and can prepare the bone autonomously [11]. TSolution One (ThinkSurgical, Inc., Fremont, CA) is an example of a fully active robot which was built based on the ROBODOC technology.

Robotic THA Execution Summary

There are several steps in the robotic THA; however, this surgery can be divided into four stages.

1. Preoperative planning: The imaging of the pelvis and femur are taken to create a 3D model by a semi-automatic process called segmentation and will be used to identify the native hip anatomy and its orientation in sagittal, coronal, and axial planes. This step is important to achieve patient-specific biomechanics [1] (Fig. 40.1).

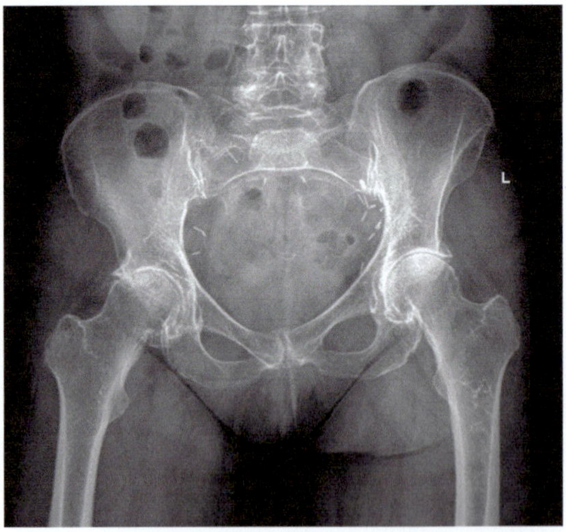

Fig. 40.1 Preoperative 2D pelvis anterior-posterior view

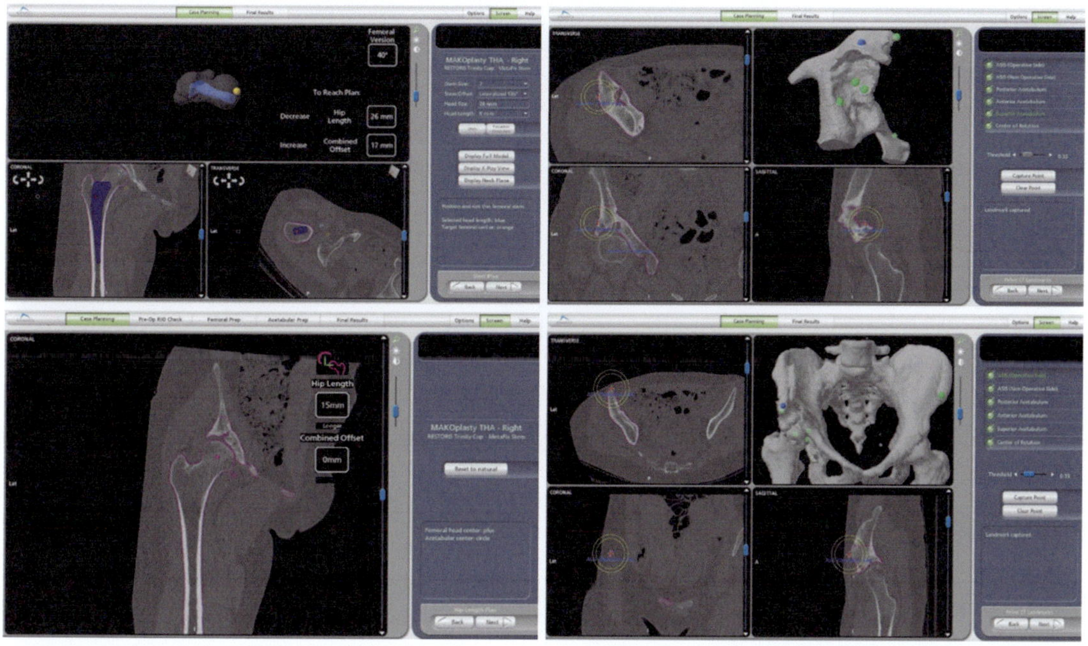

Fig. 40.2 Virtual implantation and segmentate hip model

2. In the second step, the surgeon will use the virtual implants and the 3D reconstructed and segmentate hip model to perform a virtual placement of implants and positioning to achieve desirable component version, inclination, and hip biomechanics; the software will then calculate the required depth of acetabular bone resection and the femoral osteotomy site and angles (Fig. 40.2).
3. Intraoperatively, the osseus anatomy of the acetabulum and proximal femur is mapped into the planned virtual model using an optical or mechanical tracking system for registration (Fig. 40.3).
4. The surgeon uses a robot to execute the planned virtual surgery on patient's pelvis and femur. In fully active model, surgeon will monitor bone resection while the robot acts autonomously (Fig. 40.4).

Clinical Outcome of Robotic Surgery

As the application of the robotic hip arthroplasty requires preoperative planning, previous studies on the comparison of the robotic and manual hip arthroplasty have been limited by the small cohorts. In a meta-analysis by Chen et al. [12] of the studies conducted from 2005 through 2017 intraoperative and postoperative complications between robotic versus manual THA were compared. There were 1516 patients included in these studies (522 robotic vs. 994 conventional THA). Intraoperative complications that included femoral fractures had significantly higher rate in manual cases; however, postoperative complications that included infection, nerve palsy, deep vein thrombosis, and dislocation were fairly similar between robotic versus manual THA [12]. In addition, robotic surgery resulted in better cup and stem positioning and patients demonstrated higher rate of heterotopic ossifications. The postoperative clinical outcome measured by Japanese Orthopaedic Association Score, Harris Hip Score, Merle d'Aubigne Hip Score, Western Ontario and McMaster Universities Osteoarthritis indicated that there was no significant difference between robotic and manual approach. Radiographic data analyses showed insignificant difference in leg length discrepancy; however, cup positioning was performed more optimally by the application of robotic

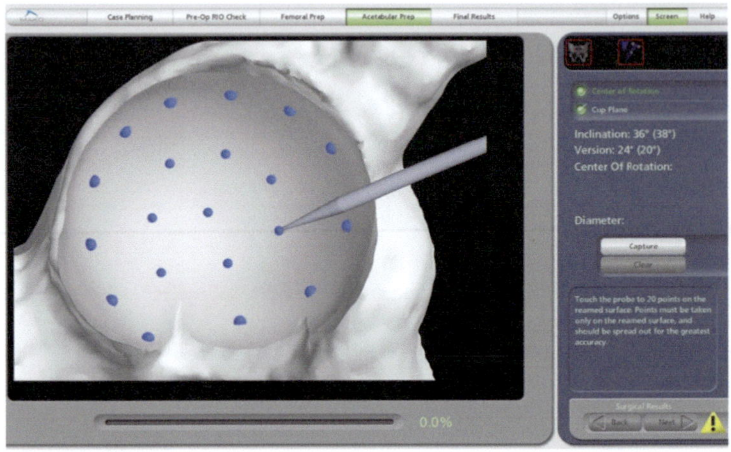

Fig. 40.3 Registration of osseus anatomy with the 3D reconstructed model

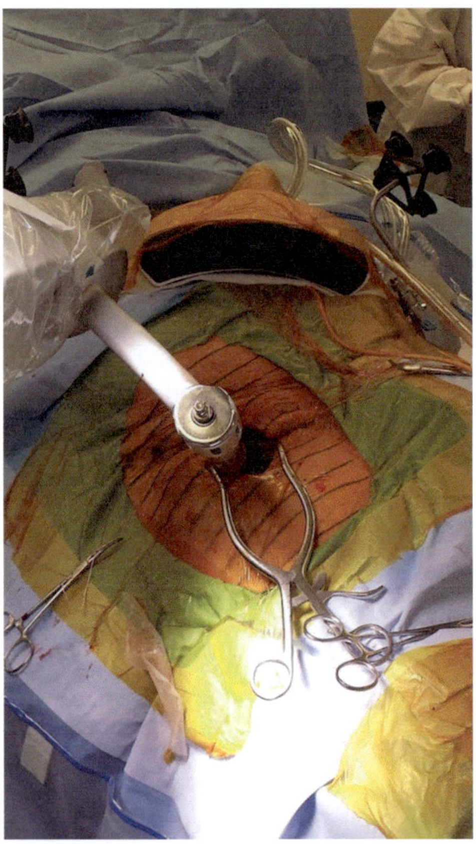

Fig. 40.4 Intraoperative implementation of robotic arm to ream the acetabular cup using the haptic technology of MAKO

technology. Cup positioning and optimal component placement within the margin of the safe zone (5–25 degrees anteversion and 30–50 degrees inclination) decrease the risk of dislocation, instability, and revisions. Surgeons who utilized manual THA operated within shorter time; however, this decrease in surgical time was not statistically significant between the robotic and the manual group. Surgical learning curve particularly in robotic surgery might be a significant factor in reducing surgical time; however, further research is required to address the effect of learning curve in reducing surgical time in robotic surgery. Only two investigations in the meta-analysis assessed blood loss and only one study indicated lower blood loss in the robotic group while the second study did not find any significant differences between the surgical approach.

Risks & Limitations of Robotic Surgery

Some patients may interpret the usage of robots in hip replacement as the lack of proper human oversight resulting in an increase in litigations following robotic surgery particularly in earlier cases [13]. In addition, inadvertent soft tissue injuries to the abductor mechanism and femoral fractures have been reported as a concern in fully active robotic systems and have resulted in several litigations against the manufacturers [14]. Greater trochanteric fractures have also been documented in MAKO cases due to the large cannulated screw being placed into the tip of the trochanter. These litigations have resulted in hesitations among surgeons and healthcare entities to fully utilize robotic THA [1].

In addition, another major concern with robotic hip replacement is the recent reports on the correlation of lumbopelvic motion and the previously identified Lewinneck "component placement safe zone". The historical target of 40 degrees of inclination and 20 degrees of anteversion did not improve hip stability [15, 16]; therefore, identifying patient-specific safe zone may be critical to achieve desirable outcome in robotic hip replacement.

In addition, fully active robotic THA is not developed for acetabular reaming or acetabular cup placement. Therefore, optimal combined version cannot be achieved and executed by the application of robotic surgery.

Another limitation of active robotic THA is the inability to adjust the surgical plan intraoperatively; however, this issue is less critical in semi-active robots. The ability to adjust the plan is critical in surgeries as the surgeons might need to alter predefined surgical plans in response to the unforeseen changes during the operation such as instability, poor bone quality, and occurrence of a fracture. In these situations, the surgeon halts the use of the robotic system and must complete the bone cutting by using the manual instruments. Manufacturers are utilizing artificial intelligence to address this issue and in the future active robotic surgeries may become capable of changing the treatment plan intraoperatively [2]. In addition, mechanical failure during the operation is a significant issue at this stage. Previous studies indicated up to 18% of the robotic surgery cases would need a manual intervention to be completed [17].

Direct Anterior Approach and Robotic Hip Replacement

While robotic surgery is beneficial to improve component placement accuracy, the supine positioning of the patient during the anterior approach correlates with improved implant position [2]. Based on the author's surgical experience during FDA validation lab for MAKO, no significant difference was documented in the outcome of the surgery between robotic-assisted cases versus manual instrument cases. However previous studies indicated implant component positioning difference between robotic versus manual instruments in posterior approach hip replacement [3].

Learning Curve in Robotic Hip Replacement

The learning curve is highly variable among surgeons and since most surgeons have some level of experience with the robotic platform for other procedures such as partial or full knee replacement. In such cases, 5–10 cases are usually required to establish a good workflow. Experience with general computer navigation also reduces the learning curve.

However, surgeons specifically newly practicing ones should be cautioned about "stacking of learning curves". It is important that a less experienced surgeon avoid stack learning curves by avoiding the application of newer techniques such as anterior approach, placement of a new implant, and utilizing robotic assistance. Hip replacement is a complex procedure, therefore surgeons should utilize new surgical techniques or equipment in a stepwise approach by achieving competency in utilizing each approach or instrument before utilizing a new one.

Costs

High cost of robotic system hardware is a major discouraging factor that reduces the usage of this technology in THA cases. Training of the surgical team, updating the system to the most current version, purchasing disposable equipment used specifically for these surgeries, and the need to recalibrate the system are some of the factors that increase the cost of operating robots. In addition, manual surgeries have significantly less costs that certainly improve the cost-efficiency of such surgeries compared to robotic THA. On average, a robotic platform will add between $600 and $1500 additional cost per case. In addition, the surgical time is another factor that can significantly increase the cost of robotic THA. In the United States, 18% of GDP is spent on healthcare, therefore any new technology has to be cost neutral. With most robotic platforms being a closed platform (only compatible with the implants of a certain company), the cost reduction through implant price negotiation is limited. In addition, Medicare has been authorizing total hip replacement performed at the ambulatory surgery centers with a significantly less reimbursement fee schedule (at the time of writing this chapter the amount is $8800), utilizing robotically assisted hip replacement approach may not be financially viable due to a high cost of equipment pricing. Despite the initial increase in cost to perform robotic THA there is a significant benefit in utilizing this technology in THA. The application of robotic surgery would be cost-saving because of the significant reduction in instruments and required inventory during the operation. Ultimately the cost of utilizing this technology may be a defining factor in limiting the application of this technology in THA despite obvious biomechanical improvements.

References

1. Kayani B, Konan S, Ayuob A, Ayyad S, Haddad FS. The current role of robotics in total hip arthroplasty. EFORT Open Rev. 2019;4(11):618–25.
2. Dettmer M, Kreuzer SW, Malanka S. In: Rivière C, Vendittoli P-A, editors. Reproducing the hip anatomy: intraoperative planning and assistive devices (CAS, robotics), Personalized hip and knee joint replacement. Cham; 2020. p. 99–109.
3. Nodzo SR, Chang CC, Carroll KM, Barlow BT, Banks SA, Padgett DE, et al. Intraoperative placement of total hip arthroplasty components with robotic-arm assisted technology correlates with postoperative implant position: a CT-based study. Bone Joint J. 2018;100B(10):1303–9.
4. Redmond JM, Gupta A, Hammarstedt JE, Petrakos A, Stake CE, Domb BG. Accuracy of component placement in robotic-assisted total hip arthroplasty. Orthopedics [Internet]. 2016;39(3):193–9. Available from: https://doi.org/10.3928/01477447-20160404-06.
5. Mahmood SS, Mukka SS, Crnalic S, Wretenberg P, Sayed-Noor AS. Association between changes in global femoral offset after total hip arthroplasty and function, quality of life, and abductor muscle strength. Acta Orthop. 2016;87(1):36–41.
6. Rosler J, Perka C. The effect of anatomical positional relationships on kinetic parameters after total hip replacement. Int Orthop. 2000;24(1):23–7.
7. Meermans G, Van Doorn J, Kats JJ. Restoration of the centre of rotation in primary total hip arthroplasty the influence of acetabular floor depth and reaming technique. Bone Joint J. 2016;98-B(12):1597–603.
8. Lewinnek GE, Lewis JL, Tarr R, Compere CL, Zimmerman JR. Dislocations after total hip-replacement arthroplasties. J Bone Joint Surg Am. 1978;60(2):217–20.
9. Archbold HAP, Mockford B, Molloy D, McConway J, Ogonda L, Beverland D. The transverse acetabular ligament: an aid to orientation of the acetabular component during primary total hip replacement. A preliminary study of 1000 cases investigating post-operative stability. J Bone Joint Surg Ser B. 2006;88(7):883–6.
10. Murray DW. The definition and measurement of acetabular orientation. J Bone Joint Surg Br [Internet]. 1993;75-B(2):228–32. Available from: https://doi.org/10.1302/0301-620X.75B2.8444942.
11. Dungy DS, Netravali NA. Active robotics for total hip arthroplasty. Am J Orthop (Belle Mead NJ). 2016;45(4):256–9.
12. Chen X, Xiong J, Wang P, Zhu S, Qi W, Peng H, et al. Robotic-assisted compared with conventional total hip arthroplasty: systematic review and meta-analysis. Postgrad Med J. 2018;2:335–41.
13. Lang JE, Mannava S, Floyd AJ, Goddard MS, Smith BP, Mofidi A, et al. Robotic systems in orthopaedic surgery. J Bone Joint Surg Br [Internet]. 2011 [cited 2014 Jul 16];93(10):1296–9. Available from: http://www.ncbi.nlm.nih.gov/pubmed/21969424.
14. Sugano N. Computer-assisted orthopaedic surgery and robotic surgery in total hip arthroplasty. Clin Orthop Surg. 2013;5(1):1–9.
15. Tezuka T, Heckmann ND, Bodner RJ, Dorr LD. Functional safe zone is superior to the Lewinnek safe zone for total hip arthroplasty: why the Lewinnek safe zone is not always predictive of stability. J Arthroplasty [Internet]. 2019;34(1):3–8. Available from: https://doi.org/10.1016/j.arth.2018.10.034.
16. Esposito CI, Ph D, Gladnick BP, Lee Y, Lyman S, Ph D, et al. Cup position alone does not predict risk of dislocation after hip arthroplasty. J Arthroplast. 2016;30(1):109–13.
17. Siebel T, Käfer W. Clinical outcome following robotic assisted versus conventional total hip arthroplasty: a controlled and prospective study of seventy-one patients. Z Orthop Ihre Grenzgeb. 2005;143(4):391–8.

41 Problems to Solve and Potential Future Directions for Anterior Approach Total Hip Arthroplasty

Joel M. Matta

There is growing and convincing evidence that the transition to AA from posterior, lateral, and antero-lateral has been a success story of an important change in hip surgery. Surgeons switching to AA have witnessed patient satisfaction they have not seen before, with less pain, quicker recovery, minimal incidence of dislocation, and a higher incidence of replaced hips that feel normal.

Can we make AA better? Before innovation occurs the first step is the perception of shortcomings of existing techniques and technologies. This is a more difficult step than we often realize. I believe that it is almost always true that we as physicians think too highly of our current knowledge and capabilities and that those practicing some years into the future will look back at us and wonder "wow, they did that?"

The results of AA hip performed by a wide variety of surgeons by a wide variety of techniques are not consistent. The AA critics and haters point to reports of bad results and we the advocates point to the reports of good results. First, which AA methods and technologies produce the top results? Are these "top results" the maximum that can be achieved or can we do better? How can we minimize the surgeon variable? Specifically, how can we minimize result differences between high volume "virtuoso surgeons" and lower volume "normal surgeons"? How can we eliminate variability in results for any given surgeon?

I think that the most important current problem to solve is the variability in results following AA THA. I believe that the range of variability and incidence of problematic outliers for AA has been reduced as compared to hips done through posterior approach but result variability remains a problem. How do we solve this? In the chapter by Tania Ferguson and me regarding our current technique, we describe what we believe to be a currently available path to consistency that is available through existing educational pathways and existing technology. Other authors in other chapters have described their preferred methods as well as supporting reasoning. Surgeon education is an important part of the solution. Will we see clear statistical evidence to guide us toward the best existing technique(s)? I question if this will happen but the market may be our best source of truth. Individual surgeons as well as patients will drive the market. Surgeons will adopt techniques and technologies that prove most efficacious and efficient and patients will research and choose. I would reiterate however, don't try to do AA like you did PA, the intuitive methods that we have used for years for cup position, leg length and offset, as well as stability have lacked accuracy and consistency. We need to move on and move up. Technology is our friend.

J. M. Matta (✉)
Steadman Clinic, Vail, CO, USA

J. M. Matta, A. P. Sah (eds.), *Anterior Hip Replacement*,
https://doi.org/10.1007/978-3-030-91896-5_41

Even as we move toward the best existing AA methods, we may ask if the current best results are the best that can be achieved?

Keeping our scope of vision within the spectrum of AA, however we can see where improvements need to be made. We need to continue to look critically, at surgical exposure, bone instrumentation, setting and achieving accuracy goals, and implant efficacy. Operating room efficiency is another goal that is being achieved and can further improve though the goals of procedure efficacy and safety is primary.

If we are realistic regarding our anterior approach surgeries, we can say that all cases are not easy regarding exposure and access to the bone. We are at a point where we can operate all primary hips from anterior but there remain the difficult cases. Robotic orthopedic surgery has pertained to the robot doing the bone instrumentation. In this scenario, the robot may prepare the acetabulum or femur guided by a computerized plan derived from pre-operative images. I think that the other and probably more important opportunity for help from the robot is for the robot to position and hold the bone in the most ideal position for the surgeon to access it. The orthopedic table or a table attachment is the current adaptation of this concept. Future developments however of robot/mechanical control of the bone will enhance exposure and access. Particularly for big body parts like the spine and lower extremities, I think that an assistant forcefully manipulating and holding large body parts is an antiquated way to operate. The key issues supporting consideration of use of a mechanical device that holds and positions the bone are: enhancing exposure, maintaining the bone in a stable position and saving the cost of paying a human assistant to do what a device can do. The "robot" may manipulate the bone from the surface of the body or possibly most effectively by direct contact with the bone. A related issue is areas of support of the body during surgery by the operating table. It is ideal if the operating table provides the least area of contact with the skin possible. Sterility is enhanced and options for skin access for incisions are increased when the contact areas between the skin and table are minimized. When I hear that AA on a standard operating table with human extremity manipulation is possible, I agree but we need to move on to improvements.

There are several steps of bone preparation/instrumentation: The neck cut, acetabular preparation, and femoral preparation. I am not aware that we have an accurate, widely accepted method to guide the neck cut. In a way this is OK because the neck cut can be an approximation. The neck cut is thereby later adjusted (further shortened). However with this scenario, making it initially too long is OK but initially too short can lead to problems. I have experimented with a number of prototype neck-cutting guides but not to my satisfaction. I keep coming back to just looking that the pre-op x-ray and templating and then looking at the neck and making an intuitive cut but there must be a better way. There must be a better way, especially to achieve the goal of minimizing variability between surgeons as well as minimizing variability between cases done by an individual surgeon.

Proper reaming of the acetabulum is an underestimated problem. Finding the combination of ideal center or rotation, acetabular cup size, and obtaining a reamed cavity that will grip the cup are problems that have not been solved to the extent that consistent results are achieved. My own observation of post-op x-rays following acetabular reaming with a robot indicates that the current robot does not consistently produce the desired result.

It is interesting that with traditional manual bone instrumentation, acetabular reaming and femoral broaching, that the bone guides the tools. The reamer is centered by the shape of the acetabulum and the broach is guided by the internal femoral contour. On the other hand, the concept of the robot is that the robot machines and instruments the bone in a preprogrammed way and resists guidance from the bone. Which concept is correct? For the bone to guide the instrument or for the instrument to follow a programmed direction? There may be a place for both and if the robot is to become truly useful we may need to rethink how it works. I think another current problem with the robot is that it is assumed that the robot can work accurately on bone that is not secured in place. I don't think that the best accuracy can be achieved by the robot with the current situation where the bone it is working on is an unsecured moving target.

The dramatic reduction in the incidence of post-operative dislocation with AA has not only reduced the incidence of re-admission and re-operation, it has also opened the door for new thinking. Posterior approach practices like soft tissue tensioning, increasing offset and upsizing the acetabulum to accommodate bigger ball heads, have become unnecessary. The new focus driven by AA is toward accurate restoration of normal hip biomechanics and more anatomic acetabular sizing. To achieve accurate hip biomechanics some AA surgeons still rely entirely on traditional methods for cup position, leg length and offset including bony landmarks, shuck test, range of motion tests, mechanical guides, feeling the ankles, etc. I believe however that the variability and outliers inherent in these intuitive techniques will lead to their demise. No assembly process can be performed consistently and accurately without reliable quantitative measures. The x-ray is the final judge of restoration of cup position, leg length and offset. Computer guidance utilizes x-ray data to guide accuracy by means of a computer-generated virtual reality and then a post-op x-ray is taken for confirmation. The other form of computer guidance is the use of software for quantitative assessment of fluoroscopic images taken in real-time during surgery. The bottom line, however, is that increased accuracy will provide patient benefits and quantitative assessment by innovative technology is essential.

Other problems remain that are not addressed in detail in this text. These problems include infection, DVT, and post-operative pain. I would say that AA has had a positive effect in combating these problems but improvements still need to be made.

Positive change and innovation in hip surgery is part of our current exciting and positive environment. We cannot assume however that our current healthcare environment that facilitates this will continue. In fact, even our current regulatory and legal environment presents increasing challenges for innovation. Capitalism and The Market drive positive change and innovation. The positive change to AA THA was driven by The Market: what patients wanted and what surgeons found gave them the best results and attracted patients. This change happened in spite of opposition by "hip experts" and editorial boards. The same is true for creation and adoption of innovative technologies. Market forces and market incentives are necessary. It is my impression that dominance of socialized medicine has stifled innovation in the effected countries. No profit, no motivation, no innovation. When there is not a financial motivation to attract patients (profitable fee for service) there is reduced motivation to improve what the provider offers. When prices are fixed there is a loss of incentive for product innovation. Socialistic efforts to create and design economies have consistently failed. Economic evolution trumps economic creationism. The US healthcare economy by itself must be larger than the GDP of the majority of countries. Relying on regulators and planners cannot bring the benefits of a healthcare market economy. Think: evolution vs creationism. The unstoppable positive *evolution* and innovation that a market, healthcare or otherwise produces, cannot be the result of *creation* and design. A profitable medical market economy is the path to innovation, improved outcomes and cost savings. For continued positive evolution in hip surgery to occur, the proper environment is essential. We have a mission to provide top care to our patients and to continue to innovate to improve. Like it or not, I believe that in order to accomplish our primary mission of excellence for patients through innovation we must also join the fight against the current misguided efforts of purportedly omniscient government regulators and planners.

Index

J. M. Matta, A. P. Sah (eds.), *Anterior Hip Replacement*, https://doi.org/10.1007/978-3-030-91896-5

MIX
Papier aus verantwortungsvollen Quellen
Paper from responsible sources
FSC® C105338

If you have any concerns about our products,
you can contact us on
ProductSafety@springernature.com

In case Publisher is established outside the EU,
the EU authorized representative is:
Springer Nature Customer Service Center GmbH
Europaplatz 3, 69115 Heidelberg, Germany

Printed by Libri Plureos GmbH
in Hamburg, Germany